Sidman's Neuroanatomy

A Programmed Learning Tool

SECOND EDITION

Sidman's Neuroanatomy

A Programmed Learning Tool

SECOND EDITION

Douglas J. Gould, PhD
Associate Professor, Division of Anatomy
The Ohio State University College of Medicine
Columbus, Ohio

Jennifer K. Brueckner, PhD
Associate Professor
Department of Anatomy and Neurobiology
University of Kentucky College of Medicine
Lexington, Kentucky

Wolters Kluwer | Lippincott Williams & Wilkins
Health

Philadelphia • Baltimore • New York • London
Buenos Aires • Hong Kong • Sydney • Tokyo

Acquisitions Editor: Crystal Taylor
Managing Editor: Kelley Squazzo
Senior Marketing Manager: Valerie Sanders
Production Editor: Beth Martz
Design Coordinator: Stephen Druding
Compositor: Aptara

Second Edition

351 West Camden Street
Baltimore, MD 21201

530 Walnut Street
Philadelphia, PA 19106

Printed in the United States of America

9 8 7 6 5 4 3 2 1

Library of Congress Cataloging-in-Publication Data

Gould, Douglas J.
Sidman's neuroanatomy : a programmed learning tool / Douglas J. Gould, Jennifer K. Brueckner.—2nd ed.
p. cm.
ISBN-13: 978-0-7817-6568-8 (alk. paper)
ISBN-10: 0-7817-6568-4 (alk. paper)
1. Neuroanatomy—Programmed instruction. I. Brueckner, Jennifer K., 1970-
II. Sidman, Richard L. Neuroanatomy. III. Title.
QM451.S5 2008
611'.8—dc22

2007033285

DISCLAIMER

Care has been taken to confirm the accuracy of the information present and to describe generally accepted practices. However, the authors, editors, and publisher are not responsible for errors or omissions or for any consequences from application of the information in this book and make no warranty, expressed or implied, with respect to the currency, completeness, or accuracy of the contents of the publication. Application of this information in a particular situation remains the professional responsibility of the practitioner; the clinical treatments described and recommended may not be considered absolute and universal recommendations.

The authors, editors, and publisher have exerted every effort to ensure that drug selection and dosage set forth in this text are in accordance with the current recommendations and practice at the time of publication. However, in view of ongoing research, changes in government regulations, and the constant flow of information relating to drug therapy and drug reactions, the reader is urged to check the package insert for each drug for any change in indications and dosage and for added warnings and precautions. This is particularly important when the recommended agent is a new or infrequently employed drug.

Some drugs and medical devices presented in this publication have Food and Drug Administration (FDA) clearance for limited use in restricted research settings. It is the responsibility of the health care provider to ascertain the FDA status of each drug or device planned for use in their clinical practice.

To purchase additional copies of this book, call our customer service department at **(800) 638-3030** or fax orders to **(301) 223-2320**. International customers should call **(301) 223-2300**.

Visit Lippincott Williams & Wilkins on the Internet: http://www.lww.com. Lippincott Williams & Wilkins customer service representatives are available from 8:30 AM to 6:00 PM, EST.

To my wife, Marie, for her love, encouragement, support, and above all, her patience; to my daughters, Maggie and Lulu, for all of the joy they bring. (DJG)

To my dear parents, John and Rheba, whose love, encouragement, and support have sustained me both professionally and personally. (JKB)

Preface

The first edition of *Neuroanatomy: A Programmed Text*, Volume 1, was published over 40 years ago by Drs. Richard and Murray Sidman, with the goal of creating a two-volume set that would function as a neuroanatomy tutorial using a programmed-learning strategy. Although Volume 2 was never completed, the longevity of Volume 1 stands as a testament to the legendary and innovative work of those involved in the original project.

This second edition of the text, *Sidman's Neuroanatomy: A Programmed Learning Tool*, extends the content of the first edition to include critical topics such as the basal nuclei (ganglia), extrapyramidal pathways, cerebellum, diencephalon, and special senses and completes the authors' original goal of creating a comprehensive neuroanatomy tutorial. Much of the original material has been retained with minor modifications, including updated terminology, appropriate clinical scenarios, and fresh artwork. We have worked diligently to integrate new material seamlessly, with the goal of remaining true to the programmed-learning philosophy and style. The book will lead the reader through the fundamentals of neuroanatomy in a step-by-step fashion, as might be done by an actual instructor, with each step building on the one before. To use the book most effectively, you should proceed in numbered sequence, working your way through at your own pace.

While we have worked hard to ensure accuracy, we appreciate that some errors and omissions may have escaped our attention. We would welcome your comments and suggestions to improve this book in subsequent editions.

Acknowledgments

The authors would like to thank:

The original authors of and contributors to *Neuroanatomy: A Programmed Text*, Volume 1. They created a time-tested staple of neuroanatomy education that we hope we have done justice in revision.

The faculty and student reviewers of the book proposal and manuscript:

Faculty: David Lopes Cardozo, PhD; James Culberson, PhD; Kathleen M. Klueber, PhD; Farrel Robinson, PhD; Anthony Salvatore, PhD; Mark Seifert, PhD; R. Shane Tubbs, PhD; Michael Yard, BS, PhD (cand)

Students: Gopika Banker; Amir Ghaferi; Erica Grimm; James Kong; James Pinckney, II; Shilpa Shah; Simant Shah

The individuals at Lippincott Williams & Wilkins who were involved in this revision, including Crystal Taylor, Kelley Squazzo, and Valerie Sanders. Their patience, organization, and cooperation made the creation of this book an outstanding experience.

All of the senior neuroanatomy experts who we have informally consulted with in hallways, on the telephone, and via email. Without your expertise, this revision would not have been possible.

Contents

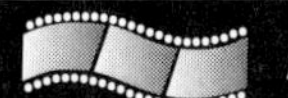

Animations

Online neuroanatomical animations listed at the end of each Part.

I CEREBRUM

1 Surface of the Brain I

1.1. Examine the surface of the cerebral cortex and note the grooves, or *sulci*. The deepest and longest groove on the lateral surface of the cerebral cortex is the ____________ ____________.

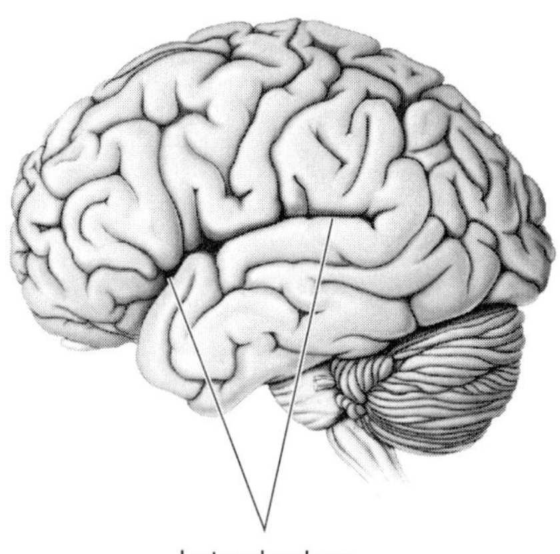

1.2. In the 17th century, the French anatomist Francois Sylvius first recognized the __lateral__ sulcus as a horizontal groove separating the __temporal__ lobe inferiorly from the frontal and parietal lobes superiorly.

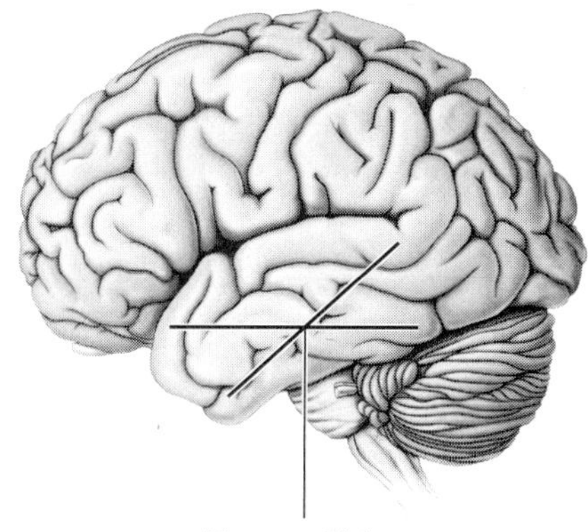

1.3. On the diagram provided, locate and label the major groove running horizontally just superior to the temporal lobe.

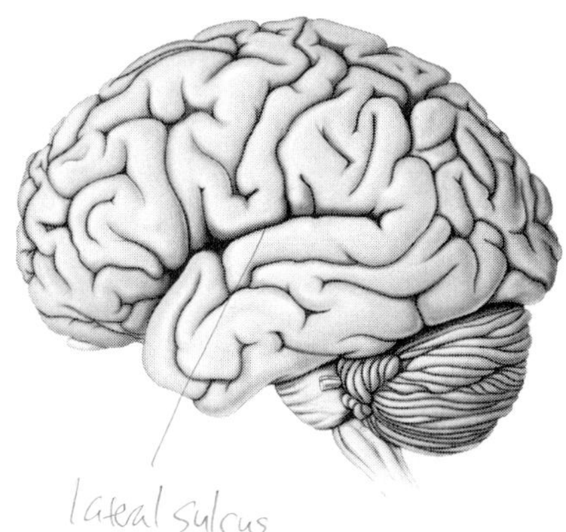

1.1A. lateral sulcus (also known as the Sylvian fissure)

1.2A. lateral; temporal

1.3A.

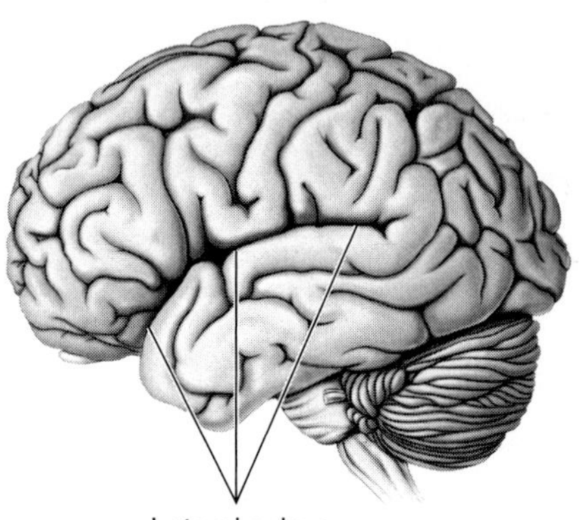

1.4. Identify and label the superior temporal sulcus, located parallel and inferior to the lateral sulcus.

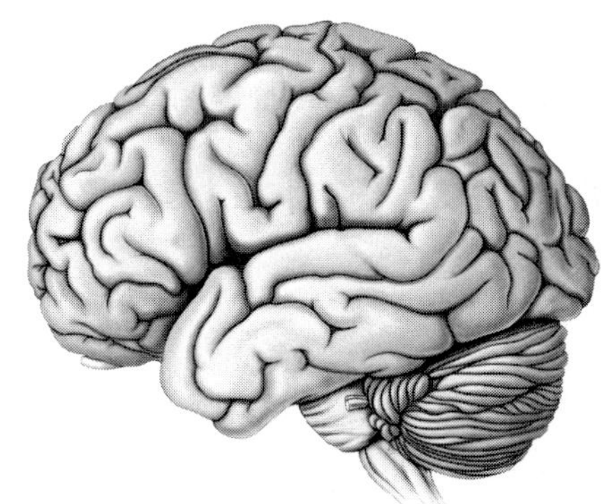

1.5. To locate the superior temporal sulcus, connect the three dots on the diagram and label the sulcus.

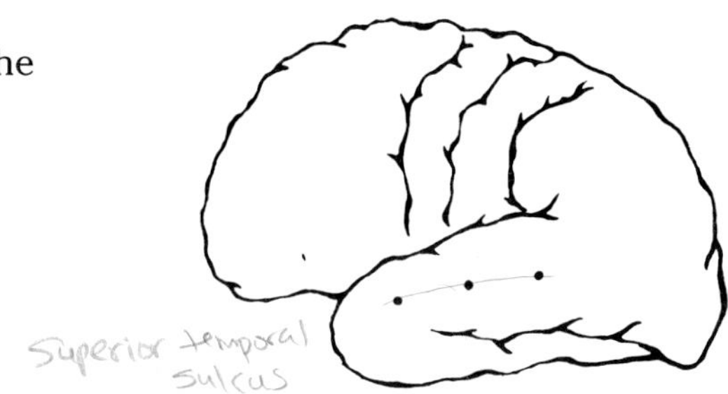

1.6. The preceding diagrams showed the left side of the cerebral cortex; this diagram shows the right side. Draw and label the superior temporal sulcus.

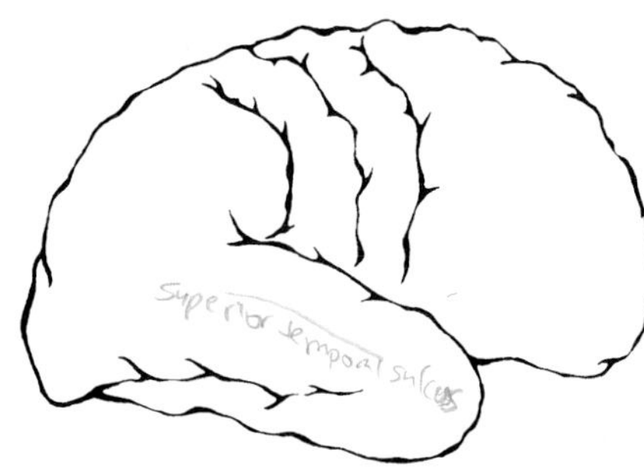

1.7. The superior __temporal__ sulcus takes its name from its location on the __superior__ part of the temporal lobe.

1.8. The lateral sulcus is deeper than the sulcus immediately inferior and parallel to it, termed the __superior__ __temporal__ sulcus.

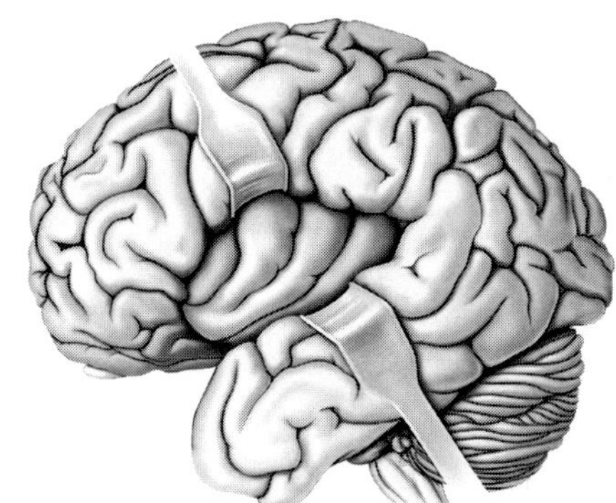

1.4A.

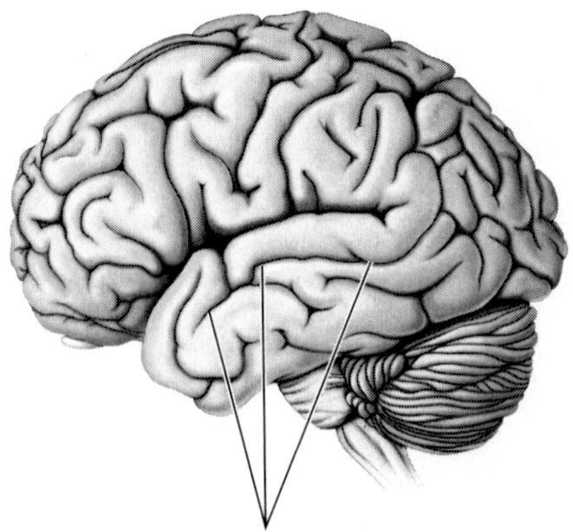

1.5A.

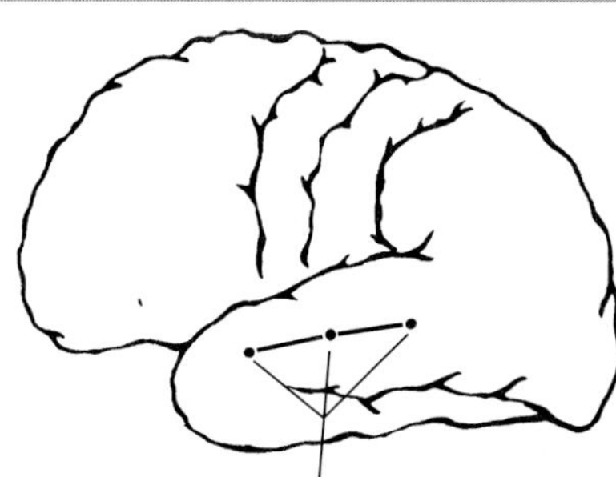

1.6A.

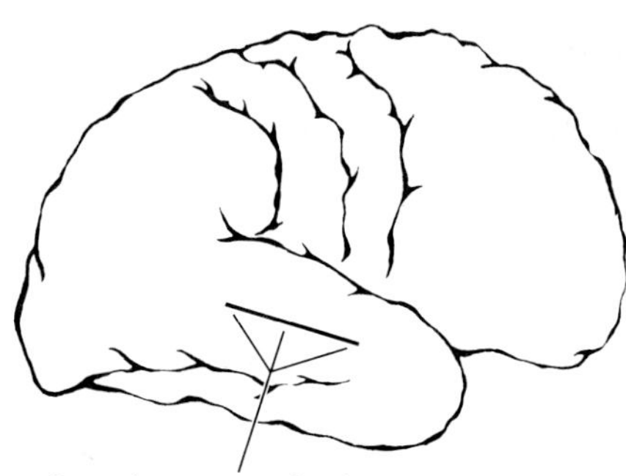

1.7A. temporal; superior

1.8A. superior temporal

1.9. The lateral sulcus is deeper than the superior temporal sulcus.

1.10. The worm-like convolutions of the cortex are *gyri* (singular is *gyrus*). Each gyrus is bounded by sulci.

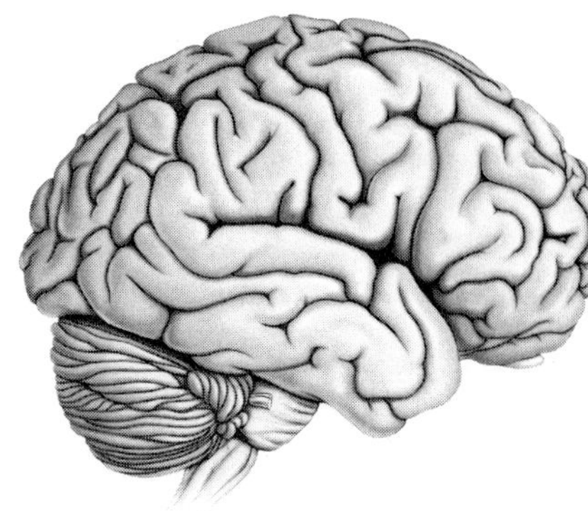

1.11. The grooves on the cortex are called sulci; the convolutions between the grooves are called gyri.

1.12. The lateral sulcus and the superior temporal sulcus enclose a gyrus between them.

1.13. Adjacent gyri appear to be separated on the surface of the cortex, but as the diagram shows, the surface is actually infolded, and adjacent gyri are continuous at the base of each sulcus.

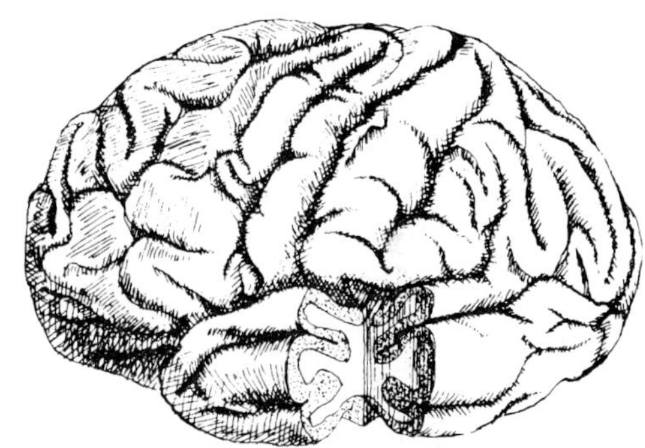

1.14. More than half of the surface of a gyrus is hidden from view in the walls of two adjacent sulci. On the cut surface, blacken the hidden portions of the gyrus labeled "G." The most superior region of the area you blackened is hidden in the wall of the superior temporal sulcus; label this sulcus on the diagram.

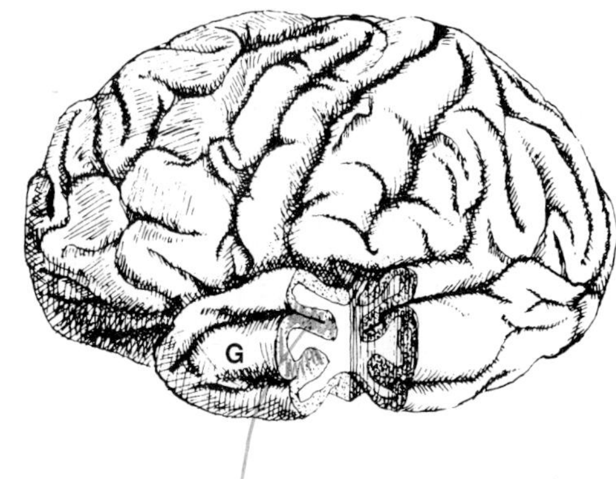

1.9A. lateral; temporal

1.10A. gyrus

1.11A. sulci; gyri

1.12A. gyrus

1.13A. continuous

1.14A. sulci; superior temporal

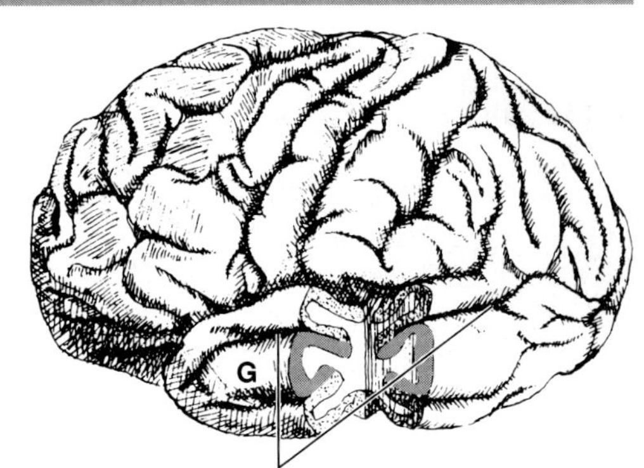

1.15. Inferior to the lateral sulcus, the superior temporal gyrus forms the superior part of the ___temporal___ lobe. Label the gyrus with its name.

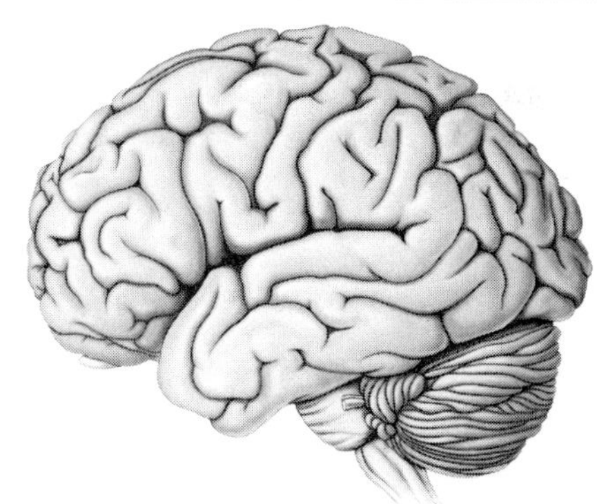

1.16. On the diagram, label the:

lateral sulcus
superior temporal sulcus
superior temporal gyrus.

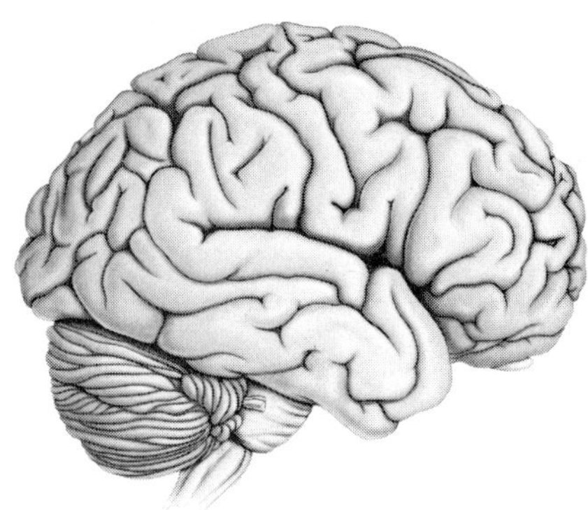

1.17. Inferior to the lateral sulcus is the ___temporal___ lobe.

1.18. The cerebral cortex has other lobes in addition to the temporal lobe. One of these other lobes, named for its location in the *frontal* portion of the brain, is the ___frontal___ lobe.

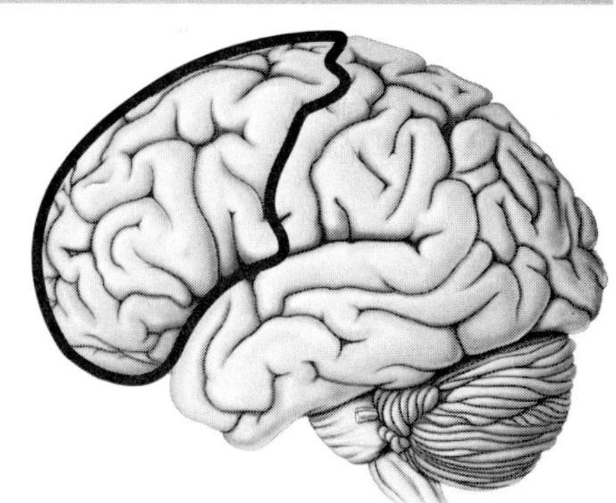

1.19. Three parallel sulci run from the superior surface of the cortex inferiorly to the lateral sulcus. Locate these three sulci, and draw a single circle around the group of them on the diagram (they are located between the broken lines).

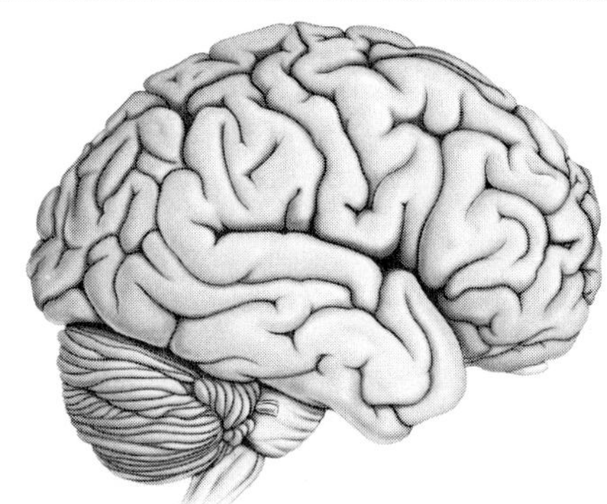

1.15A. temporal

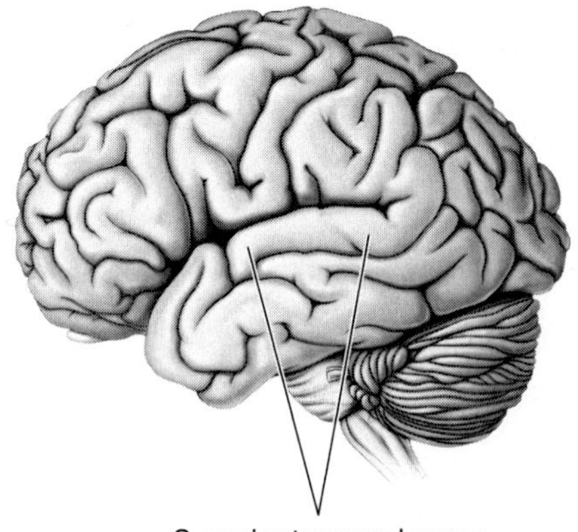

1.16A.

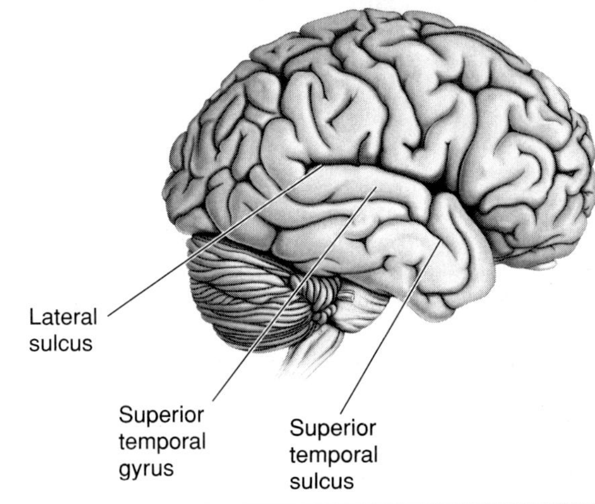

1.17A. temporal

1.18A. frontal

1.19A.

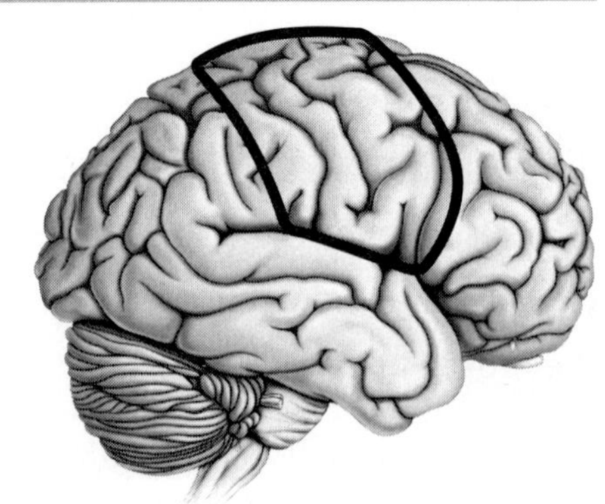

1.20. The central sulcus forms the posterior boundary of the ____________ lobe.

1.21. The three sulci enclose two ________.

1.22. The two gyri on either side of the central sulcus are logically named the precentral and ________ central sulci.

1.23. The gyrus between the central and precentral sulci is the ________central gyrus.

1.24. Of the two gyri bordering the central sulcus, the one in the frontal lobe is the ____________________ gyrus.

1.25. The gyrus posterior to the central sulcus is the ____________________ gyrus. The gyrus just anterior to the central sulcus is the ____________________ gyrus.

1.26. The gyrus farthest posterior on the frontal lobe is the ____________________ gyrus.

1.27. The lobe directly posterior to the frontal lobe is the parietal lobe. The postcentral gyrus is in the ____________ lobe.

1.20A. frontal

1.21A. gyri

1.22A. postcentral

1.23A. precentral

1.24A. precentral

1.25A. postcentral; precentral

1.26A. precentral

1.27A. parietal

1.28. On the lateral surface of the cortex, the sulcus dividing the frontal from the parietal lobe is the ________ sulcus. Indicate this sulcus with an arrow.

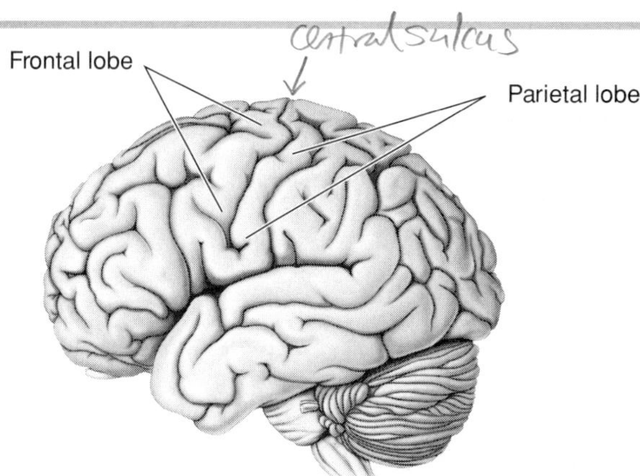

1.29. The central sulcus is the anterior boundary of the ________ lobe.

1.30. On passing posteriorly from the precentral gyrus of the ________ lobe, one reaches the ________ lobe. With an arrow, indicate the boundary between these two lobes.

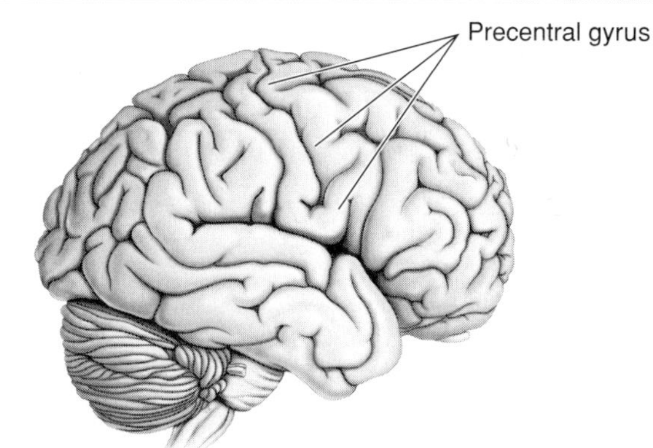

1.31. The most anterior gyrus of the parietal lobe is the ________ gyrus.

1.32. The central sulcus is fairly constant from brain to brain. Label the central sulcus with a "C" on both sides of this brain, viewed from ________.

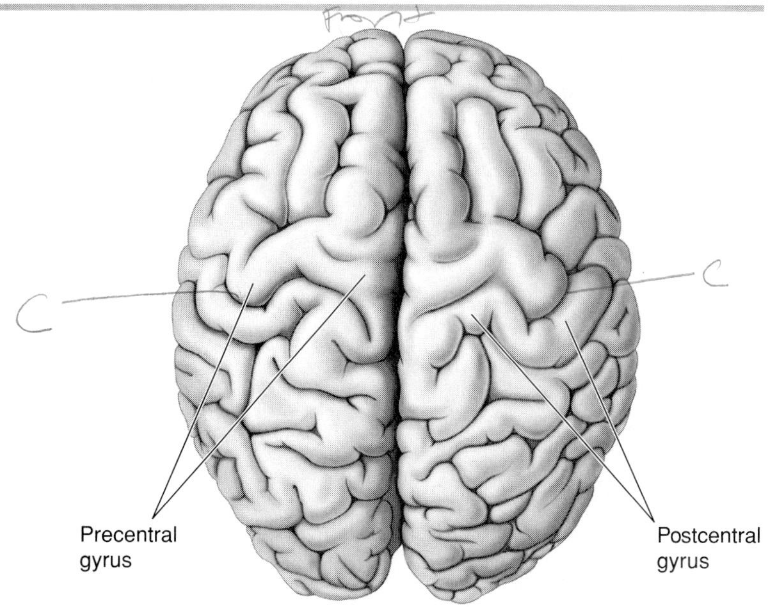

1.28A. central

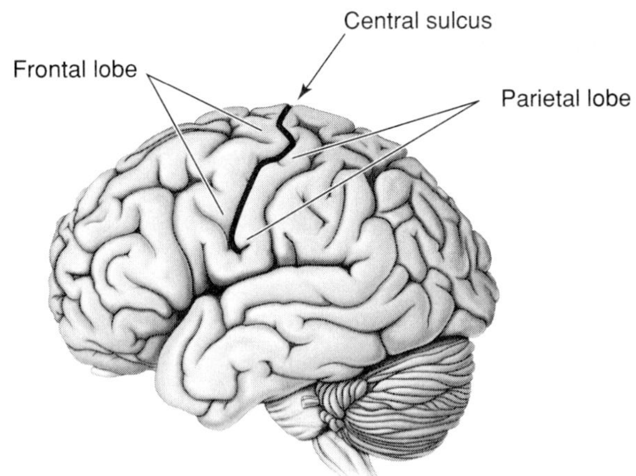

1.29A. parietal

1.30A. frontal; parietal

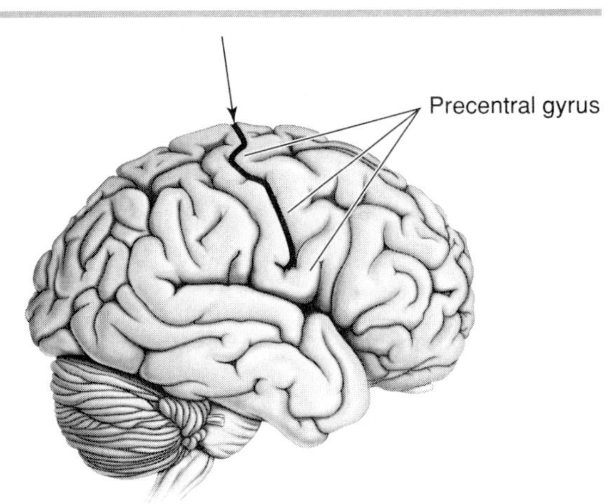

1.31A. postcentral

1.32A. above

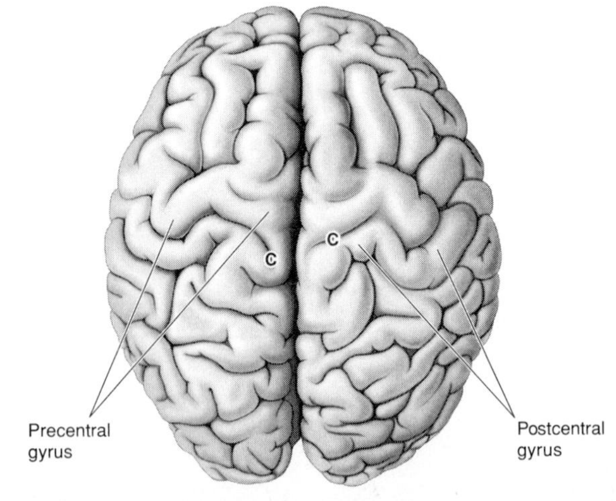

1.33. Label the three sulci that delineate the precentral and postcentral gyri.

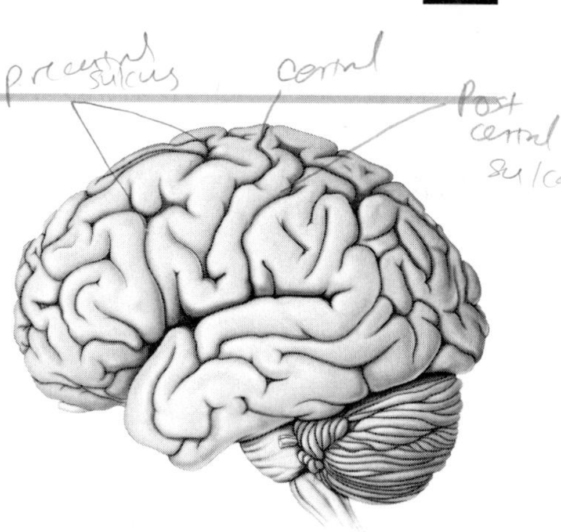

1.34. Connect the labels with the appropriate structure. With each labeled gyrus, write the name of the lobe in which it is located.

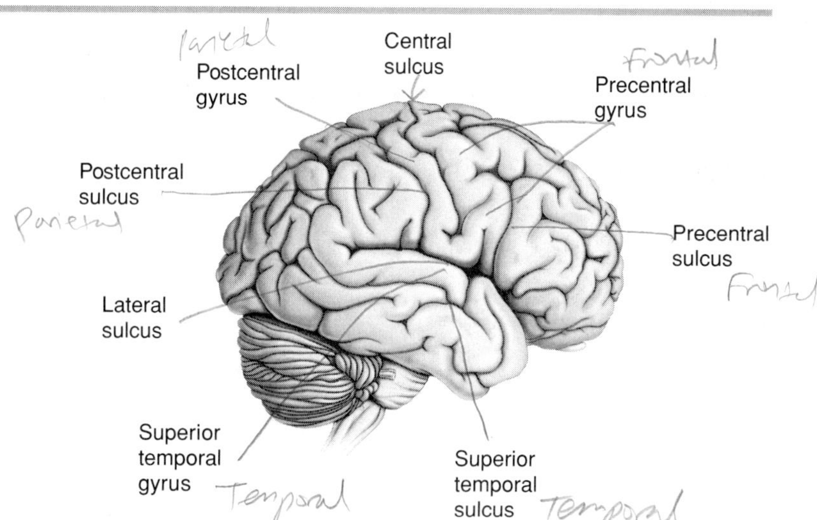

1.35. Label the cortical components to which lines have been drawn on the diagram.

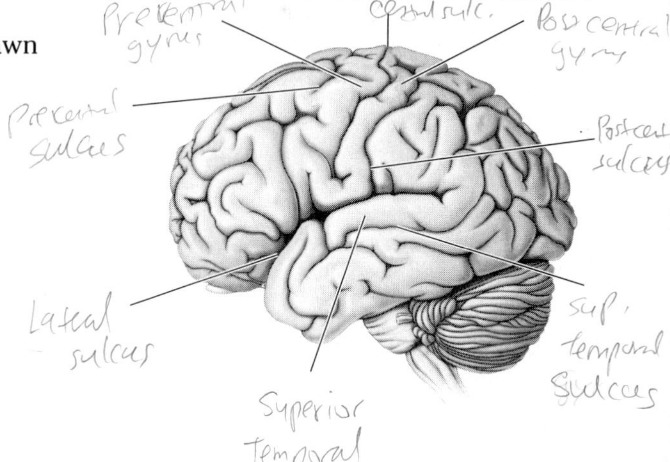

1.33A.

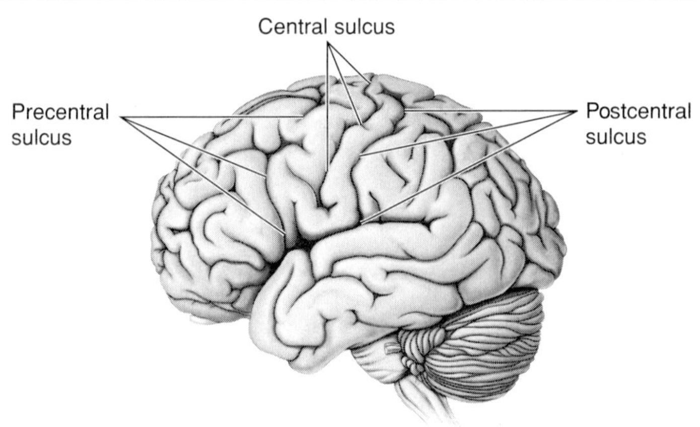
Central sulcus
Precentral sulcus
Postcentral sulcus

1.34A.

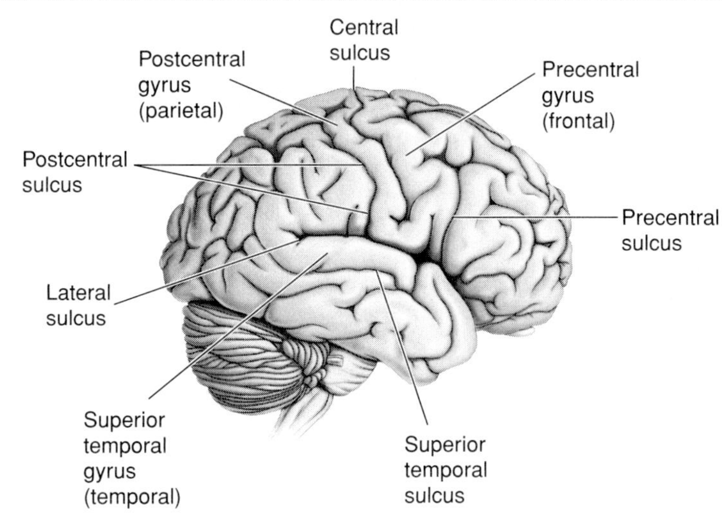
Central sulcus
Postcentral gyrus (parietal)
Precentral gyrus (frontal)
Postcentral sulcus
Precentral sulcus
Lateral sulcus
Superior temporal gyrus (temporal)
Superior temporal sulcus

1.35A.

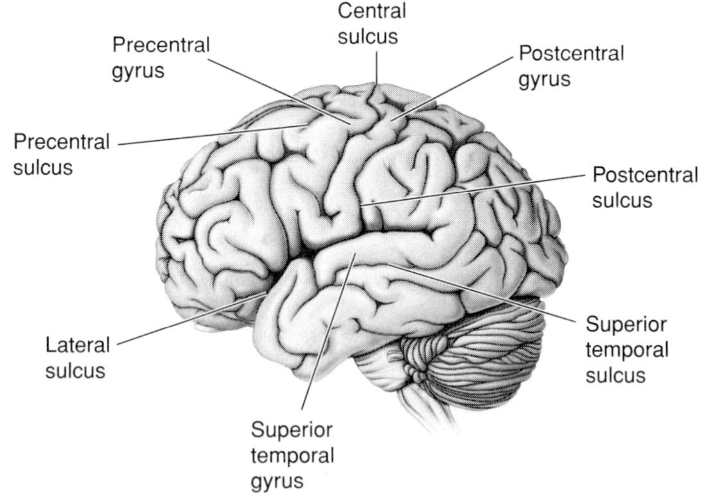
Central sulcus
Precentral gyrus
Postcentral gyrus
Precentral sulcus
Postcentral sulcus
Lateral sulcus
Superior temporal sulcus
Superior temporal gyrus

2 Surface of the Brain II

2.1. The anterior end of the cortex is part of the frontal lobe; the opposite end of the cortex is part of the occipital lobe. Label these two lobes on both views.

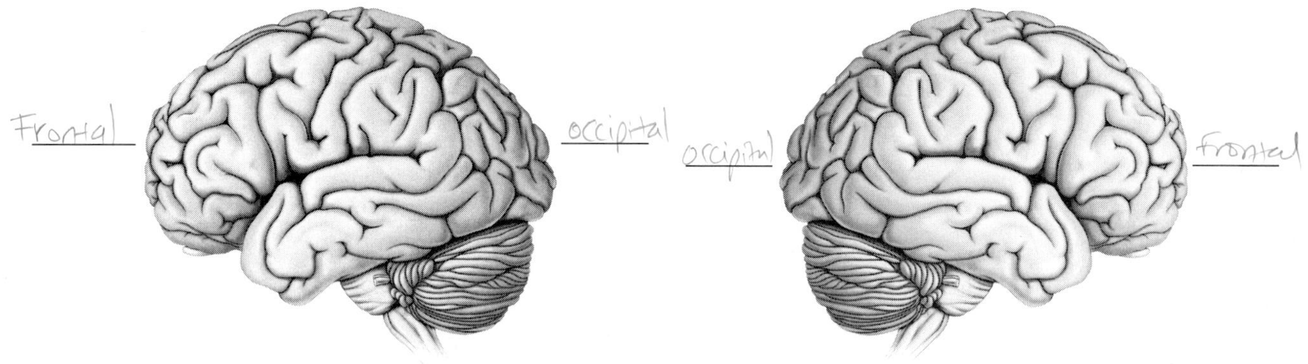

2.2. The two extreme ends of the cortex are often referred to as poles, the frontal ________ and the ________ ________.

2.3. The ________ sulcus extends over the superior surface of the brain and runs a short distance on the medial surface. As it turns over the top, the sulcus is closer to the ________ pole than to the opposite pole.

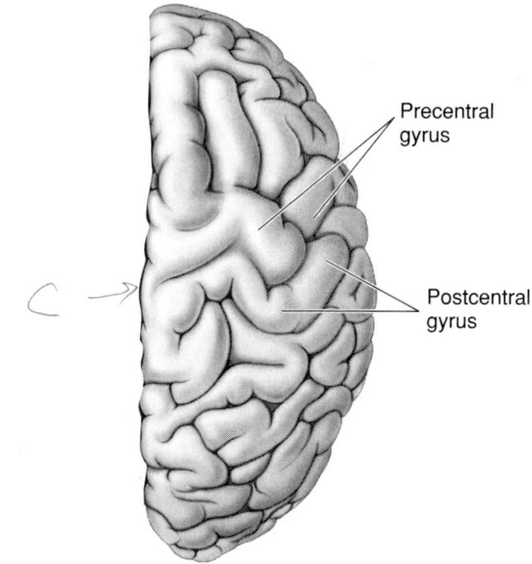

2.1A.

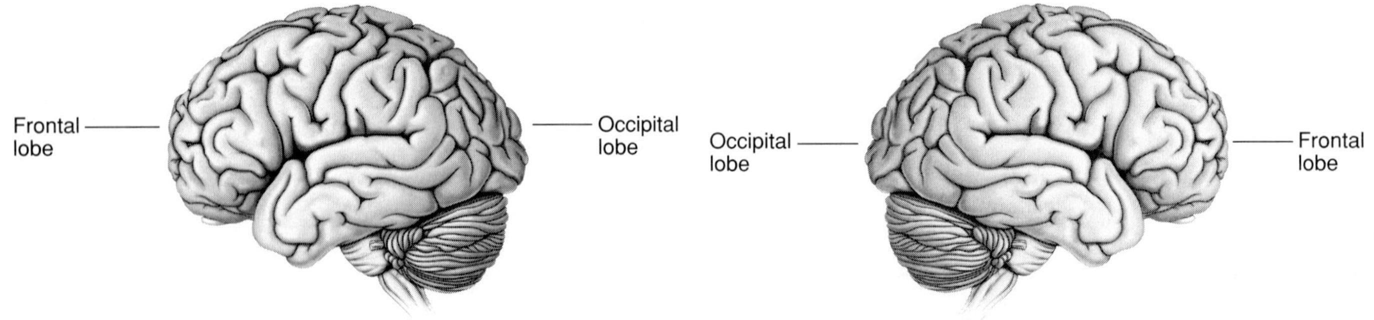

2.2A. pole; occipital pole

2.3A. central; occipital

2.4. Although most of the boundaries are imprecise, the cortex is conventionally divided into four lobes. Locate and label them on the diagram.

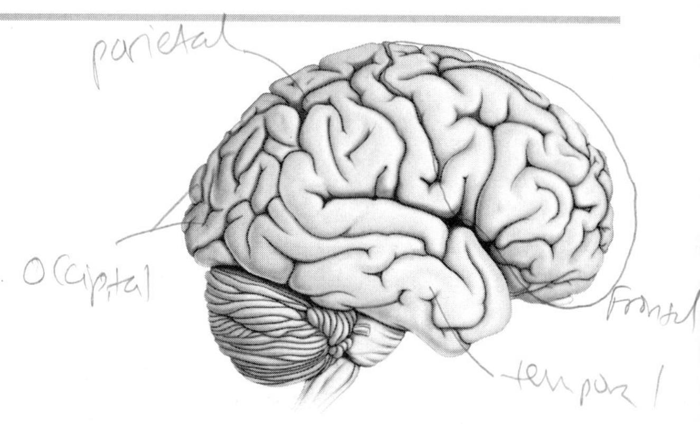

2.5. The occipital pole of the cortex is at the ________ ior end of the occipital lobe; the precentral gyrus lies ________ ior to the central sulcus; at the anterior end of the frontal lobe is the ________ ________. Most of the temporal lobe lies ________ ior to the parietal lobe; the lateral sulcus lies ________ ior to the superior temporal sulcus.

Superior

Posterior

Anterior

Inferior

2.6. Identify the frontal pole with arrows. A course traced from the frontal pole over the superior surface of the cortex will pass from the ________ lobe to the ________ lobe to the ________ lobe.

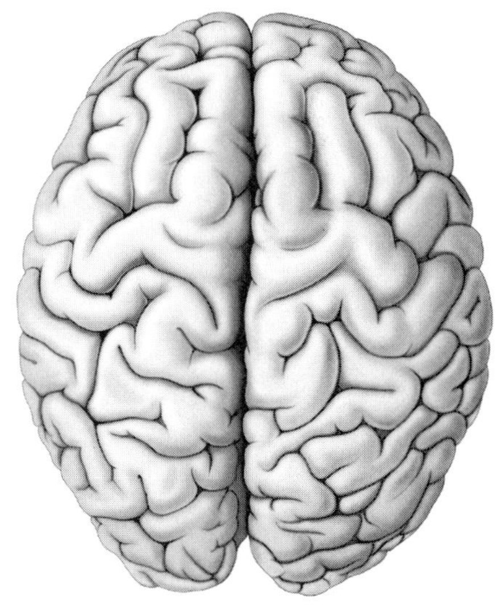

2.4A.

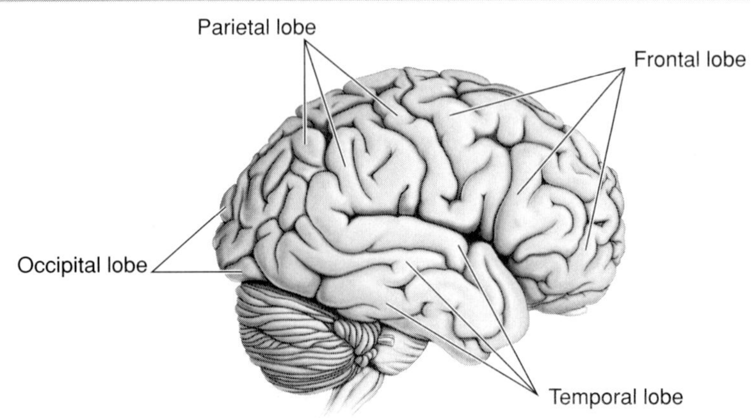

2.5A. posterior; anterior; frontal pole; inferior; superior

2.6A. frontal; parietal; occipital

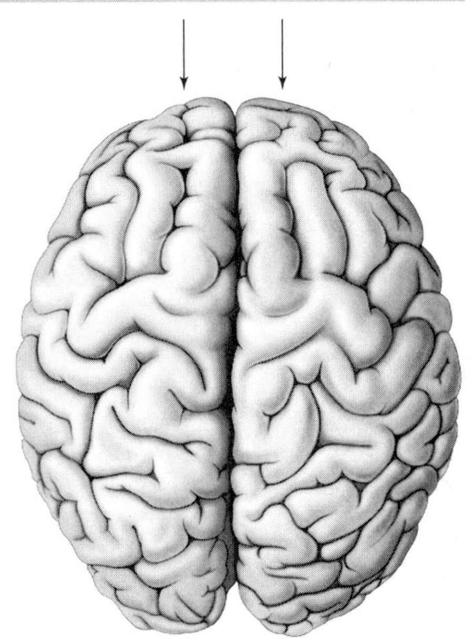

2.7. The parietal lobe is bounded anteriorly by the frontal lobe, posteriorly by the occipital lobe, and inferiorly by the temporal lobe.

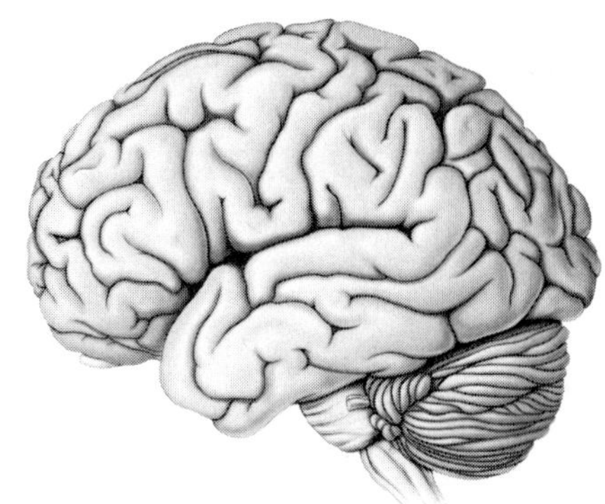

2.8. The boundary between parietal and frontal lobes is the Central sulcus.

2.9. Much of the border between the parietal and temporal lobes is indefinite and forms a zone (shaded on the diagram) called the parieto- temporal area.

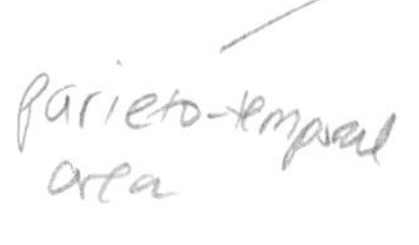

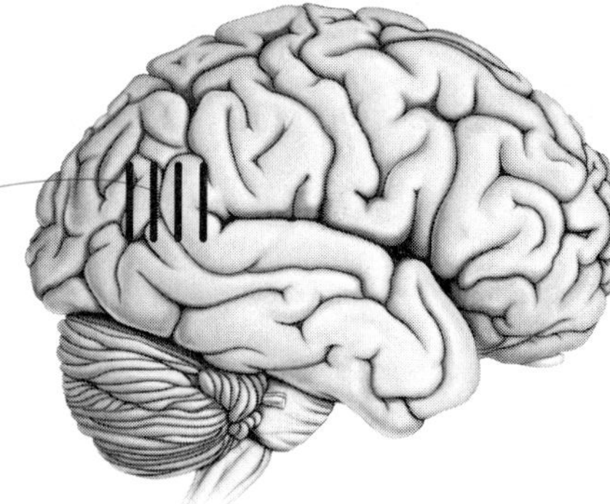

2.10. There are other indefinite borders (shaded in) on the lateral aspect of the brain in addition to the parieto-temporal area. There are the parieto- occipital and temporo -occipital transition areas.

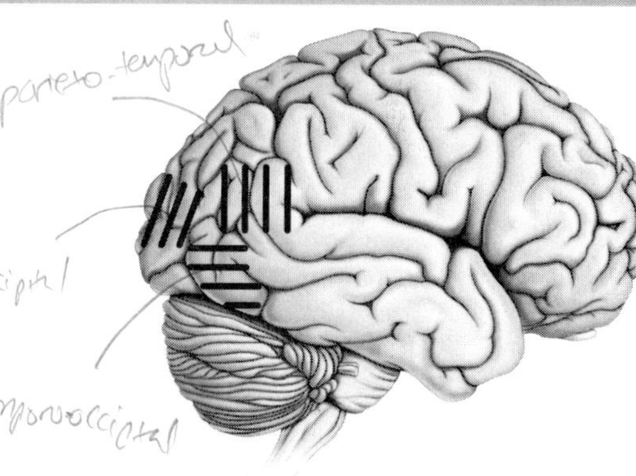

2.11. On the lateral surface of the brain, the parietal, occipital, and frontal lobes appear to be continuous.

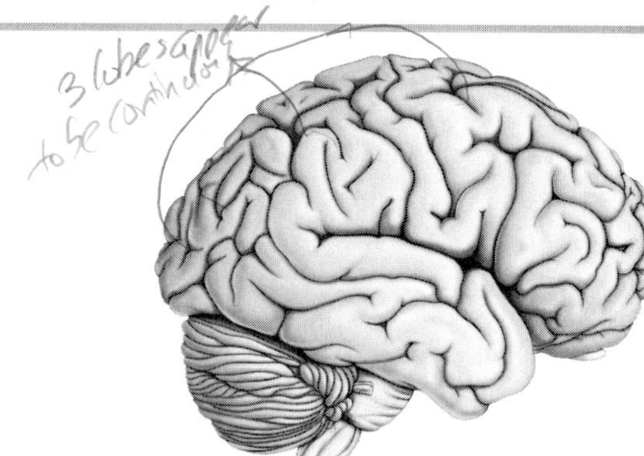

2.7A. frontal; occipital; temporal

2.8A. central sulcus

2.9A. temporal

2.10A. parieto-occipital; temporo-occipital

2.11A. frontal; parietal; occipital

2.12. This diagram shows that a line connecting the preoccipital notch and the parieto-occipital sulcus forms the anterior boundary of the occipital lobe on the lateral surface of the cortex.

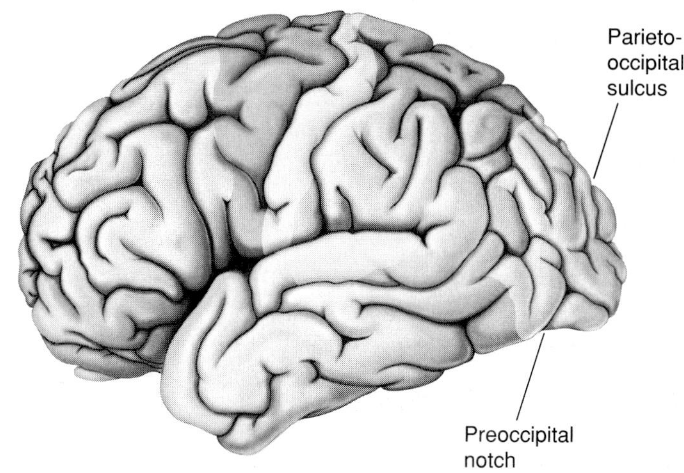

2.13. The parieto-occipital sulcus and preoccipital notch are not prominent on the lateral surface of most brains. On the diagram, shade in the approximate extent of the occipital lobe.

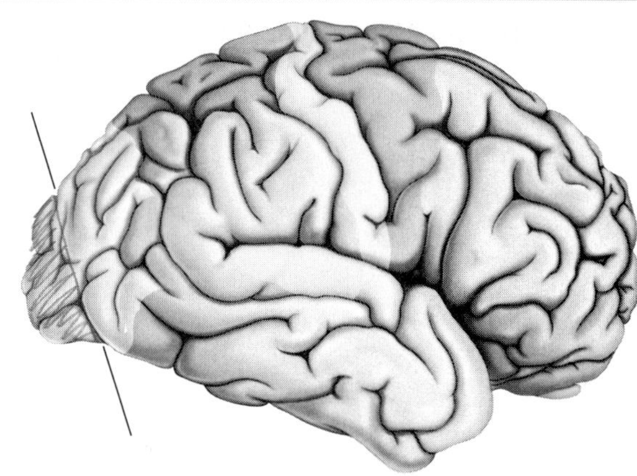

2.14. On the lateral surface of the cortex, the occipital lobe is the small est in area of all of the cortical lobes.

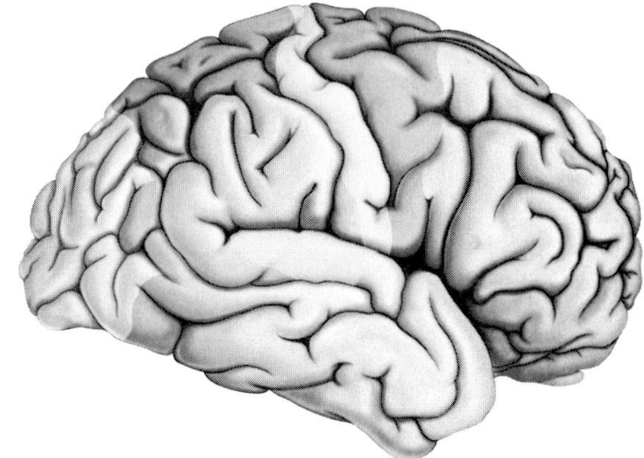

2.12A. <u>occipital</u>

2.13A.

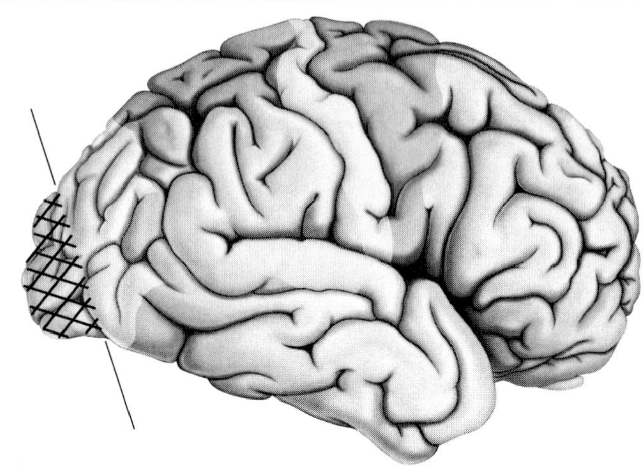

2.14A. <u>small</u>est

2.15. Trace the parieto-occipital sulcus from the lateral surface over the superior aspect of the brain to the medial surface. Label the arrow marking the parieto-occipital sulcus on the medial view.

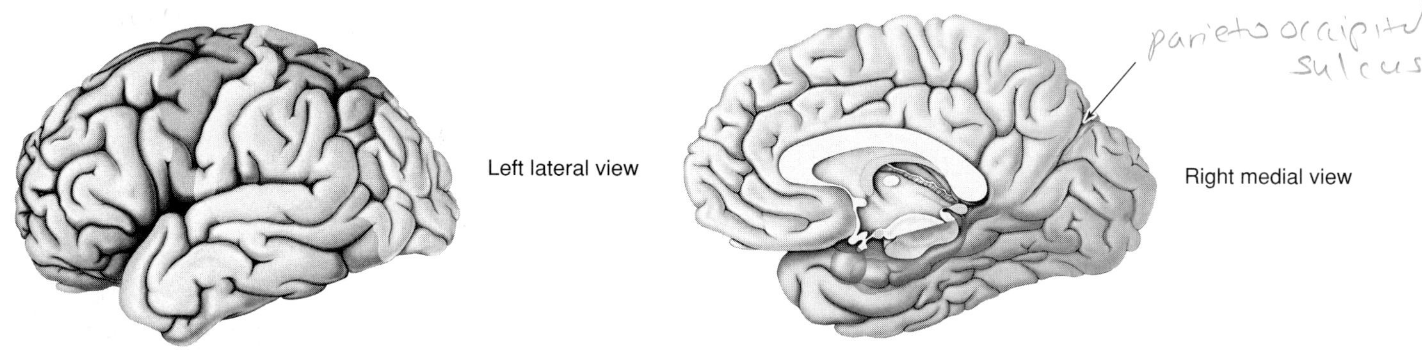

2.16. The occipital lobe is ______er in area on the medial surface than it is on the lateral surface. Label the parieto-occipital sulcus on the medial view.

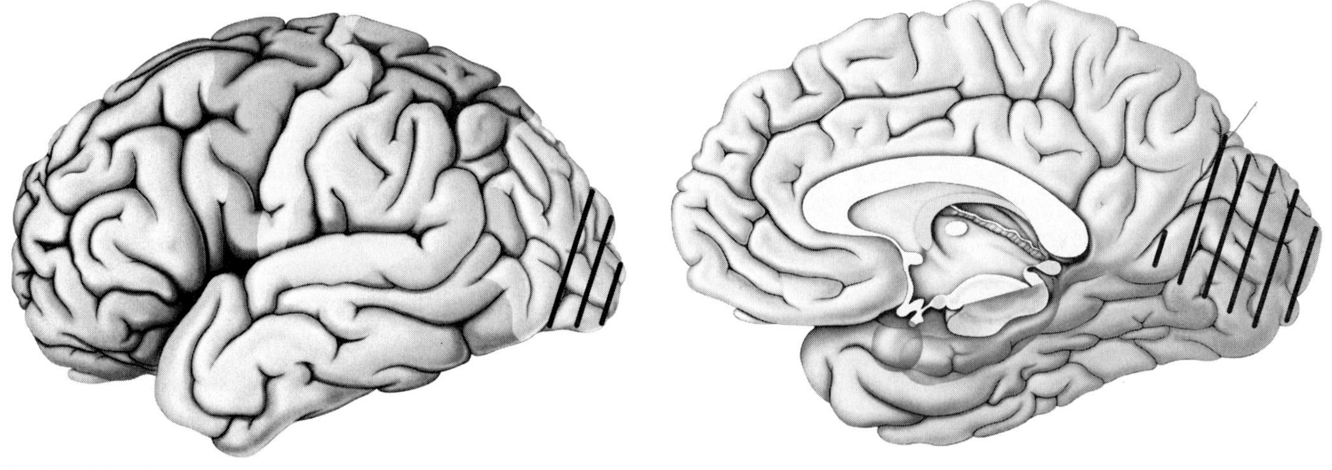

2.17. Label the prominent sulcus that forms the posterior boundary of the parietal lobe on the medial surface.

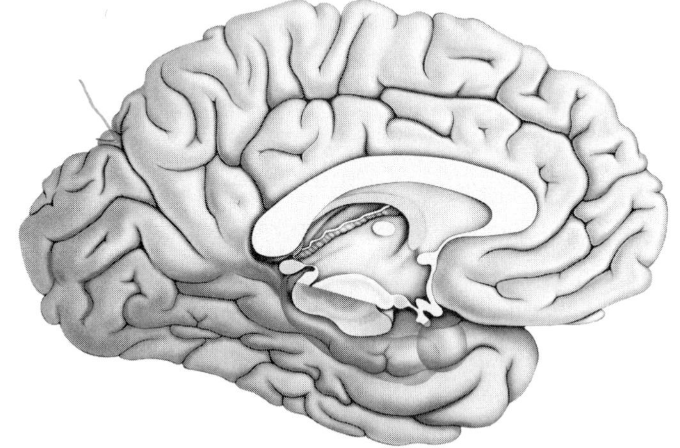

2.15A.

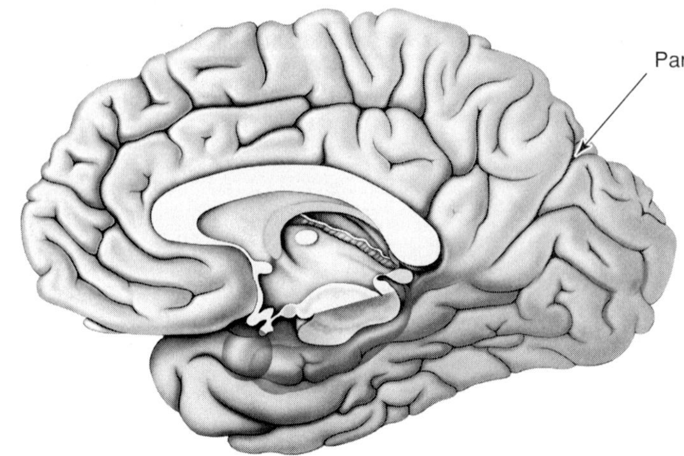

2.16A. greater

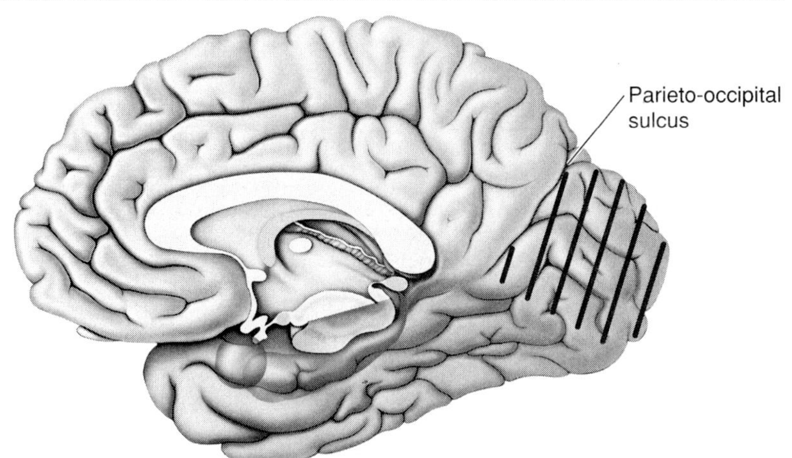

2.17A.

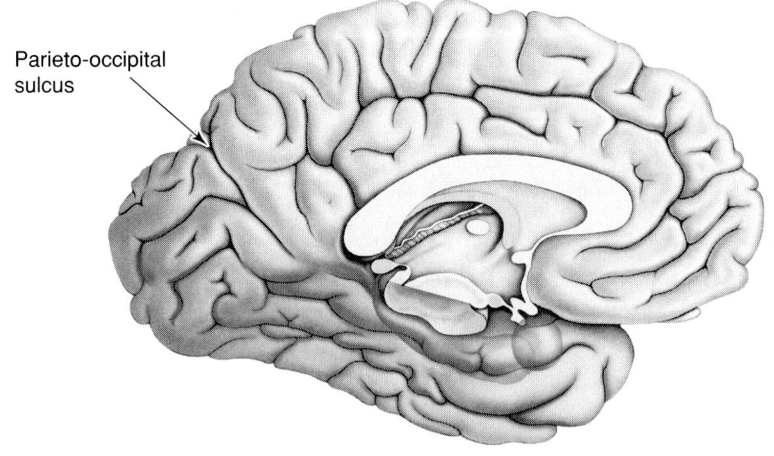

2.18. The calcarine sulcus is the other prominent landmark on the medial surface of the occipital lobe. Label the horizontally oriented calcarine sulcus on the diagram.

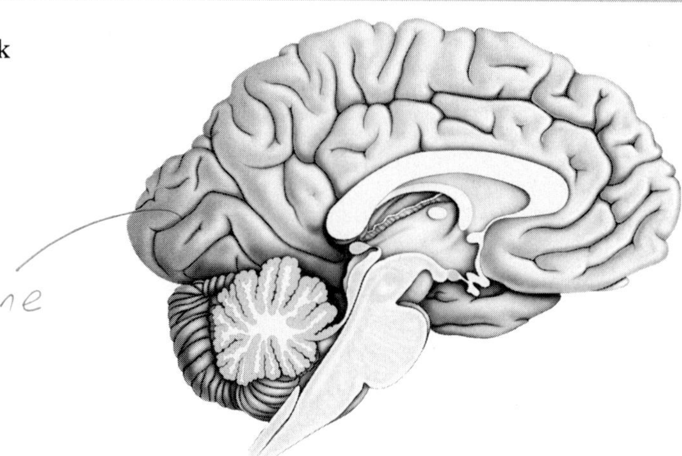

2.19. A "hard" pronunciation (as in calculus) is given to both c's in calc arine.

2.20. The part of the occipital cortex shaded on the diagram is named for the sulcus it encloses; it is called the Calcarine cortex. Label it on the diagram.

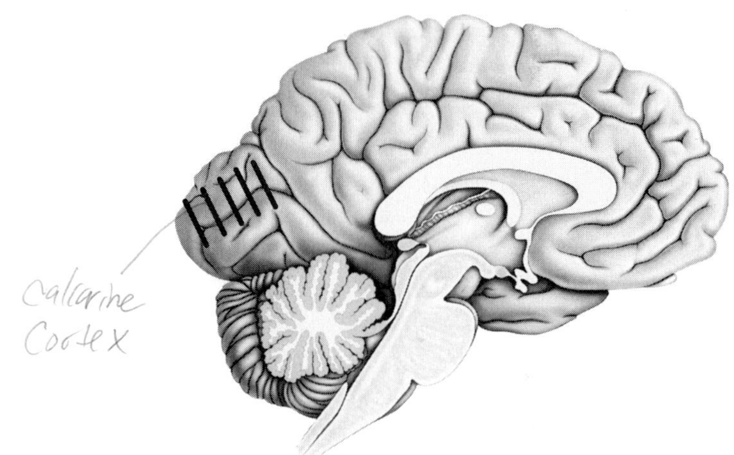

2.21. The brain is seen here from a medial-inferior view. The shaded area separates the Occipital lobe from the temporal lobe.

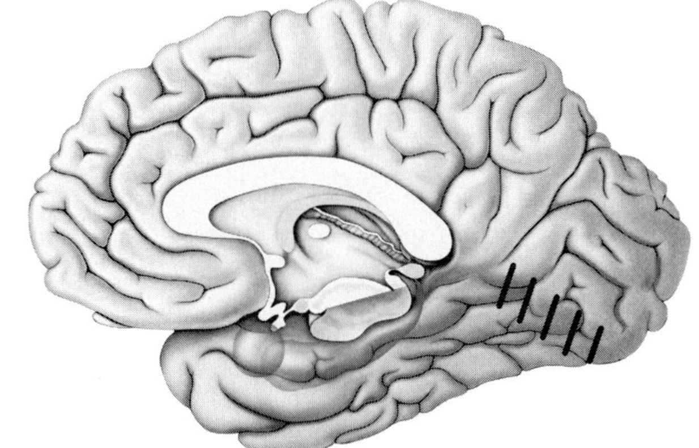

2.18A.

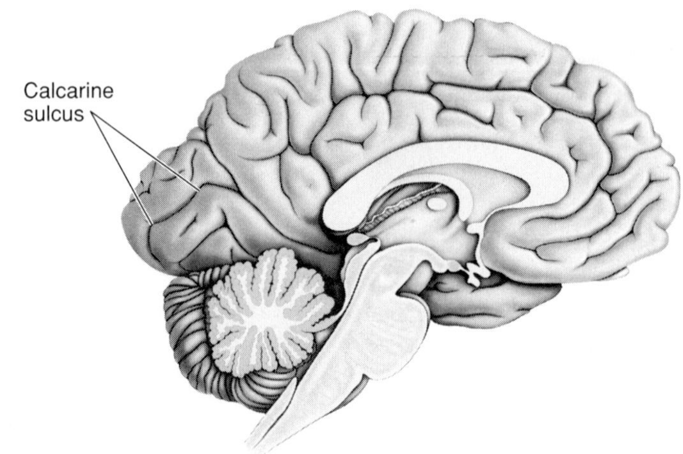

2.19A. calcarine

2.20A. calcarine

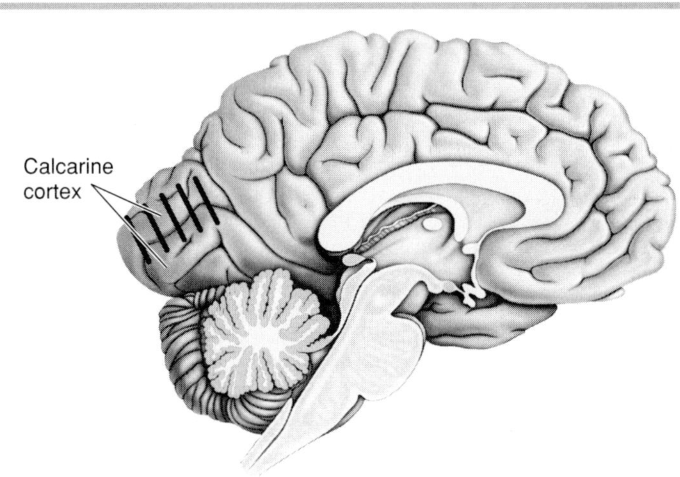

2.21A. occipital; temporal

2.22. On the medial surface of the cortex, the boundary of the parietal and occipital lobes is formed by the parieto -occipital sulcus. The calcarine sulcus lies entirely within the occipital lobe.

2.23. On the diagram, label the indicated features of the cortex in the occipital lobe.

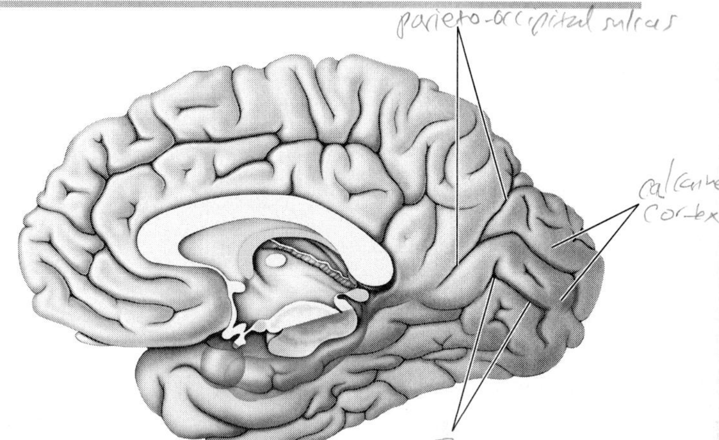

2.24. Areas of the brain are not only distinct anatomically, but they also contribute to different cortical functions (visual, auditory, somesthetic, motor, etc.). For example, if the precentral gyrus is damaged, a person may be partially paralyzed. The frontal lobe, therefore, is involved in motor function.

2.25. Refer to both diagrams to answer the following questions.

The number of primary sensory areas indicated is 3. How many motor areas? 1.

The primary auditory area is not directly on either cortical surface (medial or lateral) but is mainly out of sight on the inner sides of the Superior temporal gyrus of the temporal lobe.

The primary visual area is in the walls of the calcarine sulcus, in the occipital lobe.

The remaining primary sensory area is the Somesthetic area, located in the postcentral gyrus of the parietal lobe.

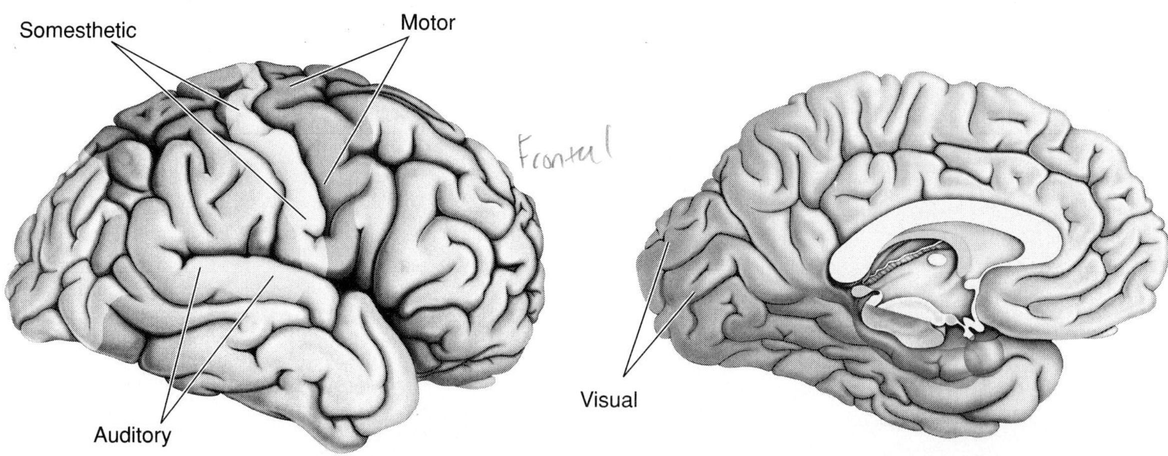

2.22A. parieto-occipital sulcus; calcarine

2.23A.

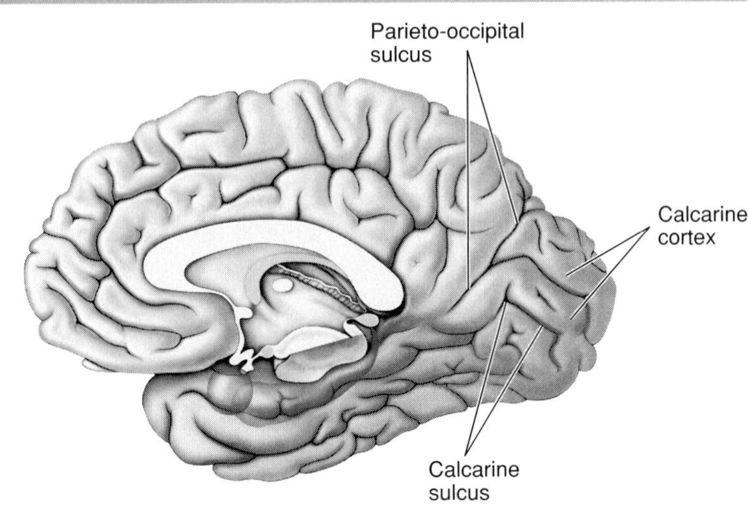

2.24A. frontal

2.25A. 3; 1

superior temporal; temporal

calcarine; occipital

somesthetic; postcentral; parietal

2.26. The specific sensory modalities such as touch, pressure, and position sense are included in the general class of som esthetic senses. On the diagram, name the general class of functions in which each of the two indicated areas is involved.

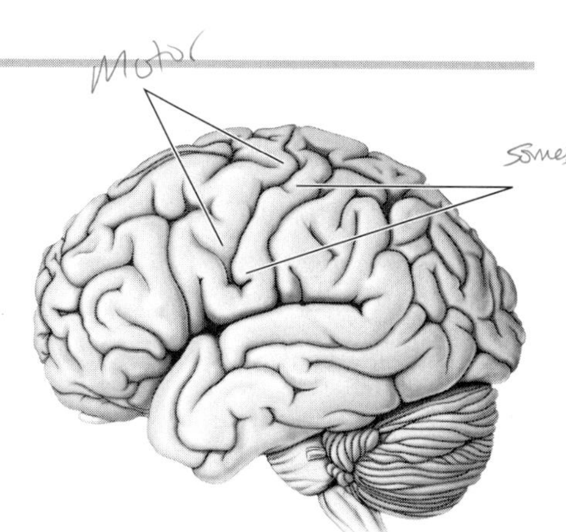

2.27. A small part of the area for primary reception of auditory information (indicated on the diagram) is barely visible on the Superior temporal gyrus. Most of the auditory area is hidden deep in the temporal lobe and can be reached by passing a finger into the lateral sulcus.

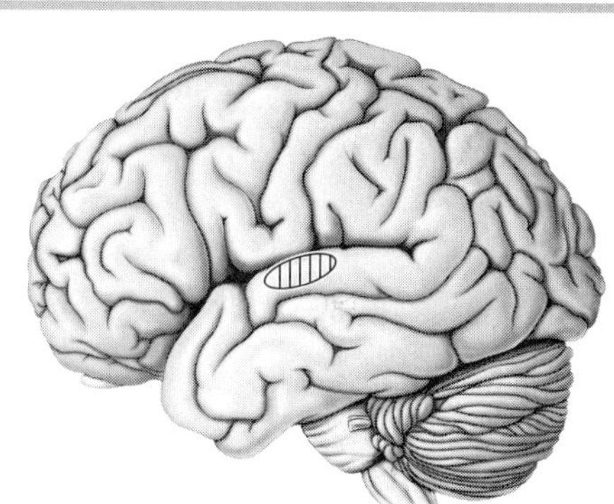

2.28. This is a view of the lateral surface of the right cerebral cortex. The primary visual area is not visible because it is almost entirely in the walls of the calcarine fissure, on the medial surface of the occipital lobe. Label the three indicated areas with the general class of functions in which each is involved.

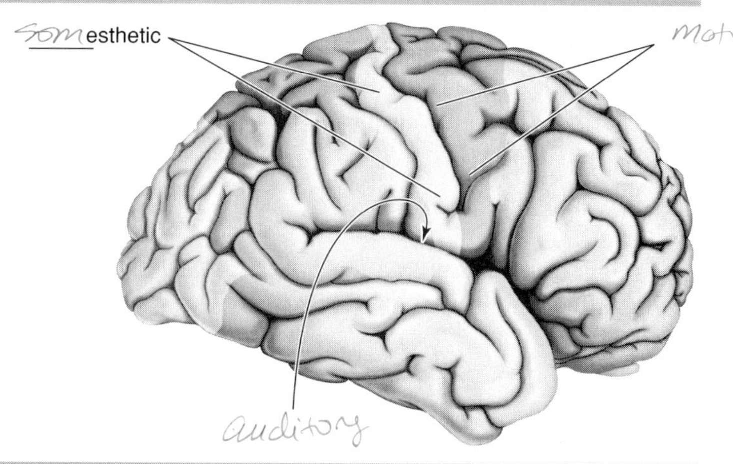

2.29. Two primary sensory areas are almost entirely in a view of the lateral surface of the cortex. These senses are vision and hearing, represented in the occipital and temporal lobes, respectively. Of the two senses, the only one represented on the medial surface of the cortex is vision.

2.26A. somesthetic

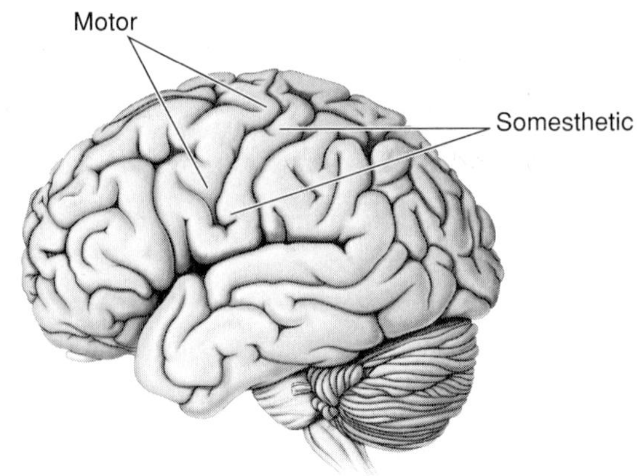

2.27A. superior temporal; lateral

2.28A. lateral; medial; occipital

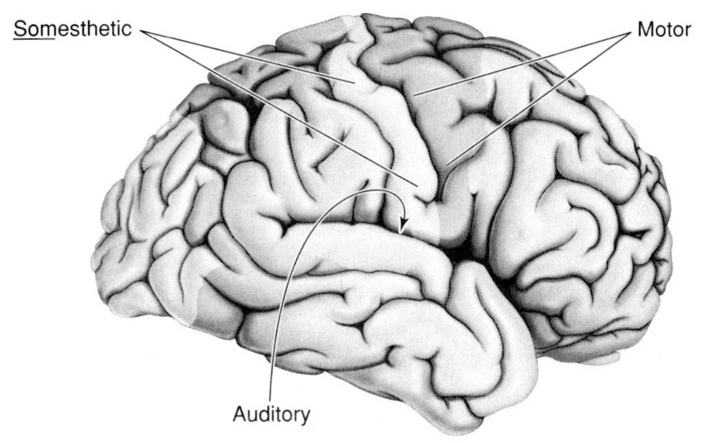

2.29A. hearing (audition); occipital; temporal; vision

2.30. A lesion that involves the territories adjacent to the central sulcus affects the general classes of motor and somesthetic sensory functions. On the diagram, locate the two gyri that are involved and label their primary functions.

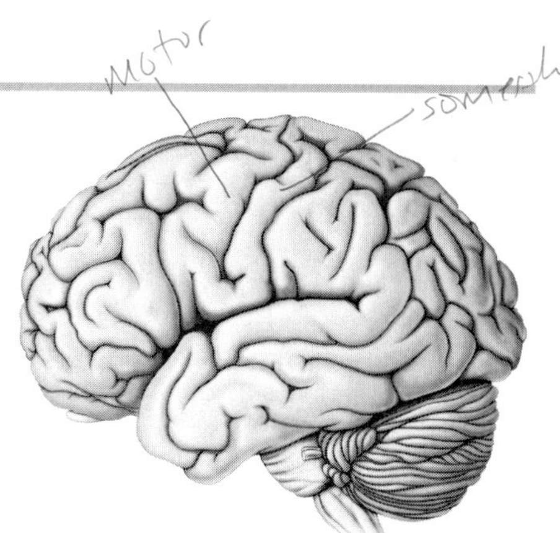

2.31. Assuming damage in the cortex, you might suspect that a paralyzed patient has a damaged frontal lobe, whereas a patient who does not respond normally to touch may have parietal lobe damage.

2.32. On the appropriate diagram, use the designated letters to indicate the sites of the primary auditory (A), visual (V), motor (M), and somesthetic (S) areas. Name the lobe in which each is located.

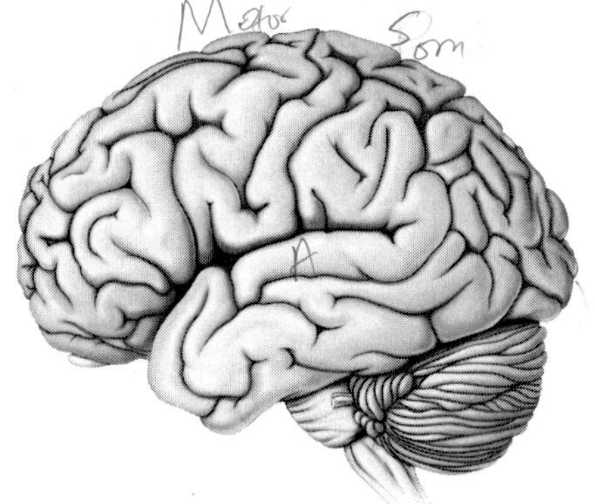

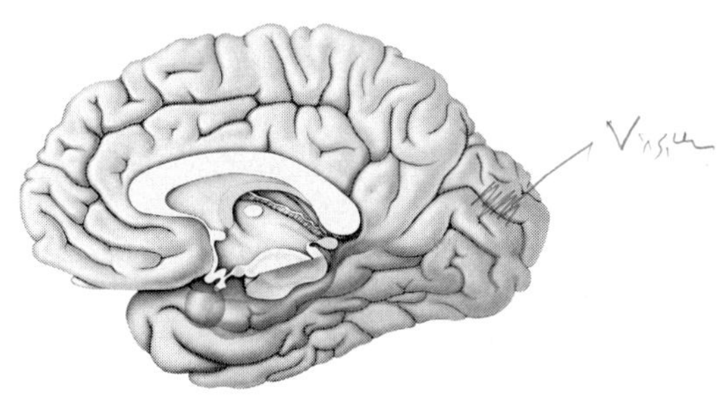

2.33. The primary motor area of the cerebral cortex is the precentral gyrus of the frontal lobe.

The primary auditory area is on the inside of the superior temporal gyrus of the temporal lobe.

The primary visual area is the calcarine cortex, bounding the sulcus of the same name, in the occipital lobe.

The somesthetic, or somatosensory, area is located in the postcentral gyrus of the parietal lobe.

2.30A. somesthetic

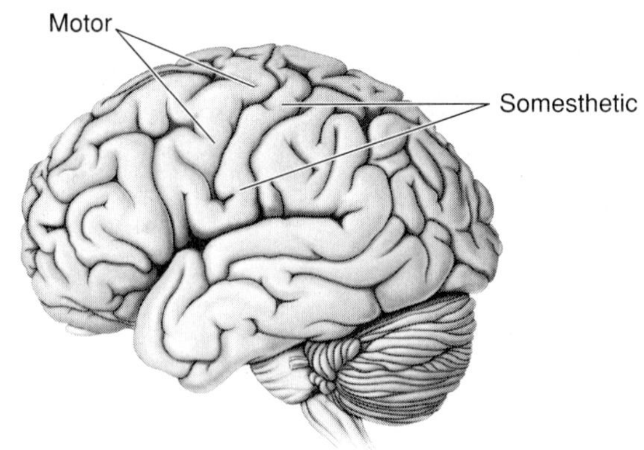

2.31A. frontal; parietal

2.32A.

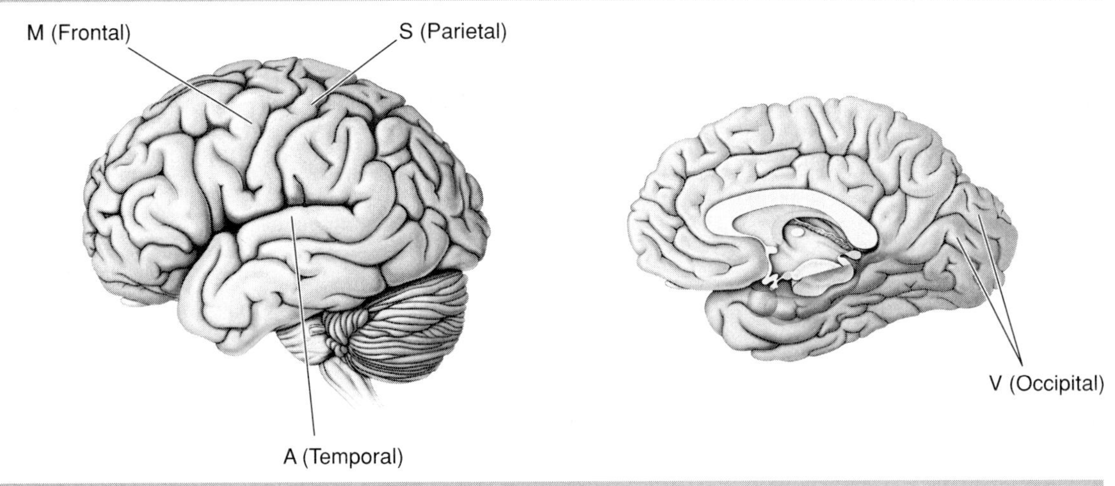

2.33A.

precentral; frontal

superior temporal; temporal

calcarine; sulcus; occipital

postcentral; parietal

2.34. On the medial view, three extensive cortical structures have a concentric arrangement. Starting with the most inferior and proceeding superiorly, these are the Corpus Callosum, the Cingulate gyrus and the Cingulate sulcus.

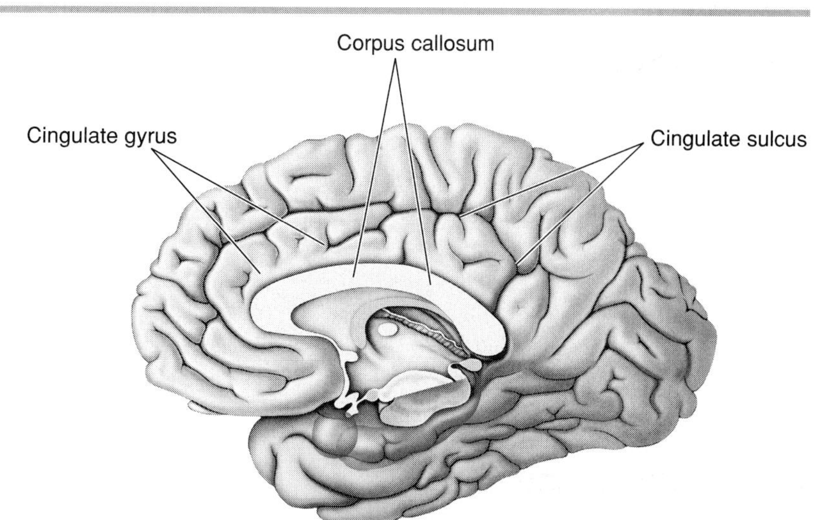

2.35. The most inferior of the concentric structures is the Corpus callosum. Indicate and label it on the diagram.

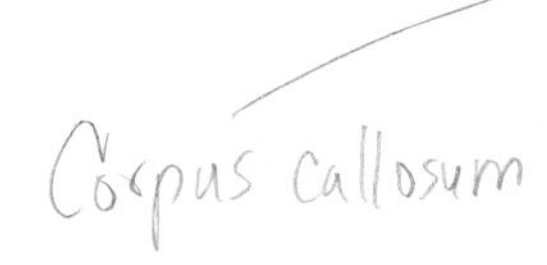

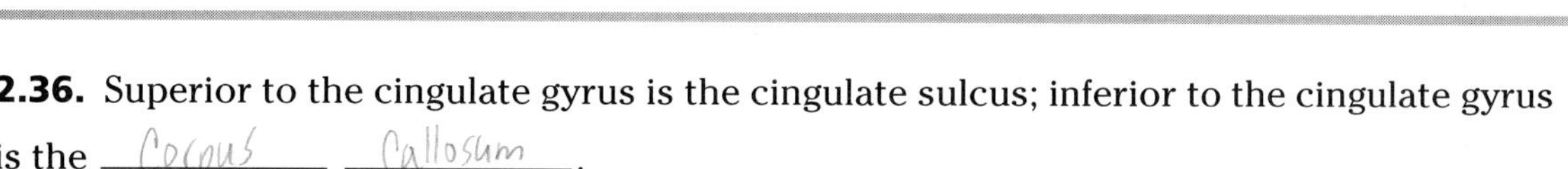

2.36. Superior to the cingulate gyrus is the cingulate sulcus; inferior to the cingulate gyrus is the Corpus Callosum.

2.37. The marginal branch of the cingulate sulcus is a reliable landmark. This groove extends from the Cing ulate Sulcus and runs along the medial surface up to the Sup ior surface of the brain.

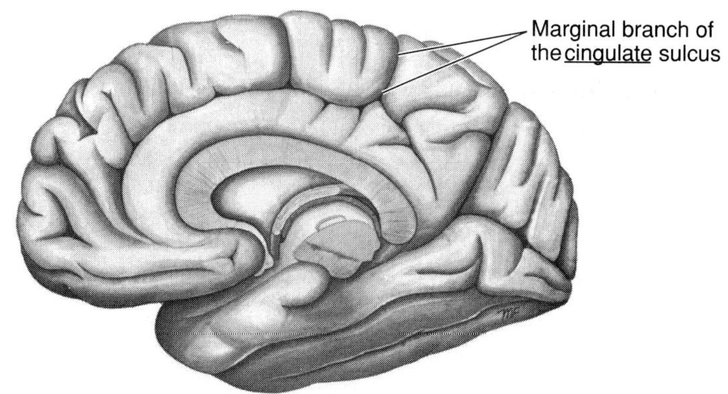

2.34A. corpus callosum; cingulate gyrus; cingulate sulcus

2.35A. corpus

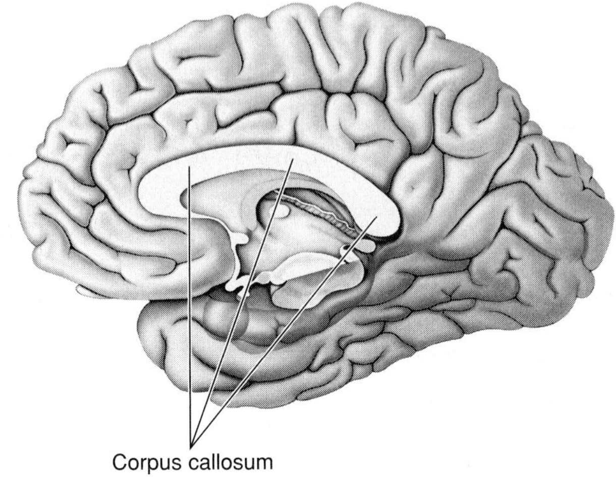

2.36A. corpus callosum

2.37A. cingulate sulcus; superior

2.38. Label the indicated structures.

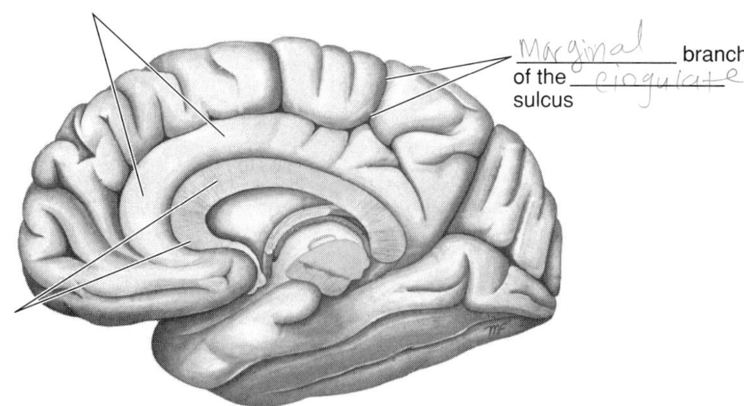

2.39. The central sulcus is visible on the medial view. It is always recognizable as the first sulcus in front of the ________ ________ of the ________ ________.

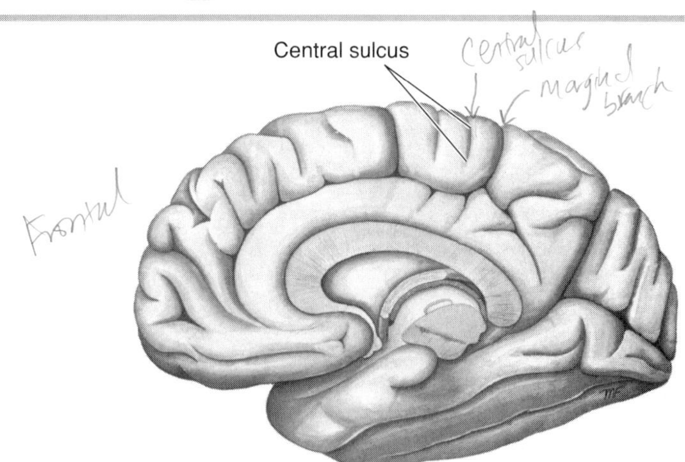

2.40. The frontal lobe is demarcated by the corpus callosum, by the lateral sulcus, and posteriorly by the ________ ________. Draw the boundaries of the frontal lobe on both views.

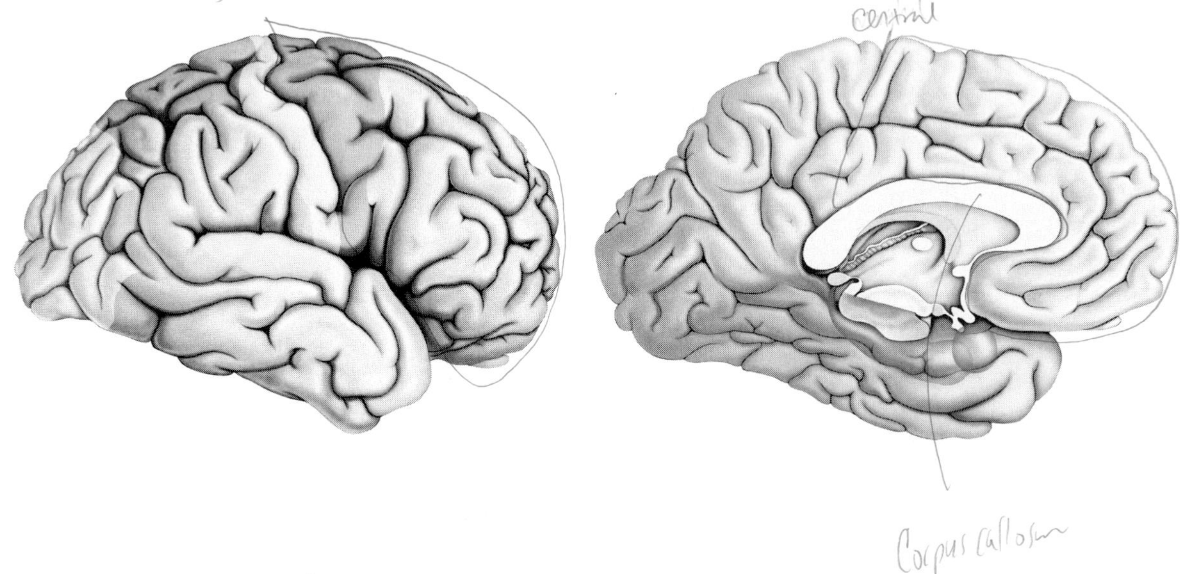

2.38A.

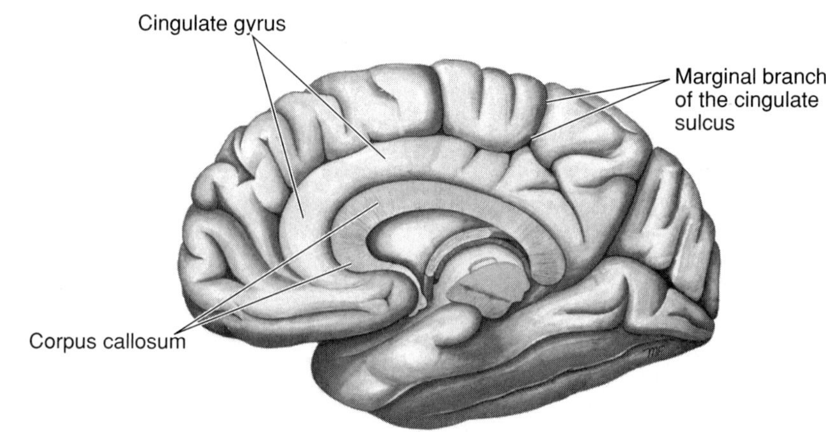

2.39A. marginal branch; cingulate sulcus

2.40A. central sulcus

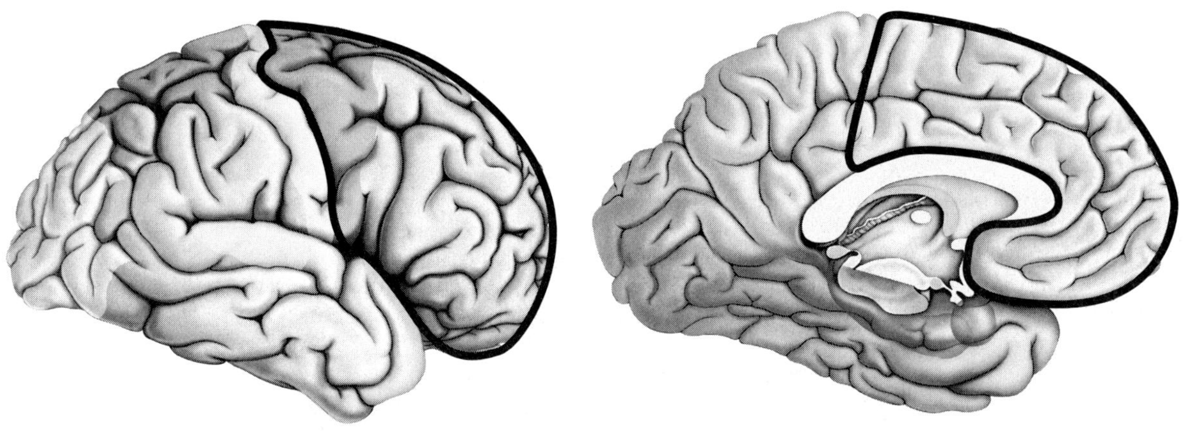

3 Divisions of the Brain and Brodmann's Areas

3.1. At the beginning of the 20th century, a German neuroanatomist named Korbinian *Brodmann* divided the cerebral cortex into 52 areas according to their histological differences. Some of these areas have distinct neurological functions and are routinely referred to clinically by their Brodmann's number.

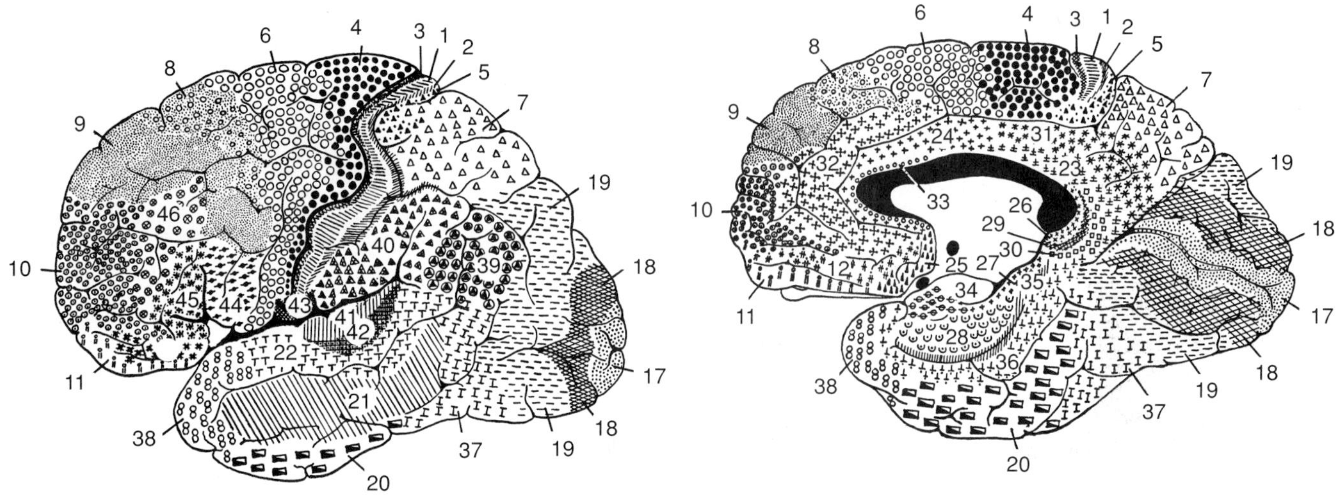

3.2. On the diagram, draw an arrow to mark the position of the *central sulcus*. The part of the cerebrum located *anterior* to this sulcus is the frontal lobe. Within this lobe, there are several key *Brodmann's areas* related to motor function. The gyrus located just anterior to the central sulcus is known as the pre central gyrus. Label it on the diagram. The posterior part of this gyrus contains the primary motor area, or Brodmann's area 4. This area generates neural impulses that control the execution of movement.

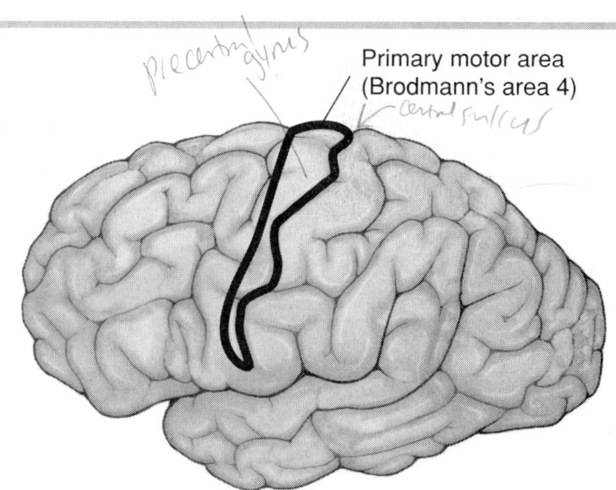

3.1A. Brodmann's

3.2A. frontal; precentral; motor; movement

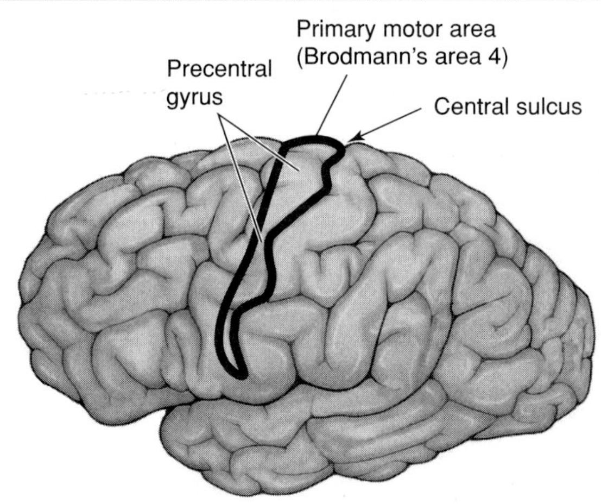

3.3. Every part of the body capable of movement is represented in the primary motor cortex, or Brodmann's area ______. The neurons controlling movement of different body regions are mapped onto the pre ______ gyrus according to their relative anatomical positions in this frontal section. For example, the motor neurons controlling movement of the foot are next to those controlling the leg in area 4. This arrangement is known as a *somatotopic* map.

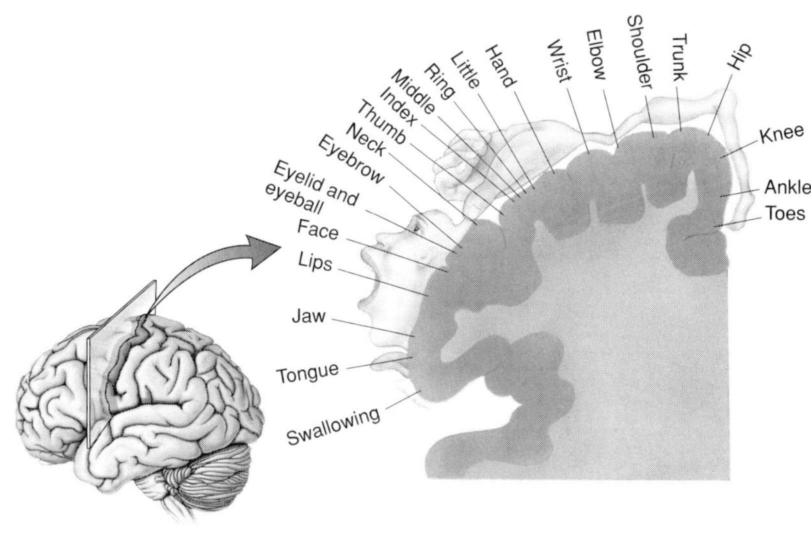

3.4. All body regions in the ______ topic map in area 4 are not represented equally. The amount of ______ central gyrus controlling a particular body part represents the amount of control that the primary ______ cortex has over that body part.

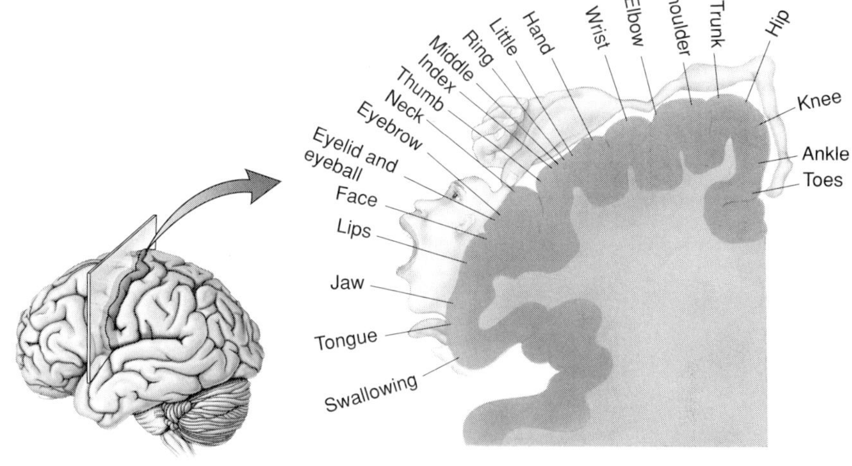

3.5. The disproportionate map of the body on the motor cortex is called the *motor homunculus*. Look at the diagram of the homunculus. The hands and fingers appear ______ than the trunk or legs because their movements require finer control and more neurons.

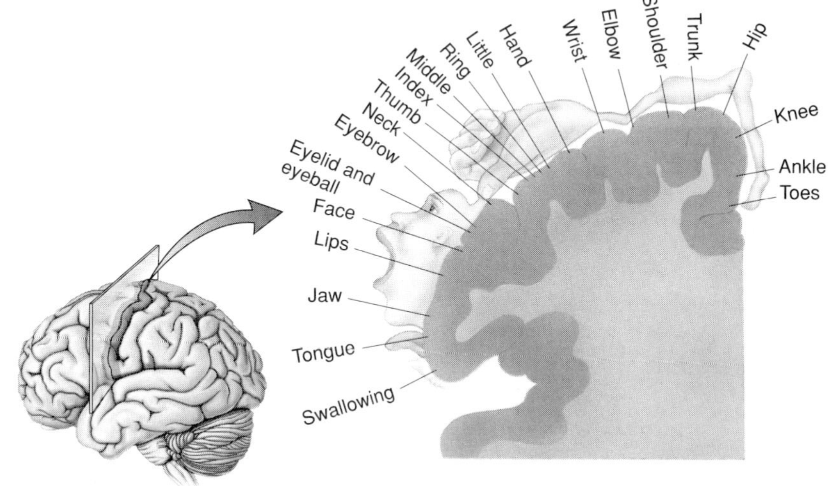

3.3A. 4; precentral

3.4A. somatotopic; precentral; motor

3.5A. larger

3.6. Each area of the body is represented in a particular area of area 4 in a somatotopic map, or motor homunculus. Stimulating the most superior part of area 4 will result in movement of the hip and trunk, while stimulating the part of area 4 closest to the lateral sulcus will result in swallowing through its activation of muscles of the pharynx and larynx.

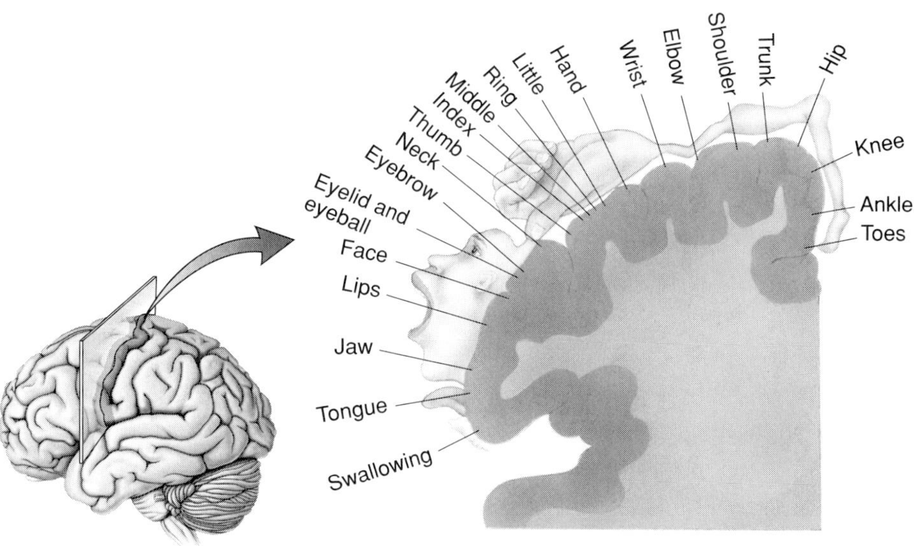

3.7. The anterior part of the precentral gyrus and adjacent superior frontal gyrus makes up *area 6* and is known as the supplementary, or *secondary motor* cortex. It stores motor activities responsible for programming the activity of area 4, or the primary motor cortex. The premotor cortex also mediates sensory guidance of movement, controlling postural muscles of the body.

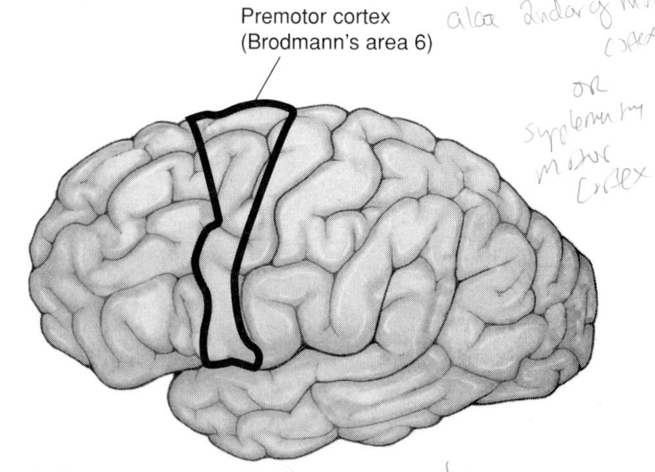

3.8. On the diagram, label areas 4 and 6. Which of these areas would execute the voluntary action of picking up a pen? 4. Which would help you position your body so that you could pick up a ball? 6.

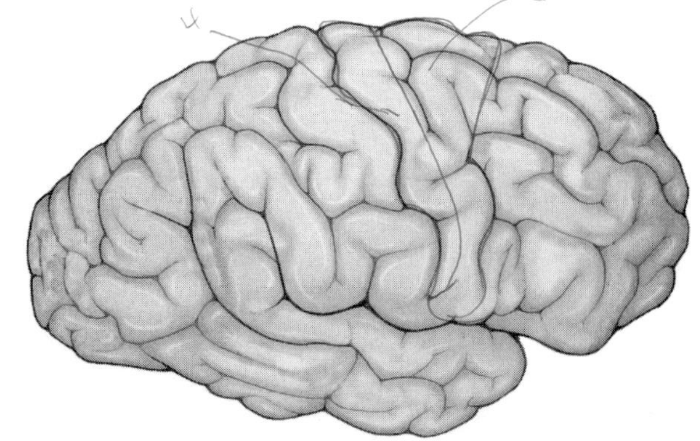

3.6A. homunculus; hip; trunk; swallowing

3.7A. precentral; supplementary; primary

3.8A. Area 4; Area 6

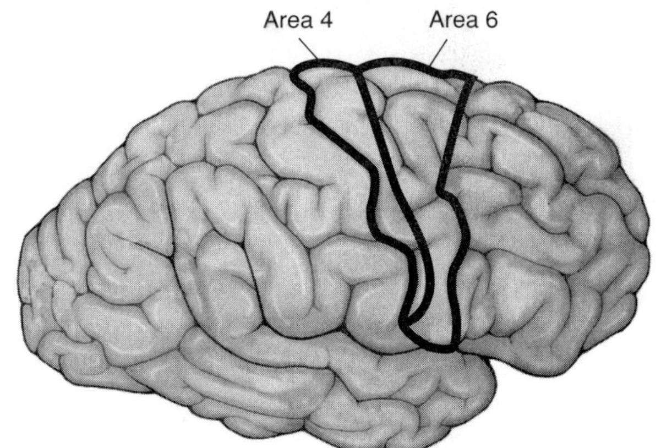

3.9. Anterior to the primary and premotor cortex, you will find area 8, which contributes to the *frontal eye field.* This area controls voluntary scanning movements of the eyes.

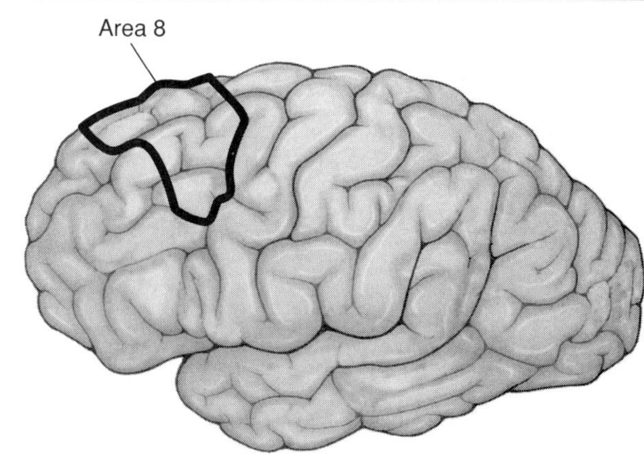

3.10. Draw a line from the Brodmann's area to its appropriate name.

Area 4	Frontal eye field
Area 6	Primary motor cortex
Area 8	Secondary motor cortex

3.11. Inferior to the frontal eye field, there is a cortical region dedicated to language production. *Broca's motor speech area* is formed by Brodmann's areas 45 and 44. On the diagram, label the primary motor cortex and premotor cortex.

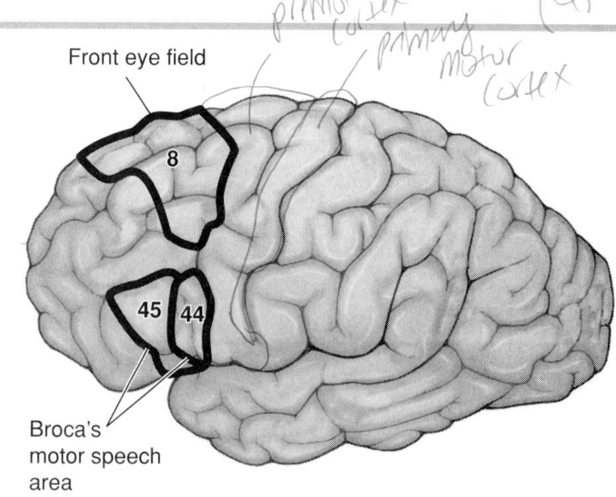

3.12. Areas 45 and 44 contain the motor programs necessary for formulating words, and they communicate with the primary motor cortex to control the muscles involved in speaking. A lesion of Broca's motor speech area produces *motor aphasia* due to difficulty in articulating words.

3.13. Broca's motor speech area is located in the frontal lobe of the cortex.

3.9A. 8

3.10A.

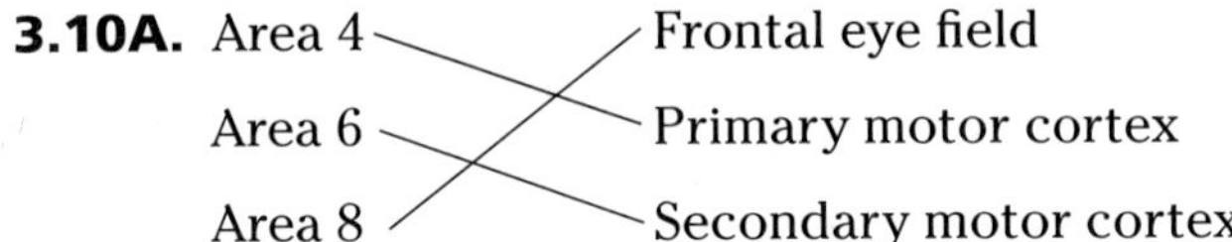

3.11A. 44; 45

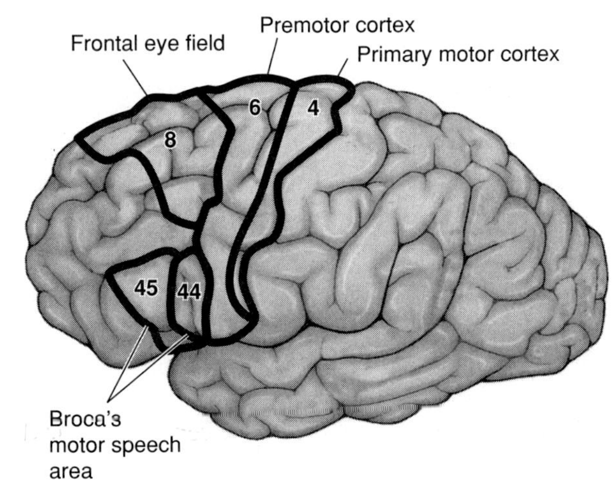

3.12A. 44; 45; Broca's

3.13A. frontal

3.14. On the diagram, label the frontal eye field and Broca's area. Anterior to these regions, identify the ____________ cortex, which includes Brodmann's areas 9, 10, 11, and 12 (area 12 is best seen on a midsagittal section of the brain, so it is not visible here).

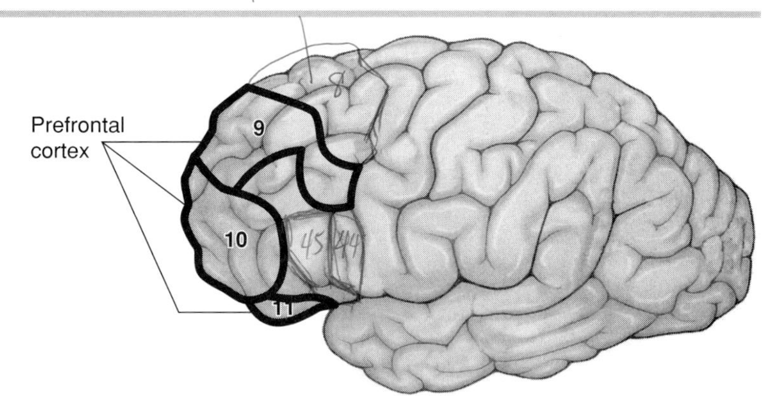

3.15. On this midsagittal section of the cortex, label the frontal and occipital poles. Shade in Brodmann's areas 9, 10, 11, and 12, which contribute to the pre __________ cortex of the __________ lobe. This cortical region is concerned with personality, motivation, planning, and judgment.

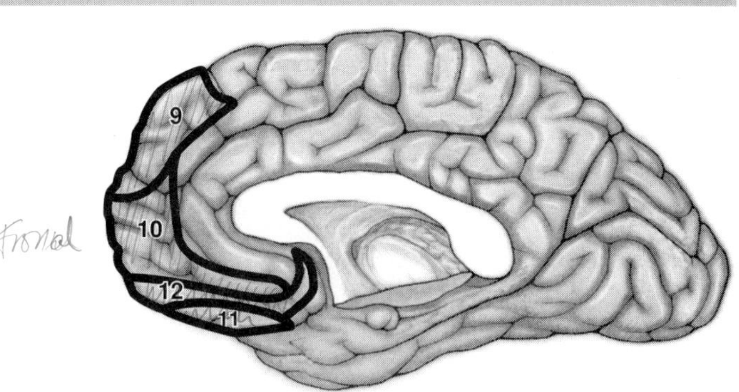

3.16. Frontal lobotomy involves removal of or damage to the pre __________ cortex and was once a common surgical procedure used to treat patients with severe behavioral problems.

3.17. Match the following clinical presentations with the site of the lesions.

____ Right upper limb weakness
____ Slow formulation of spoken words
____ Right lower facial weakness
____ Dramatic change in personality
____ Lack of conjugate eye movement to the right

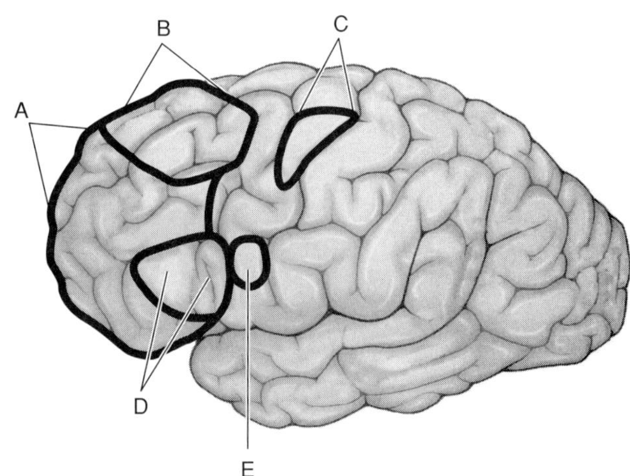

3.14A. prefrontal

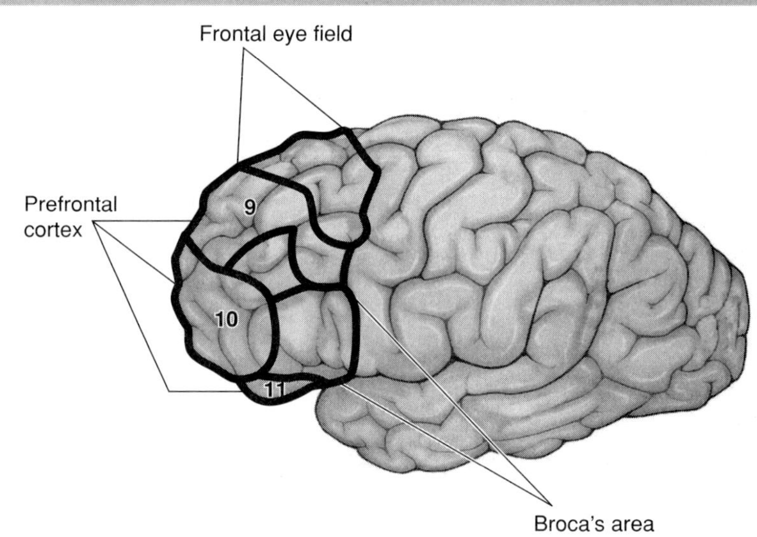

3.15A. prefrontal; frontal

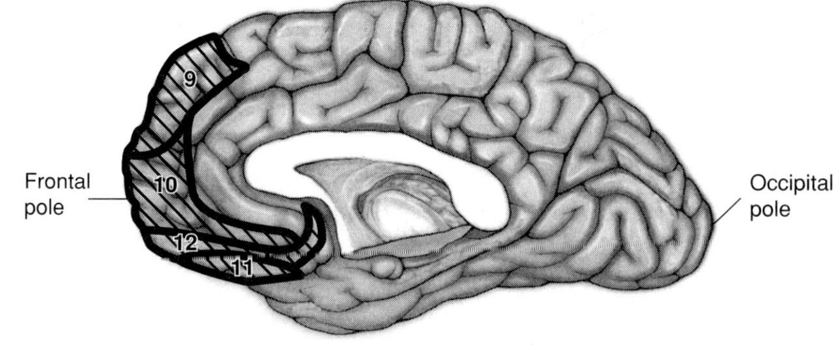

3.16A. prefrontal

3.17A.

C Right upper limb weakness

D Slow formulation of spoken words

E Right lower facial weakness

A Dramatic change in personality

B Lack of conjugate eye movement to the right

3.18. The arrow marks the position of the ________ sulcus. The part of the cerebrum located just posterior to this landmark is the ________ lobe. Within this lobe, there are several key *Brodmann's areas* involved in sensory function.

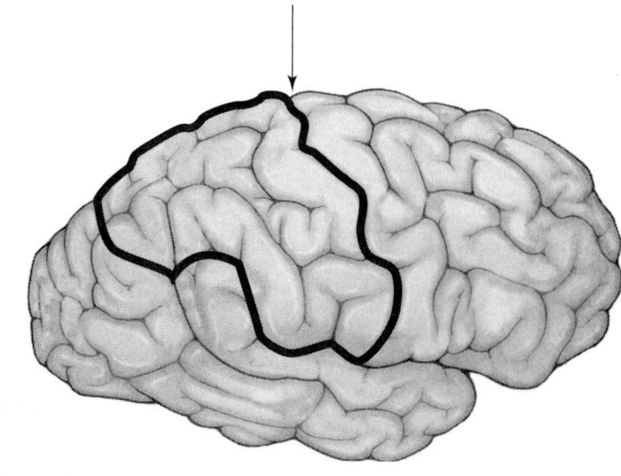

3.19. The postcentral gyrus contains the ________ cortex, formed by Brodmann's areas ______, ______, and ______. The primary somatosensory cortex receives ______ ferent information regarding tactile discrimination and position sense.

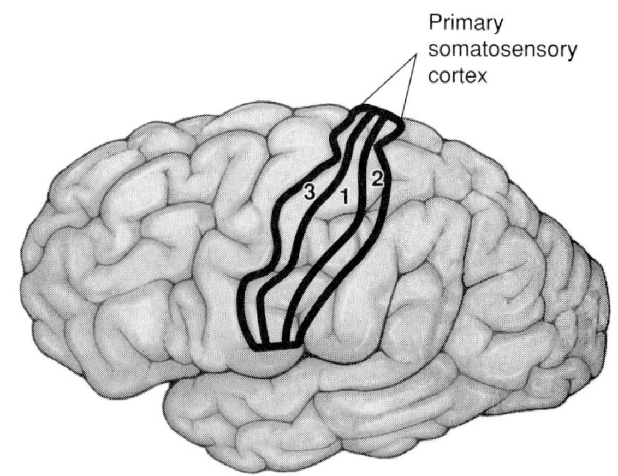

3.20. As in the primary motor cortex, the sensory fields from various parts of the body are arranged in a ________ topic map in the sensory hom ________ of the post ________ gyrus.

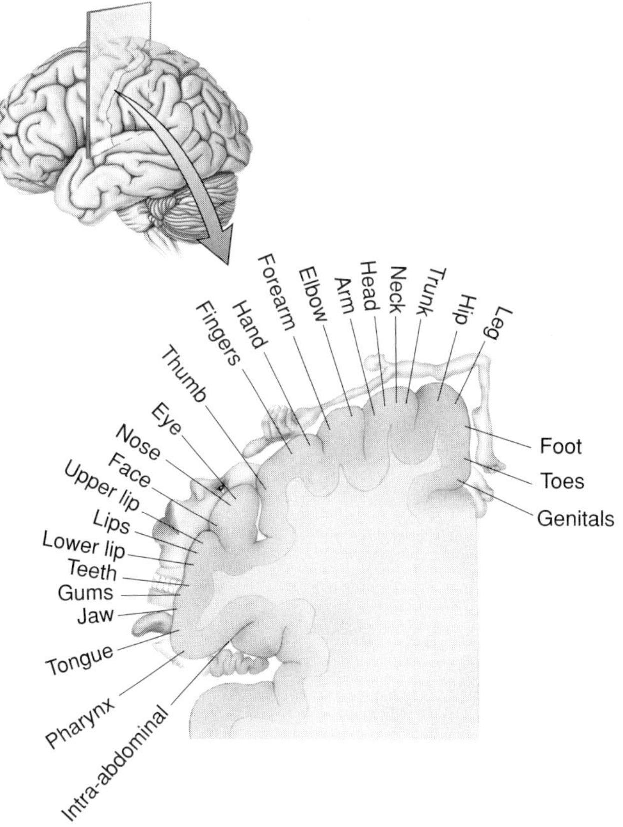

3.18A. central; parietal

3.19A. somesthetic (or somatosensory); 3; 1; 2; afferent

3.20A. somatotopic; homunculus; postcentral

3.21. Different parts of the body are not proportionately represented on the post central gyrus. Collectively, the upper limb and thorax take up as much area as the hand on the Somatotropic homunculus. The skin of the hand requires additional neurons to mediate fine, or discriminative, touch.

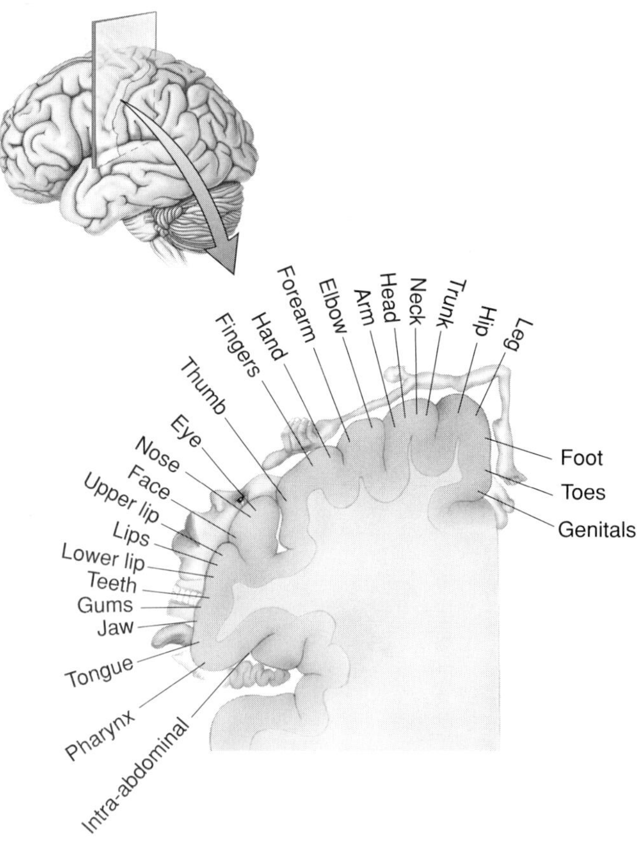

3.22. The secondary somatosensory area, or Brodmann's area 40, is part of the parietal lobe and is located posterior to the postcentral gyrus. Area 40 forms the superior border of the lateral sulcus. The sensation of pain is thought to be perceived in this region of the cortex.

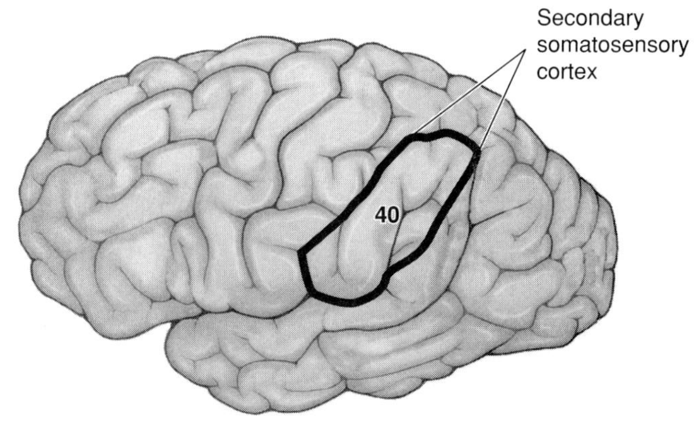

3.23. Label the primary and secondary somatosensory cortices on the diagram. Another important sensory area, the *sensory association cortex*, is located Posterior to the primary sensory cortex and Superior to the secondary sensory area. The sensory association cortex in the parietal lobe is associated with Brodmann's areas 7 and 5.

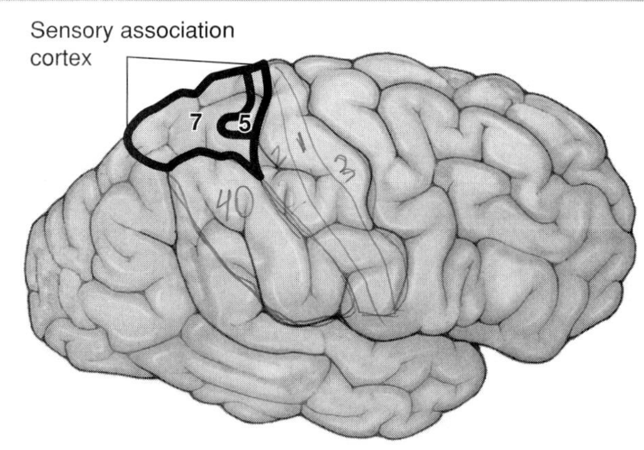

3.21A. postcentral; sensory

3.22A. 40; parietal; postcentral; lateral

3.23A. posterior; superior; parietal; 5; 7

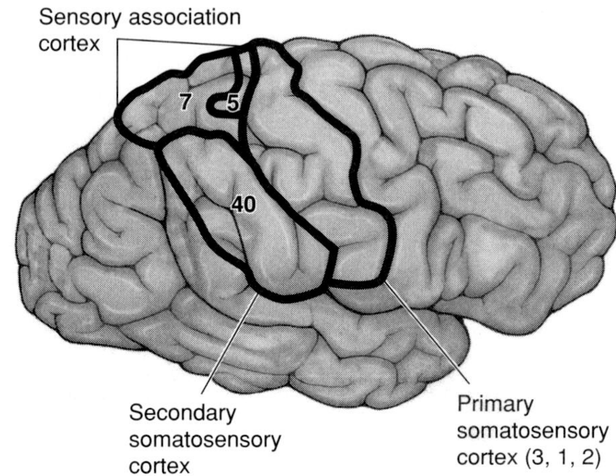

3.24. Areas 5 and 7 of the ________ ________ cortex process tactile and visual cues. Lesions of the sensory association cortex may be associated with *neglect syndrome*, in which the patient does not recognize the opposite side of the body as their own.

3.25. The occipital lobe is critical for *visual* perception and processing. On the diagram, label the *parieto-occipital sulcus* and *preoccipital notch*. A line connecting these landmarks marks the ________ boundary of the occipital lobe.

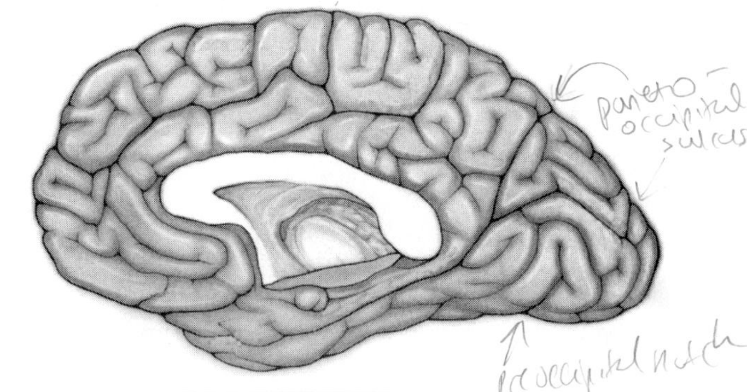

3.26. Within the occipital lobe, identify and label the horizontally oriented ________ sulcus. The primary ________ cortex, or Brodmann's area 17, surrounds this fissure. Area 17 is responsible for the perception of ________.

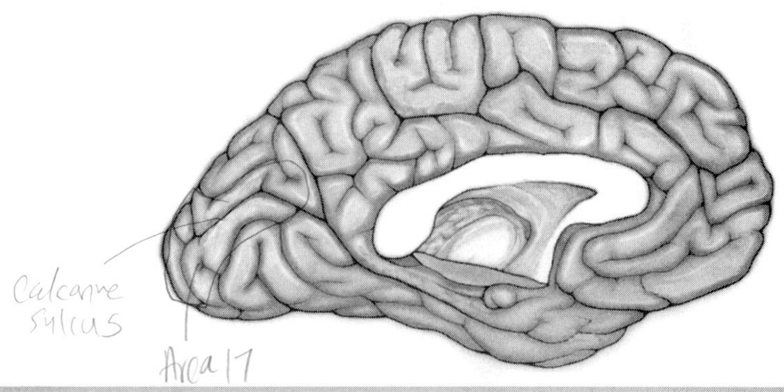

3.27. The ________ visual cortex is found in areas 18 and 19. Shade in the secondary visual cortex and label area 17 on the diagram. Areas 18 and 19 process information from the ________ cortex and interpret this information so that the brain can make sense of visual stimuli.

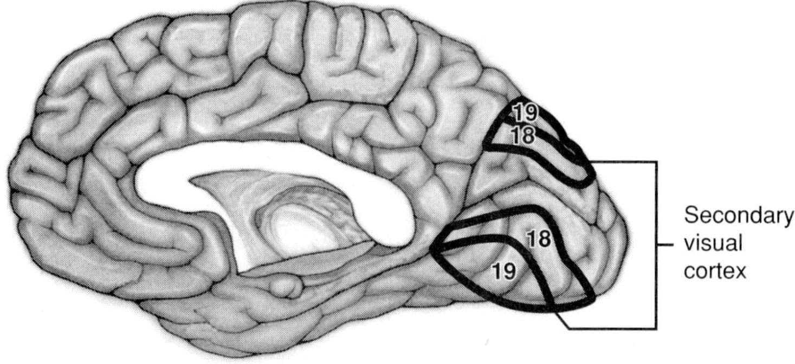

3.24A. sensory association

3.25A. anterior

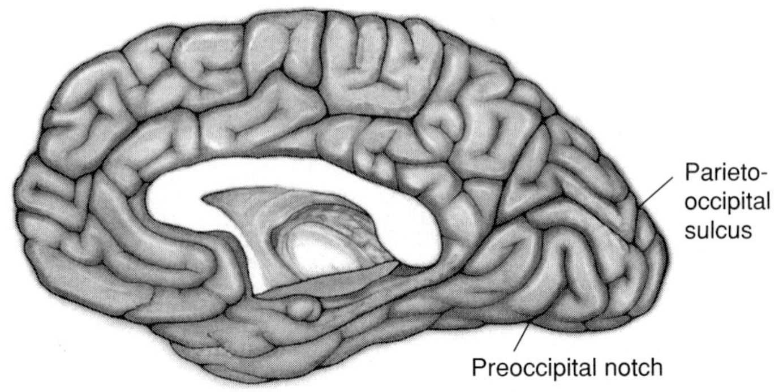

3.26A. calcarine; visual; vision

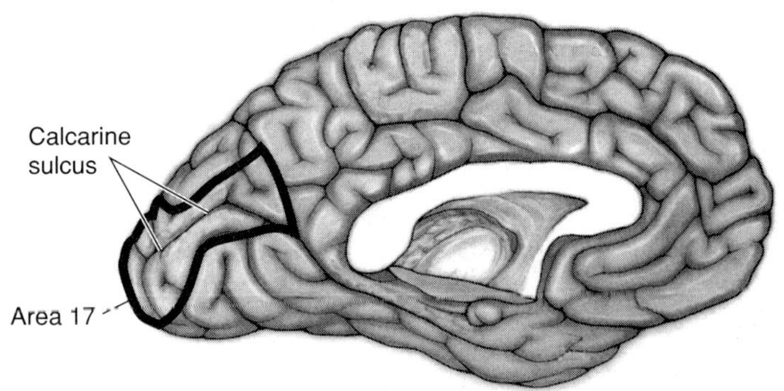

3.27A. secondary; primary visual

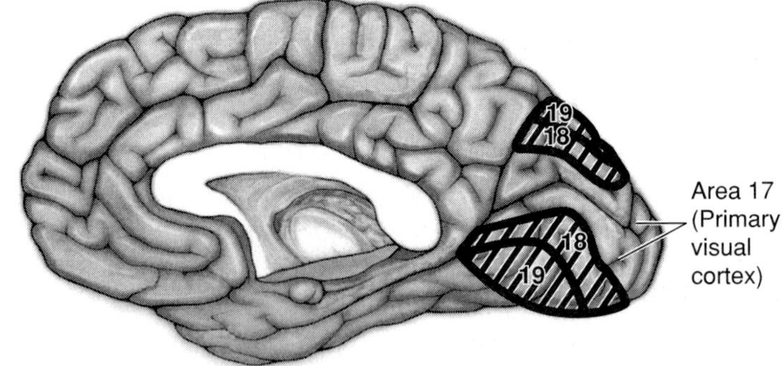

3.28. *Visual agnosia* is the failure to understand the meaning or use of an object. On the diagram, mark the cortical regions that are lesioned in this condition with an "X."

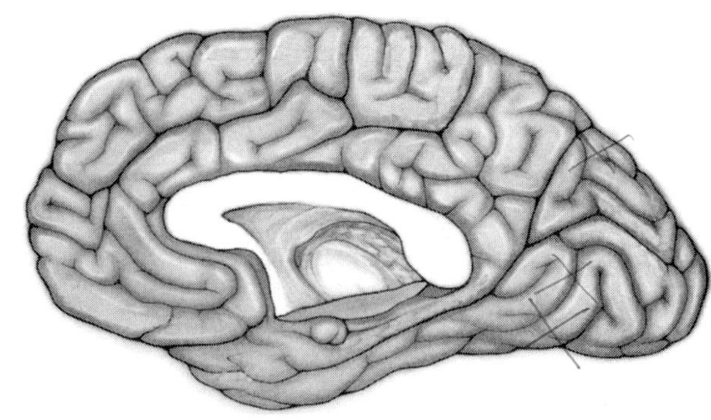

3.29. On the diagram, label the lateral sulcus. The ___temporal___ lobe is located inferior to the lateral sulcus. This region of the cerebrum processes *auditory stimuli* as well as emotions, memory, and speech.

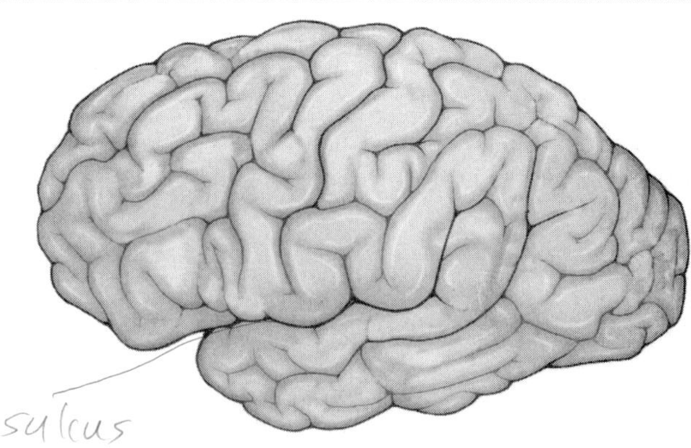

3.30. The arrows indicate the ___superior temporal___ gyrus. On the medial surface of this gyrus, *Brodmann's areas 41 and 42* represent the *primary auditory cortex.*

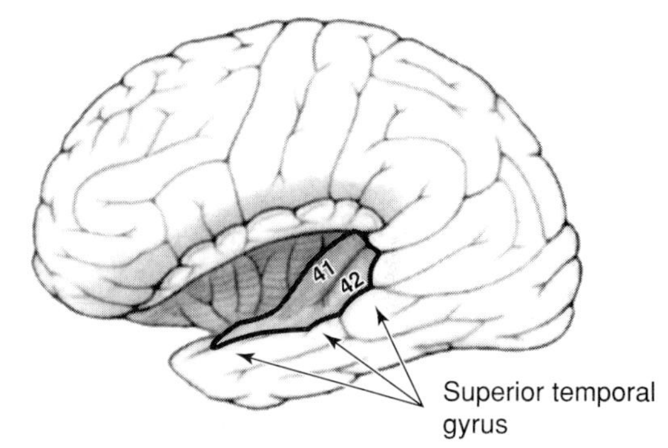

3.31. The primary auditory cortex is buried in the ___lateral___ sulcus. An alternative term for this cortical area is the transverse ___gyrus___ of Heschl.

3.28A.

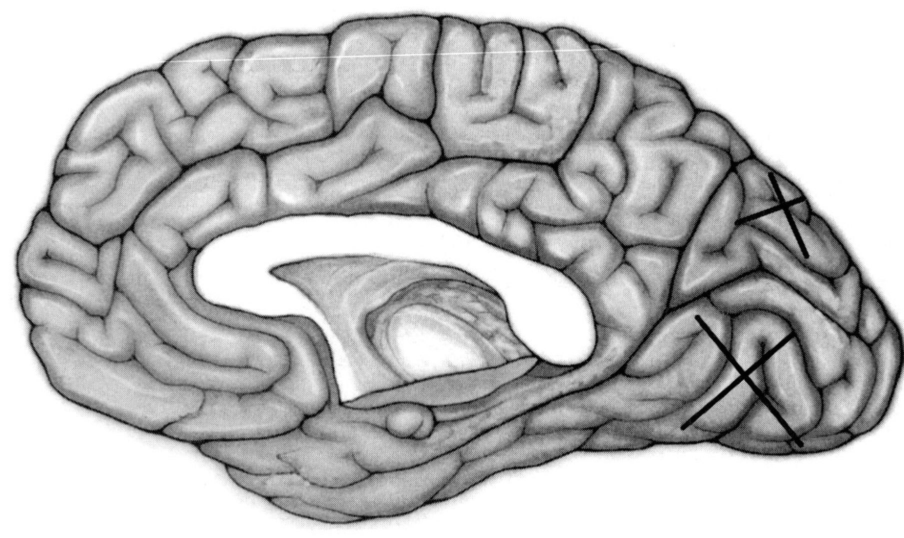

3.29A. temporal

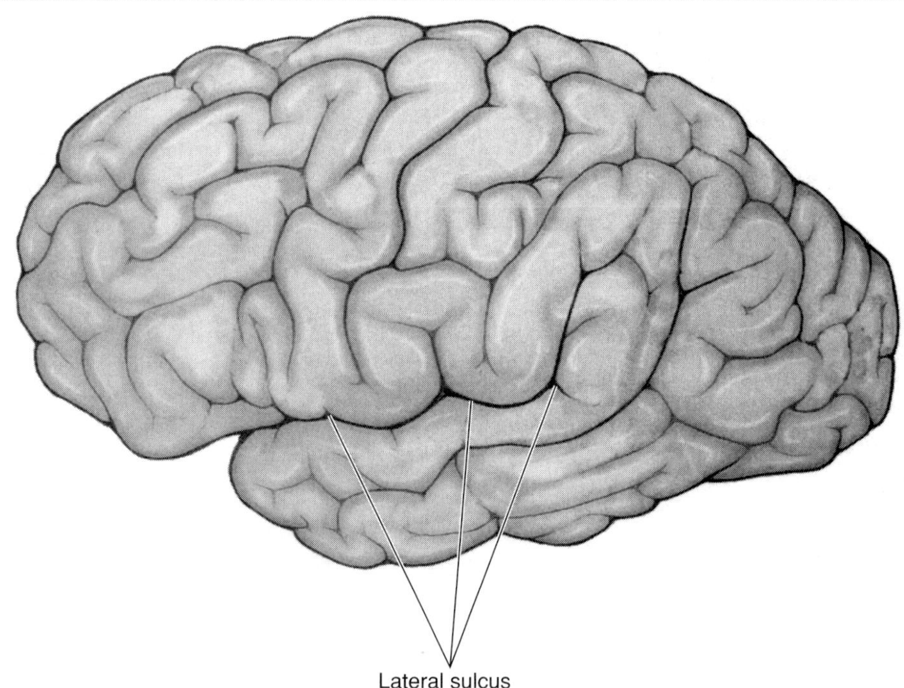

3.30A. superior temporal

3.31A. lateral; gyrus

3.32. Area 22 is outlined on the diagram. It contains both the auditory association cortex, which is critical for sound interpretation, as well as Wernicke's area, which represents the sensory speech area responsible for interpretation of both written and spoken language.

Area 22 – sound interpretation

Wernicke's area – interprets written & spoken language (sensory speech)

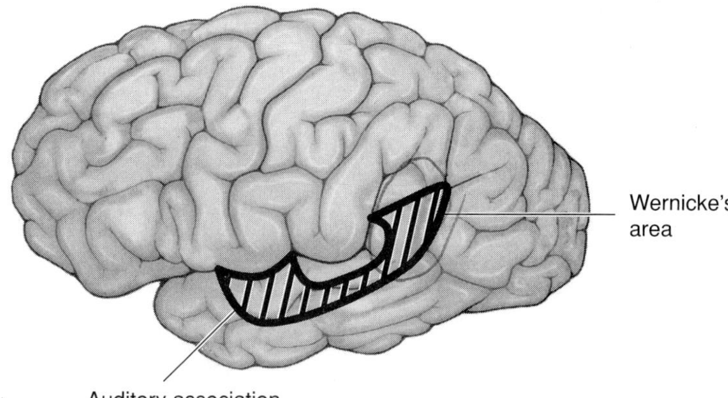

3.33. A lesion of *Wernicke's area* results in sensory aphasia, where the formulation of words is normal but the use of words is inappropriate. This is in contrast to a lesion in *Broca's area*, which produces a motor aphasia.

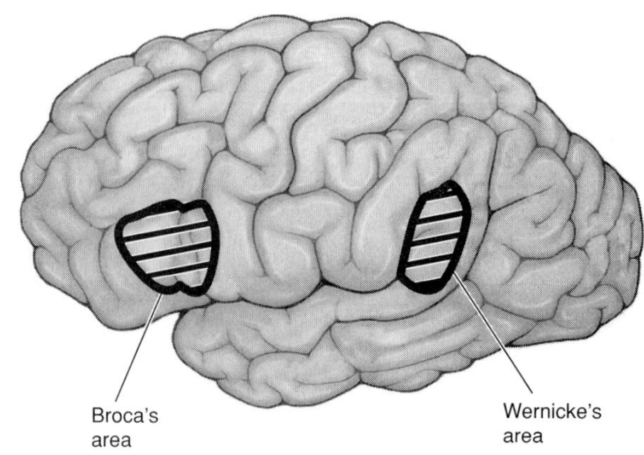

3.32A. auditory; Wernicke's

3.33A. sensory; aphasia

4 Membranes of the Brain

4.1. This figure represents a coronal section through the cranial cavity. Coronal sections divide the head into ________ and ________ regions. On the coronal section, label the skull, the gray matter, and the white matter.

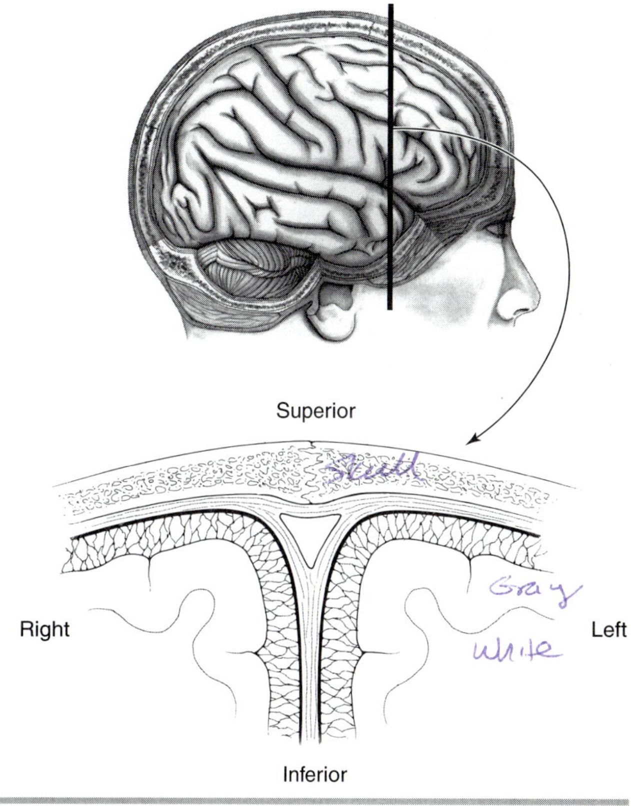

4.2. In this ________ section, you can see that the brain is surrounded by three membranes collectively called the *meninges* (Greek term for "covering"). The outermost membrane directly contacts the skull and is known as the dura ________ (Latin for "tough mother"). Deep to the dura is the ________ mater, which forms a spider web-like matrix. The innermost layer of the meninges is the ________ mater (Latin for "gentle mother"), which closely invests each gyrus of the cerebral cortex.

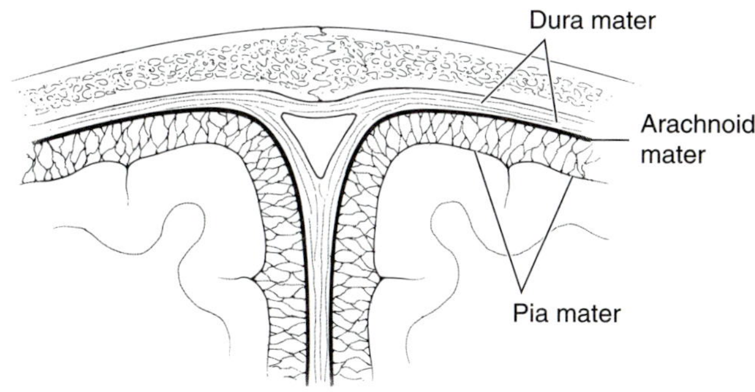

4.1A. anterior; posterior

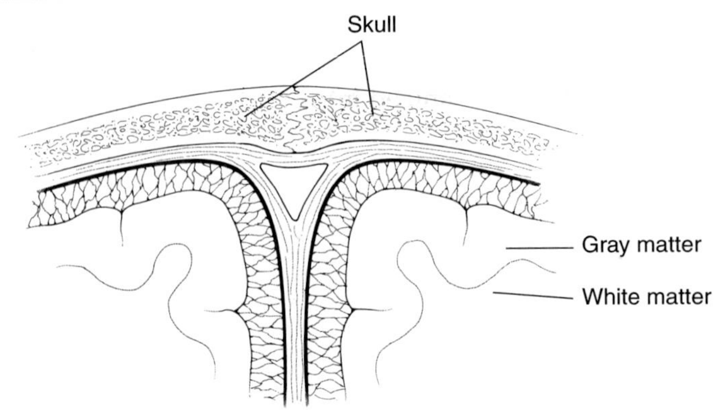

4.2A. coronal; mater; arachnoid; pia

4.3. In the cranium, the outermost layer of the meninges, the dura mater, is organized into two layers: an outer *periosteal* (or endosteal) layer and an inner *meningeal* layer. These two layers are fused together throughout most of the skull. At specific sites, however, the periosteal and meningeal layers of dura separate to form dural venous sinuses that carry blood from the brain to veins in the neck.

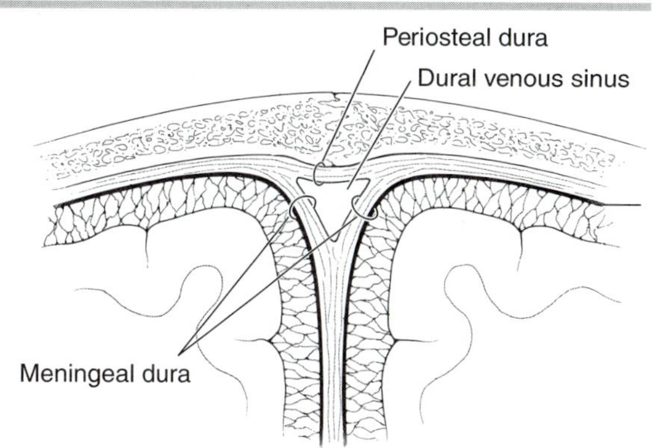

4.4. The periosteal layer of the dura mater adheres to the deep surface of the skull. A potential space lies between the dura and skull; it is known as the epi dural space because it lies above the dura mater. Rupture of a blood vessel in this space results in a life-threatening condition known as an epidural hematoma; label it on the diagram.

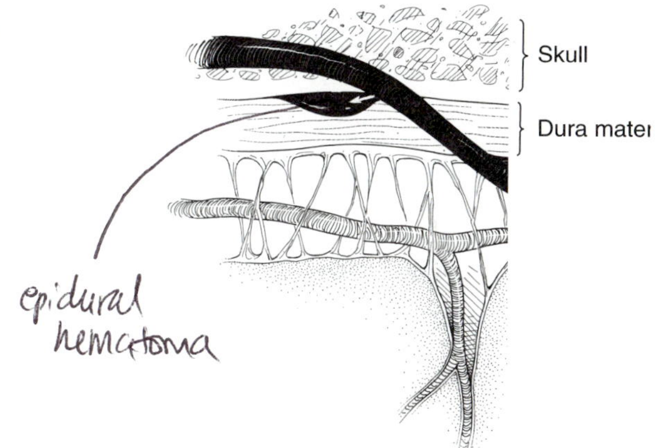

4.5. The potential space between the dura and arachnoid mater is known as the sub dural space because it is under the dura mater; label this space on the diagram. Hemorrhaging into this space creates a subdural hematoma; label it on the diagram.

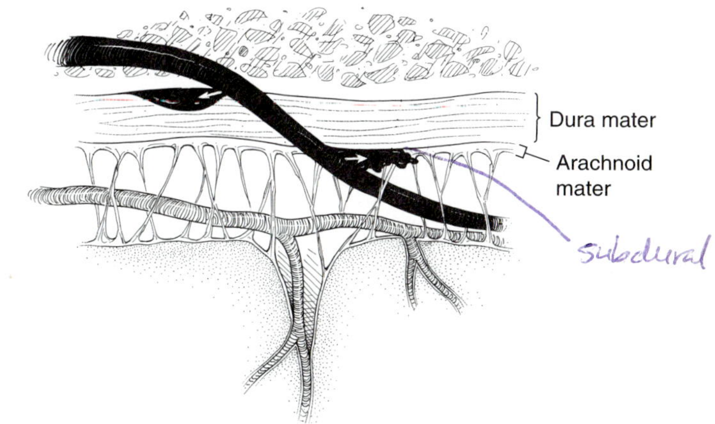

4.6. The inner layer of dura, or meningeal layer, forms four folds that partition and support different areas of the brain within the cranial cavity. Label the dural fold seen on this diagram.

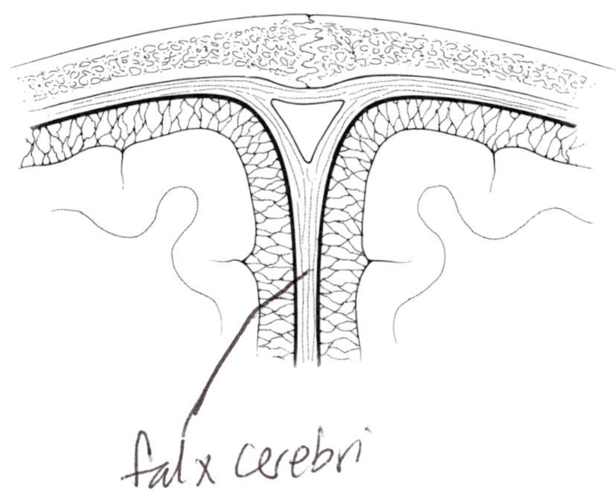

4.3A. dura; periosteal (or endosteal); meningeal; venous

4.4A. periosteal (or endosteal); epidural; epidural

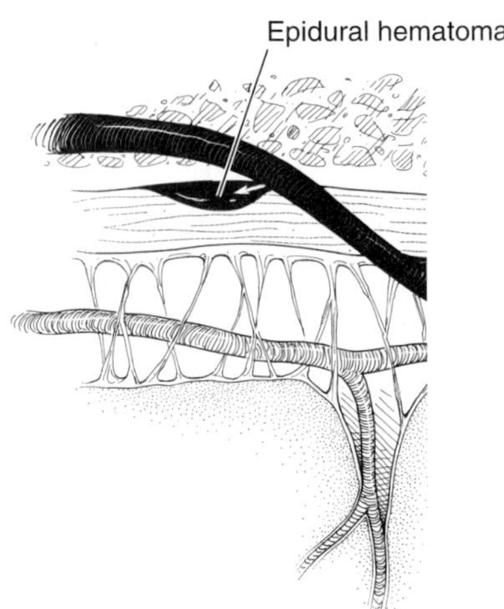

4.5A. subdural; subdural

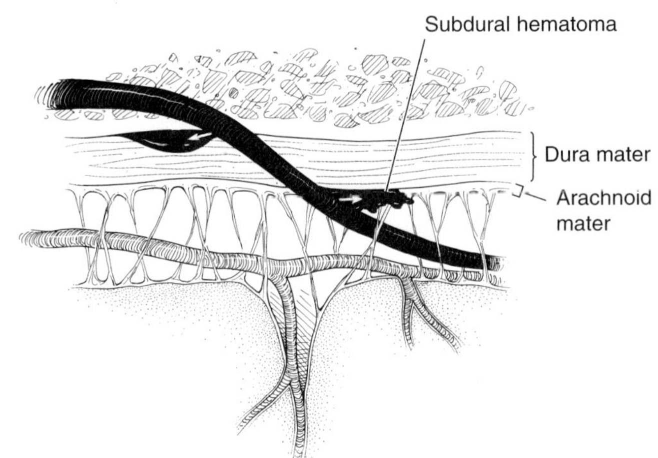

4.6A. meningeal

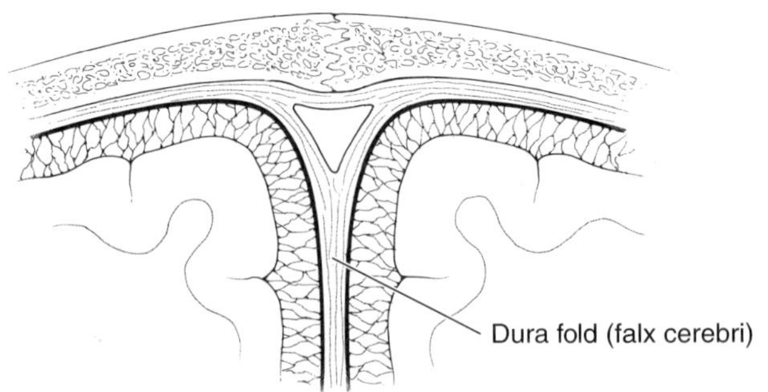

4.7. This dural fold is known as the *falx cerebri*, which separates the left and right Cerebral hemispheres. Identify and label the blood-filled space in the upper attached edge of the falx cerebri.

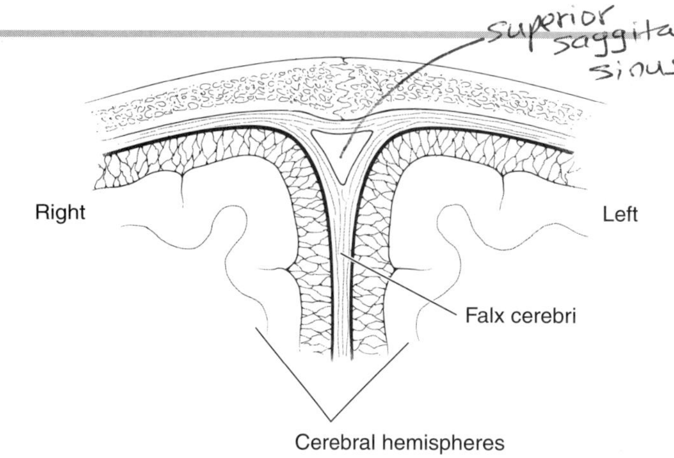

4.8. Identify and label the vertically oriented, sickle-shaped *falx cerebri* on this lateral view of cranial dural folds. It separates the left and right Cerebral hemispheres. Similarly, the cerebellar hemispheres are separated by the smaller, vertical falx cerebelli; label it on the diagram.

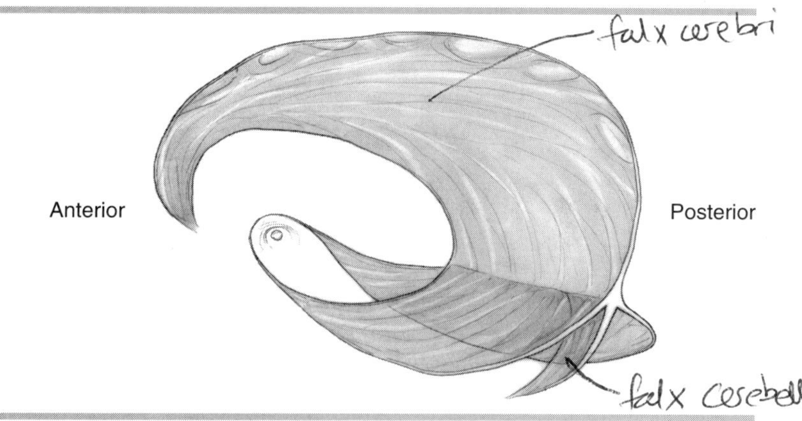

4.9. Two of the folds created by the meningeal layer of dura are oriented horizontally. The *tentorium cerebelli* is a dural fold that forms a horizontal tent over the Cerebellum, protecting it from the weight of the overlying cortex. Similarly, the diaphragma sellae forms a protective diaphragm over the *sella* turcica of the skull, which houses the pituitary gland.

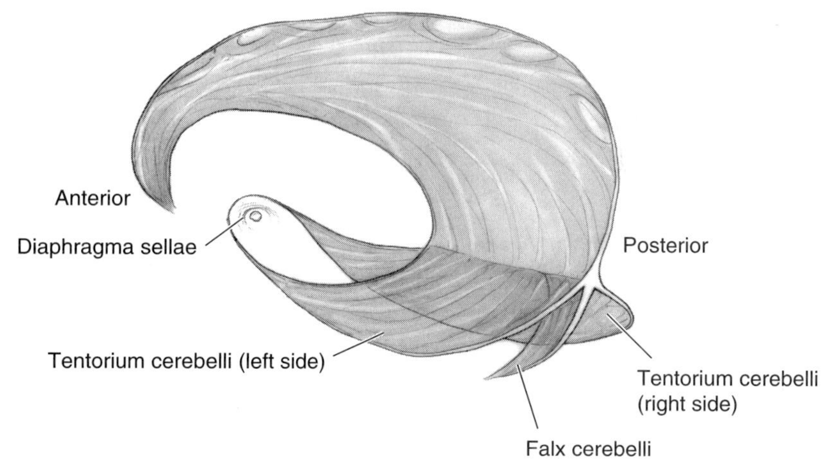

4.10. The arachnoid mater lies between the dura and the pia. The sub arachnoid space is located between the arachnoid and pia mater and is filled with *cerebrospinal fluid* (CSF).

4.7A. cerebral

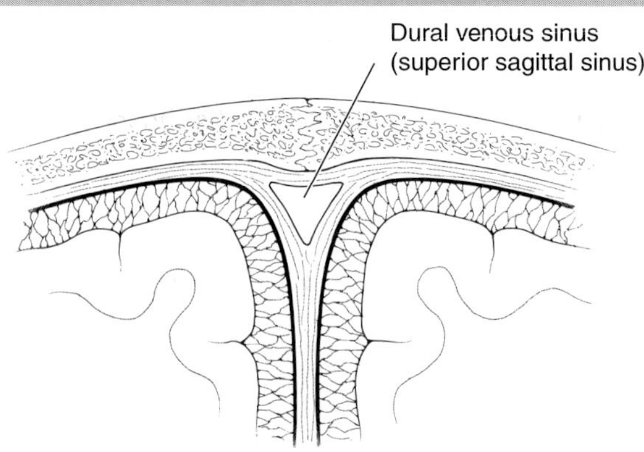

4.8A. cerebral hemispheres; falx

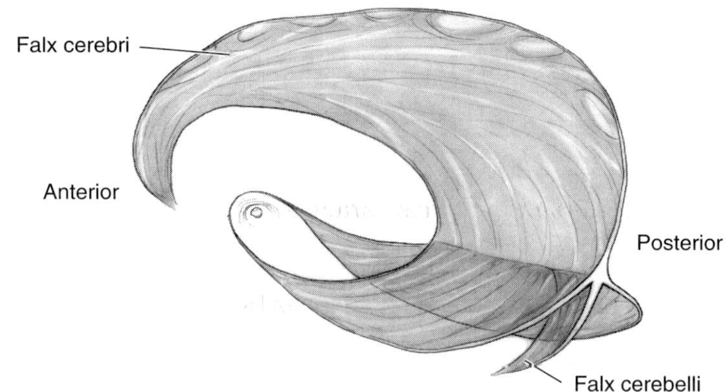

4.9A. meningeal; cerebellum; sellae

4.10A. dura; pia; subarachnoid

4.11. On this sagittal section, identify the *subarachnoid space*. At several sites in the cranial cavity, the subarachnoid space is enlarged, forming *cisterns*. *Cisterna magna* is the largest cistern and is located between the cerebellum and medulla of the brainstem.

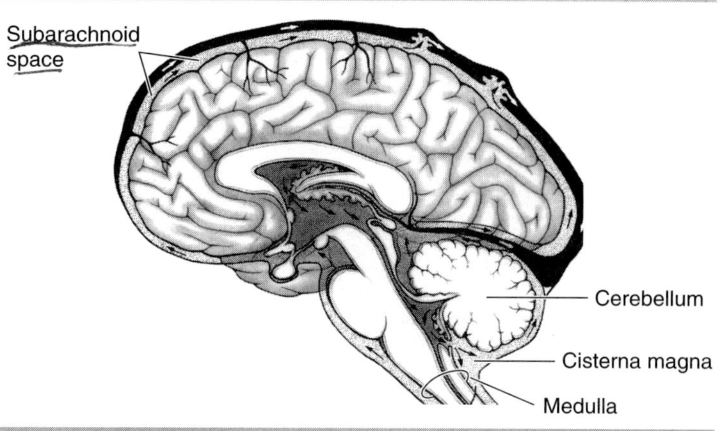

4.12. The arachnoid mater extends *arachnoid villi* into the *superior sagittal sinus*, a dural venous sinus located between the periosteal and endosteal layers of dura mater. These arachnoid villi function as one-way valves, draining CSF from the subarachnoid space into the venous blood of the superior sagittal sinus.

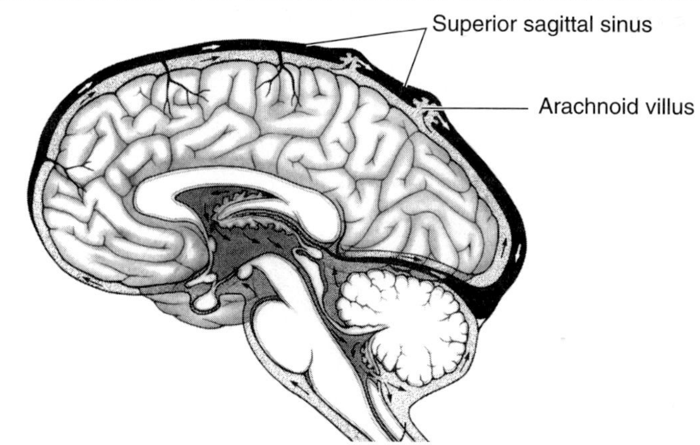

4.13. Label the *pia mater* on the diagram. It tightly adheres to the brain, extending into the sulci between gyri. The pia mater also contributes to the formation of the *choroid plexus*, which makes the CSF that circulates in the subarachnoid space.

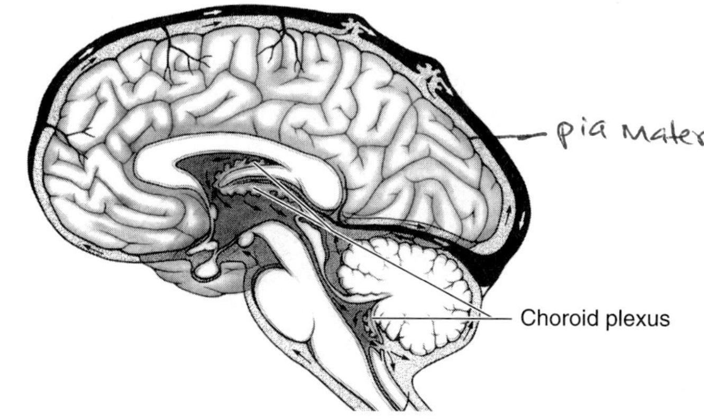

4.14. Cerebrospinal fluid is synthesized by the choroid plexus and circulates throughout the sub arachnoid space. The choroid plexus consists of capillary endothelium invested by pia mater.

4.11A. cerebellum; medulla

4.12A. dural venous; CSF

4.13A. CSF

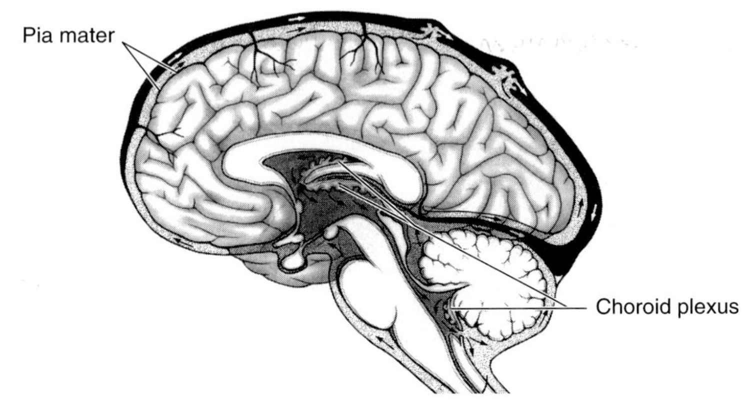

4.14A. choroid plexus; subarachnoid; pia

5 Blood Supply to the Brain

5.1. This diagram shows a ventral view of the brain and brainstem. On the figure, label the frontal pole (anterior) and occipital pole (posterior). The brain receives its arterial blood supply from two pairs of arteries: *internal carotid* and *vertebral.* Label the *left* internal carotid artery and the *right* vertebral artery on the diagram.

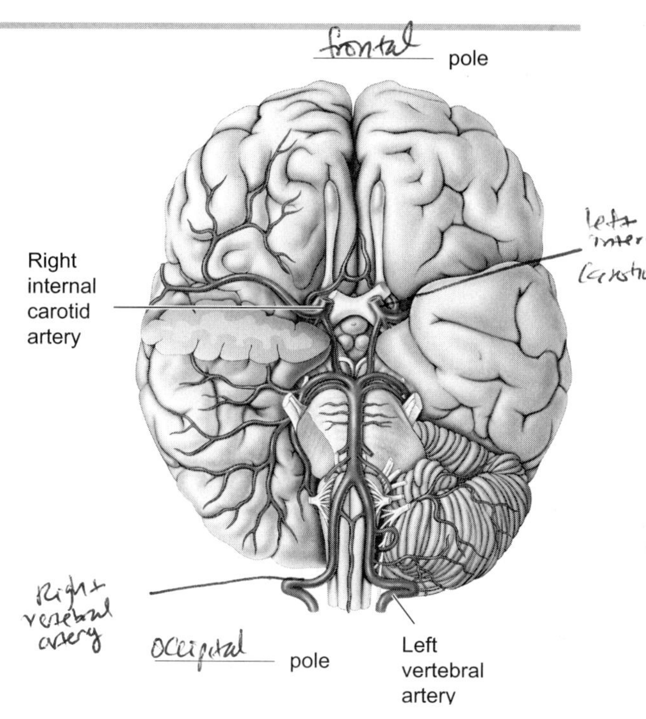

5.2. The *anterior* regions of the cerebrum receive blood from the internal carotid circulation, while the posterior parts of the cerebrum are supplied by the vertebral system.

5.3. Each internal *carotid* artery enters the base of skull at the carotid canal. It travels through a dural venous sinus known as the cavernous sinus before entering the cranial cavity where it divides into *anterior and middle cerebral arteries.*

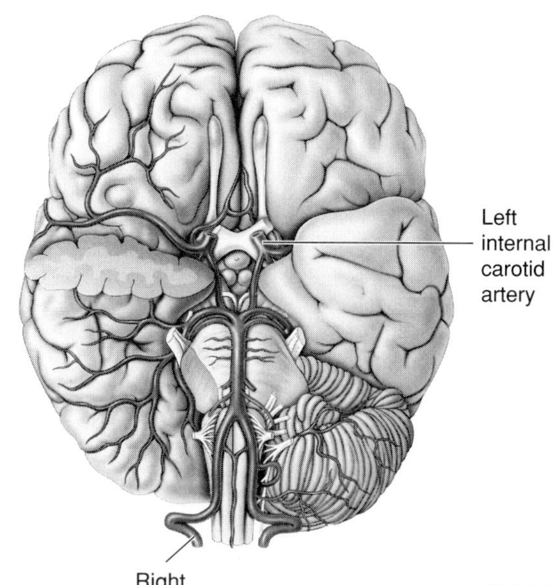

5.1A.

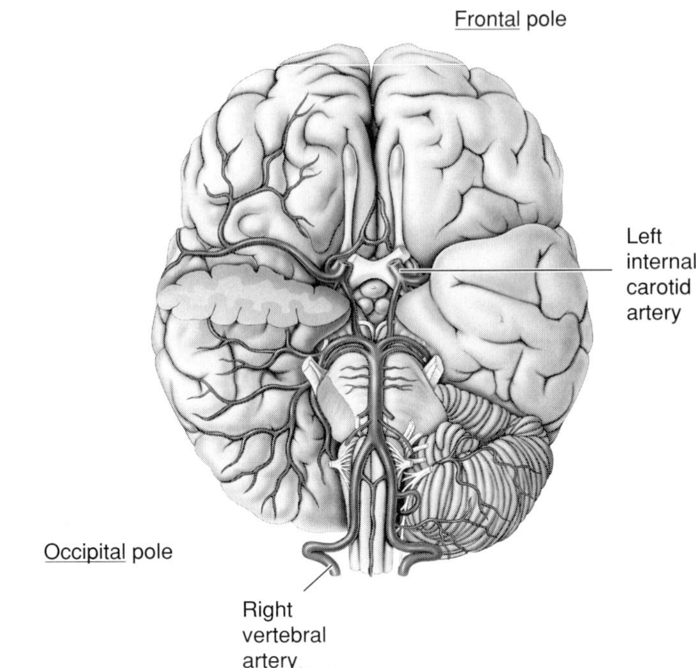

5.2A. internal carotid; posterior

5.3A. carotid; venous

5.4. The anterior cerebral artery is the smaller of the two terminal branches of the internal carotid artery. The other branch is the middle cerebral artery.

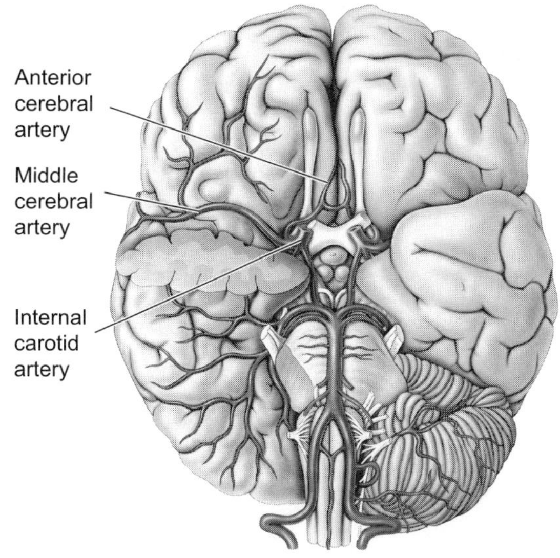

5.5. The left and right anterior cerebral arteries course anteriorly toward the frontal pole. They are united by a short anterior communicating artery. This provides an important alternate route for blood flow between the cerebral hemispheres if one of the internal carotid arteries is occluded.

Right anterior cerebral artery

Left anterior cerebral artery

Anterior communicating artery

↑ provides anastomoses btw R+L internal carotid

Internal carotid artery

5.6. The anterior cerebral artery arches posteromedially around the Corpus callosum.

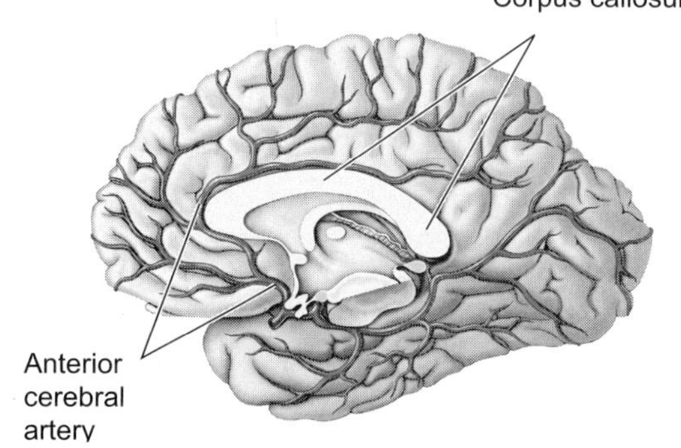

5.4A. internal; middle cerebral

5.5A. anterior communicating

5.6A. corpus callosum

5.7. The anterior cerebral artery supplies not only the medial surface of the cortex, but also extends laterally to supply the superior part of the frontal and parietal lobes.

Anterior cerebral artery → ① medial surface of cortex ② superior surface of frontal & parietal lobes

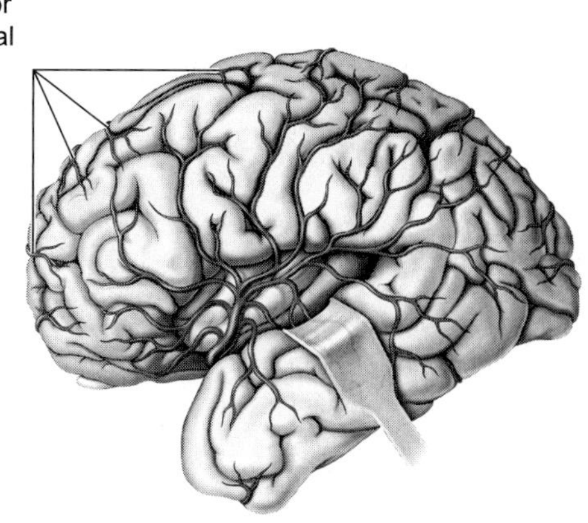

5.8. After branching off of the internal carotid artery, the middle cerebral artery travels laterally, deep to the temporal lobe.

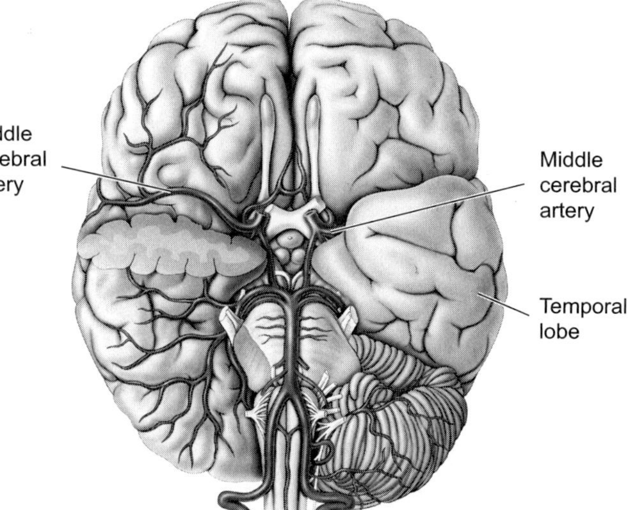

5.7A. frontal; parietal

5.8A. carotid; temporal

5.9. The middle cerebral artery passes through the _lateral_ sulcus to reach the lateral surface of the cerebrum, supplying parts of _frontal_ _parietal_, and _temporal_ lobes.

Middle cerebral artery → ① lateral surface of frontal, parietal, & temporal lobes

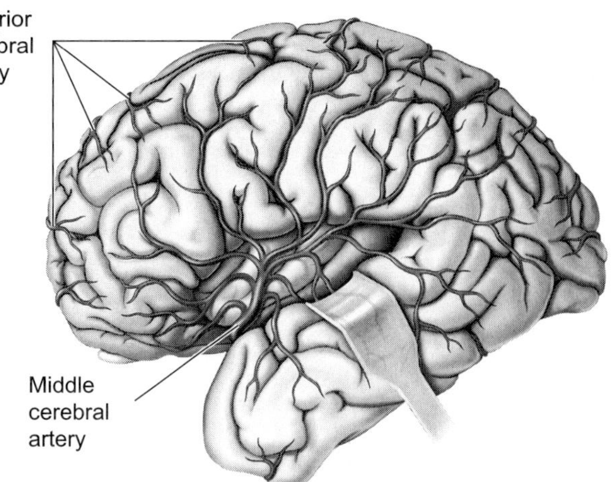

5.10. The anterior and _middle_ cerebral arteries meet on the superolateral surface of the cortex but do not anastomose. This creates a *watershed boundary*, an area that is susceptible to damage from ischemia under hypotensive conditions. Draw a line along this watershed boundary on the diagram.

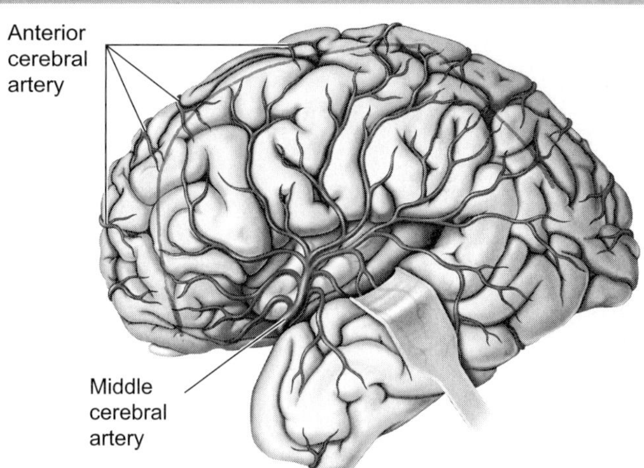

5.11. On the diagram, identify the functional areas supplied by the middle cerebral artery.

Middle cerebral artery supplies these areas.

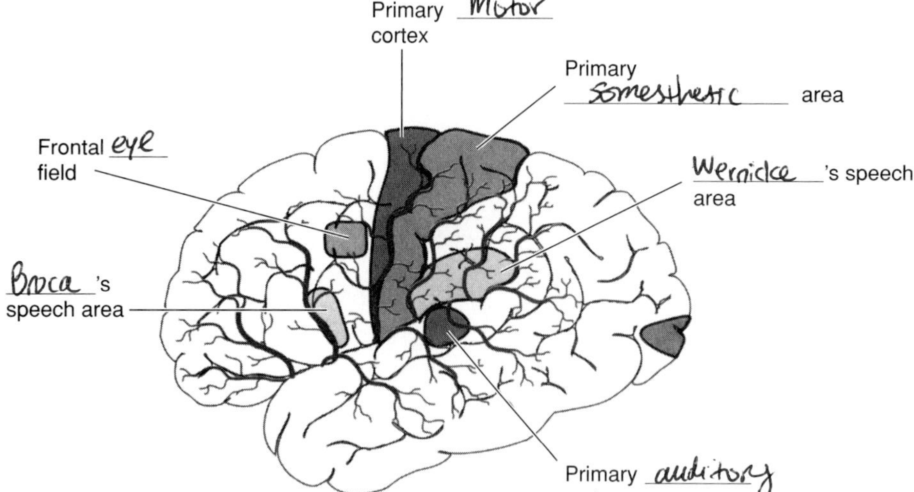

5.12. In addition to the internal carotid arteries, the two vertebral arteries contribute to the arterial blood supply of the brain and brainstem. The vertebral arteries enter the base of the skull via a large hole known as foramen _magnum_.

5.9A. lateral; frontal; parietal; temporal

5.10A. middle

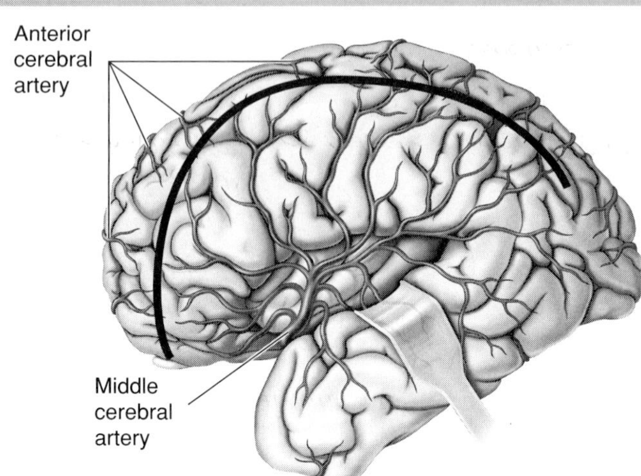

5.11A.

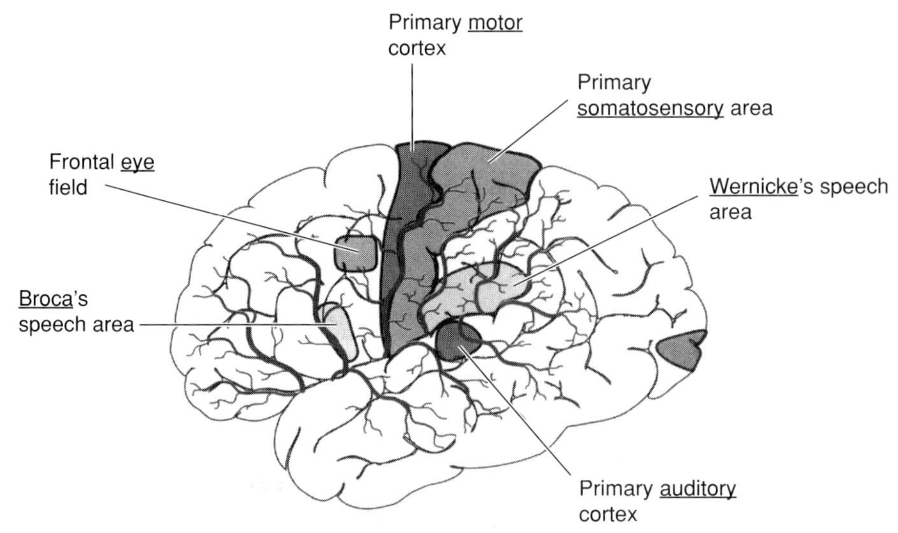

5.12A. magnum

5.13. On this ventral view of the brain, label the two *vertebral arteries*. The vertebral arteries unite ventrally at the junction of the pons and the medulla of the brainstem to form the basilar artery. The basilar artery travels superiorly along the pons and splits into two posterior cerebral arteries, which supply the inferior temporal and occipital lobes.

Posterior cerebral arteries → ① inferior temporal lobe ② occipital lobe

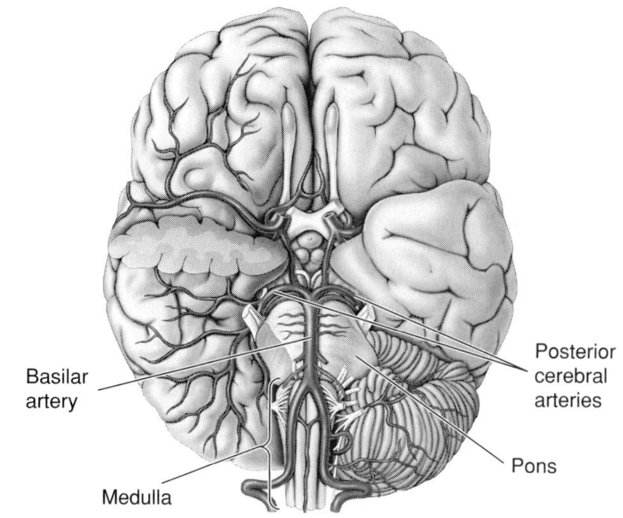

5.14. Each posterior cerebral artery is joined to the internal carotid artery via a posterior communicating artery.

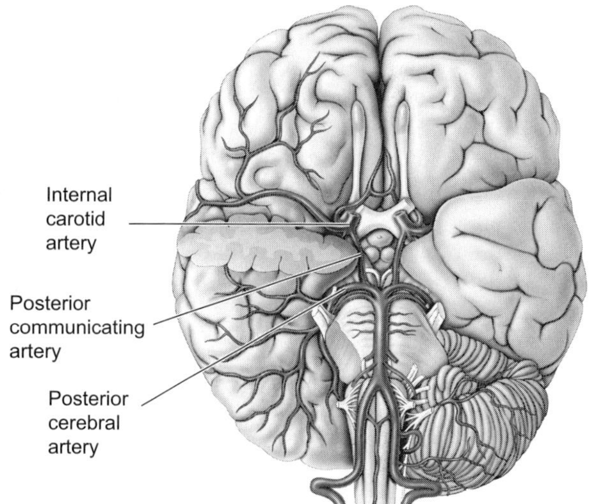

5.15. The cerebral arterial circle (of Willis) is formed by branches of the internal carotid and vertebral arterial systems. It is indicated on the diagram by a broken line. Label the vessels contributing to the circle of Willis on the diagram.

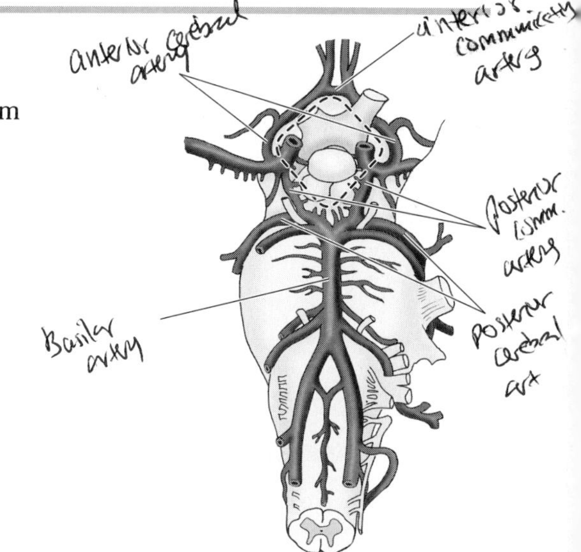

5.16. Venous blood from the brain is drained by two sets of veins, superficial and deep. Both sets of veins ultimately empty into one of the venous sinuses located between two layers of dura mater.

5.13A. pons; medulla; basilar; posterior

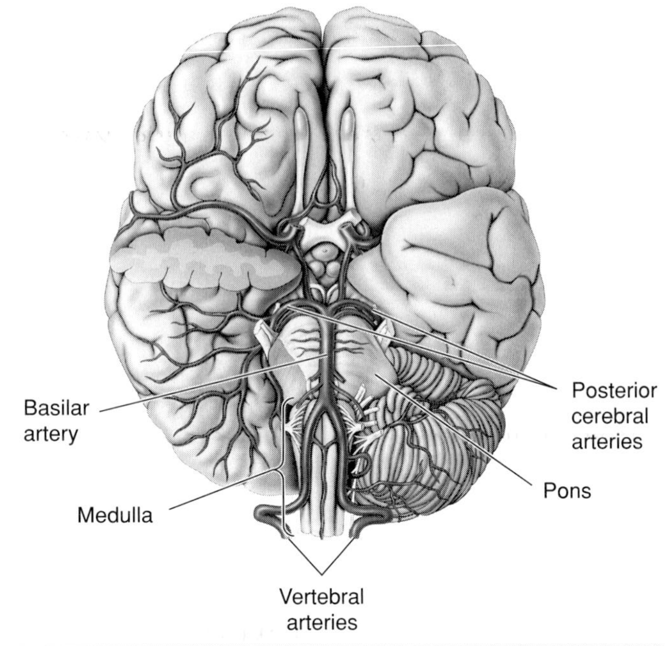

5.14A. posterior

5.15A.

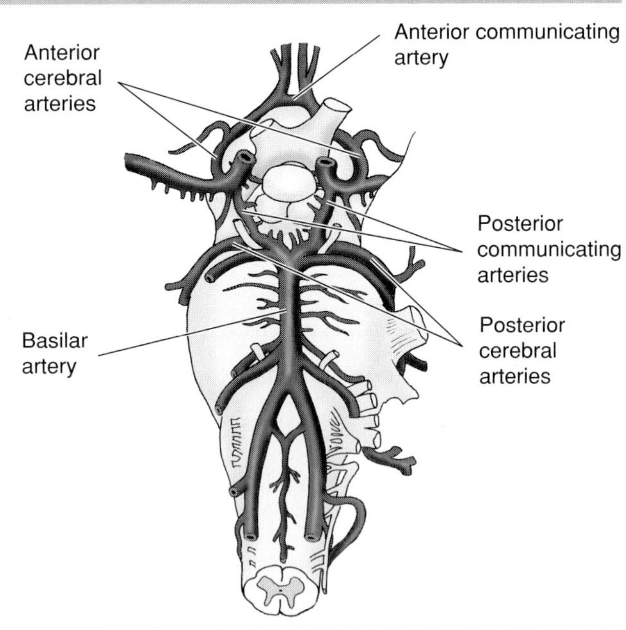

5.16A. venous sinuses; dura

5.17. The *superior sagittal sinus* is located in the upper, attached edge of the dural fold known as the falx cerebri. The superior sagittal sinus drains posteriorly toward a common collecting area called the confluence of the sinuses.

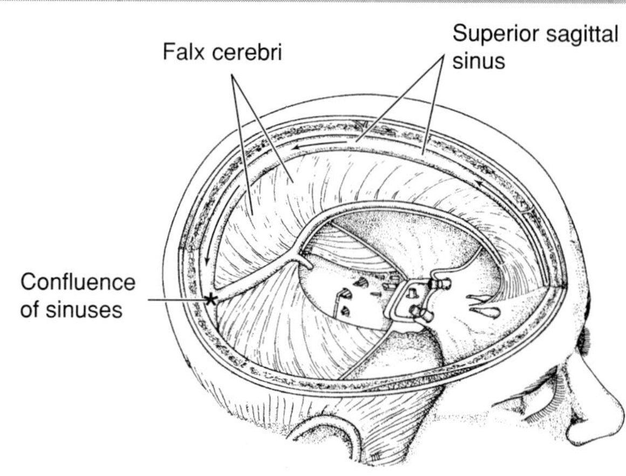

5.18. The *inferior sagittal sinus* is also associated with the falx cerebri and is located in its inferior free edge. The inferior saggital sinus drains into the straight sinus that runs through the middle of the tentorium cerebelli.

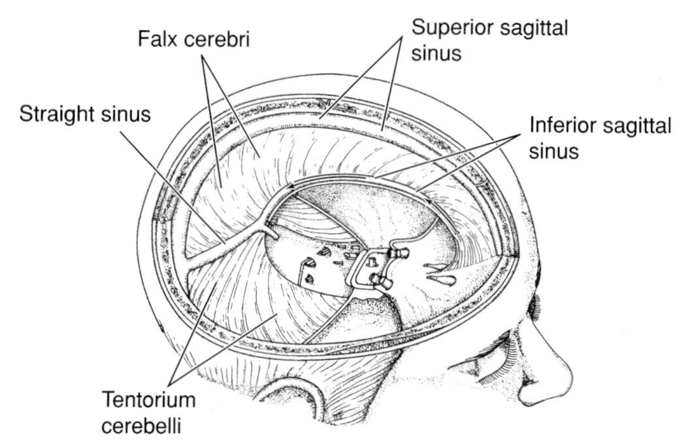

5.19. On this diagram, you are looking down into the cranial cavity, with the falx cerebri removed. Label the straight sinus on the diagram, running in midline between the left and right sides of the tentorium cerebelli. The transverse sinuses are located laterally in the attached edge of the tentorium, and they receive blood from the confluence of the sinuses (label it on the diagram).

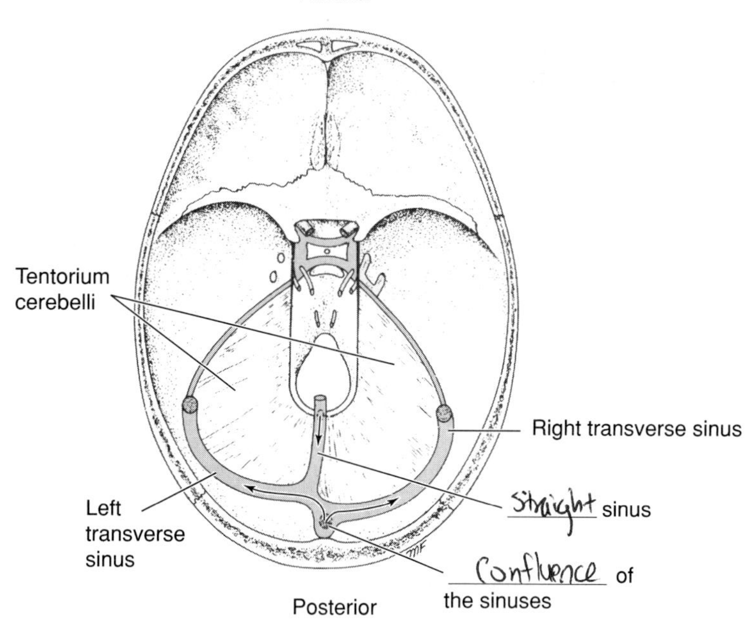

5.17A. cerebri; confluence

5.18A. cerebri; sagittal; straight; cerebelli

5.19A. cerebelli; transverse; confluence

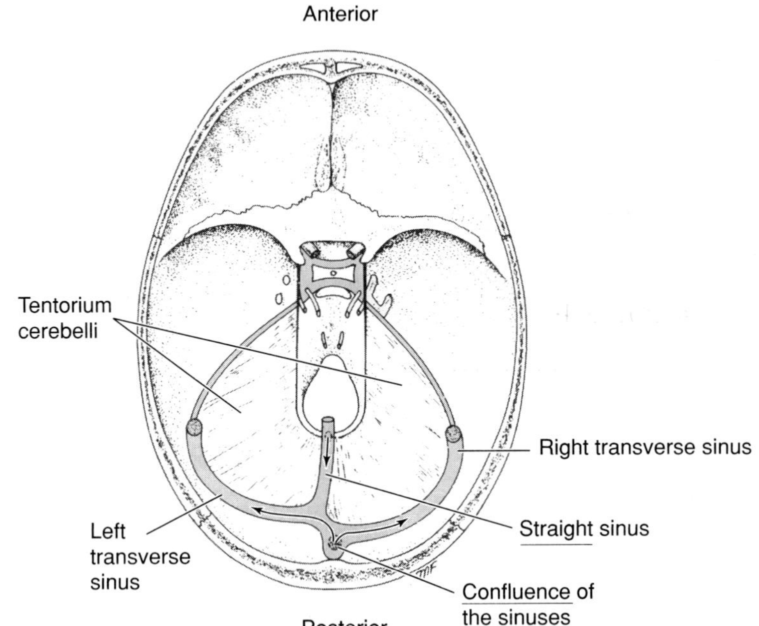

5.20. On the diagram, label the superior sagittal sinus, the confluence of sinuses, and the left transverse sinus. Each transverse sinus forms an "S"-shaped sinus anteriorly and inferiorly, the _sigmoid_ sinus, which drains into the internal _jugular_ vein.

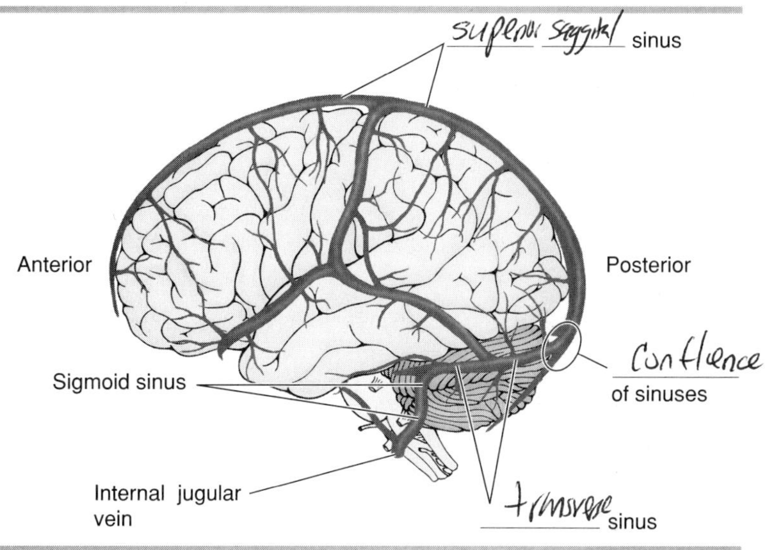

5.21. The left and right *cavernous sinuses* are positioned just lateral to the dural fold known as the diaphragma sella covering the _pituitary_ gland. Label the right cavernous sinus on the diagram. The cavernous sinuses receive blood from ophthalmic veins, superficial veins of the brain, and another dural sinus known as the sphenoparietal sinus. Each cavernous sinus empties into sinuses associated with the petrous portion or region of the temporal bone: the _petrosal_ sinuses.

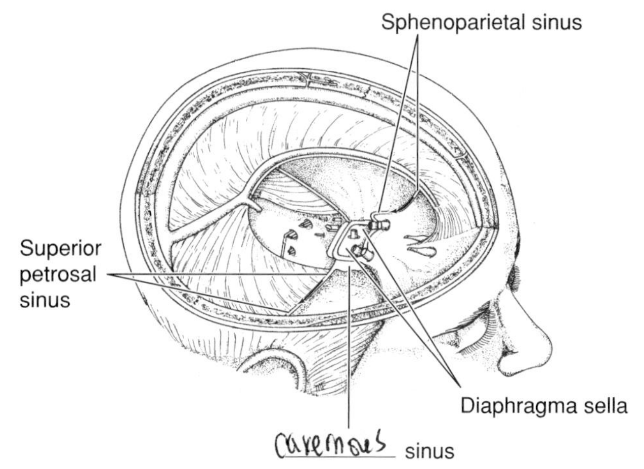

5.22. Label the dural venous sinuses indicated on the diagram.

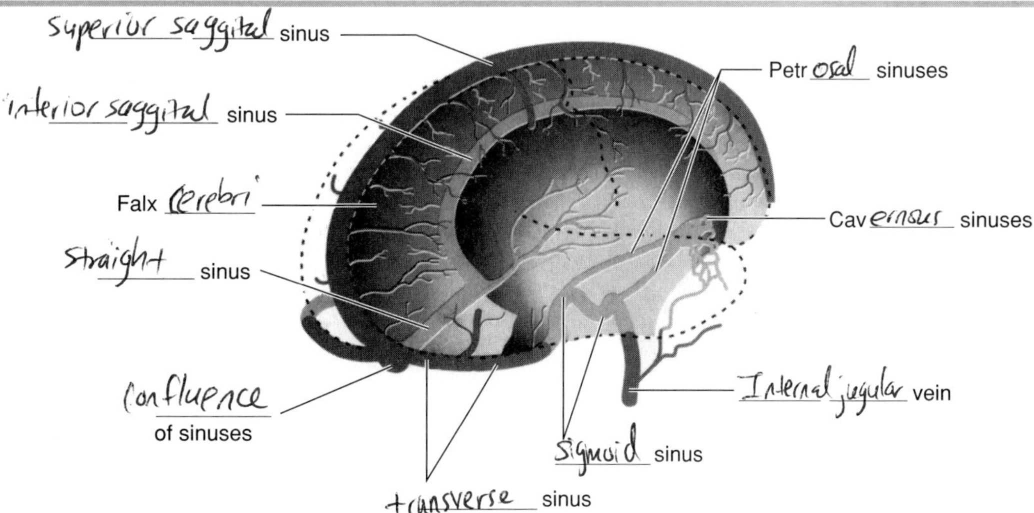

5.20A. sigmoid; jugular

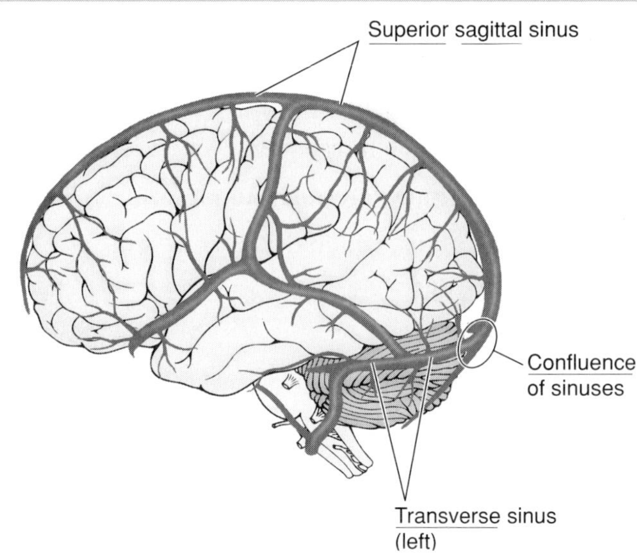

5.21A. pituitary; petrosal

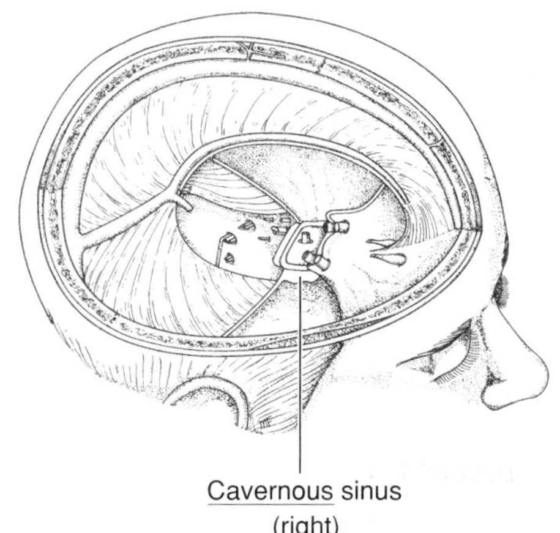

5.22A.

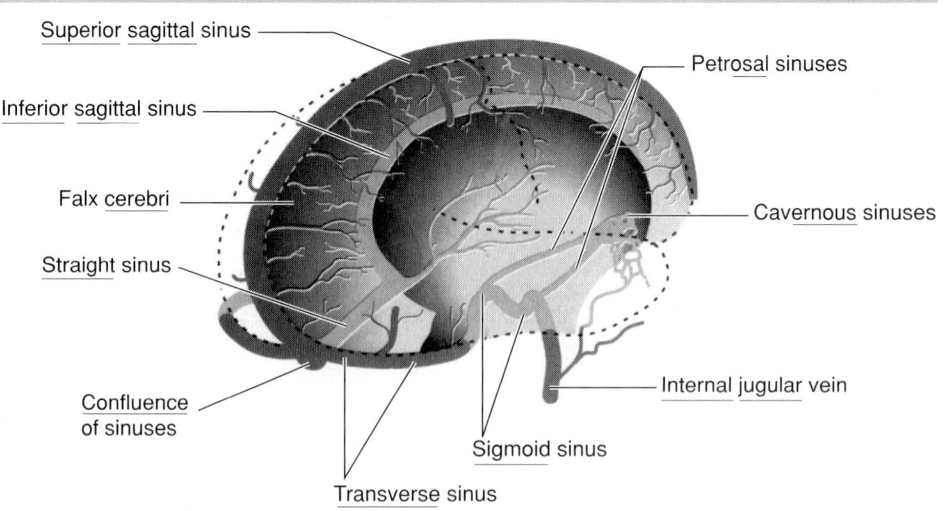

5.23. The brain is drained by two venous systems, superficial and deep. The superficial cerebral veins are associated with the lateral surface of the cortex, draining the cerebral cortex and superficial white matter. The deep cerebral veins are located on the medial cortical surface and drain the deep white matter and nuclei of the brain.

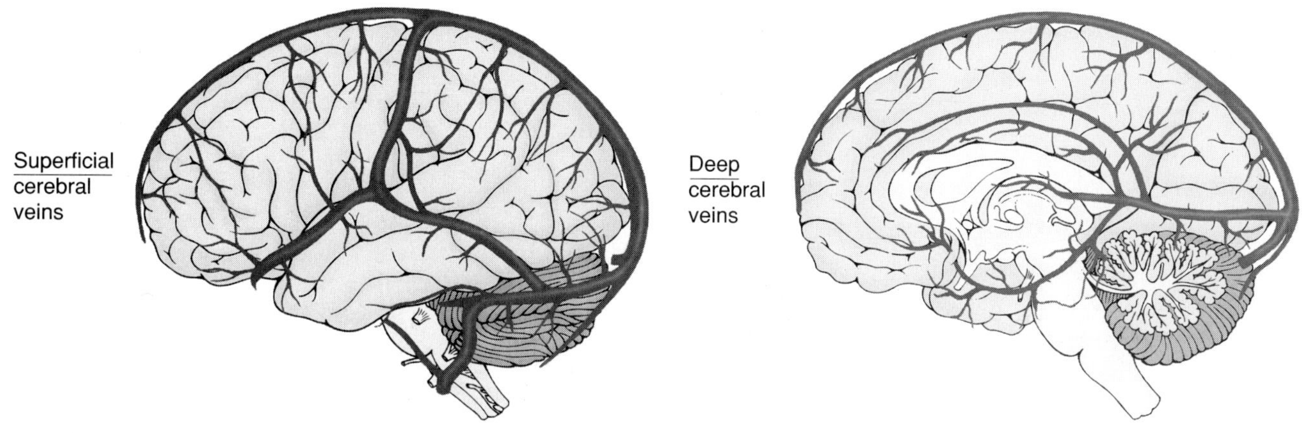

5.24. Three pairs of veins constitute the superficial cerebral venous system. The superficial Middle cerebral vein runs along the lateral sulcus in the middle of the cortex. It joins the superior anastomotic vein of Trolard, which crosses the temporal lobe of the cerebrum. The inferior anastomotic vein of Labbé crosses the temporal lobe.

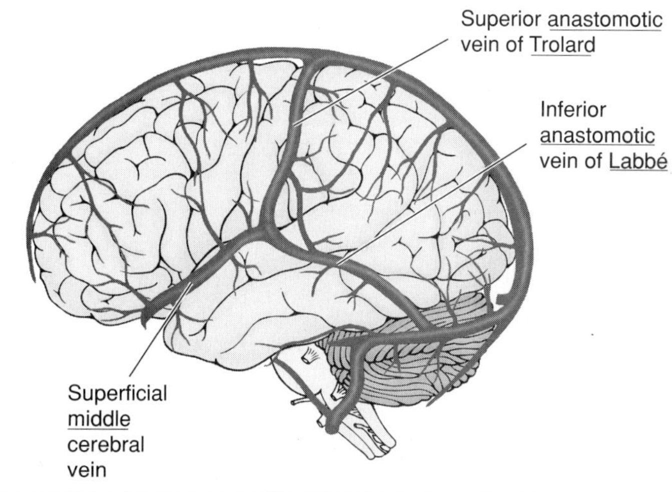

5.25. Label the superficial cerebral veins and venous sinuses on the diagram.

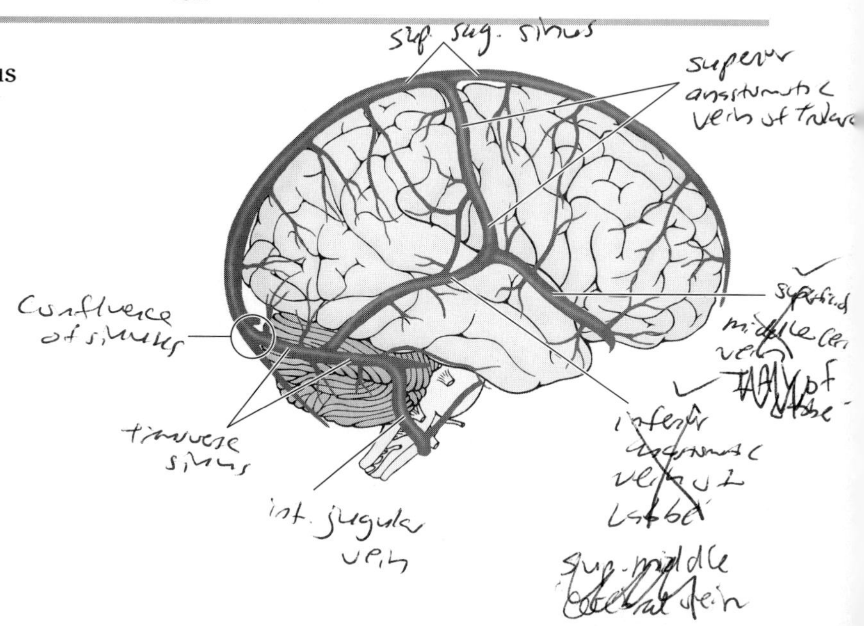

5.23A. superficial; deep; lateral; medial

5.24A. middle; anastomotic; Trolard; temporal; anastomotic; Labbé

5.25A.

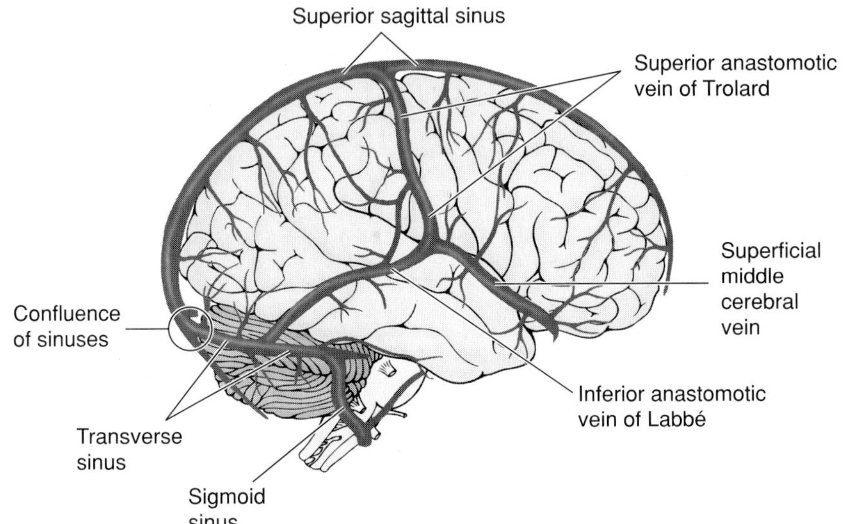

5.26. The deep cerebral venous system is formed by three pairs of veins. The *internal cerebral veins* unite to form the great cerebral vein of Galen. The great cerebral vein of Galen also receives blood from the basal vein of Rosenthal. The great cerebral vein of Galen then joins the inferior saggital sinus to form the Straight sinus, which drains into the Confluence of sinuses

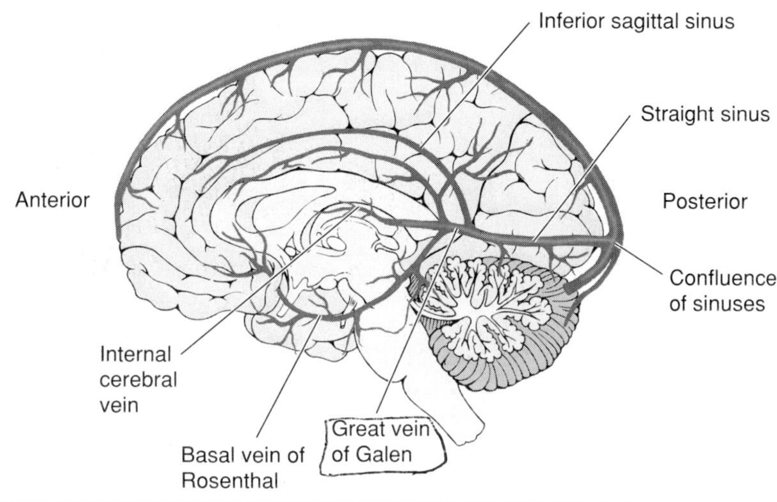

5.27. Label the deep cerebral veins and dural venous sinuses on the diagram.

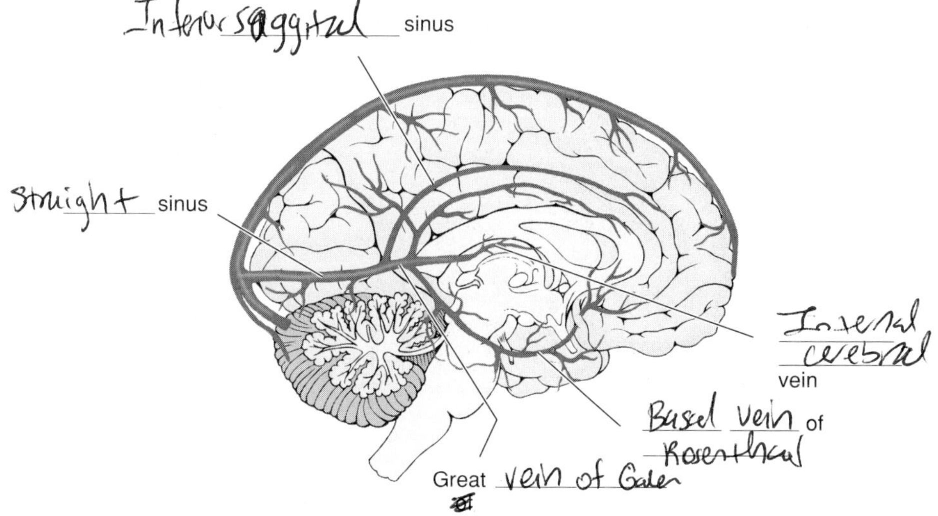

5.28. The inferior sagittal sinus joins the Great cerebral vein of Galen to form the Straight sinus.

5.26A. Galen; Galen; Rosenthal; Galen; sagittal; straight; confluence

5.27A.

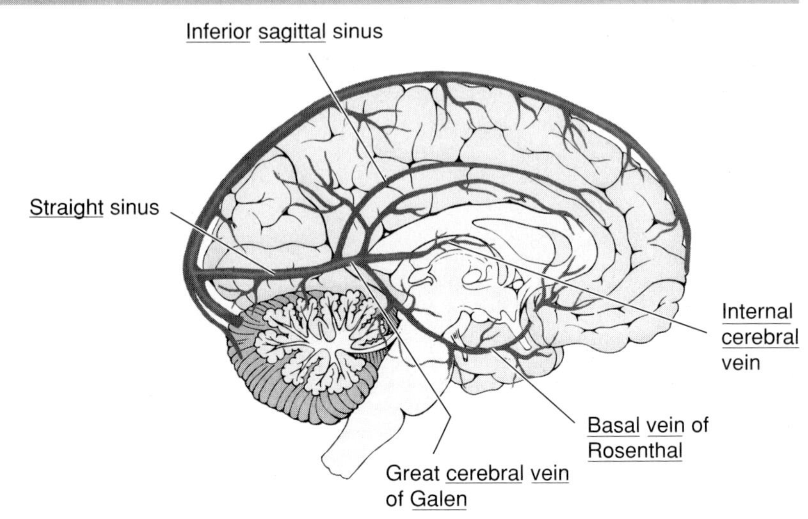

5.28A. great; cerebral; Galen; straight

6 Ventricular System

6.1. Four cavities within the brain form a continuous space known as the *ventricular system*. CSF is produced within and circulates through the ventricular system within the brain and then out into the *subarachnoid space* around the brain and spinal cord.

6.2. This diagram shows the four components of the ventricular system from a superior view. The ventricular system is composed of two lateral ventricles, a third ventricle and a fourth ventricle.

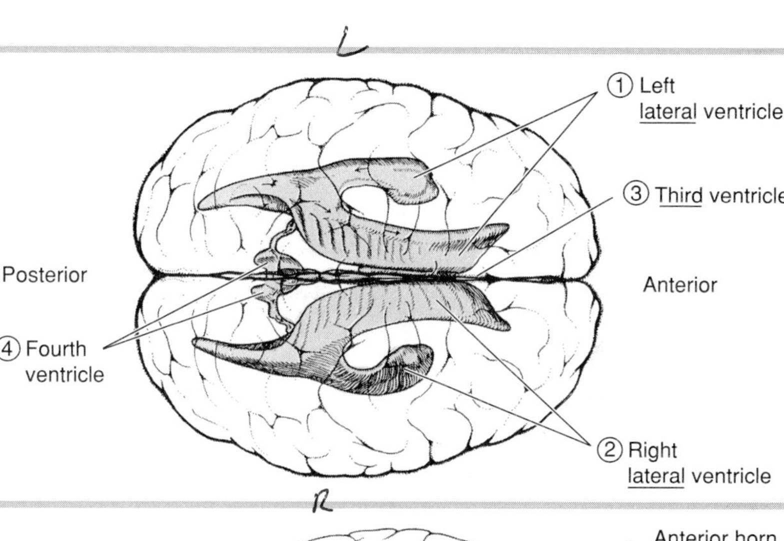

6.3. The two lateral ventricles are located *lateral* to midline and extend out into each cerebral hemisphere. The anterior horn is located in the frontal lobe; the body spans the frontal and parietal lobes, while the posterior horn extends into the occipital lobe. The inferior horn extends laterally into the temporal lobe.

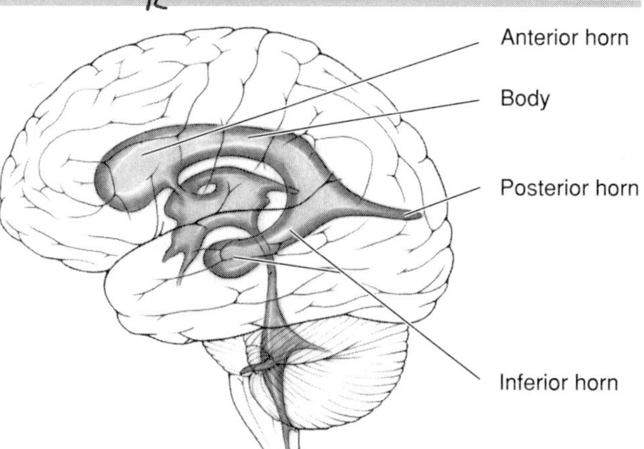

6.1A. CSF (cerebrospinal fluid)

6.2A. lateral; third; fourth

6.3A. lateral; frontal; occipital; temporal

6.4. In the lateral ventricles, CSF is synthesized by the choroid plexus. CSF flows toward the junction of the anterior horn and body of each lateral ventricle, to exit via an opening between ventricles, the inter ventricular foramen (of Monro).

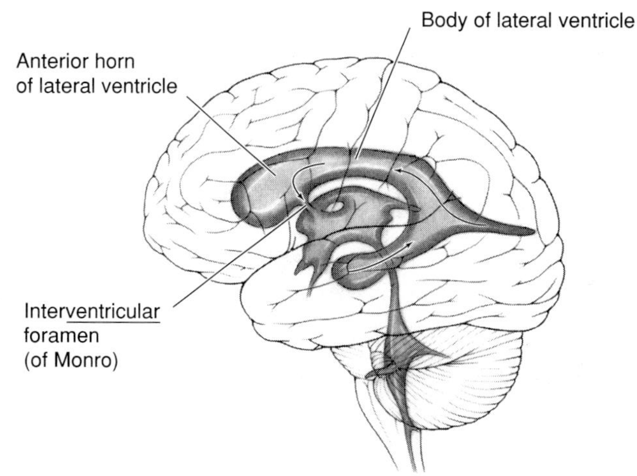

6.5. There is an interventricular foramen of Monro associated with each lateral ventricle.

6.6. You can think of the lateral ventricles as being the first and second ventricles, although they are not referred to as such. CSF drains from the lateral ventricles into the unpaired third ventricle.

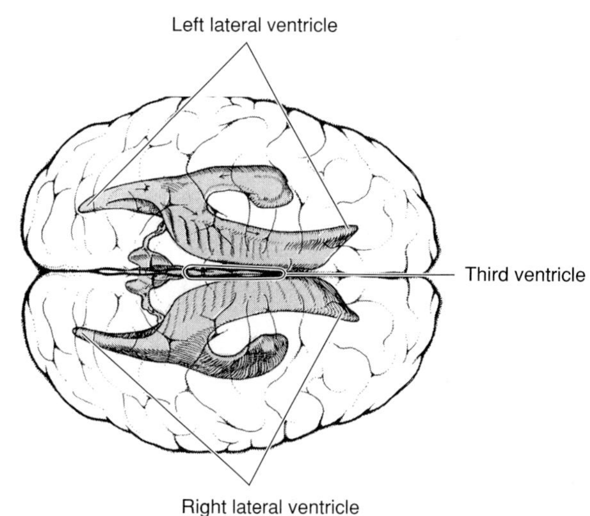

6.7. The bottom diagram represents a coronal section taken at the level shown on the upper figure. The third ventricle is a thin midline space between the two thalami. It contains choroid plexus, which produces CSF. The third ventricle is located inferior to the lateral ventricles.

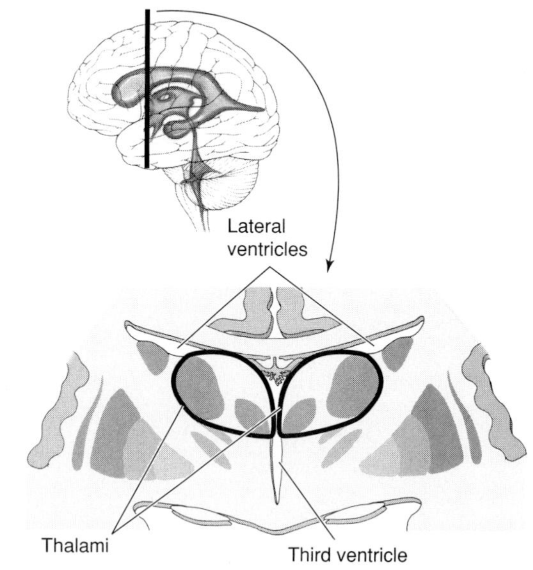

6.4A. choroid plexus; interventricular

6.5A. interventricular

6.6A. third

6.7A. thalami; choroid plexus; inferior

6.8. Label the lateral ventricles and third ventricle on this coronal section.

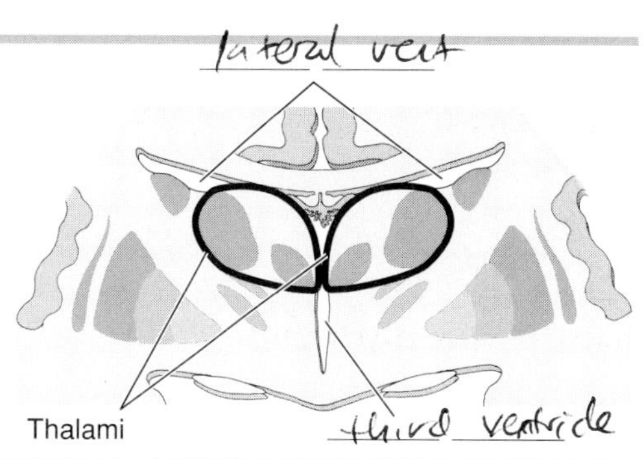

6.9. Label the third ventricle on the diagram. Inferiorly, the third ventricle narrows at the midbrain of the brainstem to drain into the cerebral aqueduct (of Sylvius). This is the narrowest part of the ventricular system, and blockage of this area results in *obstructive hydrocephalus*.

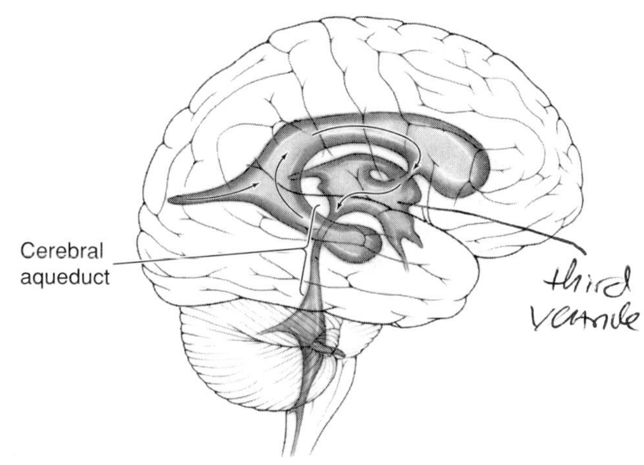

6.10. The cerebral aqueduct joins the 3rd ventricle with the 4th ventricle.

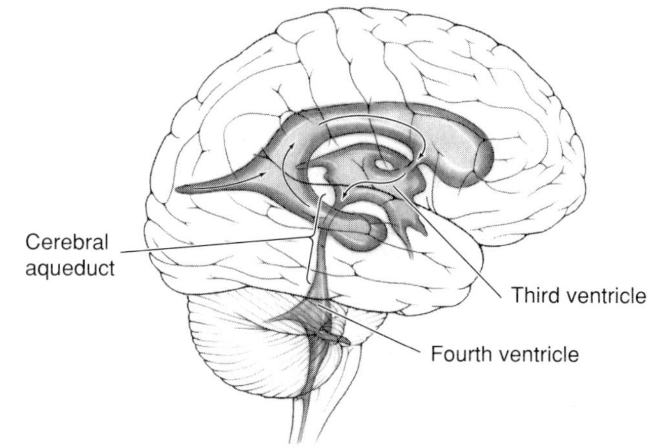

6.11. The fourth ventricle is bounded anteriorly by the pons and medulla of the brainstem and posteriorly by the cerebellum. The fourth ventricle also contains choroid plexus, which produces CSF.

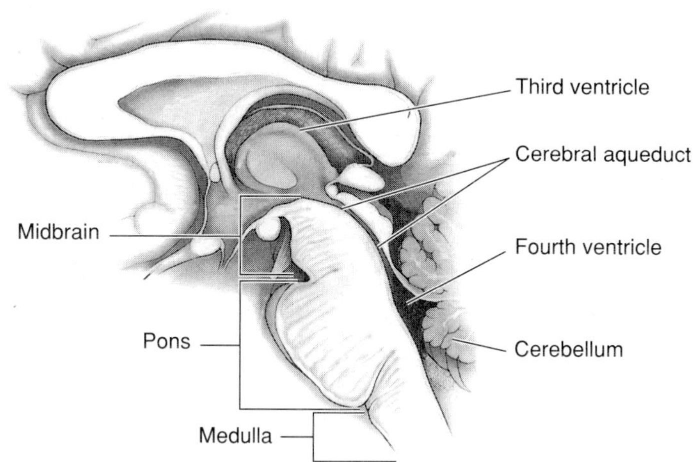

6.8A.

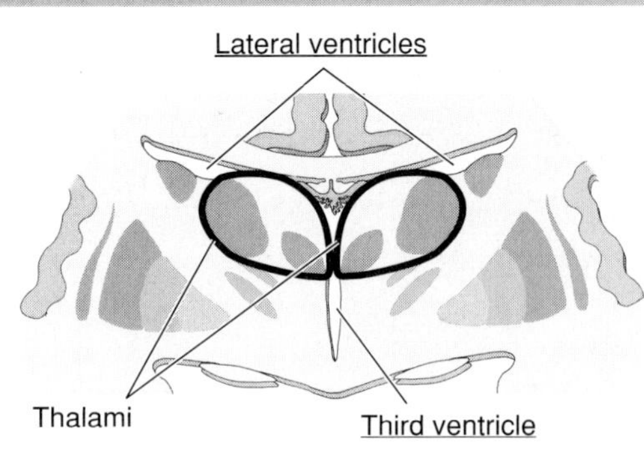

6.9A. cerebral aqueduct

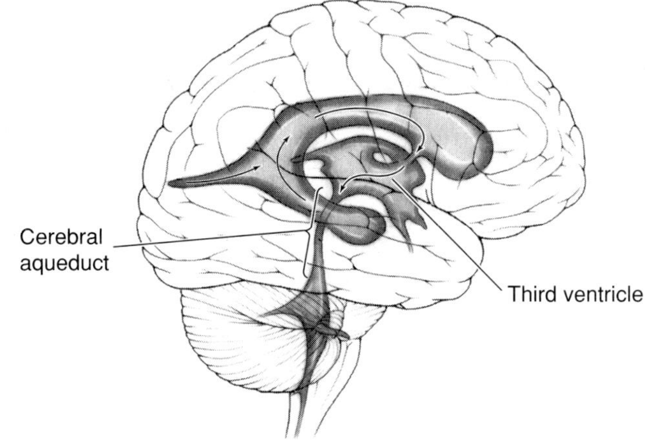

6.10A. third; fourth

6.11A. pons; medulla; cerebellum; CSF

6.12. There are four points of CSF exit from the fourth ventricle. The first is where the fourth ventricle narrows inferiorly to a point, known as the obex, and joins the central canal of the spinal cord.

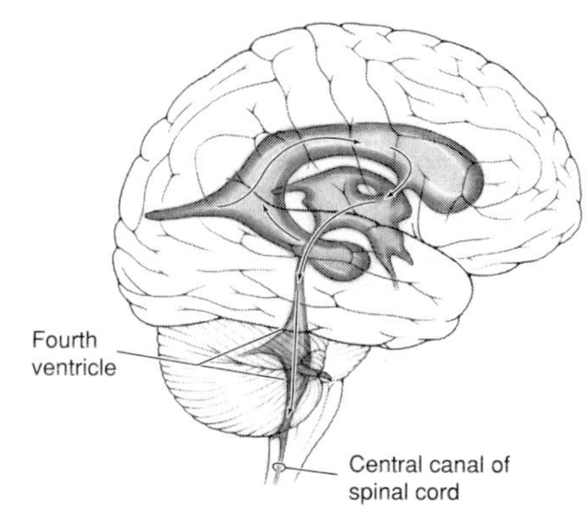

6.13. The next way that CSF can exit the fourth ventricle is via two lateral apertures (of Luschka), which open into an expansion of the subarachnoid space surrounding the lower pons, known as the pontine cistern.

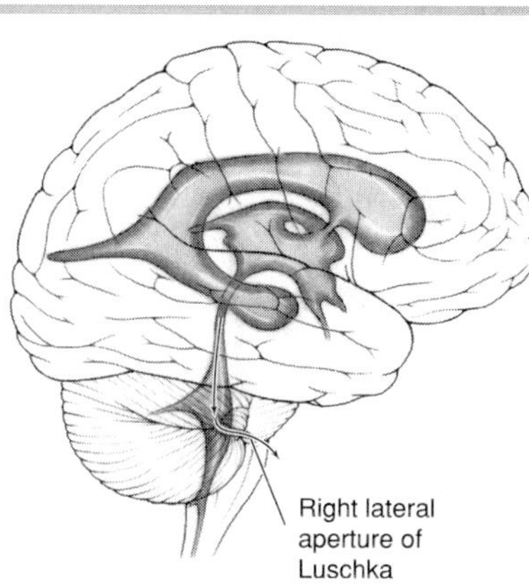

6.14. There is also a posterior midline opening, the median aperture (of Magendie), which drains into the cisterna magna.

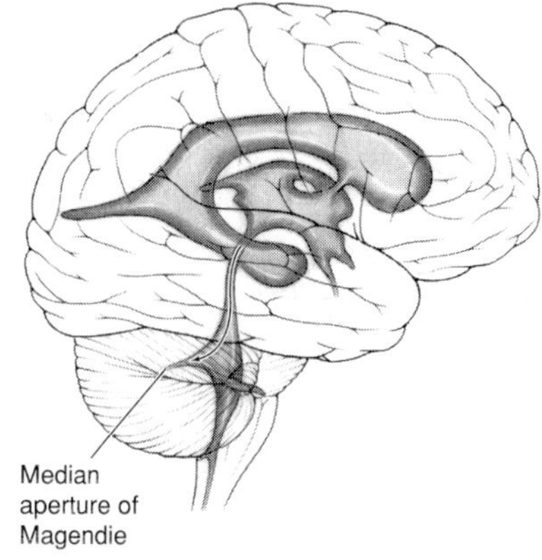

6.15. The lateral apertures and median aperture are the only communications between the ventricular system and subarachnoid space.

6.16. CSF flows into the subarachnoid space of the cranial cavity and is ultimately absorbed into dural venous sinuses by extensions of the arachnoid known as arachnoid villi.

6.17. Trace the production of CSF from the posterior horn of the lateral ventricle to the central canal of the spinal cord: Posterior horn of lateral ventricle → body of lateral ventricle → interventricular foramen (of Monro) → 3rd ventricle → cerebral aqueduct (of Sylvius) → 4th ventricle → central canal of spinal cord

6.12A. central canal

6.13A. lateral apertures; cistern

6.14A. median aperture; magna

6.15A. subarachnoid space

6.16A. venous sinuses; villi

6.17A. body; interventricular; third; cerebral aqueduct; fourth

7 The Corticospinal System: Course of Fibers from Cortex to Basal Ganglia

7.1. The anatomical pathways carrying impulses to the cortex are called *afferent* pathways. Those pathways leading from the cortex are called *efferent.* We shall soon pass from the cortex along a major ______ fferent pathway and later return via major __________ pathways.

7.2. Afferent and ______ fferent pathways carry impulses, respectively, to and ______ some reference point in the central nervous system, such as the cerebral cortex.

7.3. Sensory pathways carry impulses from sense organs toward and into the central nervous system. *Sensory* pathways are a type of __________ pathway. Motor pathways are a type of __________ pathway.

7.4. With the cerebral cortex as a reference point, a pathway carrying impulses from the thalamus toward the cortex is an __________ pathway.

7.5. With the thalamus as a reference point, an efferent pathway carries impulses in a direction ______ the thalamus __________ the cortex.

7.6. A pathway entirely confined to the central nervous system (CNS) can be afferent without necessarily being a part of a sensory system. Likewise, some pathways that connect structures within the CNS may be efferent but not necessarily ______.

7.7. The criterion for defining afferent and efferent is the __________ of impulse conduction.

7.8. The well-known *corticospinal* tract is a major efferent pathway from the cerebral cortex. It is named for its point of origin, the __________, and its point of termination, the __________ cord.

7.1A. efferent; afferent

7.2A. efferent; from

7.3A. afferent; efferent

7.4A. afferent

7.5A. from; toward

7.6A. motor

7.7A. direction

7.8A. cortex; spinal

7.9. Central nervous system pathways conducting information from sense organs toward cortex or other central structures are commonly called sensory pathways even though they are not directly connected to sense organs. Similarly, the corticospinal tract, which conducts impulses toward muscles but does not innervate them directly, is considered a ______ pathway.

7.10. The cortico ____________ tract originates in the cerebral cortex and terminates in the ____________ c ______.

7.11. The ____________ spinal tract is a motor tract. Most of its nerve cell bodies are in the ____________ lobe of the cerebral cortex.

7.12. The best defined locus of motor neurons within the frontal lobe is the ____________ gyrus.

7.13. Axons of the corticospinal tract (some several feet long) run without interruption from the cell bodies in the ____________________ gyrus to the ____________ ______. Does a given corticospinal impulse cross any synapses between cortex and spinal cord? ______

7.14. On the diagram, indicate the frontal pole of the right hemisphere of the brain with an arrow. Draw the full boundaries of the right frontal lobe and label the precentral gyrus.

7.15. Most nerve cell bodies are in the gray matter of the brain. Their axons, coated with glistening white myelin, often collect as tracts to form ______ matter.

7.16. *Nucleus* is a term designating a circumscribed collection of nerve cell bodies of the ______ matter of the central nervous system.

7.17. The thin outer layer of the cortex contains many nerve cell bodies and therefore is ______ matter.

7.9A. motor

7.10A. corticospinal; spinal cord

7.11A. corticospinal; frontal

7.12A. precentral

7.13A. precentral; spinal cord; no

7.14A.

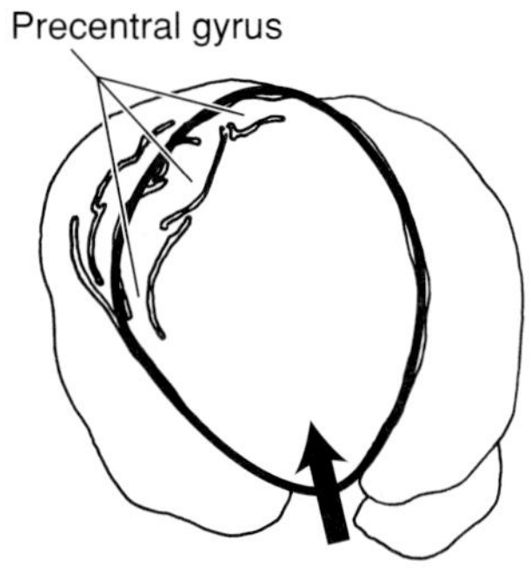

Precentral gyrus

7.15A. white

7.16A. gray

7.17A. gray

7.18. Axons of motor neurons collect in the white matter underlying the surface of the precentral gyrus to form the beginning of the ______________ tract.

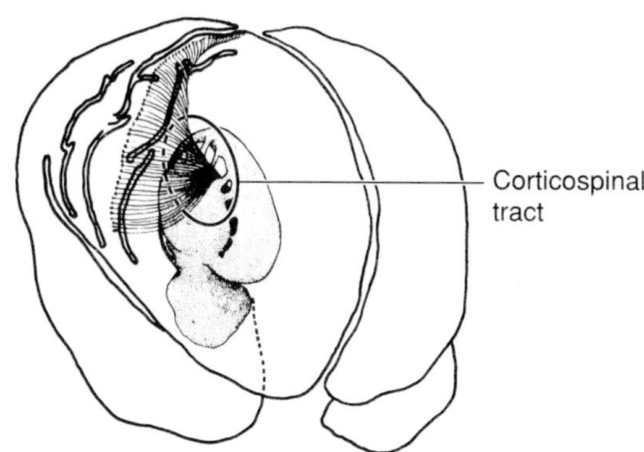

7.19. Corticospinal fibers run inferiorly from the precentral gyrus anteriorly and ______ ially; deep within the hemisphere, the fibers pass between the __________ and the __________ nuclei.

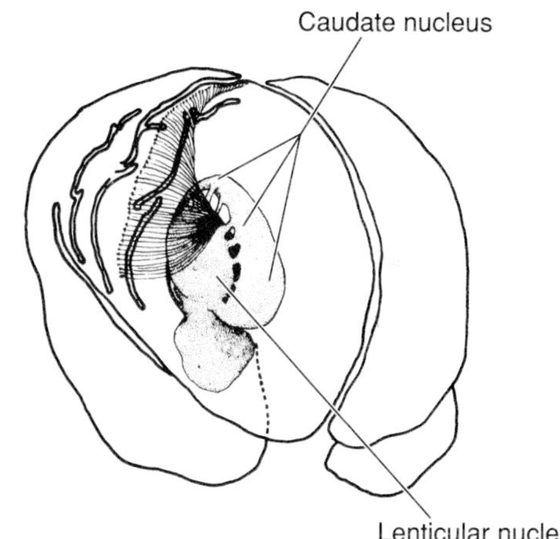

7.20. The interior of the cerebral hemispheres consists partly of white matter and partly of well-defined areas of gray matter known as the *basal nuclei.* The caudate nucleus, lenticular nucleus, and amygdala are the best known of the ______ nuclei. On the diagram, place a "C" on the C-shaped caudate nucleus. Place an "L" on the lenticular nucleus, which is located inferior to the caudate nucleus. Place an "A" on the amygdala, which is located in the temporal lobe.

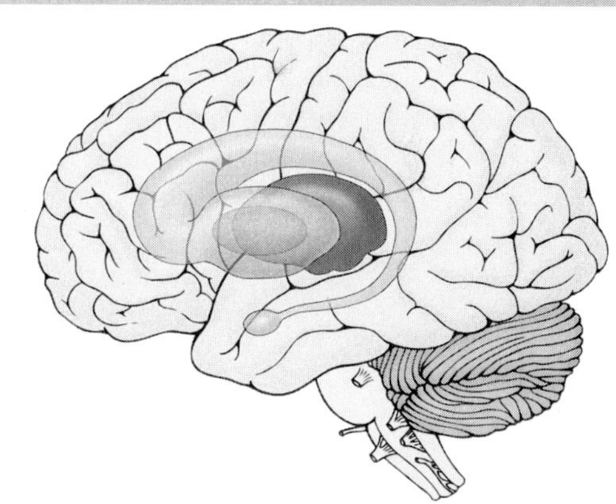

7.21. Label the appropriate ends of the brain as *anterior* (ANT) and *posterior* (POST).

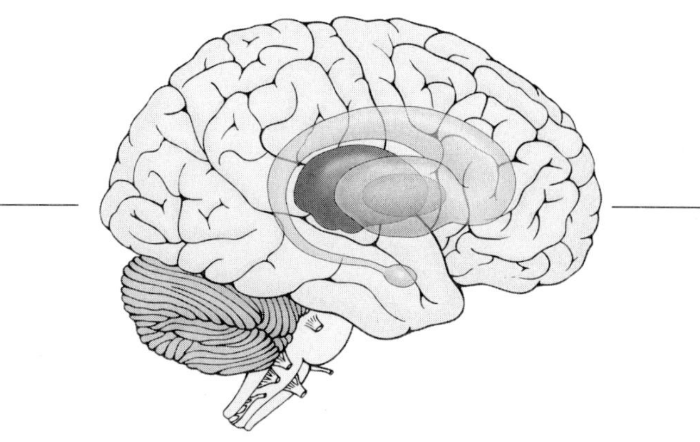

7.18A. corticospinal

7.19A. medially; caudate; lenticular

7.20A. basal

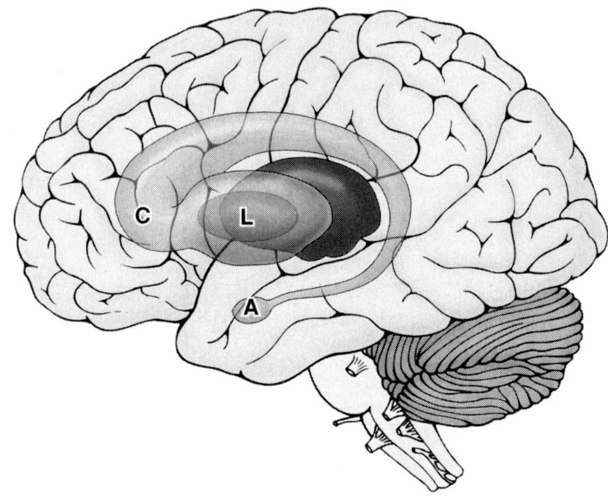

7.21A.

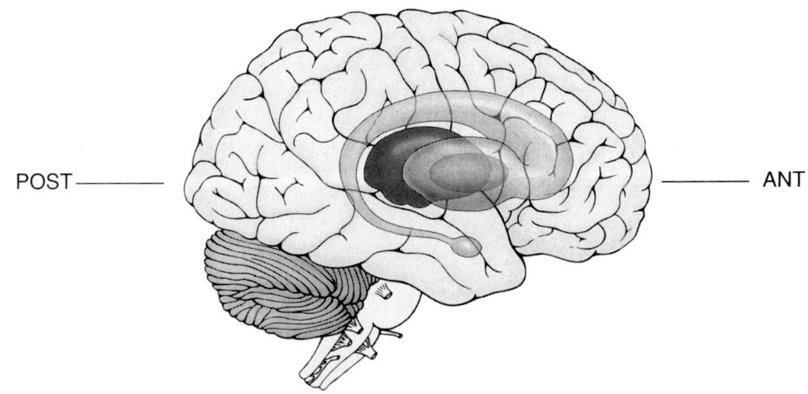

7.22. Sometimes one can best appreciate the shape of a nucleus and its relations to neighboring nuclei by abstracting it from the brain. Label the appropriate ends of the right hand diagram as ANT and POST.

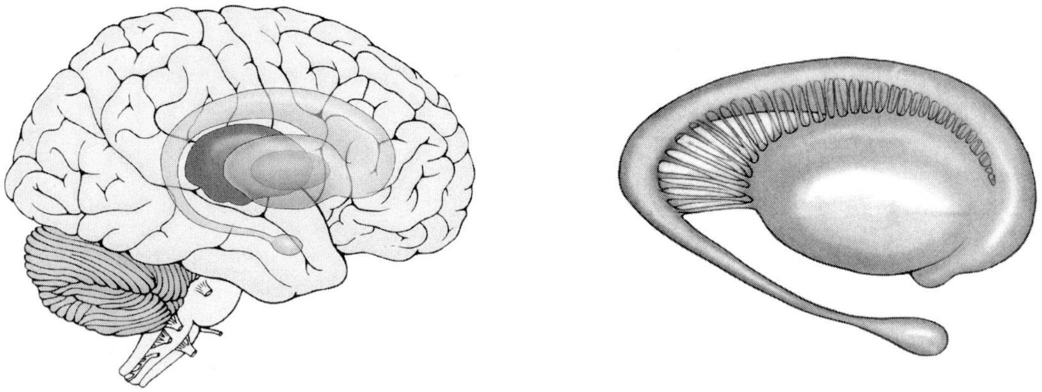

7.23. The lenticular nucleus and its associated structures are bilaterally symmetrical (one set is found in each cerebral hemisphere). Indicate with labels which diagram shows mainly the left side of the brain and which shows mainly the right.

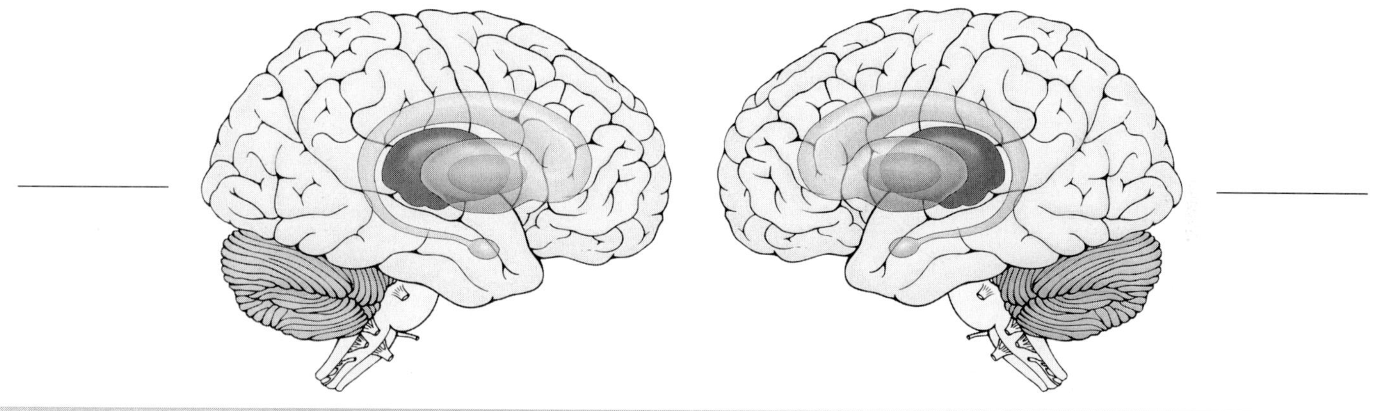

7.24. The structures in the right hand diagram have been abstracted from the ______ side of the brain. Label the right hand diagram with "ANT" for anterior and "POST" for posterior.

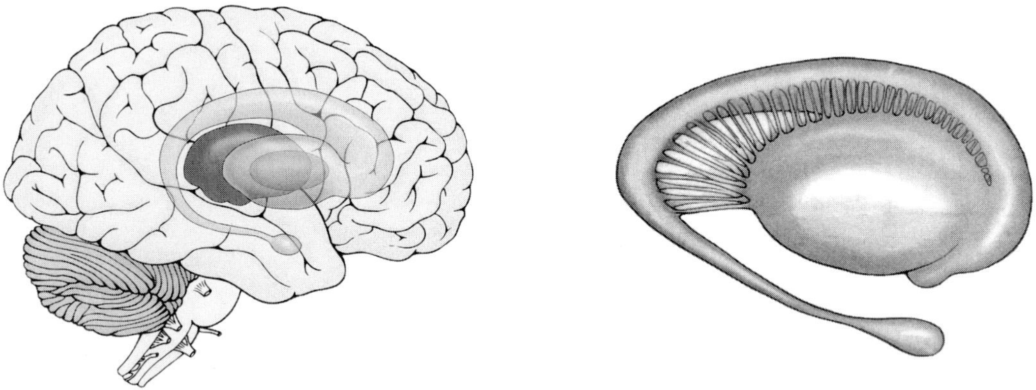

7.22A.

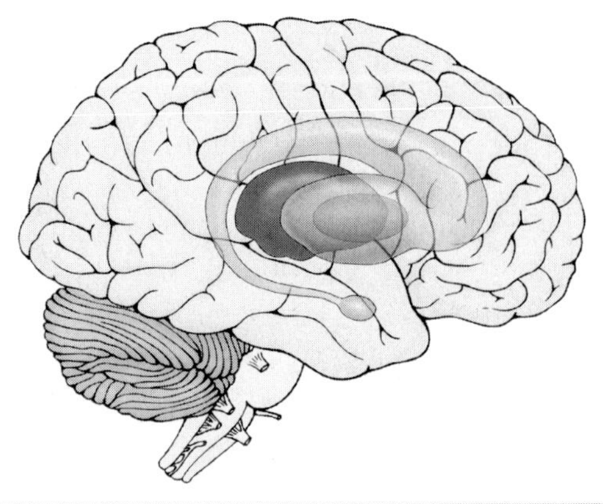

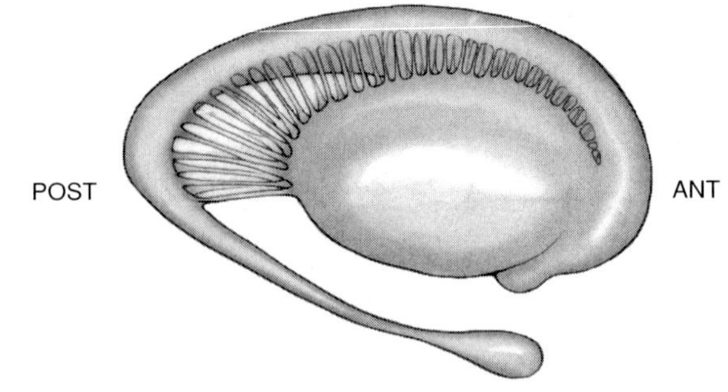

7.23A.

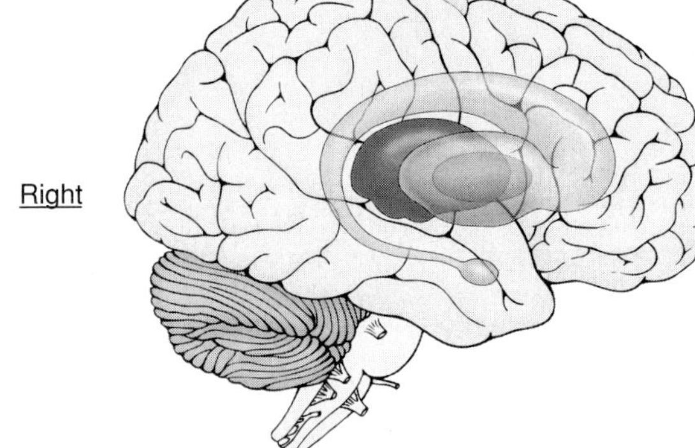

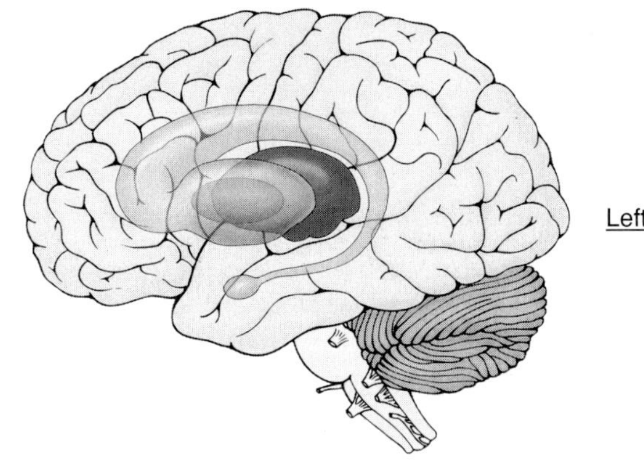

7.24A. right

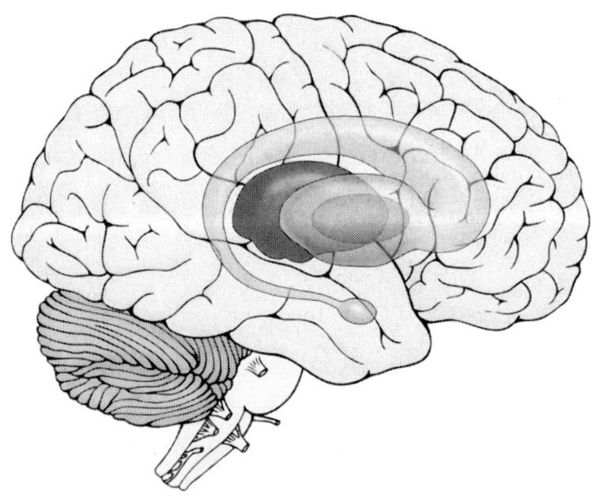

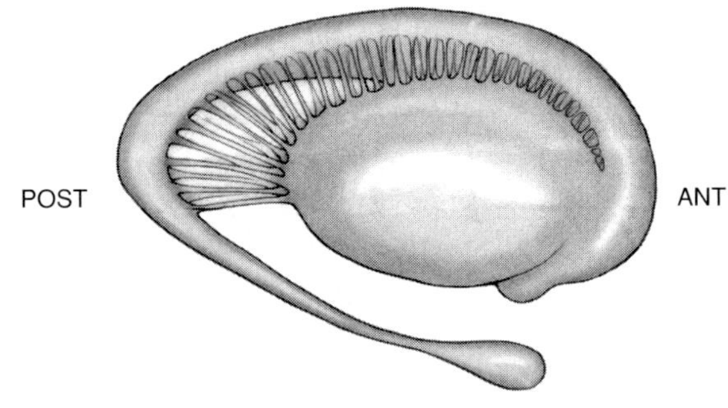

7.25. The structures in the right hand diagram are from the ______ side of the brain. Label the right hand diagram with "ANT" for anterior and "POST" for posterior.

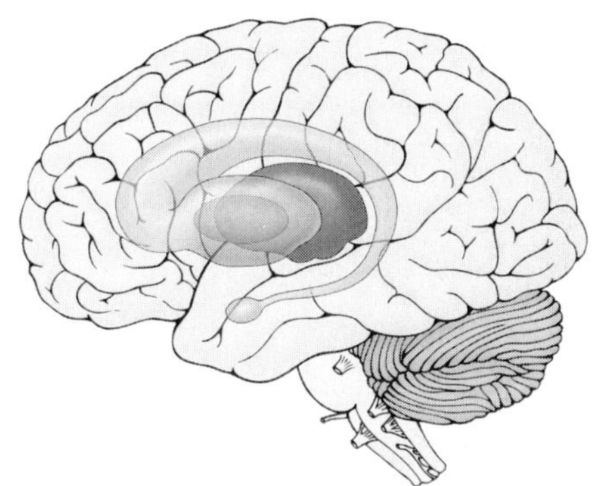

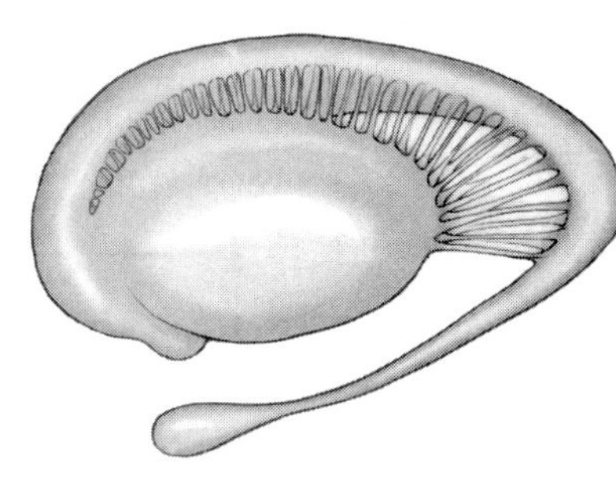

7.26. Are the structures in the right hand diagram from the same side of the brain as the structures shown in the other picture? ______. Label the right hand diagram with "ANT" for anterior and "POST" for posterior.

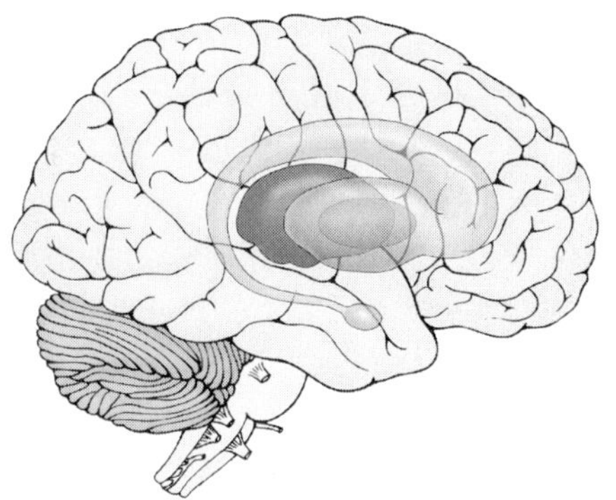

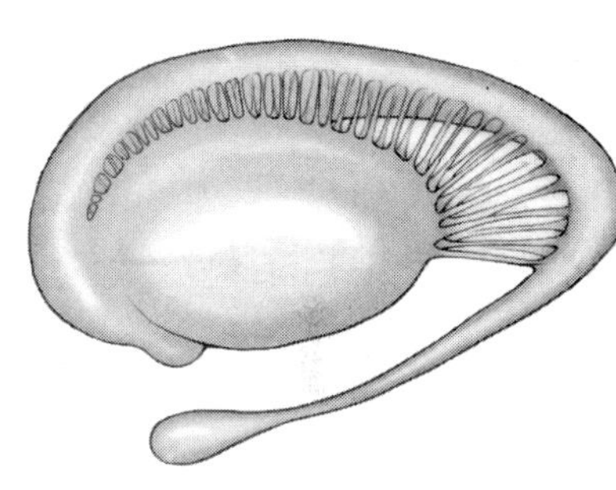

7.27. The structures in the right hand diagram are from the ______ side of the brain. Label the right hand diagram with "ANT" for anterior and "POST" for posterior.

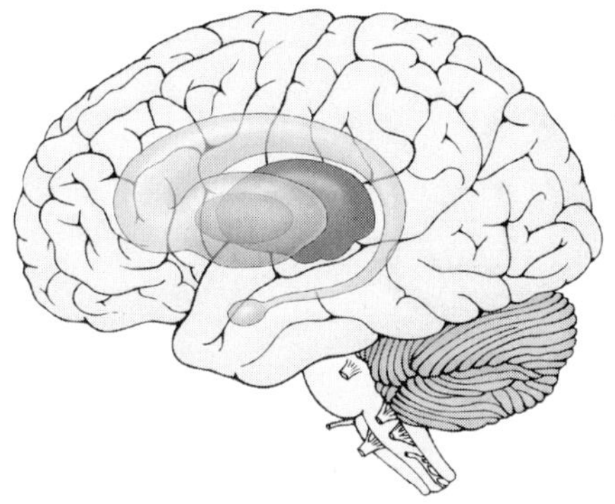

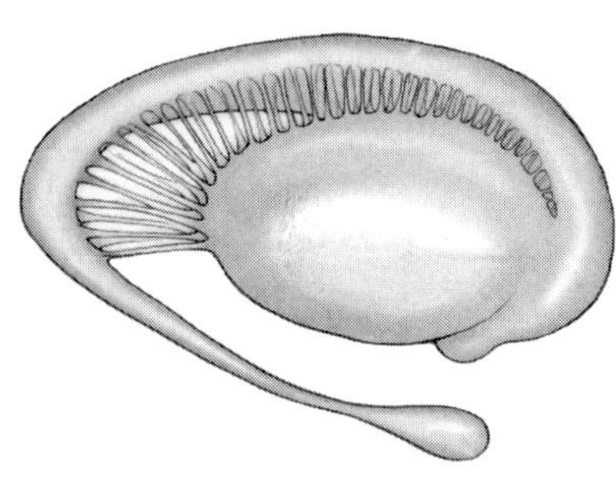

7.28. Label the three nuclei indicated on the diagram.

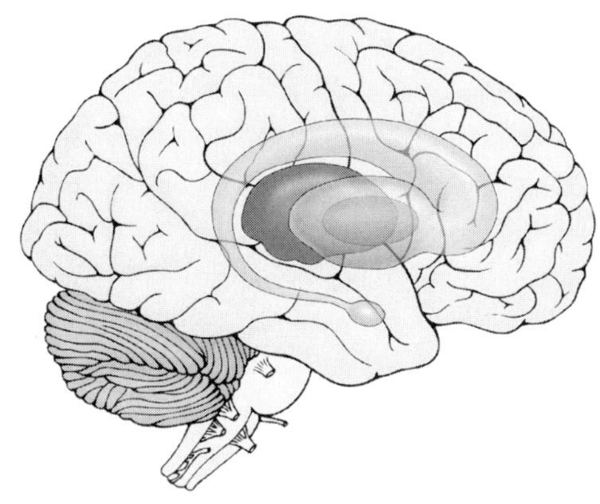

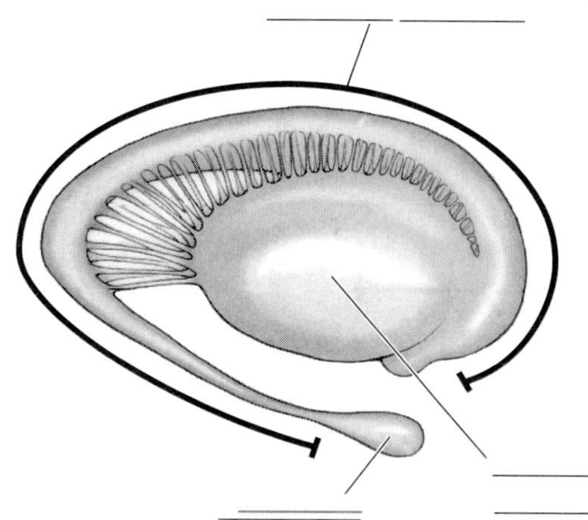

7.25A. left

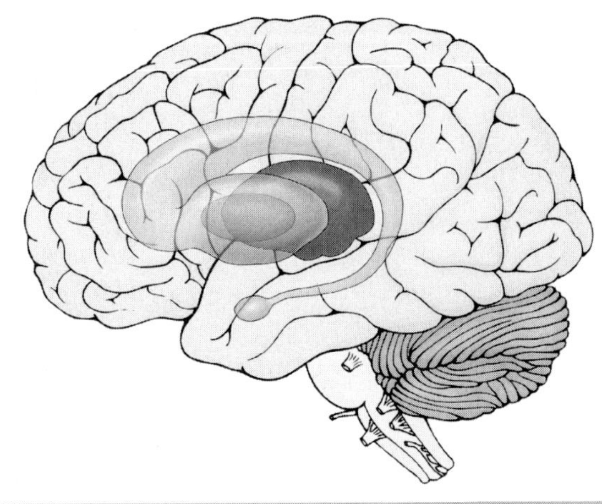

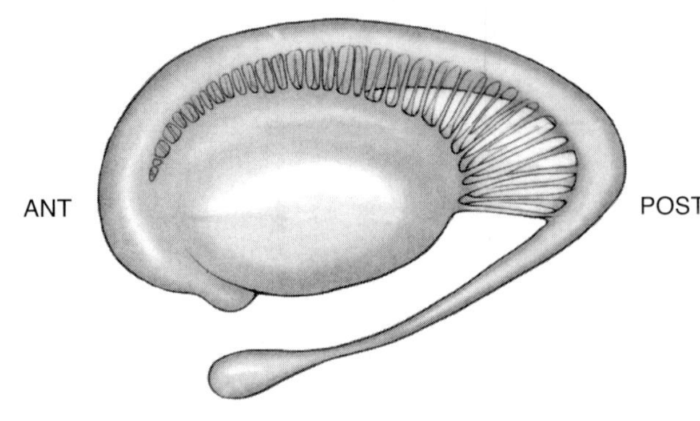

7.26A. No

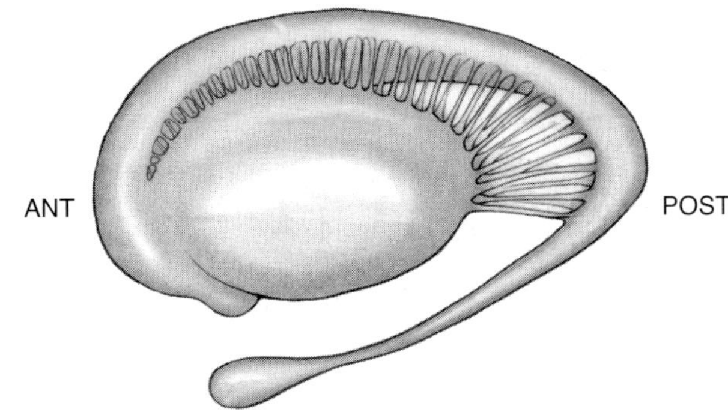

7.27A. right

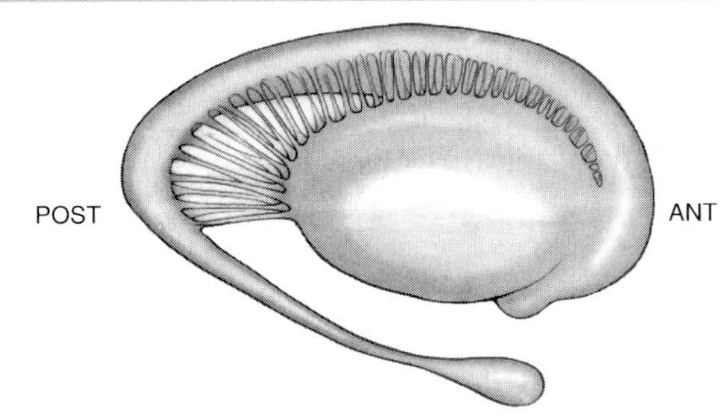

7.28A.

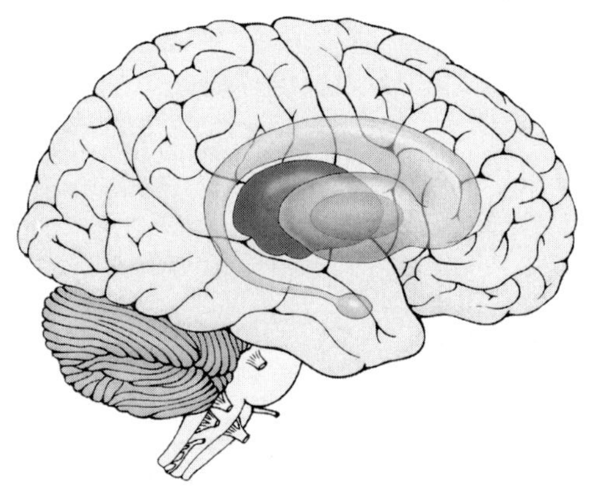

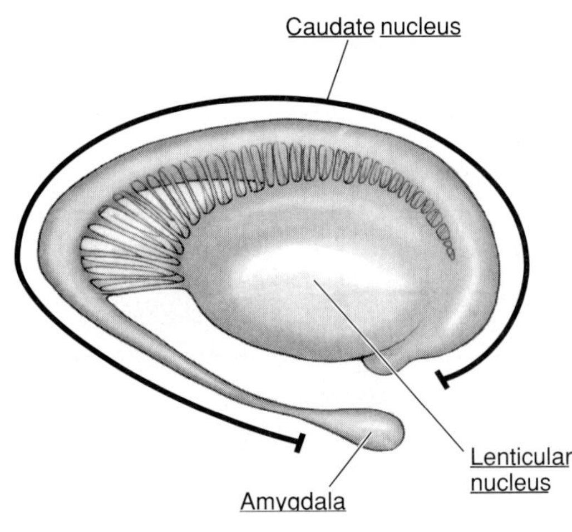

7.29. The long curving *caudal* structure is the source of the name, ______ ate nucleus. As labeled on the diagram, the nucleus is divided into how many regions? ______

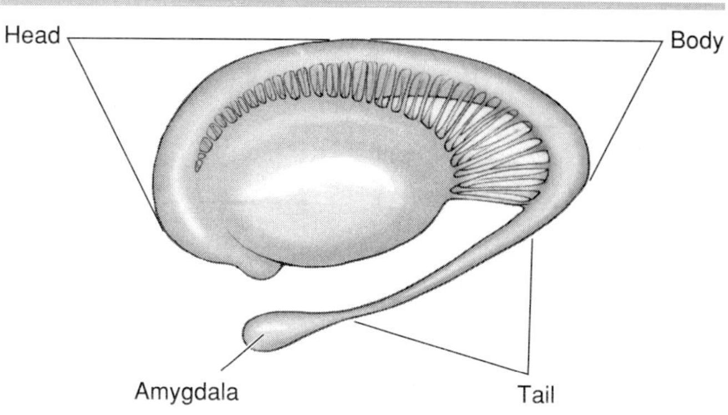

7.30. The dividing lines between the head, body, and tail of the __________ nucleus are somewhat arbitrary. Label the three regions on the diagram.

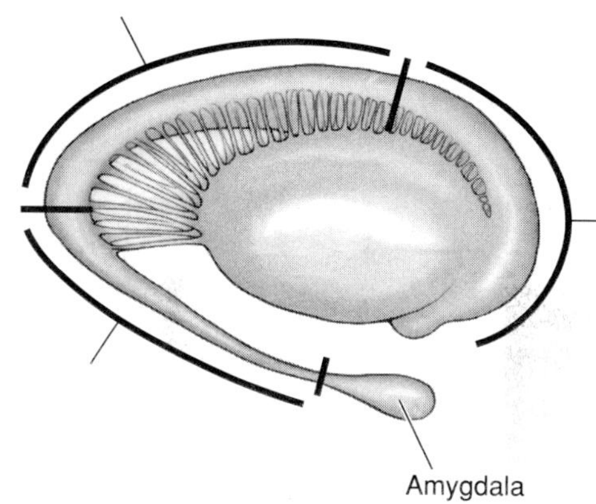

7.31. The thickest part of the caudate nucleus is its ______, located at the ______ ior end of the nucleus.

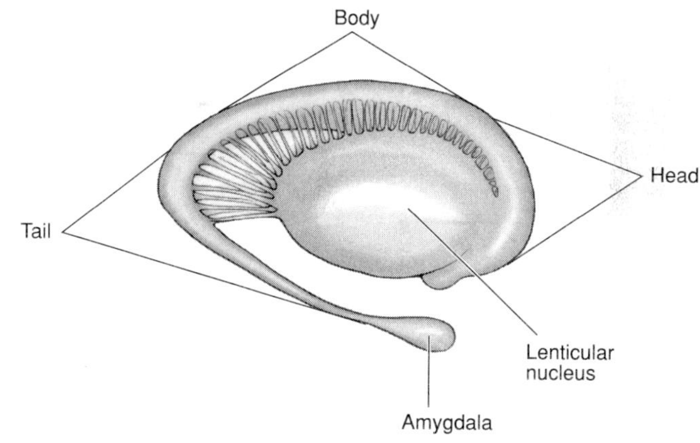

7.32. The posterior part of the caudate nucleus contains the junction of its ______ and ______.

7.33. The amygdala, another collection of nerve cell bodies, is fused posteriorly with the ______ of the caudate nucleus. The amygdala and caudate and lenticular nuclei are ______ matter.

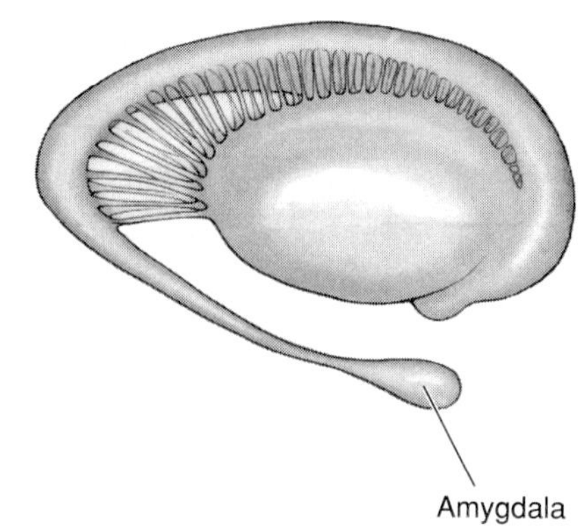

7.29A. caudate; three

7.30A. caudate

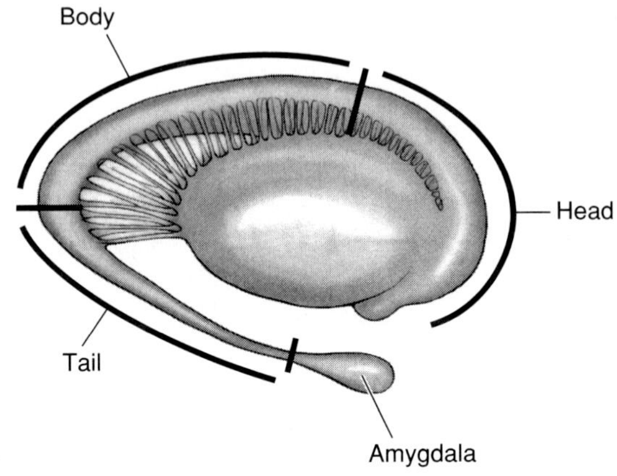

7.31A. head; anterior

7.32A. body; tail

7.33A. tail; gray

7.34. The accent is on *myg* and the *g* is pronounced hard in amyg ______.

7.35. The last two syllables of ____________ are given little emphasis and are pronounced “dah” and “lah.” Say the whole name.

7.36. Three structures in this picture contain distinct collections of nerve cell bodies. Label the structures.

________ nucleus

____ticular nucleus

____

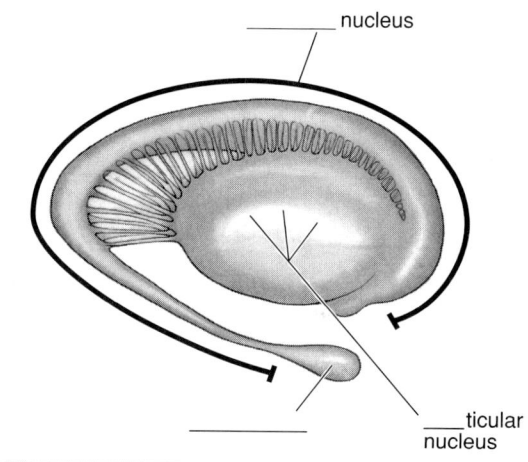

7.37. Afferent and efferent myelinated axons passing between cerebral cortex and underlying regions fill the available space between the ____________ nucleus and the ____________________ nucleus.

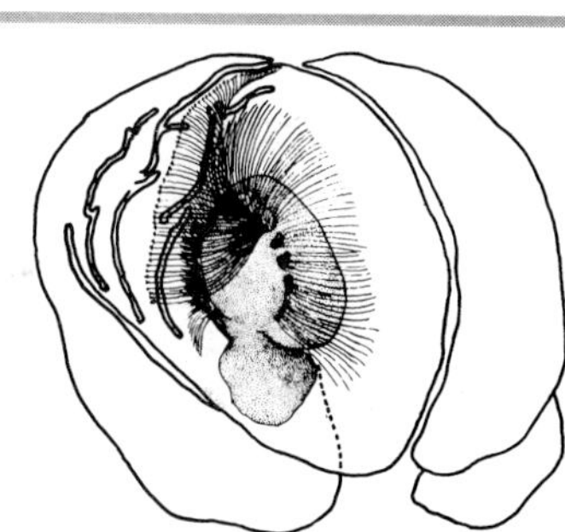

7.38. Circle the corticospinal tract just before it passes between the caudate and ____________________ nuclei.

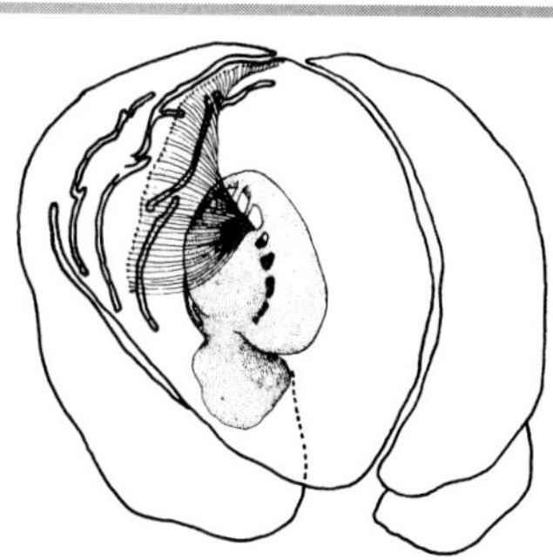

7.39. Label the indicated structures.

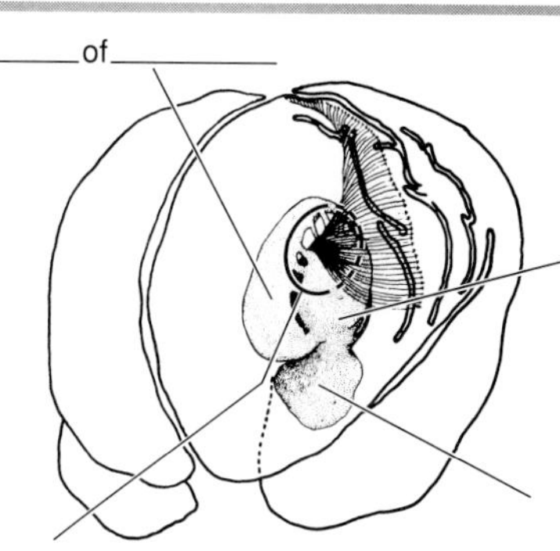

7.34A. amygdala

7.35A. amygdala

7.36A.

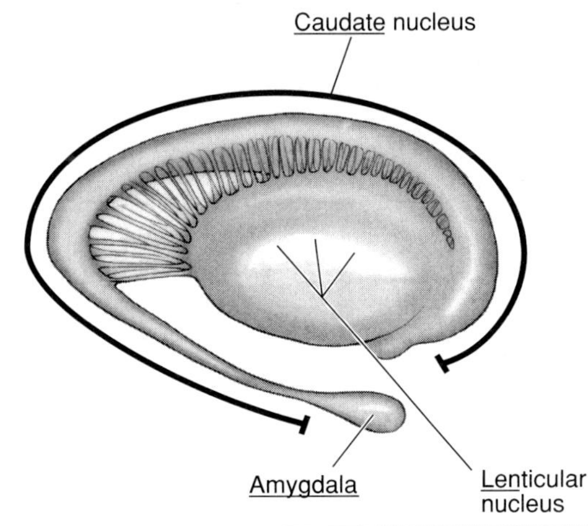

7.37A. caudate; lenticular

7.38A. lenticular

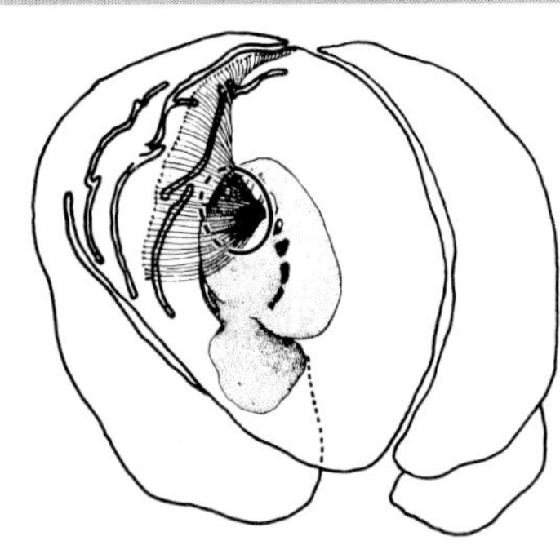

7.39A.

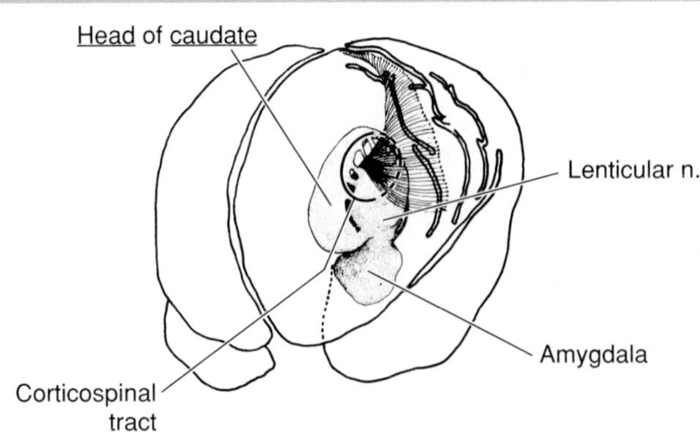

7.40. Place a "V" on the occipital pole of the left hemisphere and an "M" on the precentral gyrus. If you were viewing this specimen anteriorly, the ______ of the caudate would be closest to you.

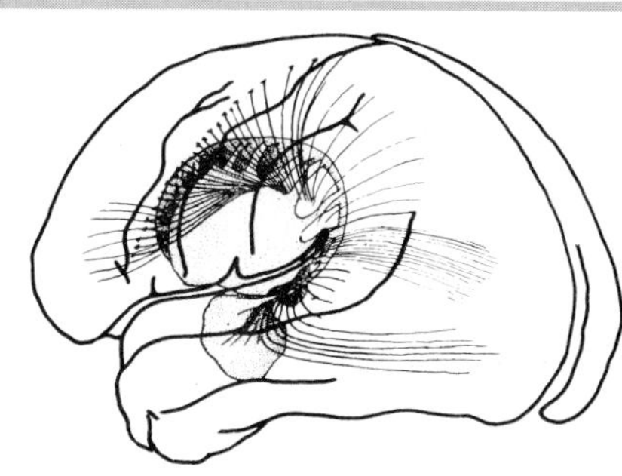

7.41. In the right hand figure, the basal nuclei are seen in ____________ view. The term nucleus is used for ______ matter.

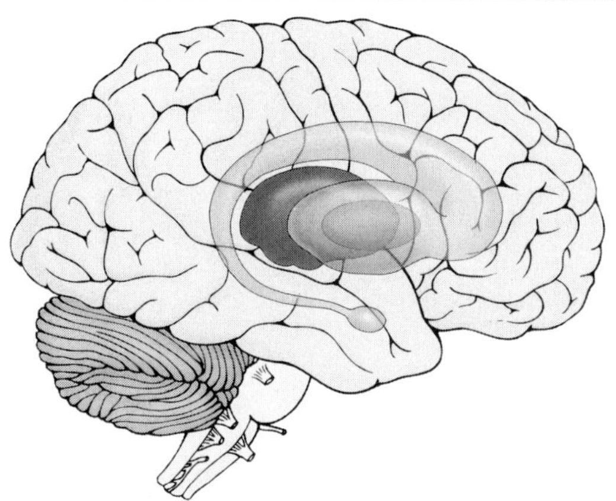

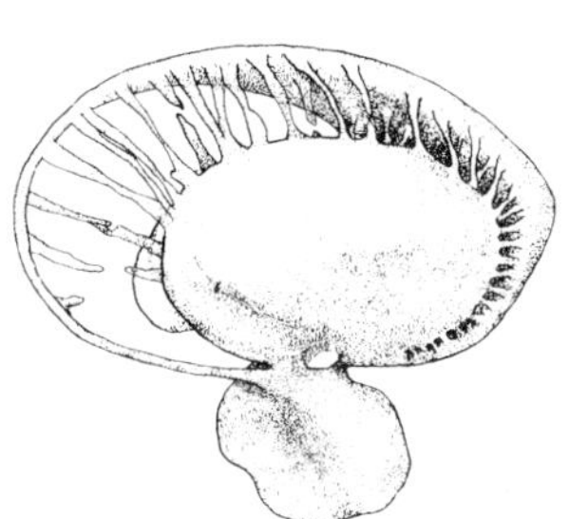

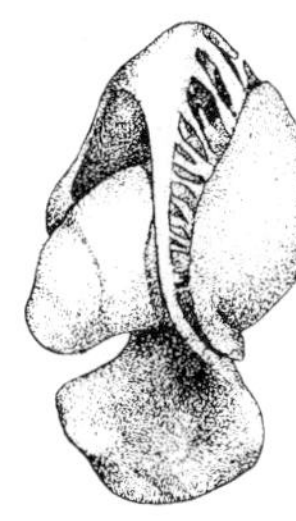

7.42. Label each view of the basal nuclei as an anterior view, posterior view, or lateral view.

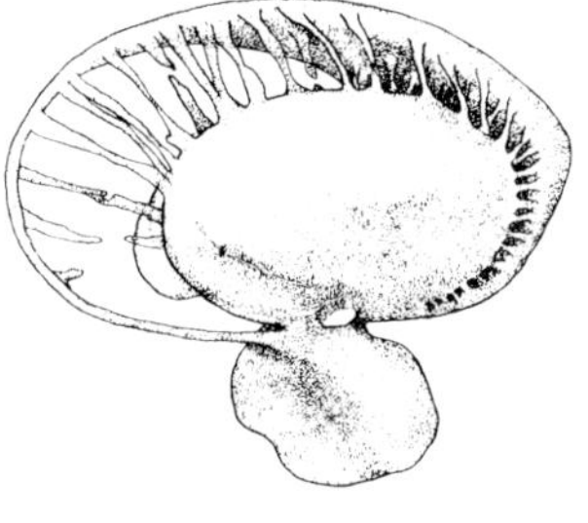

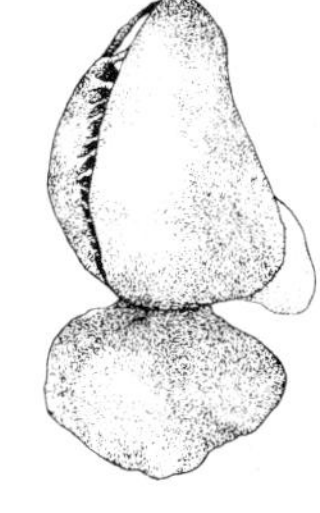

______________ view ______________ view ______________ view

7.43. From a posterior view, the lenticular nucleus has a smooth broad lateral surface and a tapered, more pointed ____________ surface.

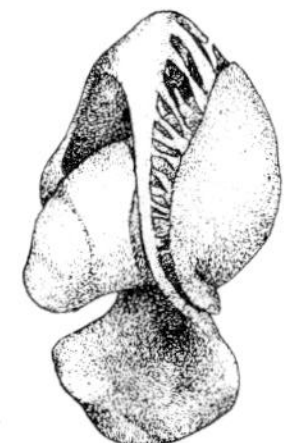

7.44. With an arrow, indicate the medial surface of the lenticular nucleus. This is a posterior view of the basal ____________ on the ______ side of the brain.

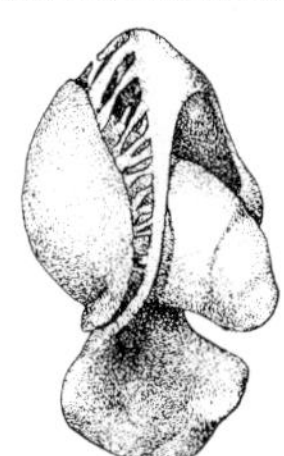

7.40A. <u>head</u>

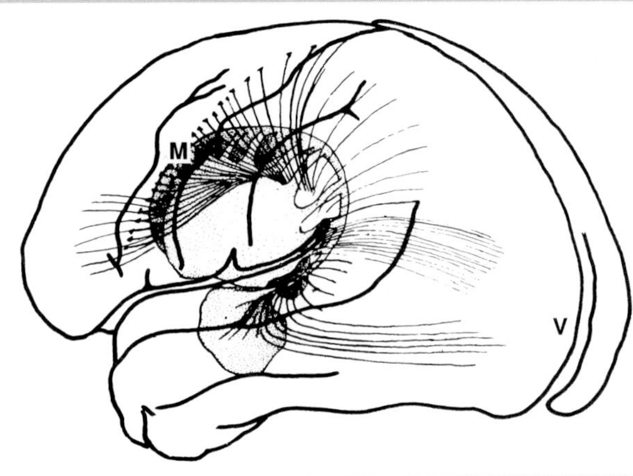

7.41A. <u>posterior</u>; <u>gray</u>

7.42A.

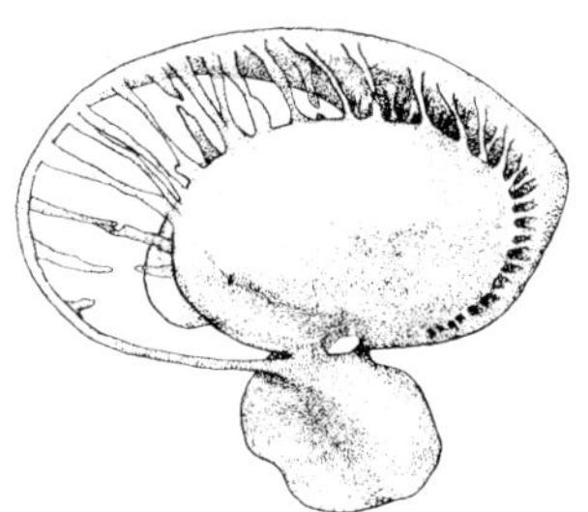
Lateral view

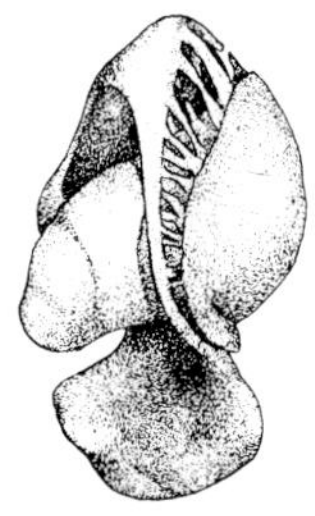
Posterior view

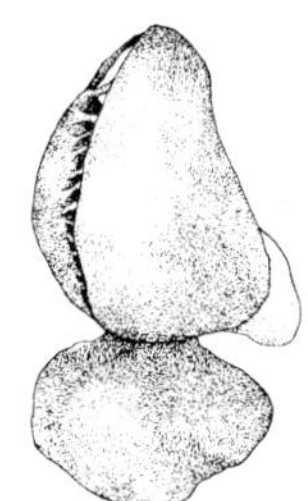
Anterior view

7.43A. <u>medial</u>

7.44A. <u>nuclei</u>; <u>left</u>

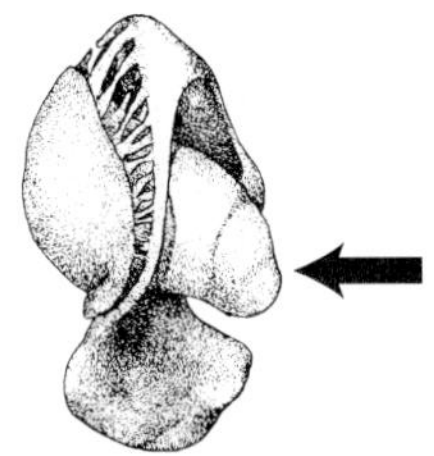

7.45. Corticospinal fibers course inferiorly along the medial surface of the ____________ nucleus.

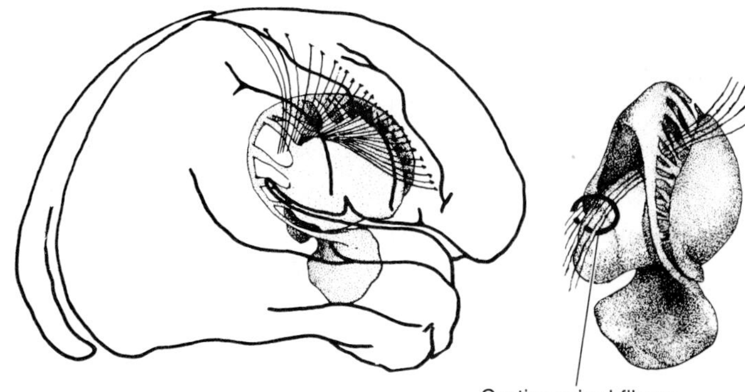

7.46. Look at the diagram. There are two parts of the ____________ nucleus. The more *pallid* medial part is the ________ ________, and the lateral part is the ________.

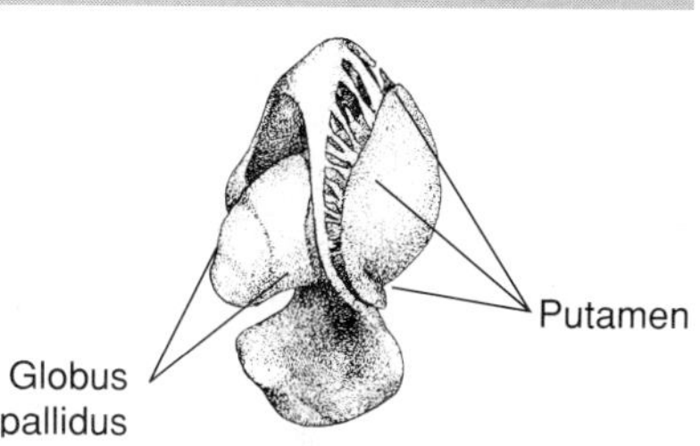

7.47. Together, the pu ________ and globus ________ make up the lenticular nucleus.

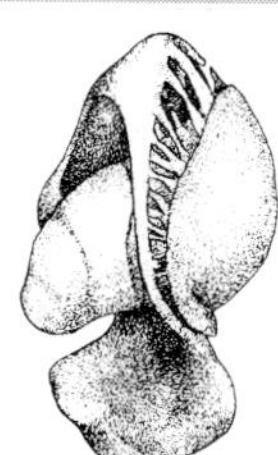

7.48. The ________ forms the lateral part of the lenticular nucleus. The ________ pallidus forms the ____ al part of the lenticular nucleus.

7.49. Label the two parts of the lenticular nucleus.

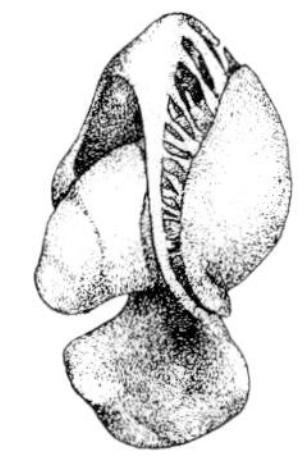

7.45A. lenticular

7.46A. lenticular; globus pallidus; putamen

7.47A. putamen; pallidus

7.48A. putamen; globus; medial

7.49A.

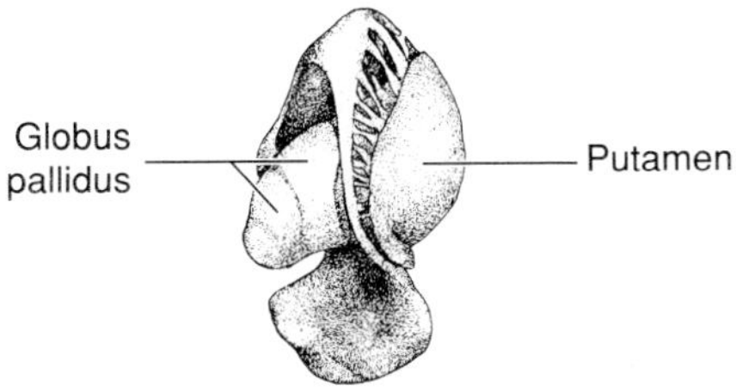

Globus pallidus

Putamen

7.50. On each view, mark the globus pallidus with an "X." The globus pallidus points slightly inferiorly but predominantly in a ____________ and ____________ direction. On each view, place a "P" on the most *posterior* part of the basal nuclei.

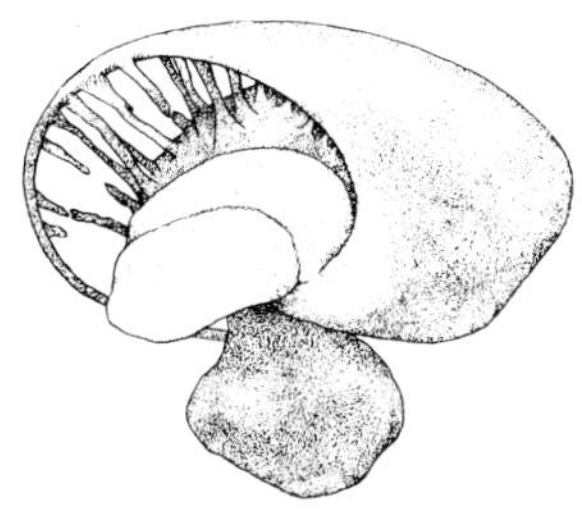

Medial view

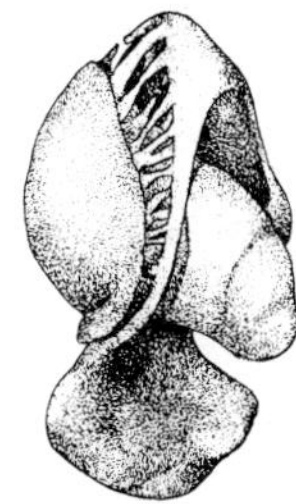

Posterior view

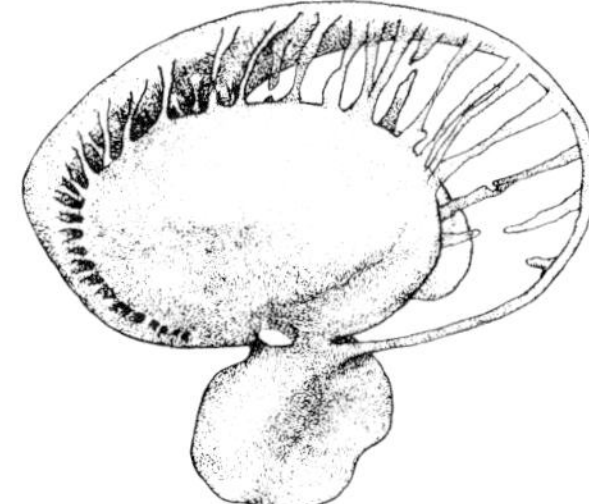

Lateral view

7.51. Place an "X" on the globus pallidus. This is a ______ al view of structures abstracted from the cerebral hemisphere on the ______ side of the brain.

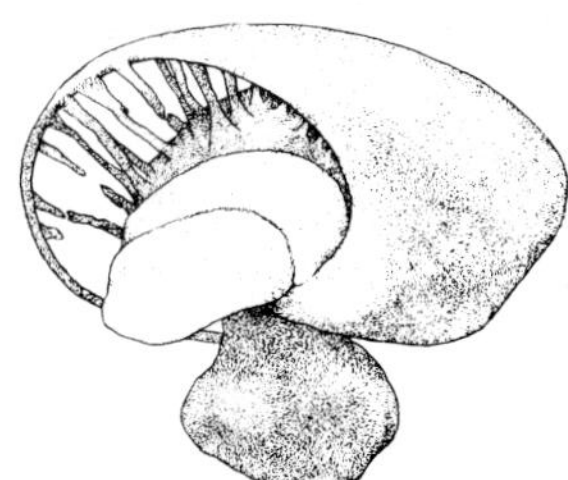

7.52. Use the basal nuclei to orient yourself with respect to this new image. Label the globus pallidus as "GP" and head of caudate as "C." This is a ______ al view of the ______ half of the brain.

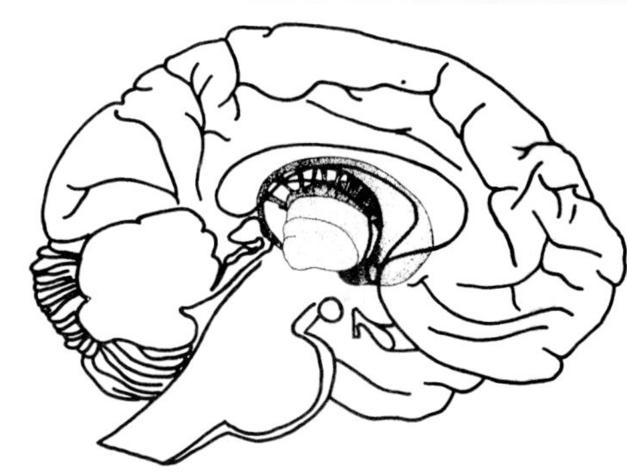

7.53. On each diagram, draw an arrow at the junction where the putamen and caudate become fused into one continuous mass and place an "A" on the amygdala. Starting with the lateral view in the left image, the basal nuclei are gradually rotated and viewed from more anterior aspects. Label the extreme right view. From which side of the brain have these structures been abstracted? ______

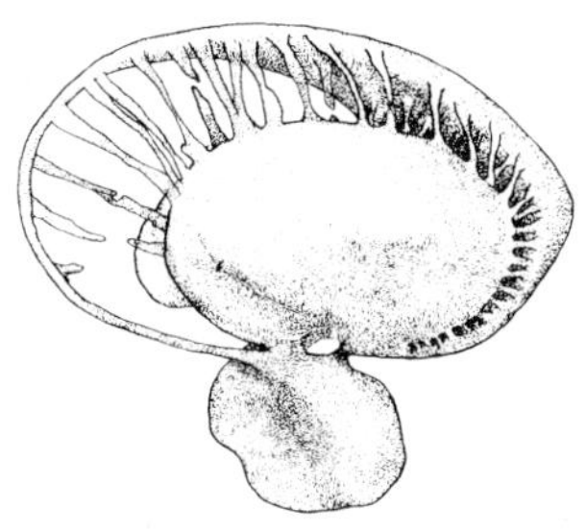

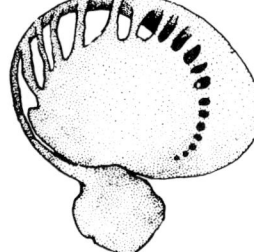

Lateral view

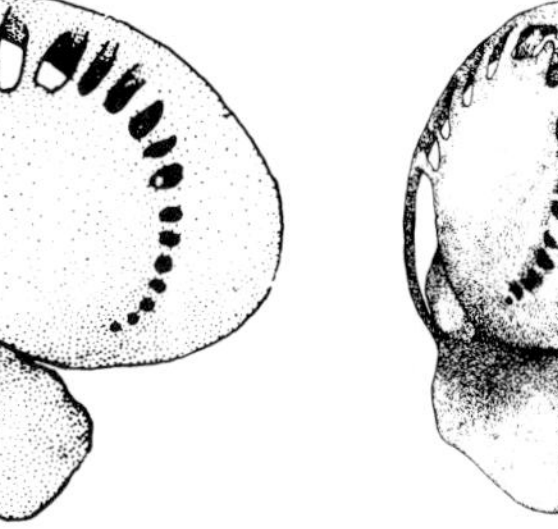

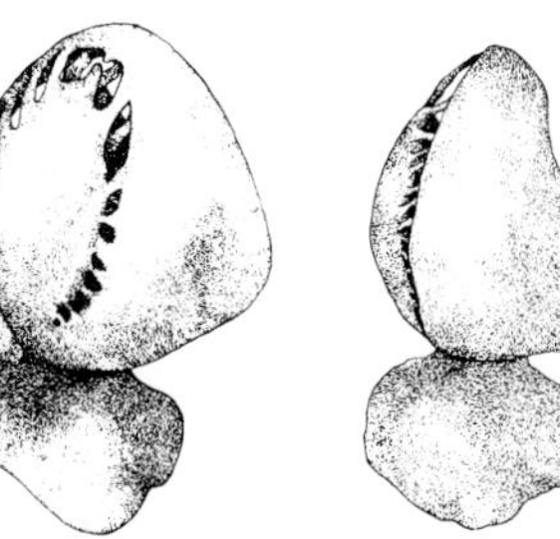

____________ view

7.50A. medial; posterior

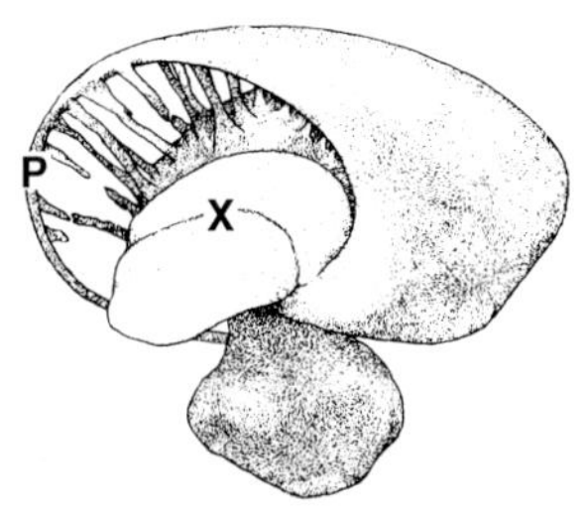

Medial view

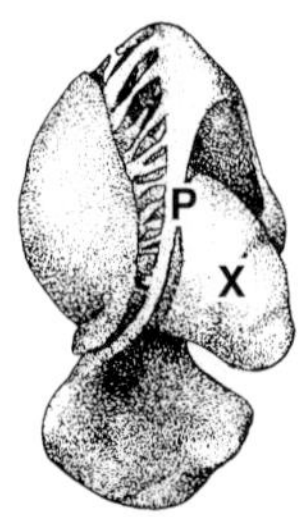

Posterior view

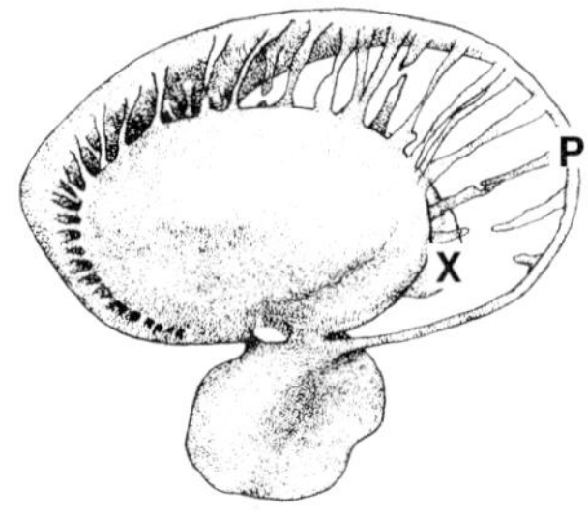

Lateral view

7.51A. medial; left

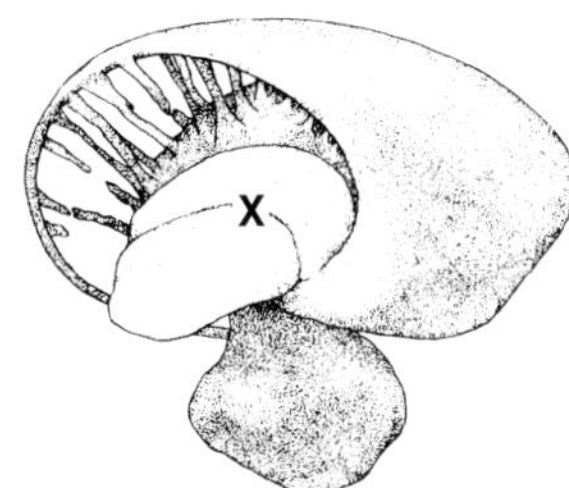

7.52A. medial; left

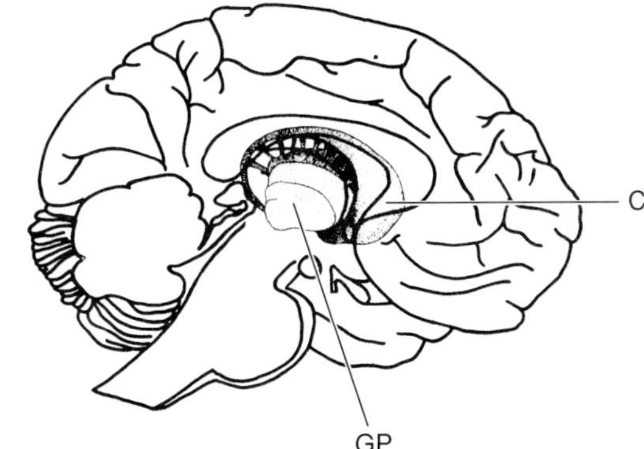

7.53A. Right

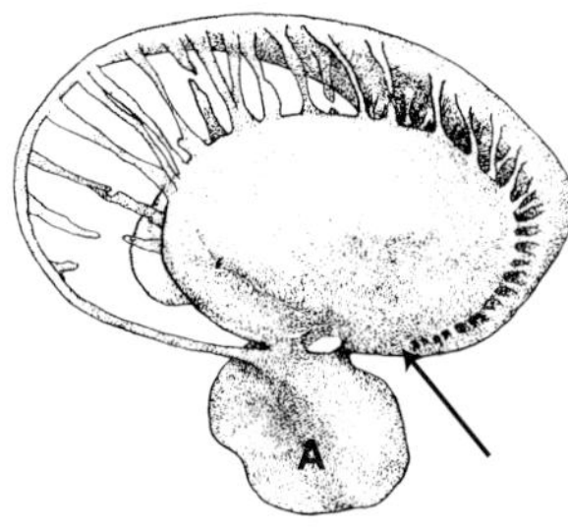

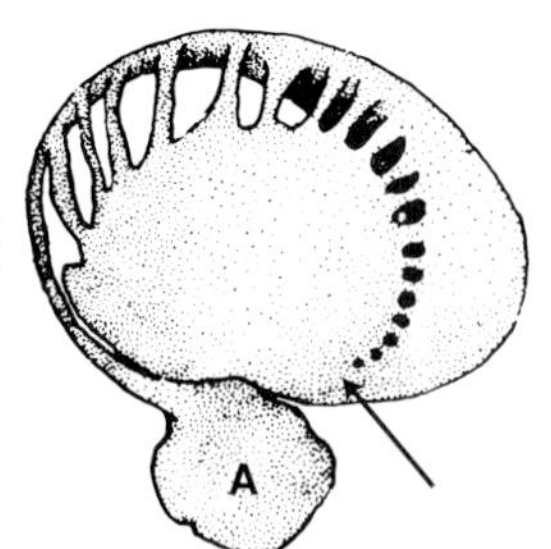

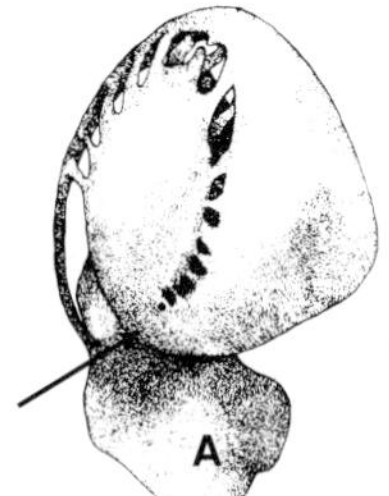

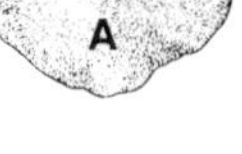

Lateral view

Anterior view

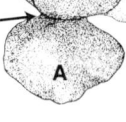

7.54. Identify the side of the brain as left (L) or right (R) on each diagram. Recall that sides are indicated with reference to the specimen, not the observer.

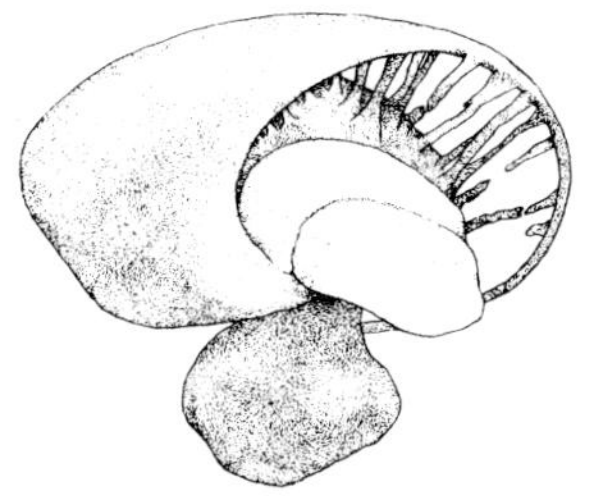
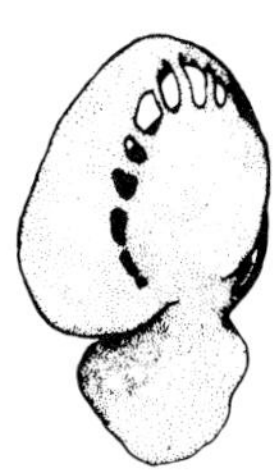
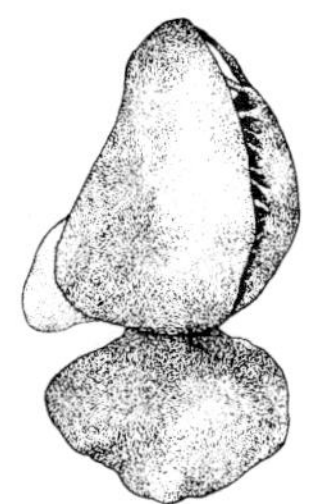
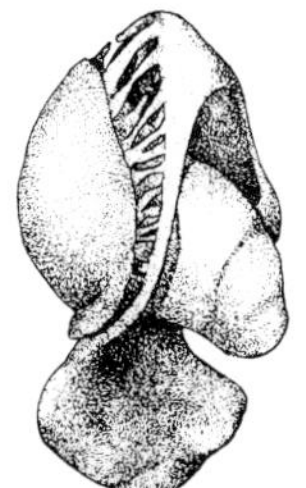
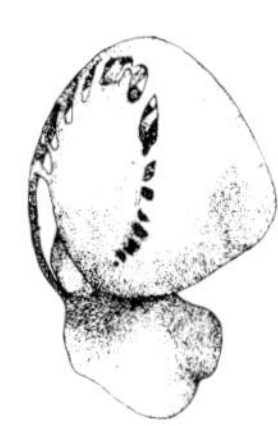

7.55. Label the surface structures indicated.

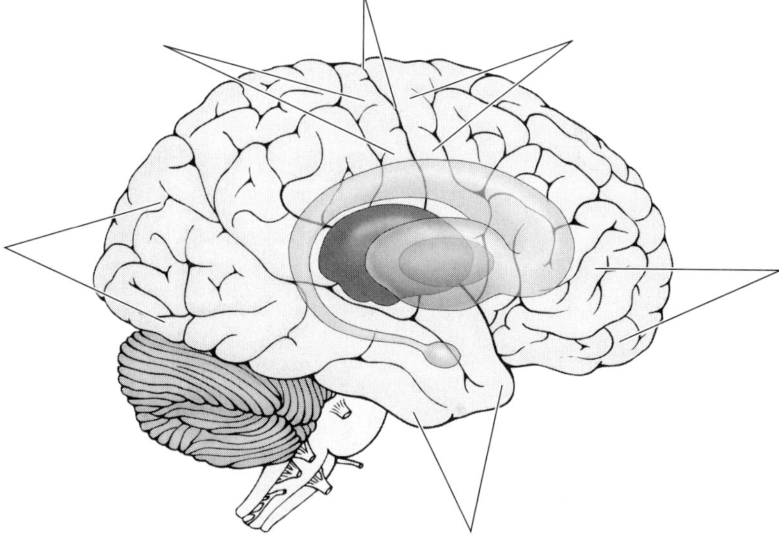

7.56. Cellular bridges connect the putamen with all parts of the ____________ nucleus.

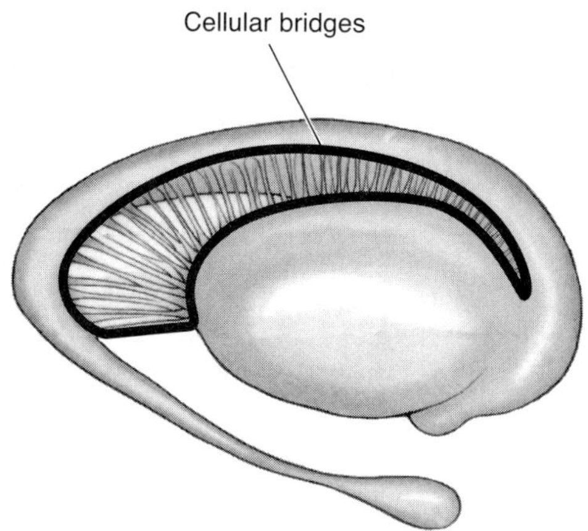

7.54A.

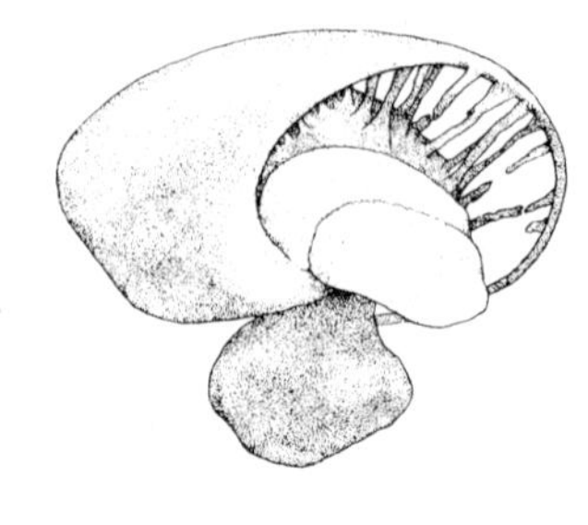

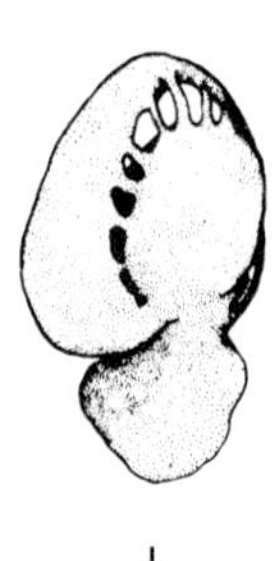

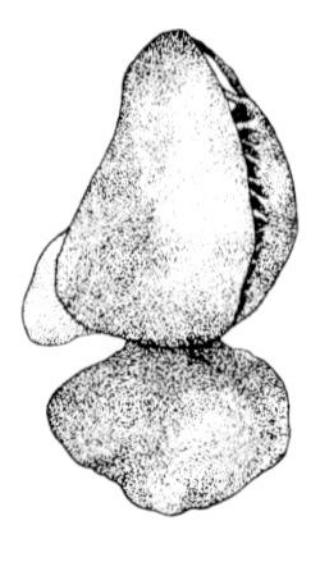

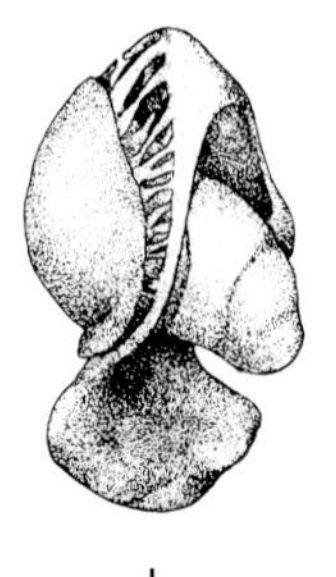

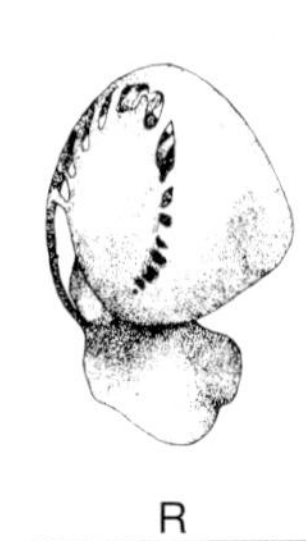

7.55A.

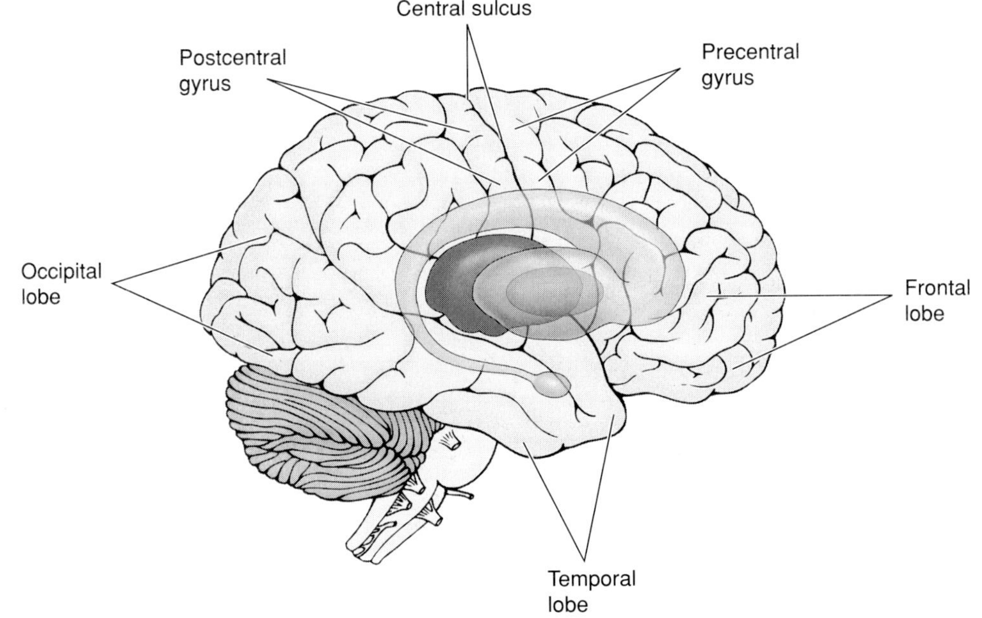

7.56A. <u>caudate</u>

7.57. Numerous fibers from the cortical surface pass between the cellular bridges that connect the caudate and putamen. Among them is a tract of fibers arising in the ________________ gyrus of the frontal lobe. Encircle and name this tract.

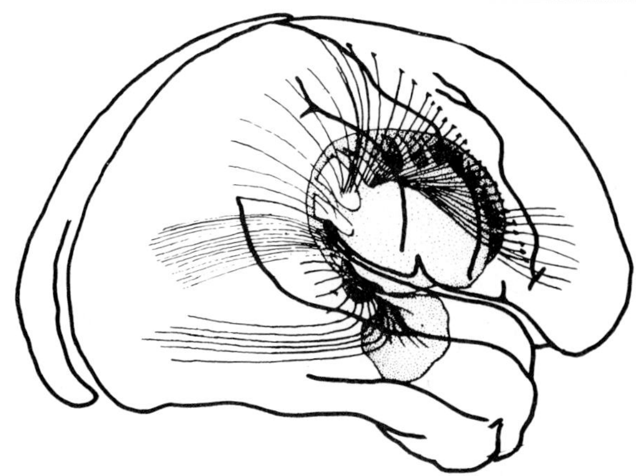

7.58. The corticospinal tract originates primarily in the ________________ gyrus, passes predominantly in a ____________ direction, and joins other myelinated fibers that separate ____________ from ____________.

7.59. In lower mammals, the caudate and putamen form one solid structure. In humans, they are incompletely separated by fibers. On both pictures, place a series of "B"s on the cellular bridges that still join the caudate and putamen in the human brain.

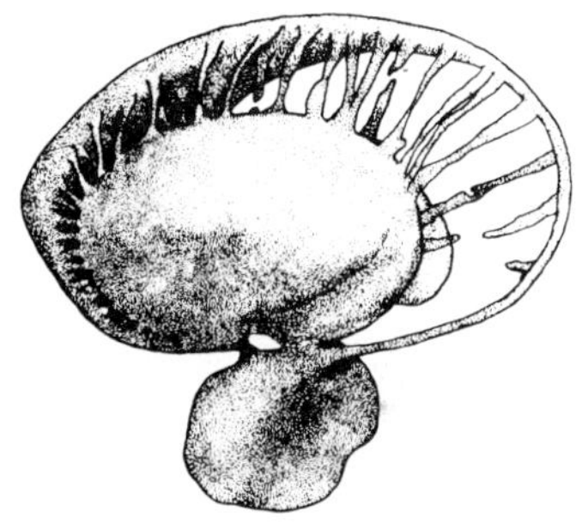

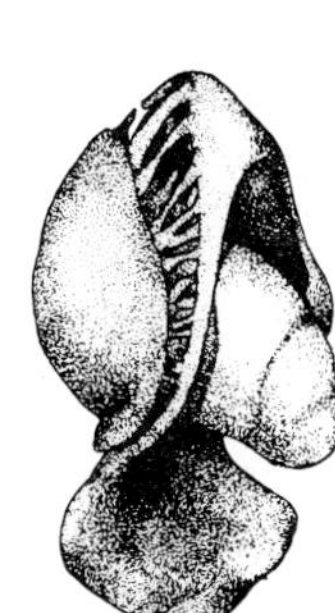

7.60. Draw a line between the appropriate items in the two columns (each item may be used more than once).

Gray matter	Cellular bridges
White matter	Globus pallidus
Most medial basal nucleus	Corticospinal tract

7.61. The putamen and globus pallidus are structurally dissimilar; however, they make up a single circumscribed mass of nerve cell bodies called the ________________ nucleus.

7.57A. precentral

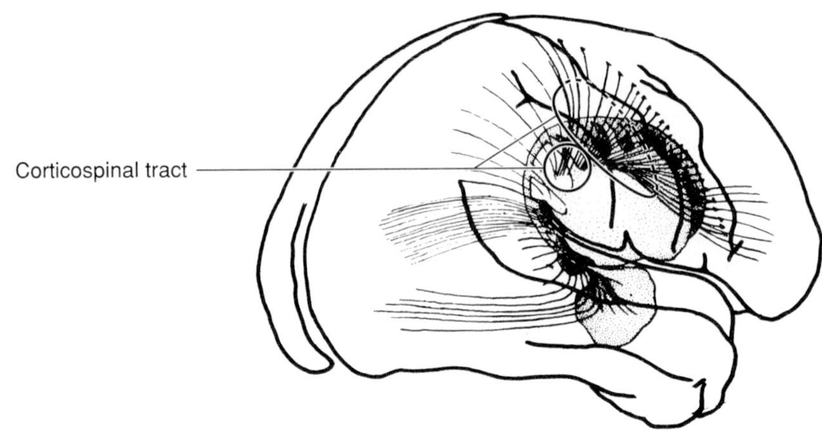

7.58A. precentral; medial (posteromedial); putamen; caudate

7.59A.

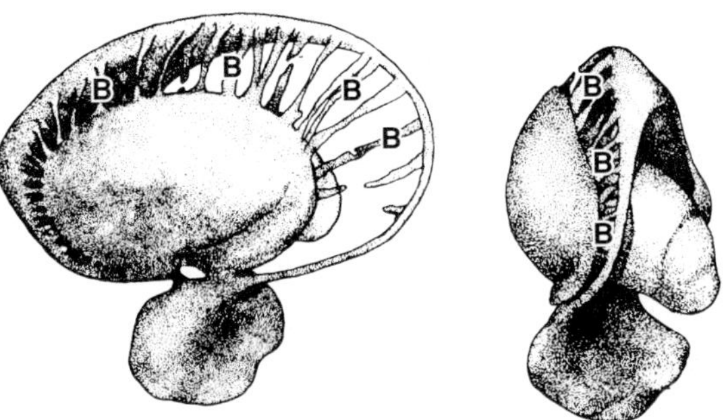

7.60A.

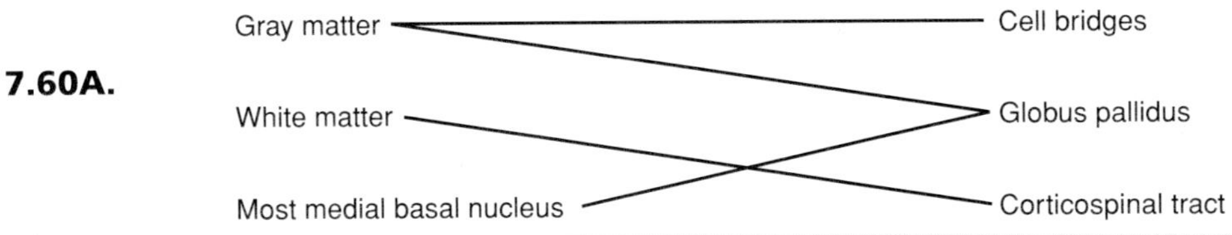

7.61A. lenticular

8 The Corticospinal System: Medial View–Internal Capsule

8.1. On the image, an "X" and "Y" have been drawn on a predominant white matter structure, the ____________ ____________. Which of the two letters is more posterior, "X" or "Y"? ______

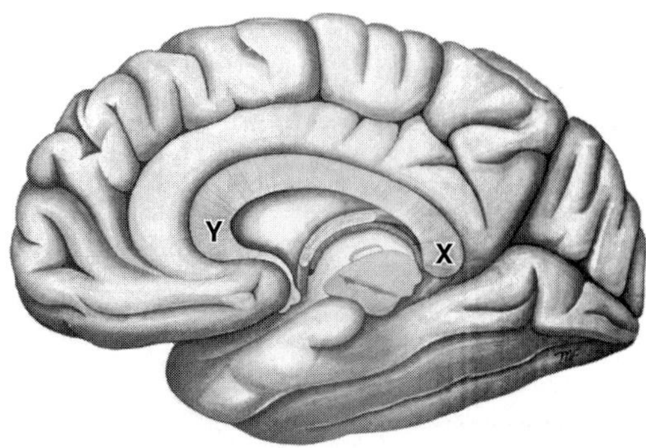

8.2. Note the orientation of the picture. Label the occipital pole (OP), corpus callosum (CC), marginal branch of cingulate sulcus (C), and the central sulcus (CS).

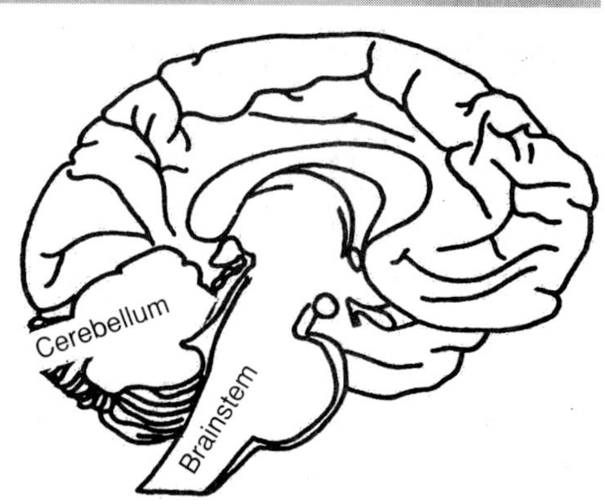

8.3. The three major regions of the brainstem are labeled on the image. From superior to inferior, they are the ____________, ______, and ____________. The thalamus of the diencephalon is located superior to the midbrain.

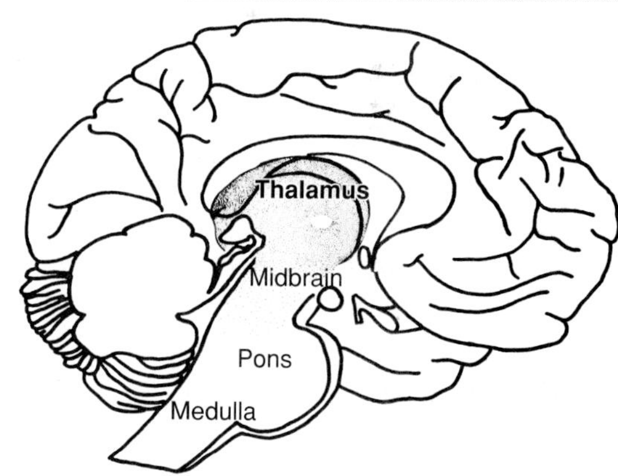

8.1A. corpus callosum; X

8.2A.

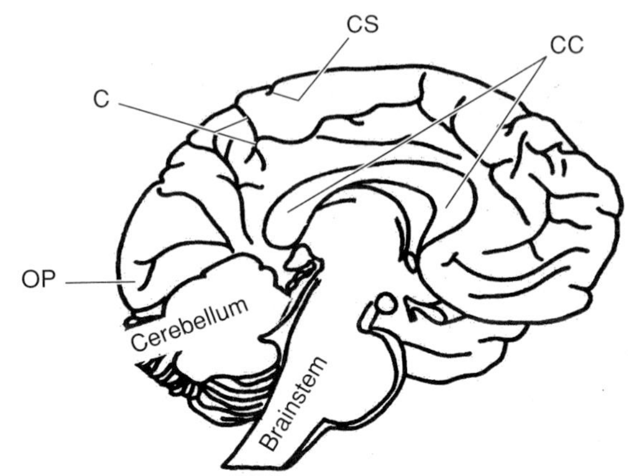

8.3A. midbrain; pons; medulla

8.4. Label the thalamus of the diencephalon with its name on the diagram.

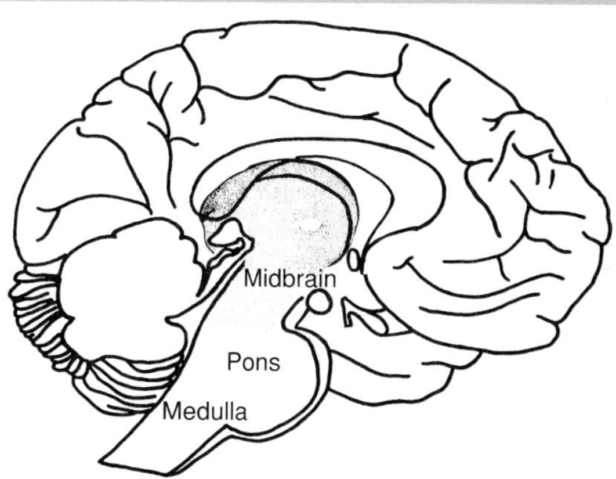

8.5. Imagine that the corpus callosum is transparent in this picture. Lateral to the posterior part of the corpus callosum is the shaded superior and ____________ ior part of the ____________.

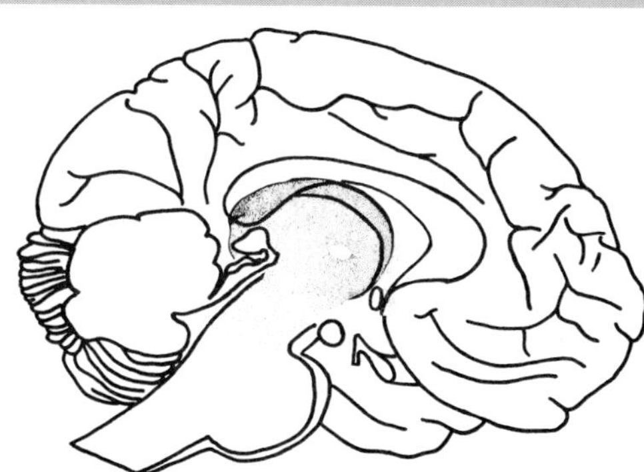

8.6. Look through the "transparent" thalamus. From your vantage point at the midline surface of the brain, you are looking in a ____________ direction. Facing you are the ______ al surfaces of the basal nuclei.

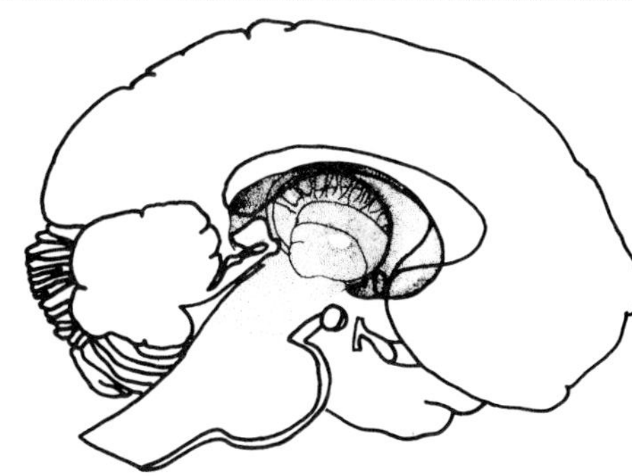

8.7. Place a "C" on the head of the caudate, a "GP" on the globus pallidus, and a "B" on the cell bridges between the ____________ and ____________.

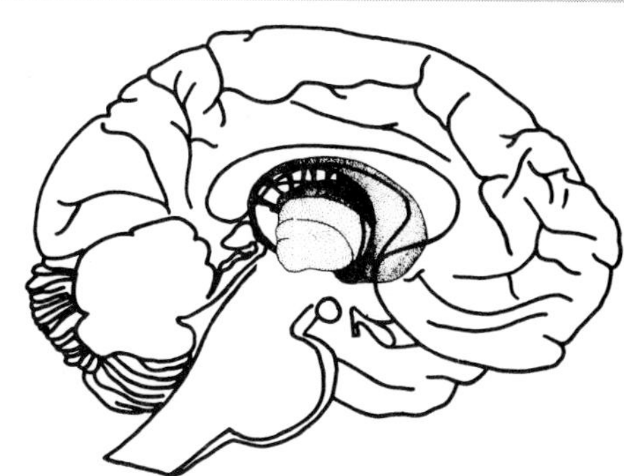

8.4A.

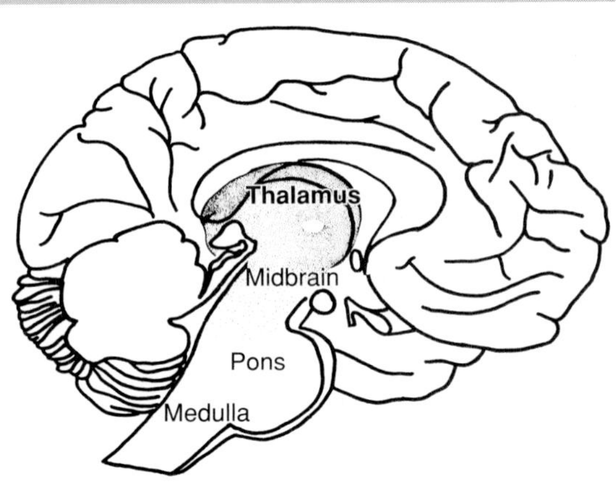

8.5A. posterior; thalamus

8.6A. lateral; medial

8.7A. caudate; putamen

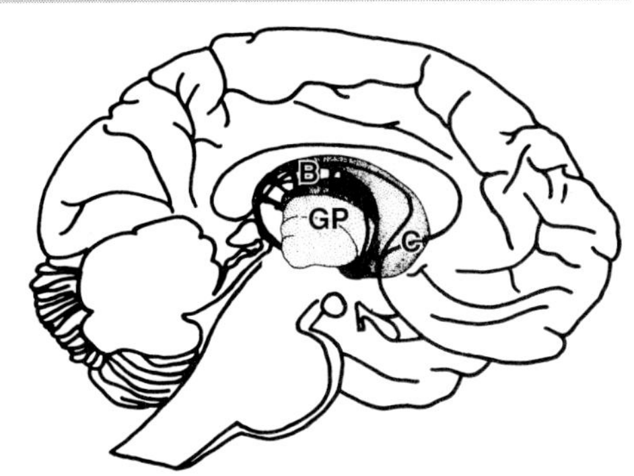

8.8. The fibers illustrated arise near the lateral surface of the brain, in the ________________ gyrus. Their course brings them ______ al to the body of the caudate, then between the cell bridges, and then ______ al to the globus pallidus.

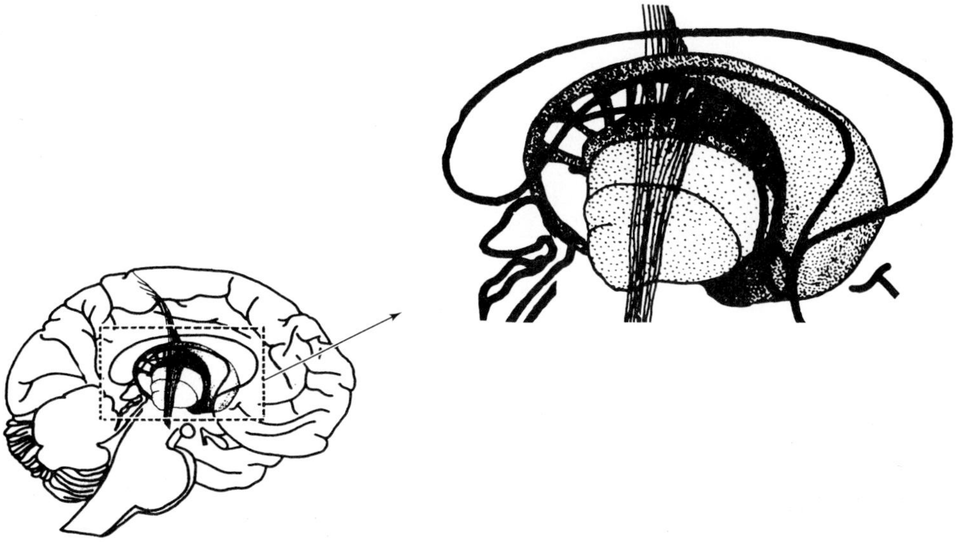

8.9. One could not see the fibers at "X" in this picture if the __________ had been drawn as a solid structure.

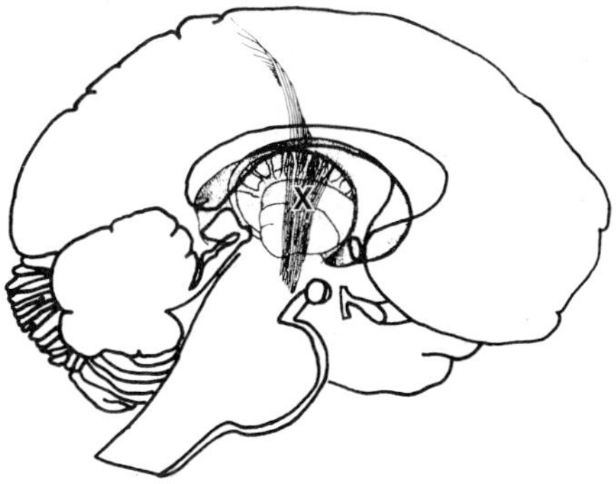

8.10. At the site marked by the "X," the fibers of the ______________ tract lie just medial (or internal) to the __________ __________ and just lateral to the __________.

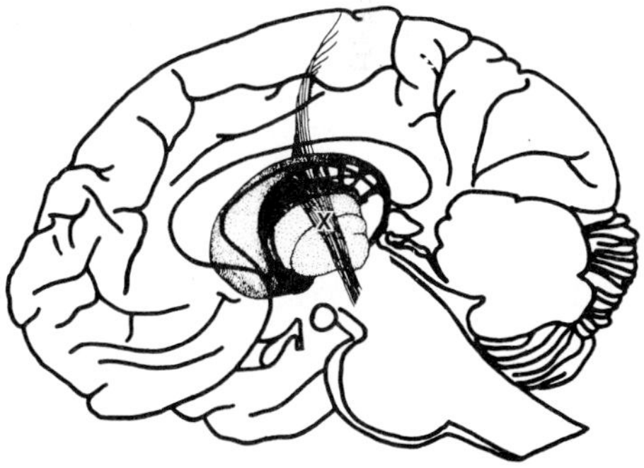

8.11. A number of tracts, among them the encircled ________________ tract, pass between the caudate and putamen and collectively form a wall (capsule) around the internal surfaces of the ________________ nucleus.

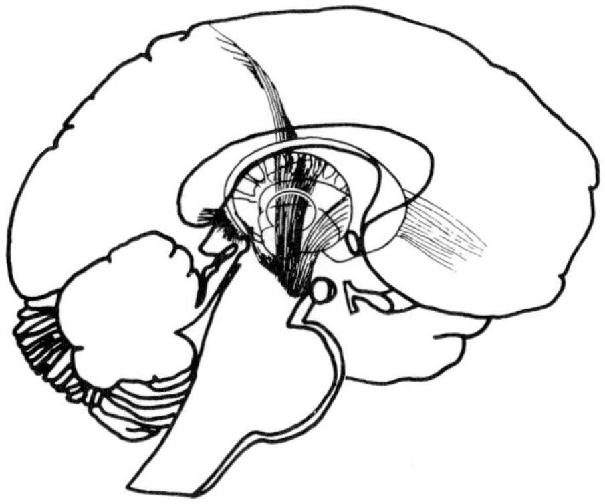

8.8A. precentral; lateral; medial

8.9A. thalamus

8.10A. corticospinal; globus pallidus (lenticular nucleus); thalamus

8.11A. corticospinal; lenticular

8.12. The fiber tracts that en*capsulate* the *int*ernal surfaces of the lenticular nucleus form the ______ ternal ______ sule.

8.13. The internal capsule would be largely hidden from view in this picture if the __________ was not transparent.

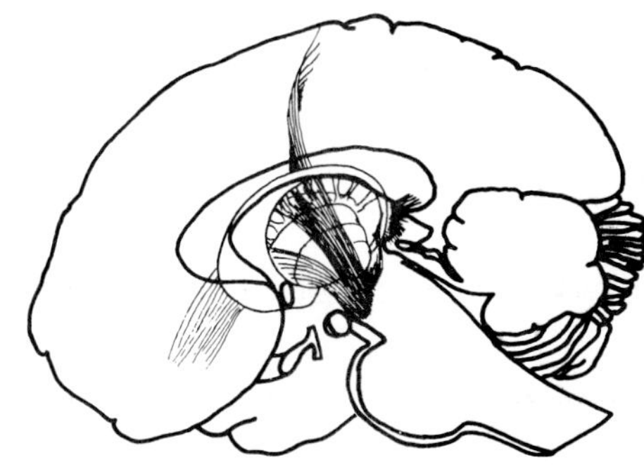

8.14. The internal capsule lies ______ al to the globus pallidus and just ______ al to the __________ .

8.15. Fibers from the cortical surface pass between the cell bridges to become part of the internal capsule. Fibers from the precentral gyrus pass between the cell bridges together with other fibers from the frontal lobe at which site, A or B? ______ Fibers from the most anterior regions of the frontal lobe pass between cell bridges at which site, A or B? ______

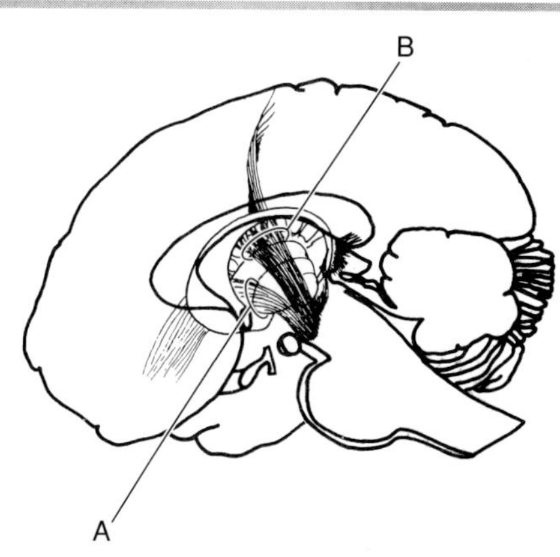

8.16. Fibers entering and exiting the more anterior regions of the frontal lobe enter more ______ ior parts of the internal capsule. On both views, place a series of "X"s to indicate the position of these fibers before they pass between the cell bridges; on the medial view, indicate their position in the internal capsule with an arrow.

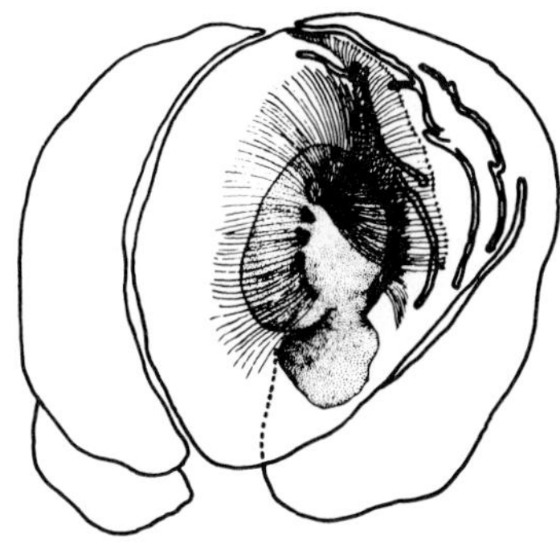

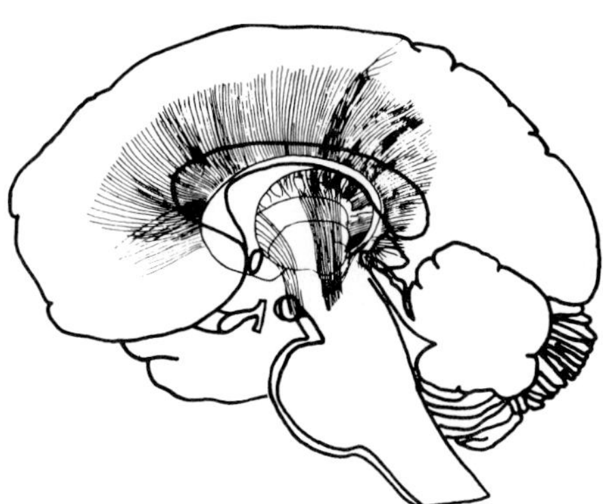

8.12A. internal capsule

8.13A. thalamus

8.14A. medial (internal); lateral; thalamus

8.15A. B; A

8.16A. anterior

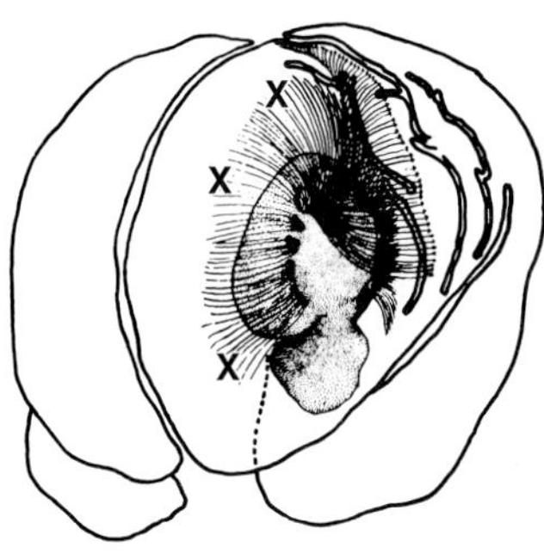

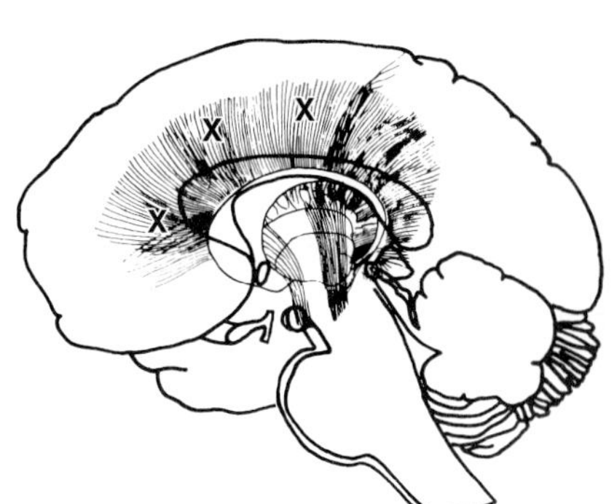

8.17. Draw a few fibers from "A," "B," and "C" on the ____________ lobe to the points where they enter the internal capsule.

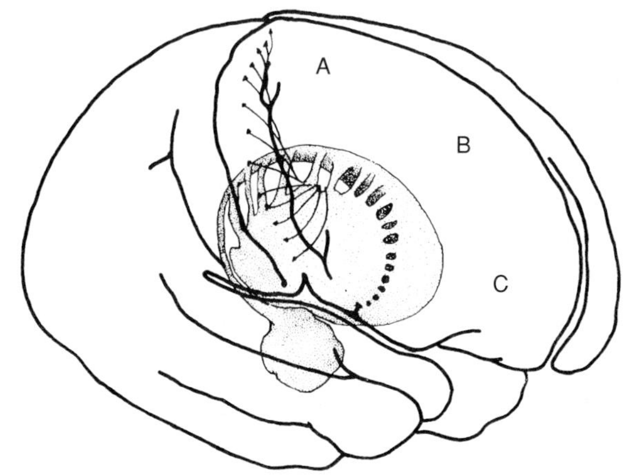

8.18. Many of the fibers illustrated are efferent with respect to the cortex. Many others are afferent. The tract marked "M" is ______ ferent.

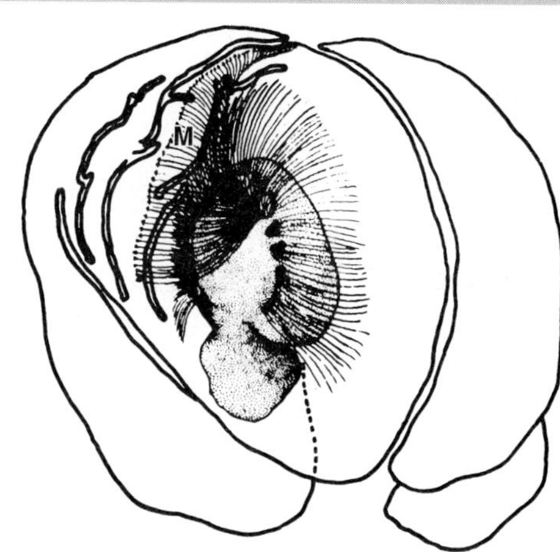

8.19. Fibers of the internal capsule coat parts of the ______ al surfaces of both components of the lenticular nucleus: the ____________ and the ____________ ____________.

8.20. In addition to the corticospinal tract, efferent tracts labeled on the diagram as "A" and "C" arise in the ____________ and ____________ lobes of the cortex.

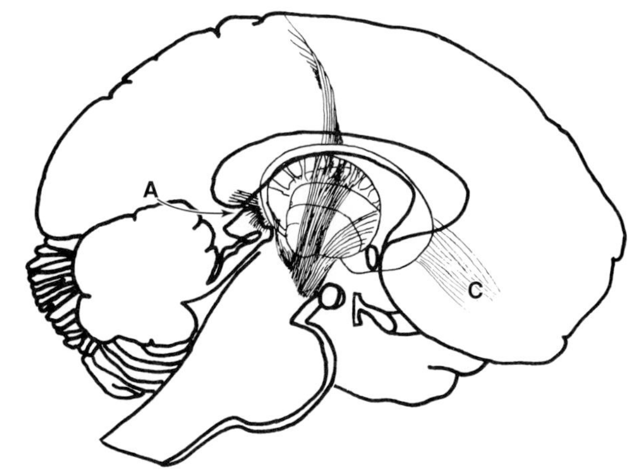

8.17A. frontal

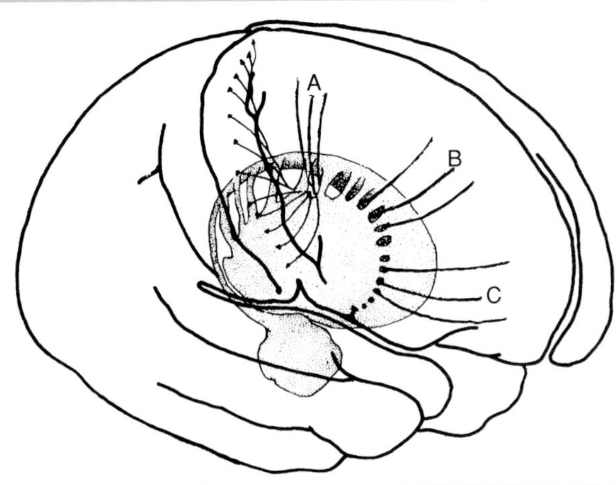

8.18A. efferent

8.19A. medial; putamen; globus pallidus

8.20A. occipital; frontal

8.21. Efferent fibers from the parietal and temporal lobes follow a course posterior and inferior to the lenticular nucleus to enter the ______ erior part of the internal capsule.

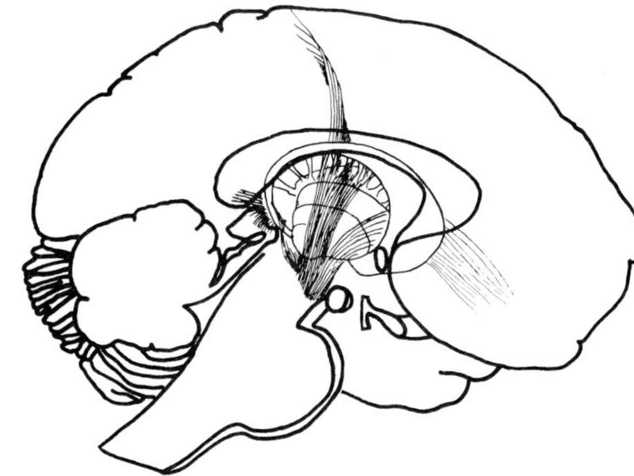

8.22. The tracts at "A," "B," and "C" are ______ ferent with respect to the cortex.

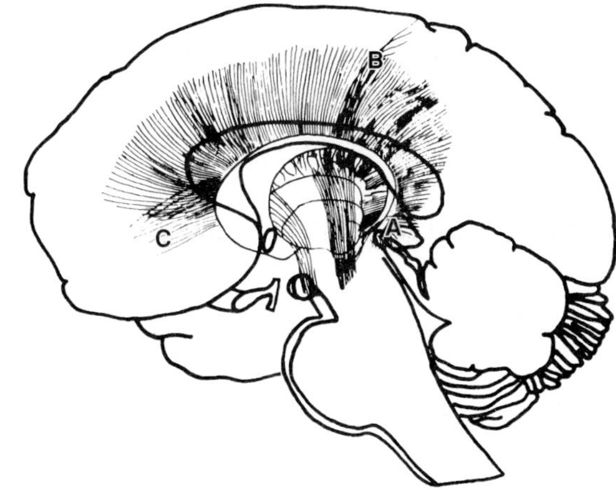

8.23. Some fibers passing into the internal capsule pass from cortex and terminate in the basal nuclei. Additional large numbers of fibers arise from cell bodies in the thalamus and pass upward to the __________, __________, __________, and __________ lobes of the cortex.

8.24. Like the lenticular nucleus, the outermost part of the precentral gyrus is ______ matter. The internal capsule is ______ matter because it contains axons with __________ sheaths.

8.25. Fibers of the internal capsule that terminate in the surface gray matter of the cortex originate in the __________. Fibers that arise in the cortical gyri, enter the internal capsule, and terminate in basal nuclei or lower centers are ______ ferent with respect to cortex.

8.21A. posterior

8.22A. efferent

8.23A. frontal; parietal; temporal; occipital

8.24A. gray; white; myelin

8.25A. thalamus; efferent

9 The Corticospinal System: Introduction to Horizontal Sections

9.1. The diagram shows a brain with a small portion sliced off of the top. The horizontal section exposes _____ matter that lies deep to the surface gray matter.

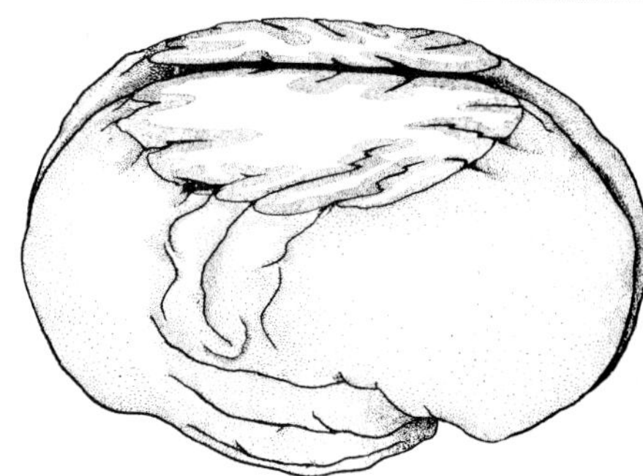

9.2. Point to the frontal pole with an arrow. On the *lateral* surface of the brain, indicate and label the gyrus in which most of the cell bodies of the corticospinal tract lie.

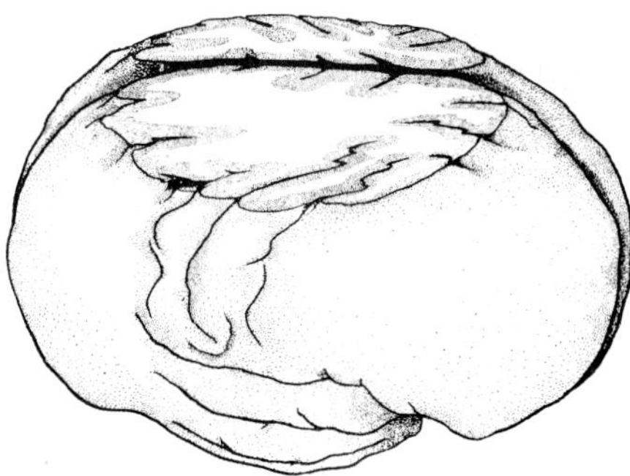

9.3. The white matter extends into the gyri formed by the convolutions of the cerebral cortex. Place an "X" on the white matter of the postcentral gyrus of the right hemisphere.

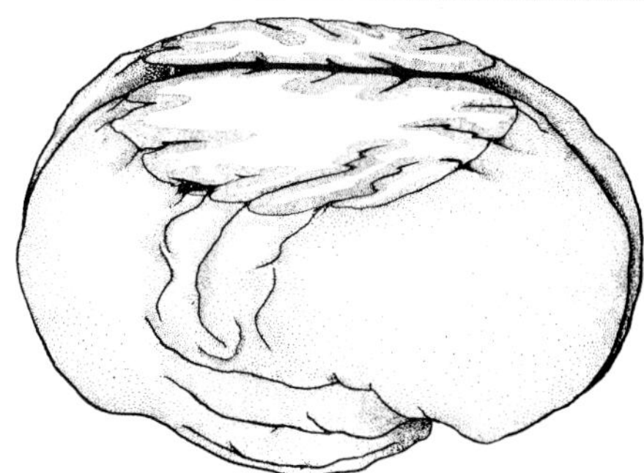

9.4. Label the indicated structures.

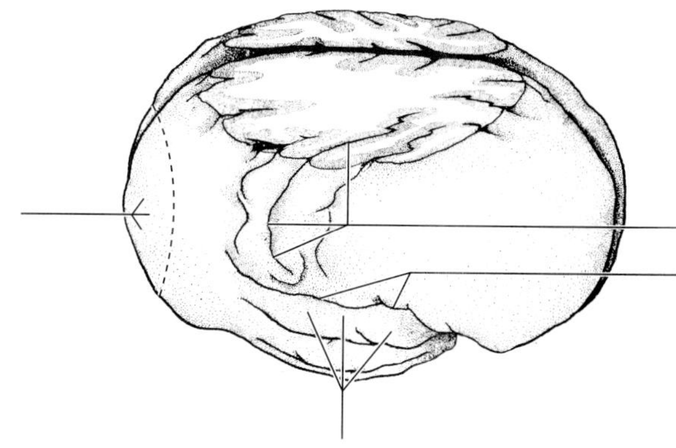

9.1A. <u>white</u>

9.2A.

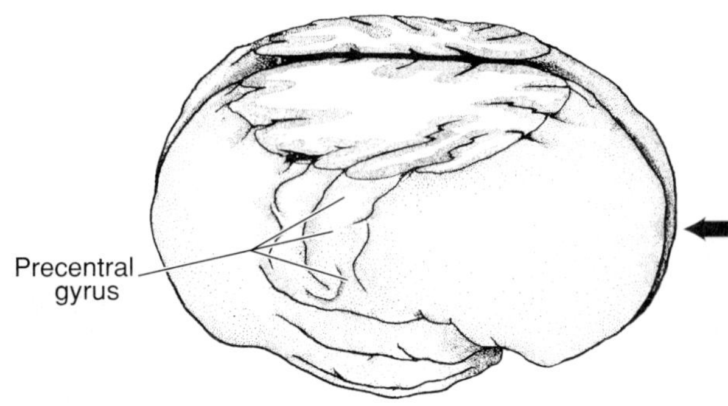

9.3A.

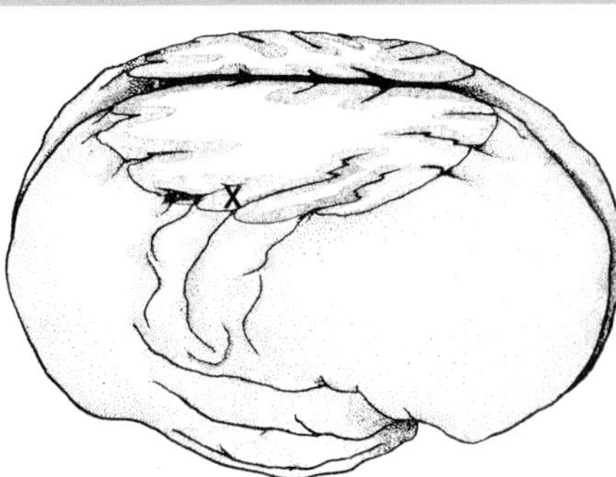

9.4A.

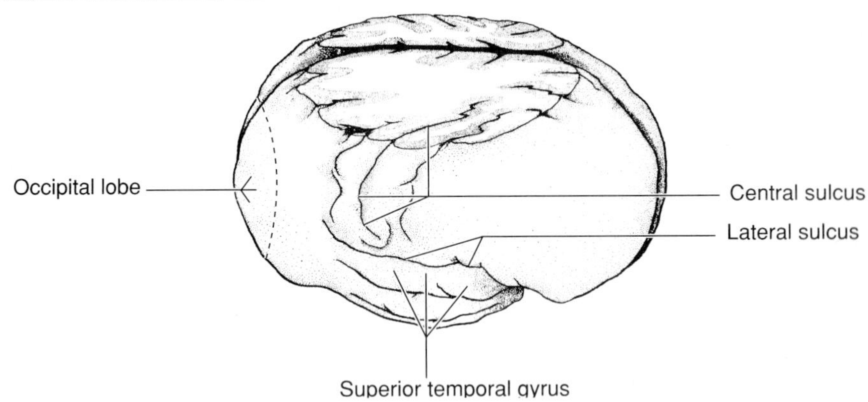

9.5. Label the indicated structures.

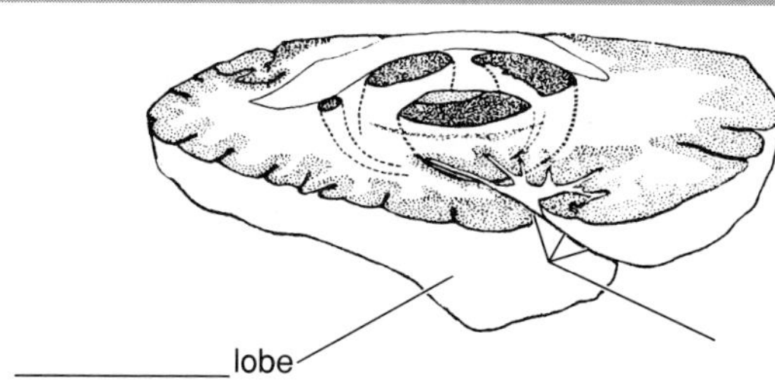

9.6. This diagram shows more tissue cut from one hemisphere than the other. The deeper (inferior) cut is on the ______ side of the brain.

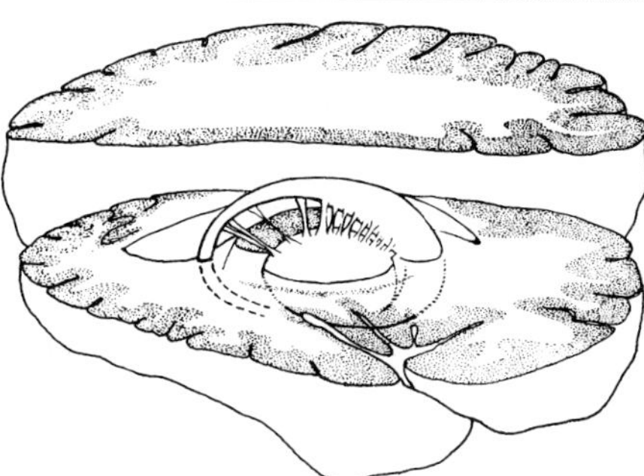

9.7. Draw an arrow to the part of the lateral fissure exposed by the horizontal section.

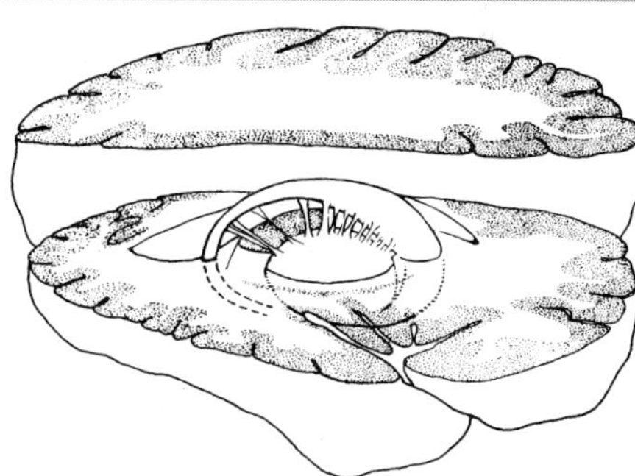

9.8. The horizontal section exposes some structures deep to the surface of the cortex. Two of these are drawn projecting above the cut surface: the elongated one is the __________ nucleus, and the other is the __________.

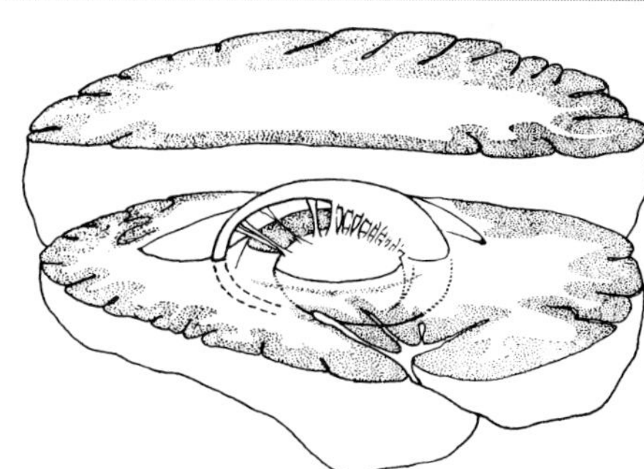

9.5A.

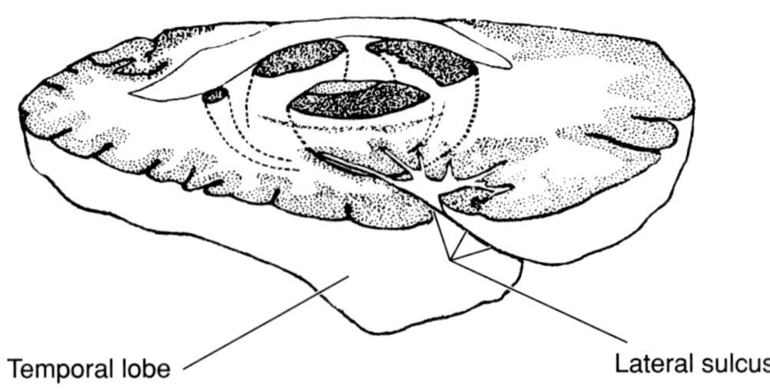

9.6A. right

9.7A.

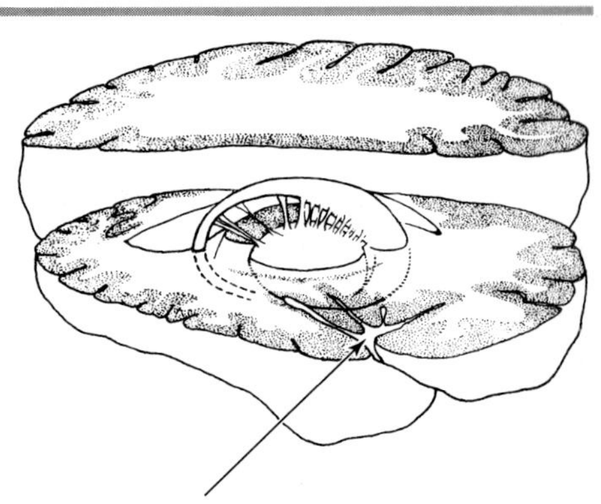

9.8A. caudate (body of caudate); putamen (lenticular nucleus)

9.9. Place an "S" on the caudate head below the cut surface. The part of the caudate that is entirely above the cut surface is its ______.

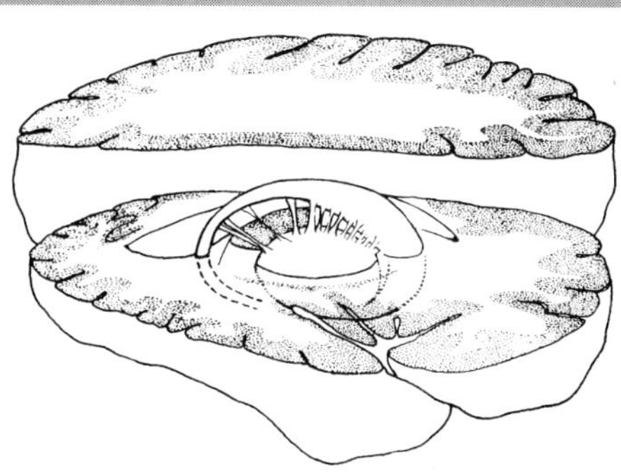

9.10. In the right diagram, the caudate nucleus is sectioned in two places. One sees a cut through the small ______ of the caudate and a larger cut across the caudate near the arbitrary junction of its ______ and ______.

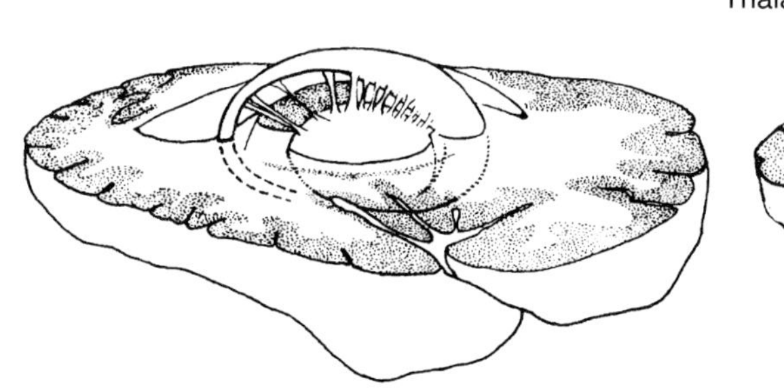

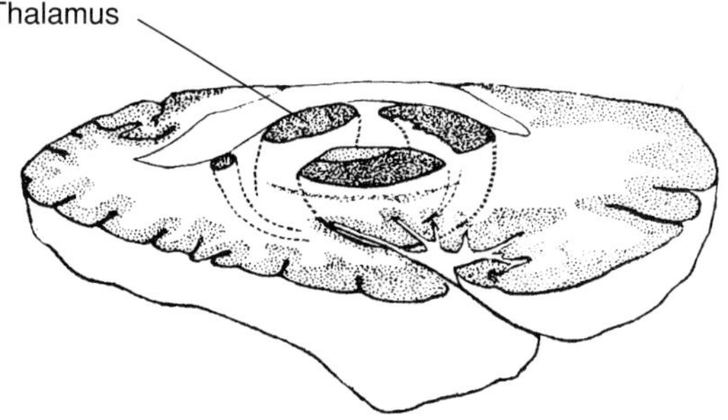

9.11. Indicate and label the *cut surfaces* of the head and tail of the caudate nucleus.

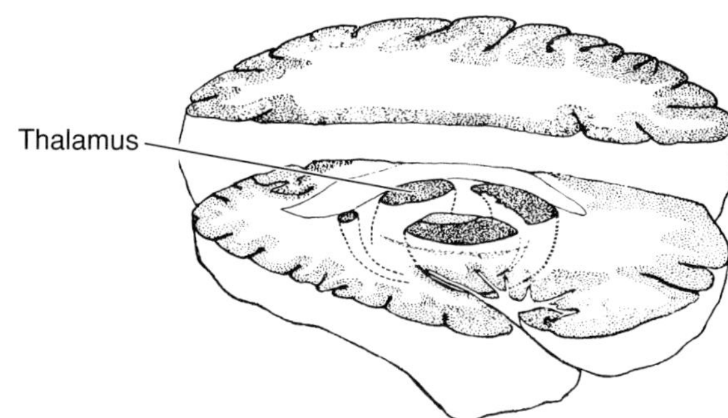

9.12. Label the thalamus. Dotted lines outline some of the structures beneath the cut surface. Indicate with an arrow the site where the caudate and putamen become directly fused together.

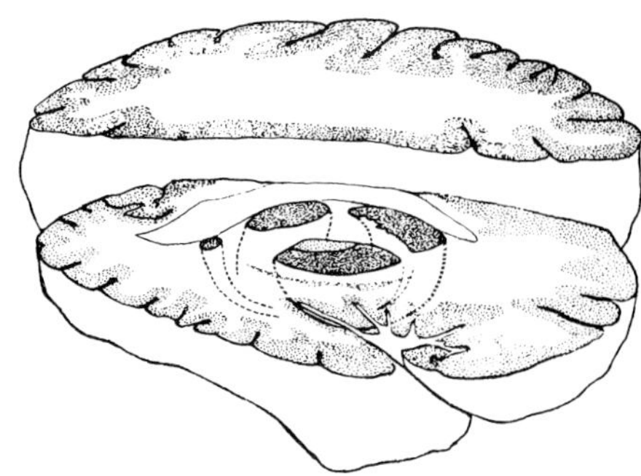

9.9A. <u>body</u>

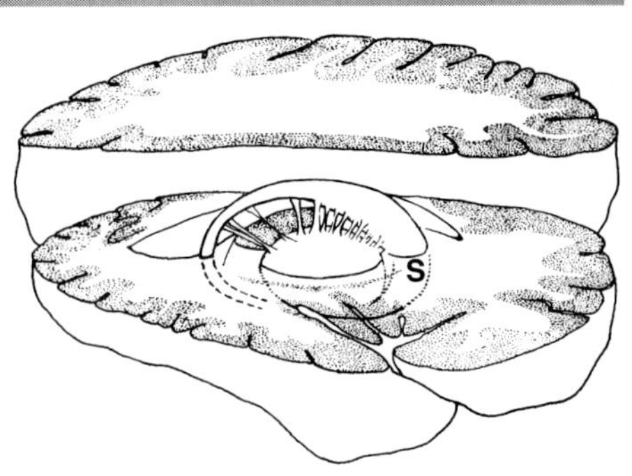

9.10A. <u>tail</u>; <u>body</u>; <u>head</u>

9.11A.

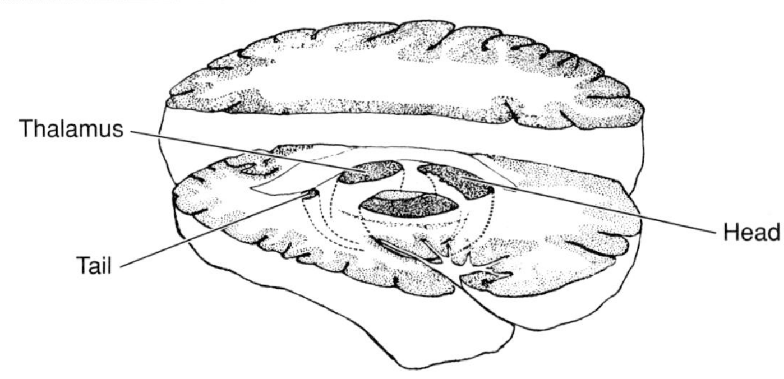

9.12A.

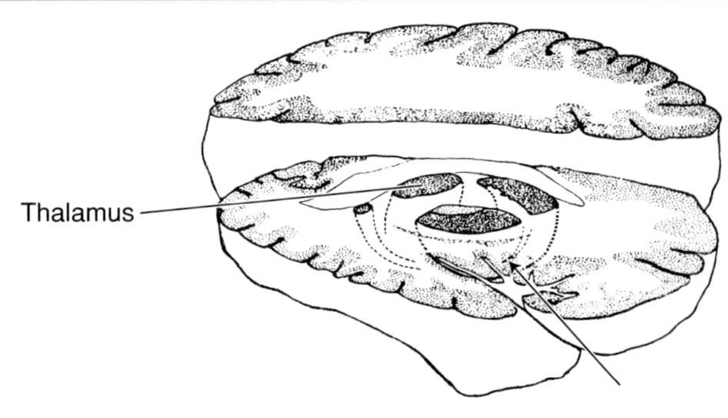

9.13. Identify and label the two parts of the lenticular nucleus that are visible *at the cut surface*.

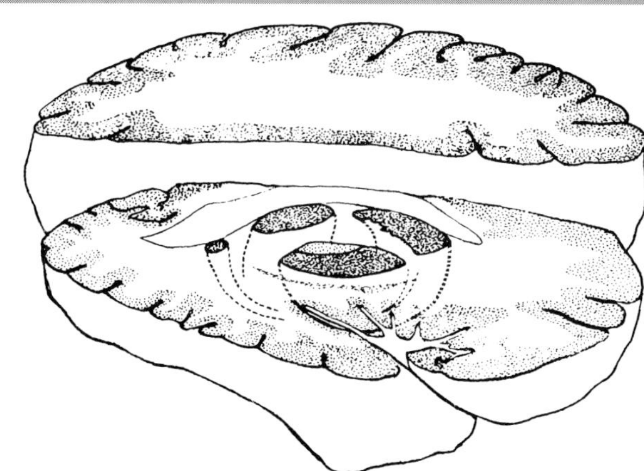

9.14. In the lower diagram, structures below the cut surface are no longer shown. Indicate and label on the cut surface of each diagram the horizontal sections of putamen (P), globus pallidus (GP), head (H) of caudate, and tail (T) of caudate.

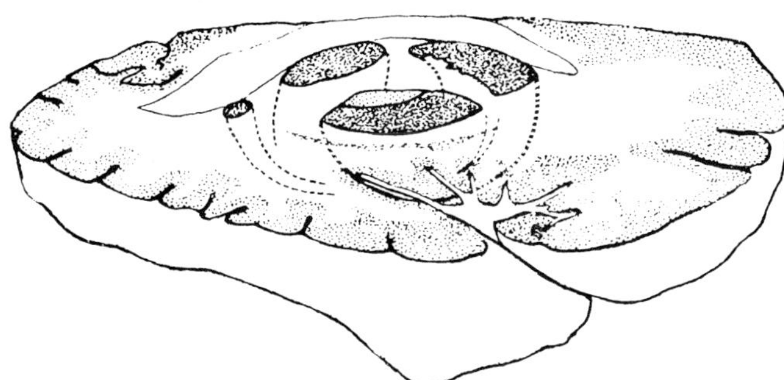

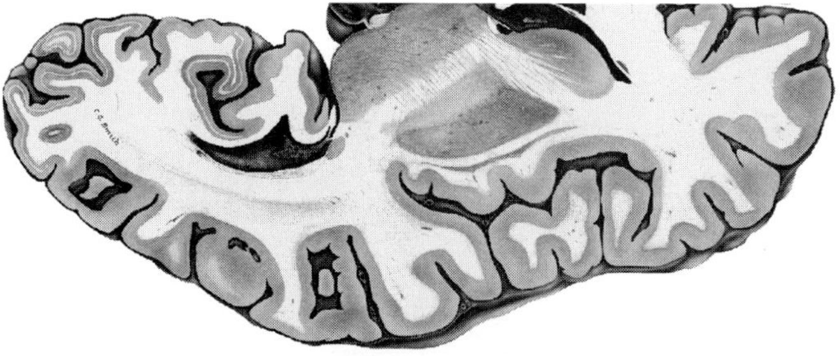

9.15. The globus pallidus points in a ______ al and somewhat __________ ior direction. It points toward another gray matter structure, the __________.

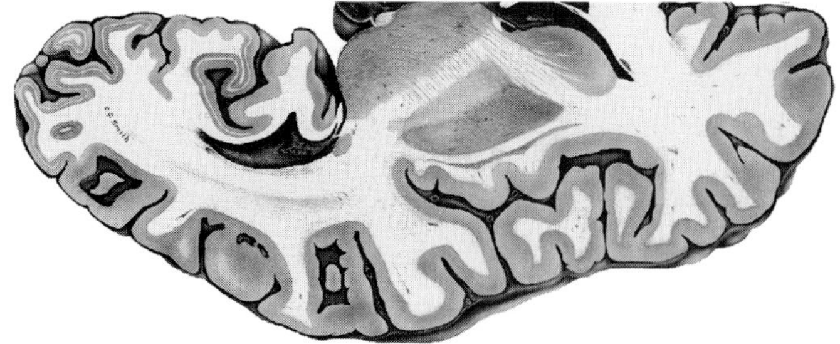

9.13A.

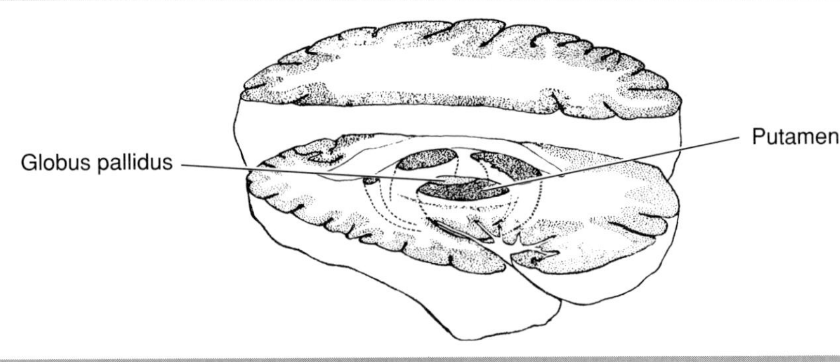

9.14A.

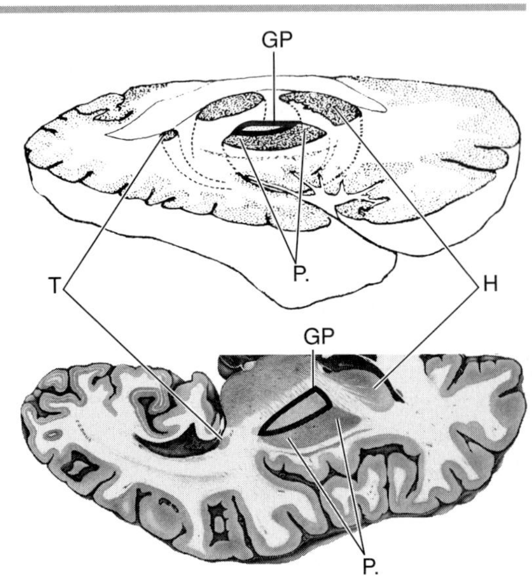

9.15A. medial; posterior; thalamus

9.16. The two diagrams are the same, rotated 90° apart. On each diagram, label the frontal lobe, the *horizontal* section of the lateral sulcus and the lenticular nucleus.

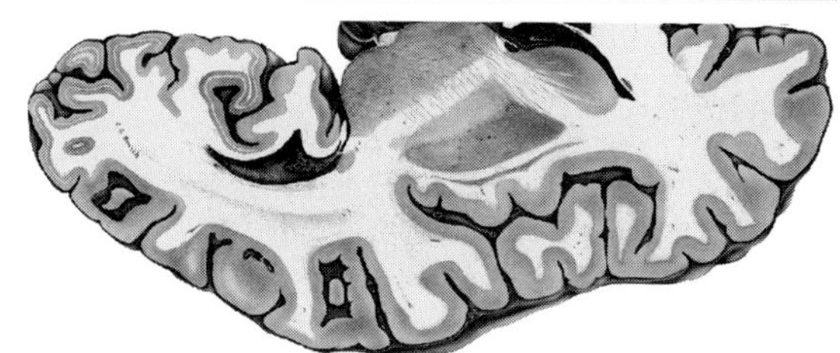

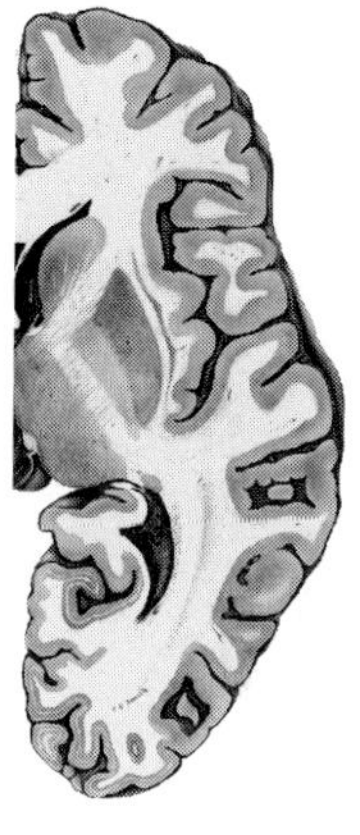

9.17. Draw a border around the cut section of the lenticular nucleus. Geometrically, it is shaped roughly like a ____________.

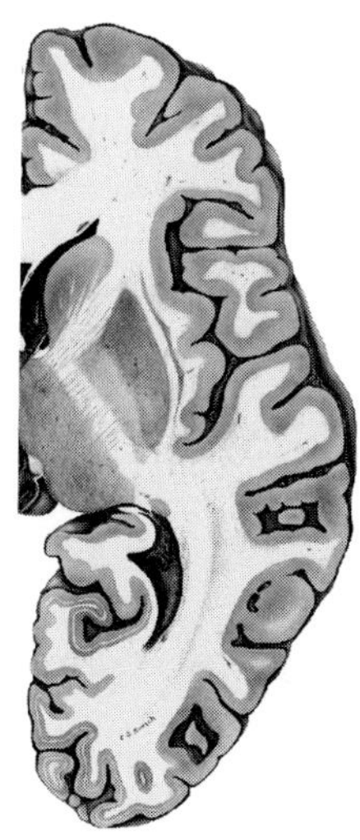

9.18. The globus pallidus points medially and in a ____________ direction. Draw the border around the globus pallidus.

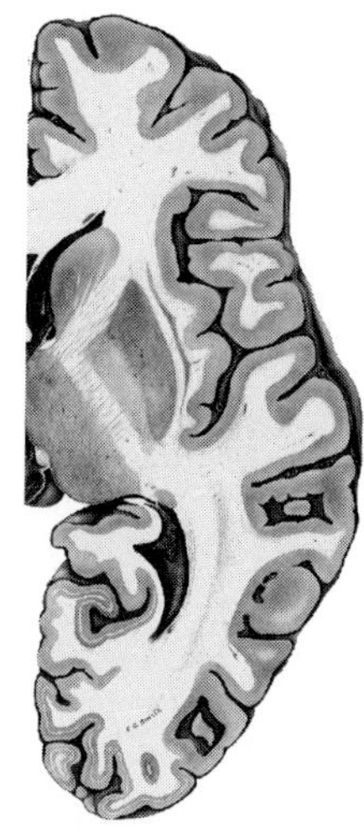

9.16A.

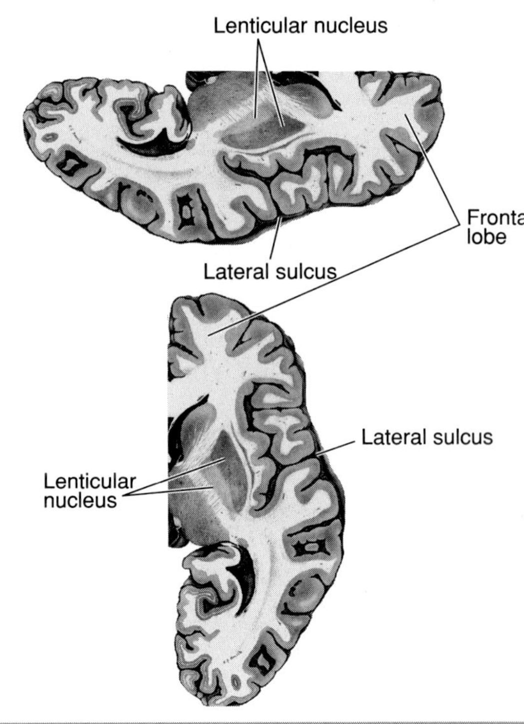

9.17A. triangle (lens)

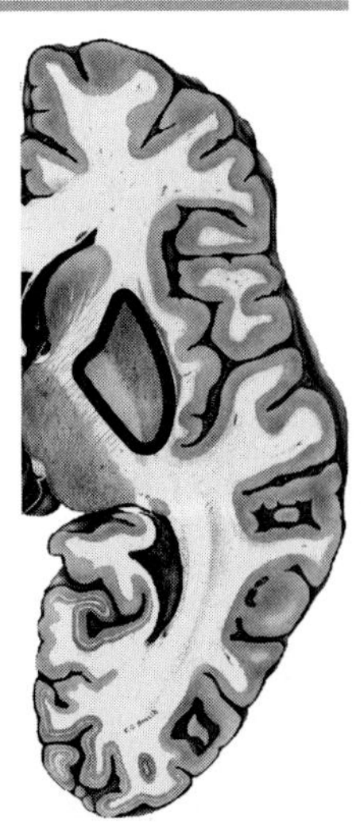

9.18A. posterior

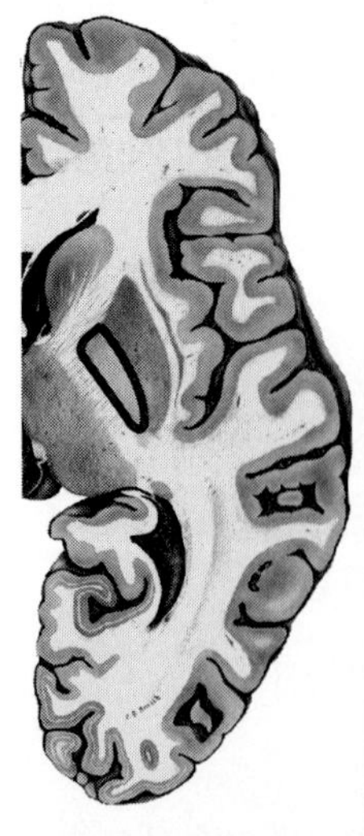

9.19. Label the structures indicated. Check the one that is more anterior.

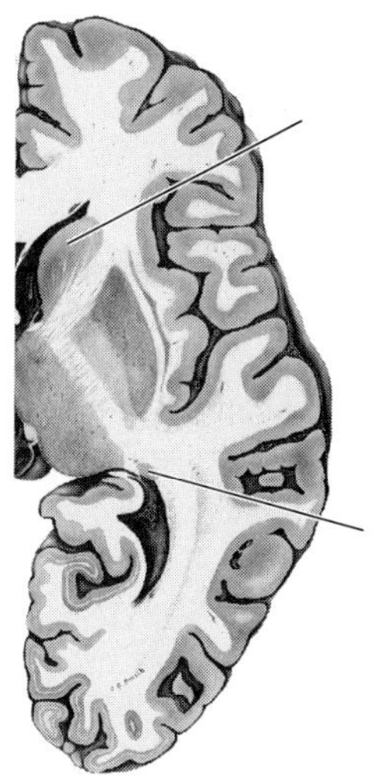

9.20. Draw a line connecting the most posterior point on the lenticular nucleus to the most posterior extension of the lateral sulcus on the cut surface. Place an "X" on the thalamus.

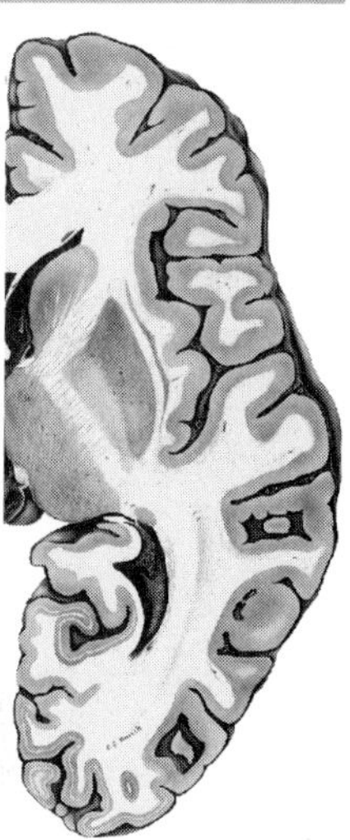

9.21. This is a horizontal section through both hemispheres at a slightly different level from the previous one. In the right hemisphere, label the frontal lobe, lateral sulcus, and lenticular nucleus.

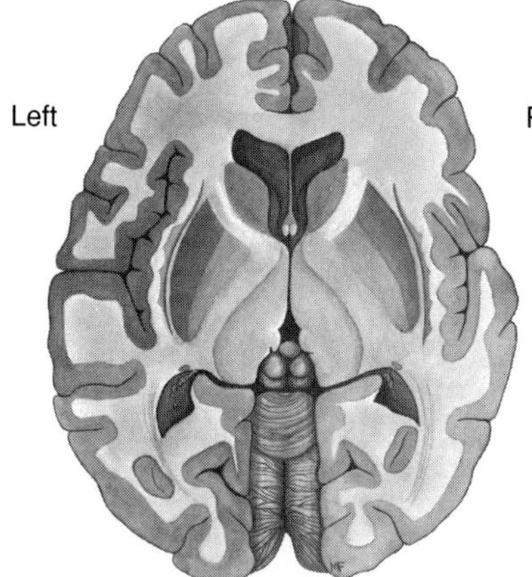

9.19A.

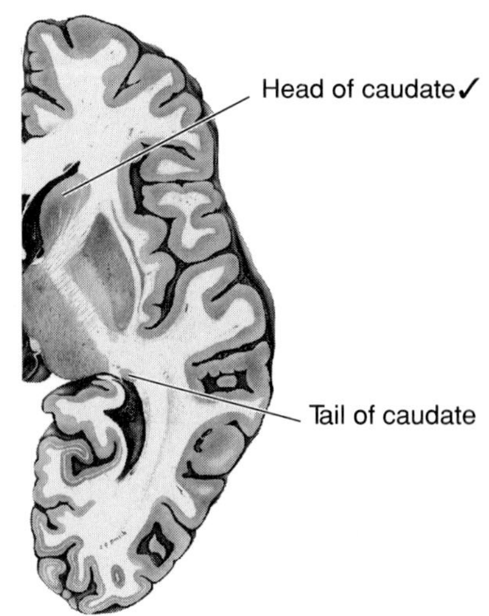

9.20A.

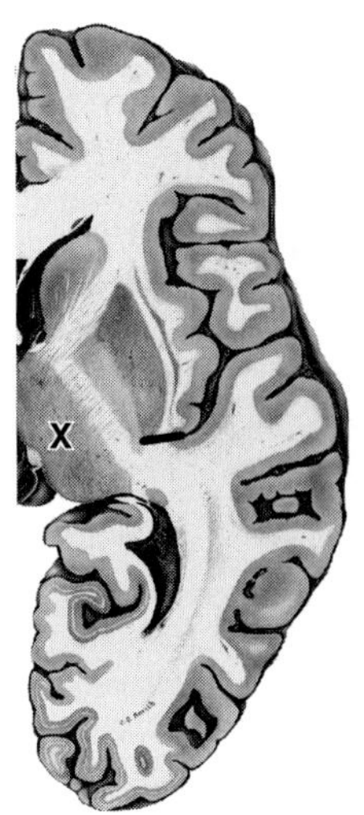

9.21A.

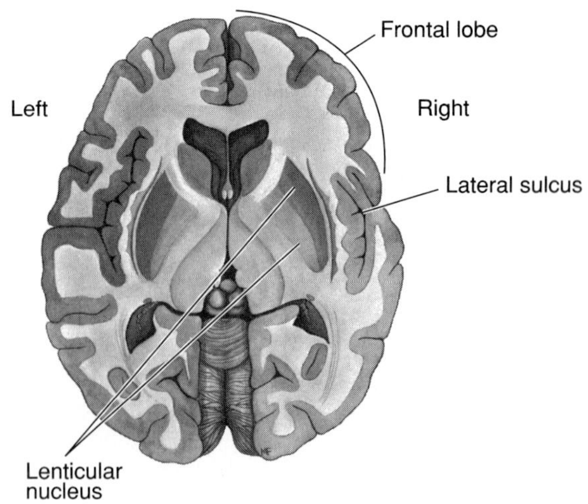

9.22. Draw the border around the lenticular nucleus on both sides of this horizontal section. The most lateral surface is called the external surface. The two internal surfaces are encapsulated by the __________ __________.

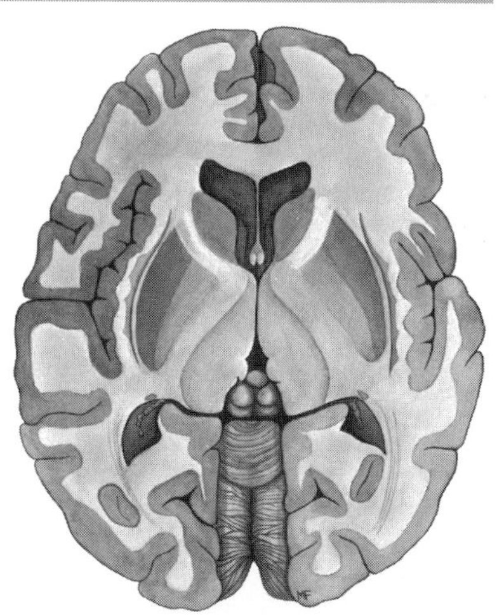

9.23. The lateral part of the lenticular nucleus is structurally different from the medial part. On the right side of this horizontal section, label the two parts with their names and draw the boundary between them.

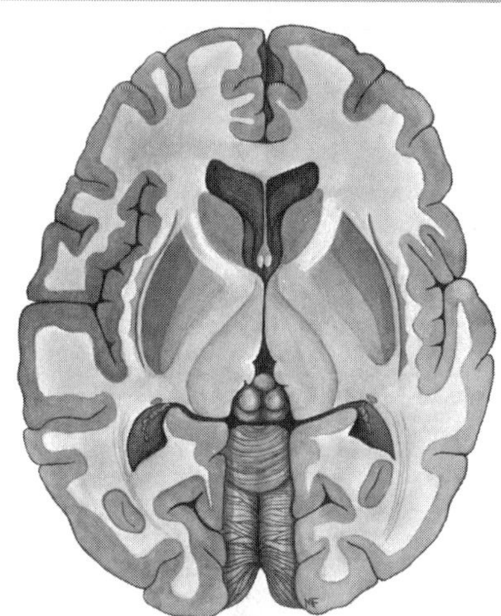

9.24. The caudate and putamen are partially separated by the __________ __________. The tail of the caudate is much __________ in size than the head and is located more __________ iorly. Label the head and tail of the caudate on both halves of the sectional figure.

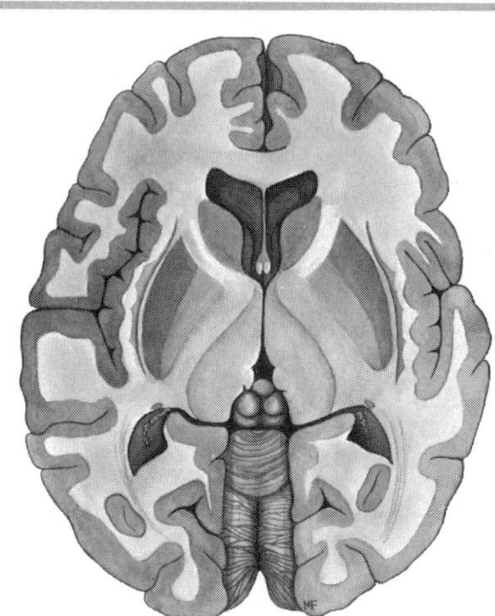

9.22A. internal capsule

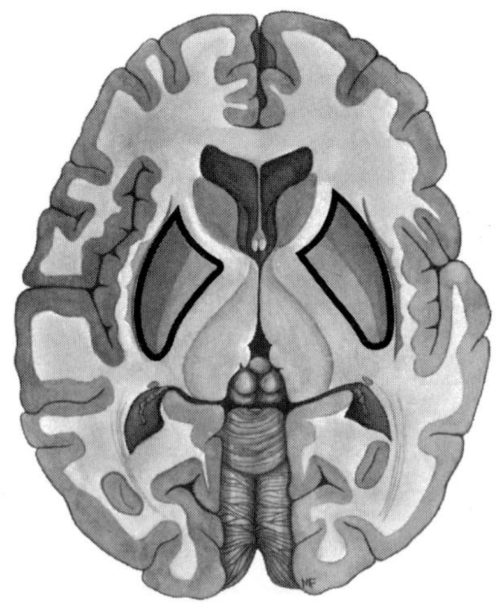

9.23A.

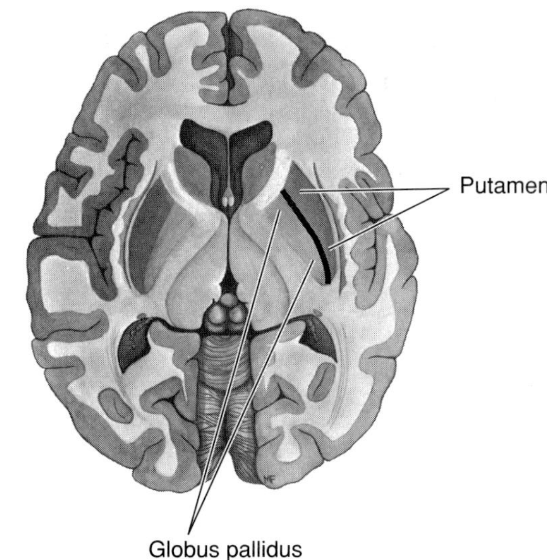

9.24A. internal capsule; smaller; posteriorly

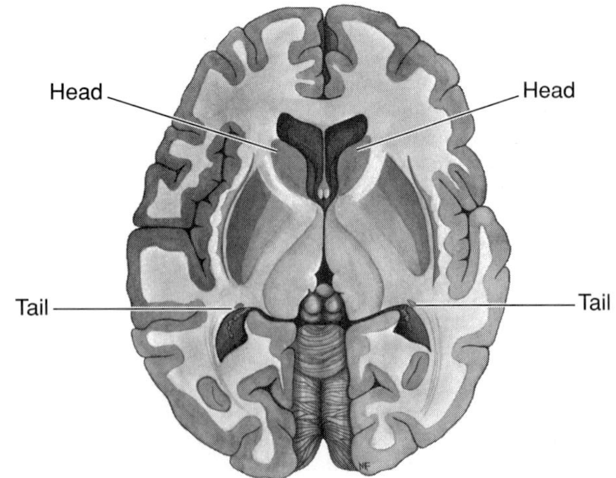

10 The Corticospinal System: White Matter Structures in Relation to Basal Nuclei

10.1. Bridges of cells connect the caudate and putamen. Running between and past these bridges are fibers of the corticospinal tract from the frontal lobe as well as other fibers to and from all lobes. The fibers collectively form the ____________ ____________.

10.2. The cell bridges, like the caudate and putamen, are composed of ______ matter; the internal capsule is ______ matter.

10.3. A thin horizontal section (35 microns thick) shows a few cell bridges between the caudate and putamen (see "B" in the left hand picture). Imagine the concentration of bridges in 10 successive thin sections, all superimposed (total thickness of 0.33 mm). The diameter of each bridge is actually smaller, and the number of such bridges is much ____________, than is illustrated in the right hand picture.

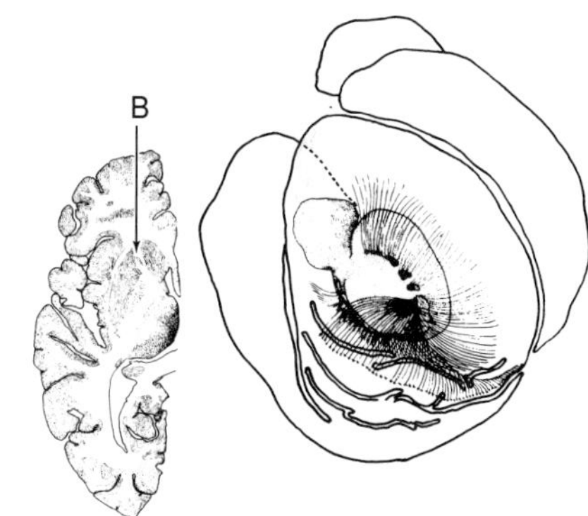

10.4. The white matter that runs along the surface of the globus pallidus is the ____________ ____________.

10.5. The internal capsule is bent by the tip of the globus pallidus to form an anterior limb and a posterior limb. Label each limb on the diagram.

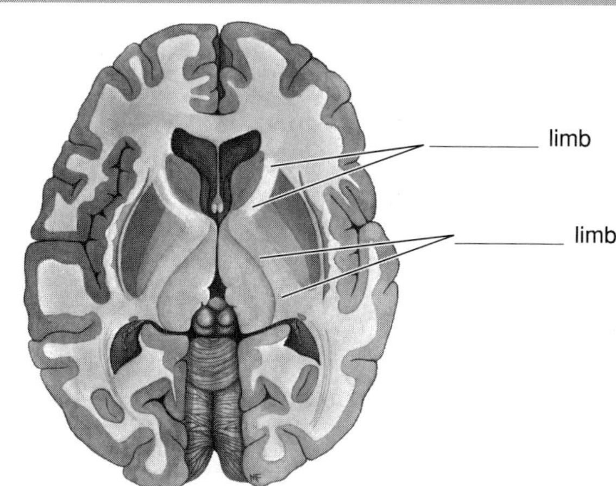

10.1A. internal capsule

10.2A. gray; white

10.3A. greater

10.4A. internal capsule

10.5A.

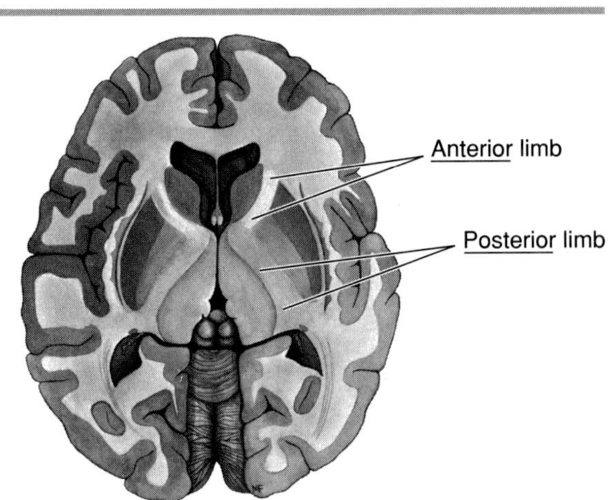

10.6. The two limbs are joined at the "knee" or genu of the internal capsule. Label the three parts of the internal capsule: anterior limb, posterior limb, and genu.

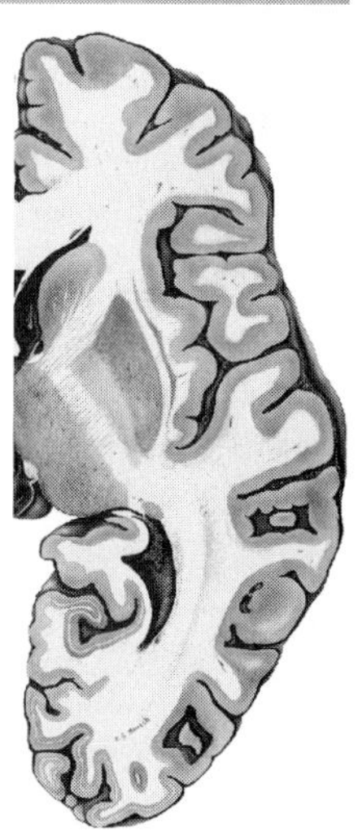

10.7. A horizontally cut surface through the basal ganglia and internal capsule is drawn on the right hand picture. Between the two pictures, draw lines connecting the corres-ponding parts of the internal capsule: genu, anterior limb, and posterior limb.

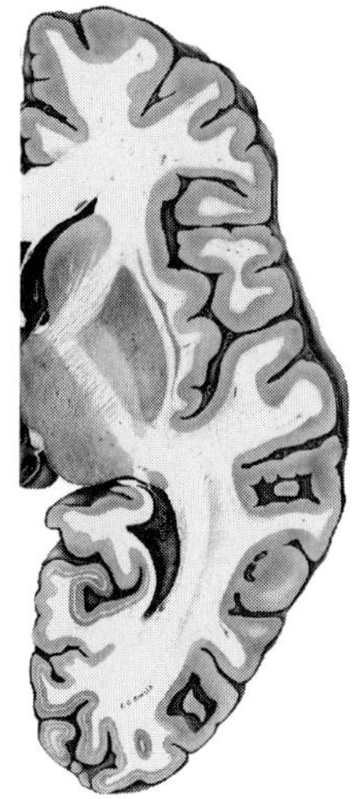

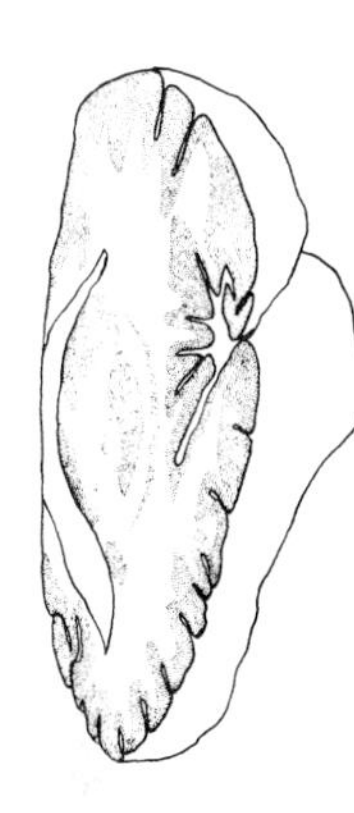

10.8. The diagrams illustrate the ____________________ tract passing down in the ____________ limb of the internal capsule. On both pictures, label the *anterior* limb of the internal capsule.

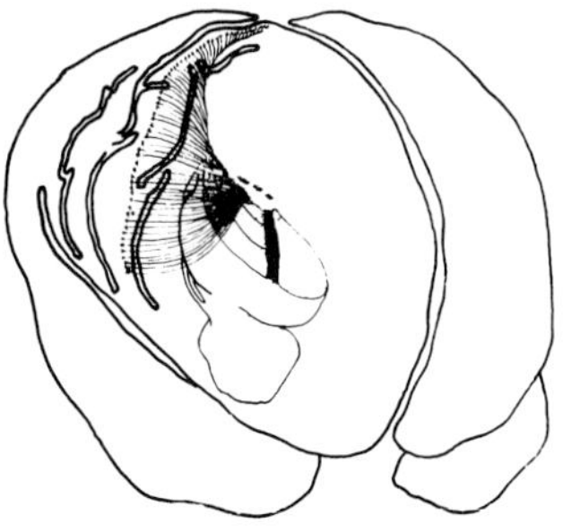

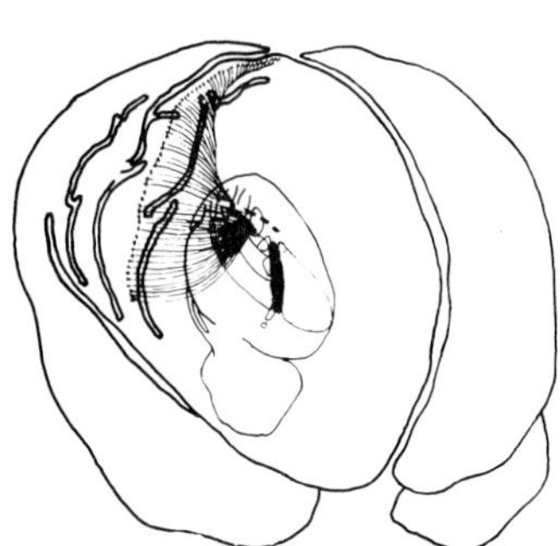

10.6A.

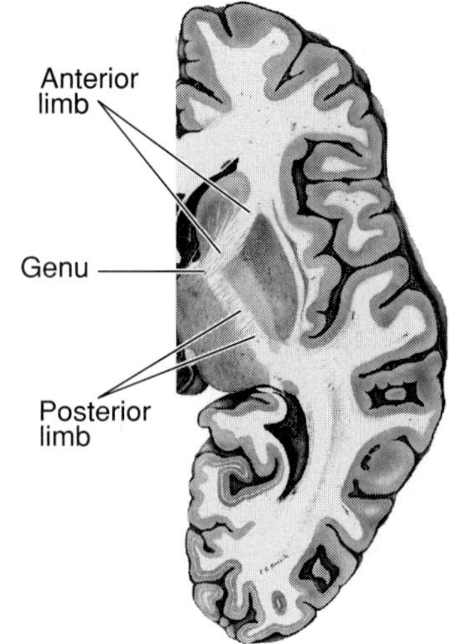

10.7A.

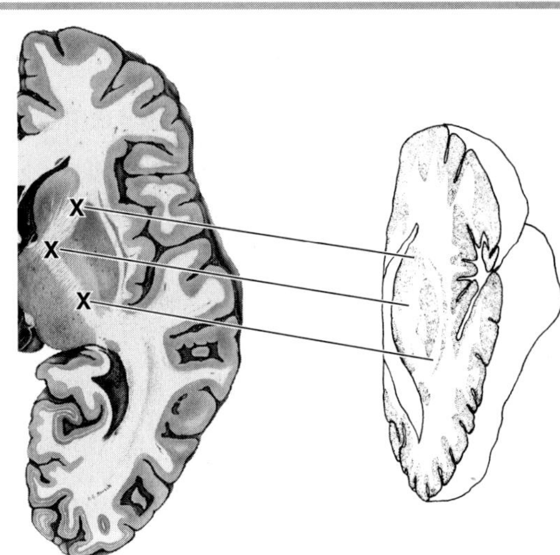

10.8A. corticospinal; posterior

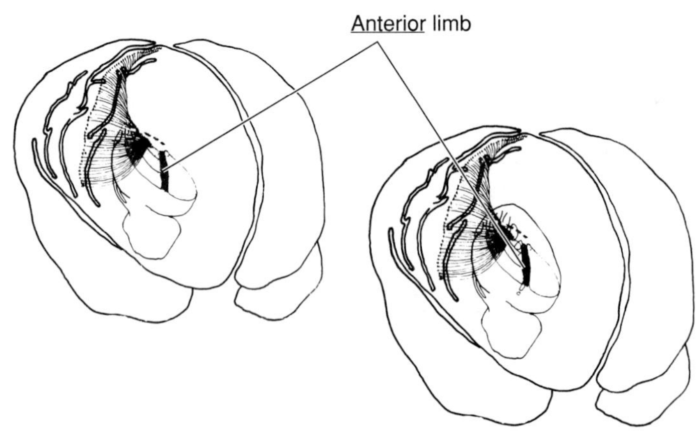

10.9. The brain has been rotated. Indicate and label the three parts of the internal capsule with their names.

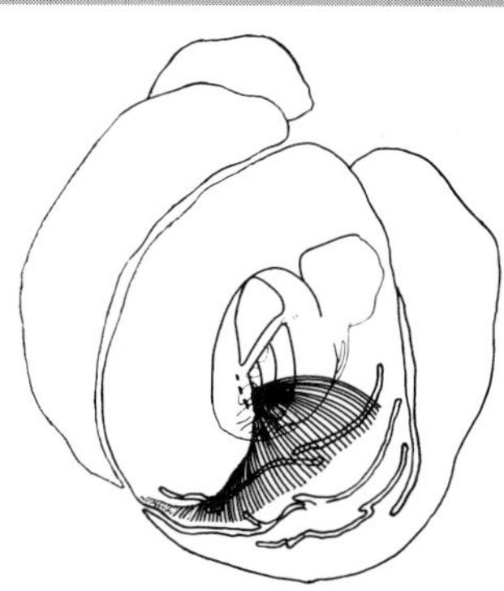

10.10. Blacken the approximate area where the corticospinal fibers pass through the internal capsule.

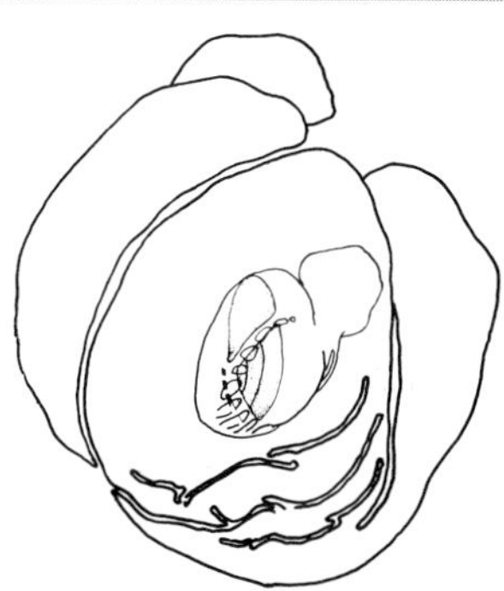

10.11. On both sides of the section, number the three regions of the internal capsule as 1, 2, and 3, beginning anteriorly. Blacken the approximate area where the corticospinal fibers pass through the internal capsule.

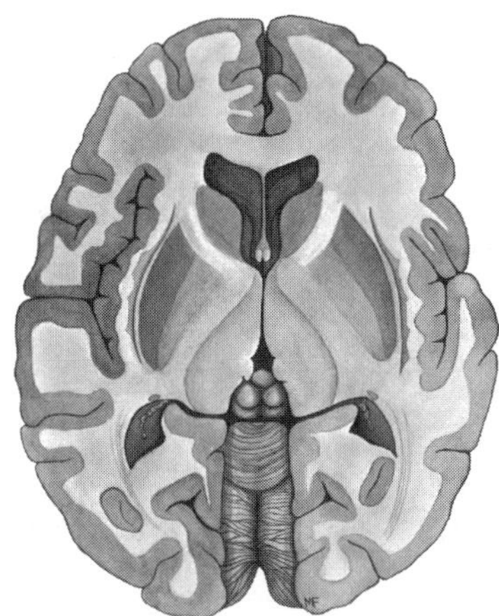

10.12. The arrow in the anterior limb of the internal capsule points to a cell ___________ connecting the ___________ with the ______ of the caudate nucleus.

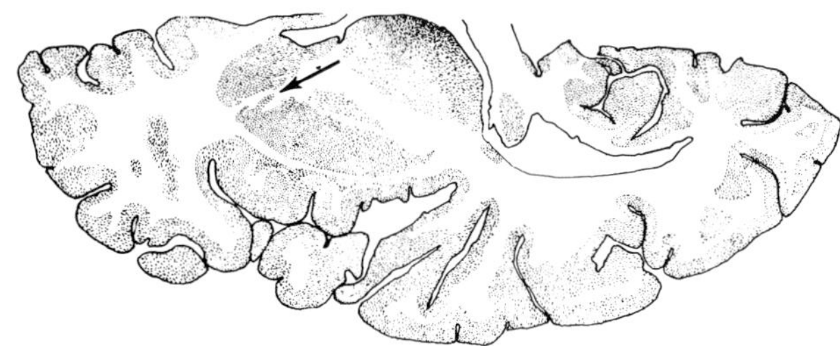

10.13. In addition to the corticospinal tract, other fiber tracts pass between the cell bridges into the ________________ ___________ to connect the surface of the cerebral cortex with deeper structures.

10.9A.

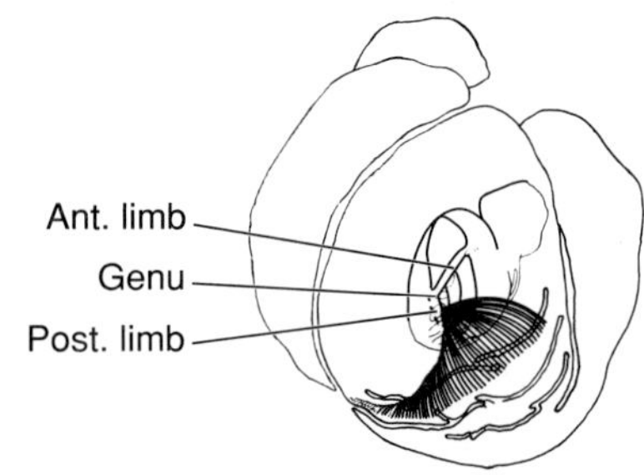

10.10A.

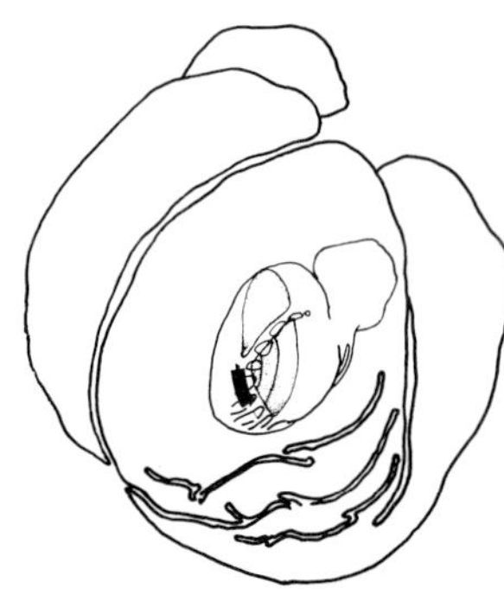

10.11A.

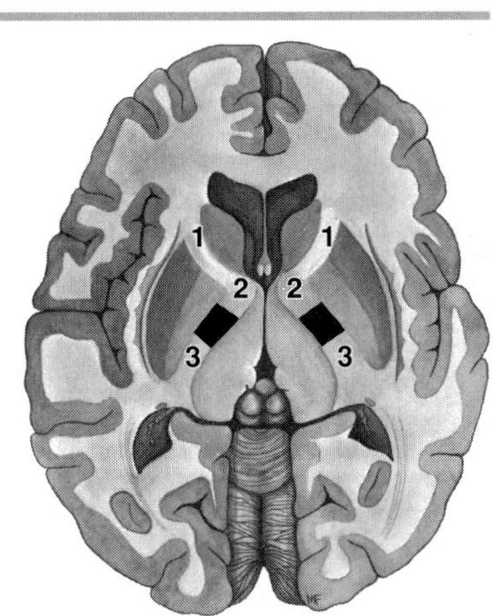

10.12A. bridge; putamen; head

10.13A. lenticular nucleus

10.15. On each diagram, with the corticospinal fibers as a guide, place a "G" *between* the caudate and putamen at the approximate position of the genu of the internal capsule.

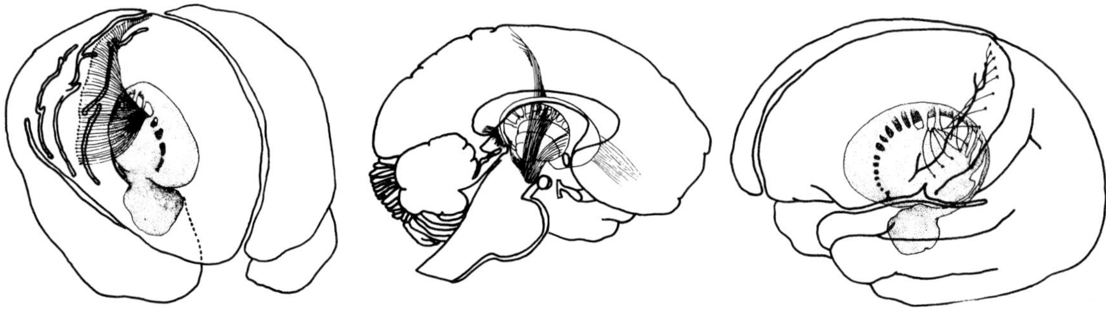

10.16. With the main exception of the corticospinal tract, the frontal lobe is connected to deeper structures via the ____________ limb of the internal capsule; posterior parts of the cortex send or receive fibers via the ____________ limb.

10.17. Superior to the caudate, there are densely packed white matter tracts. Many myelinated fibers of this white matter converge toward the internal capsule, forming a crown of fibers radiating outward from the basal nuclei. Collectively, these fibers are named the ____________ ____________.

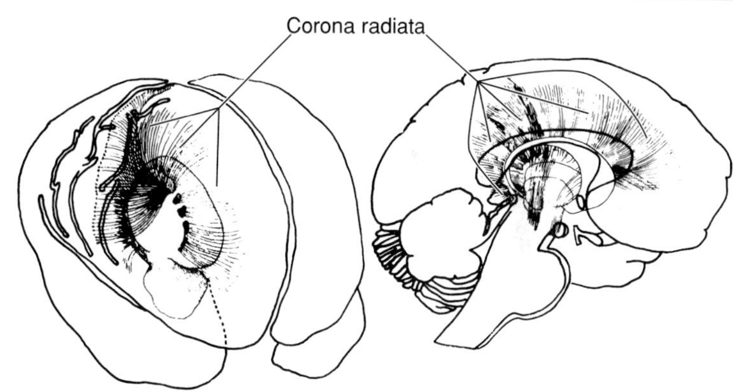

10.18. The myelinated fibers radiating between the internal capsule and the superior, anterior, posterior, and lateral areas of cortex collectively make up the corona ____________.

10.19. Afferent fibers running from the thalamus toward the cortex pass in succession through the ____________ capsule and ____________ ____________.

10.15A.

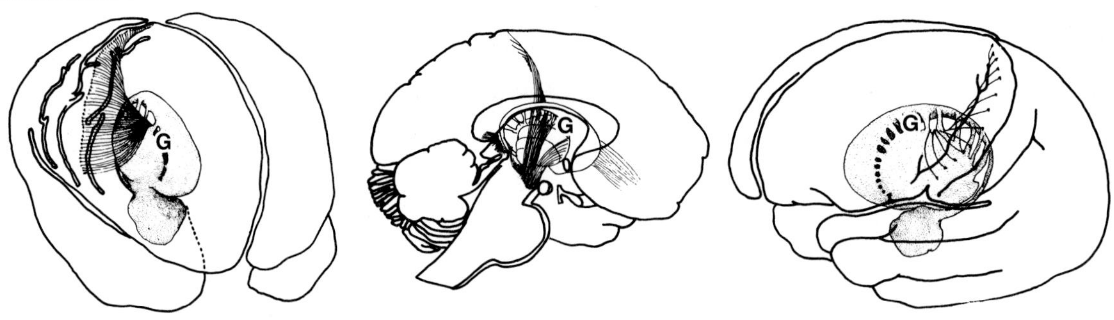

10.16A. anterior; posterior

10.17A. corona radiata

10.18A. radiata

10.19A. internal; corona radiata

10.20. As the fibers of the corona radiata are traced medially past the lenticular nucleus, they turn inferiorly in the ____________ ____________; at this point, a horizontal section through the brain cuts them in ____________________ section.

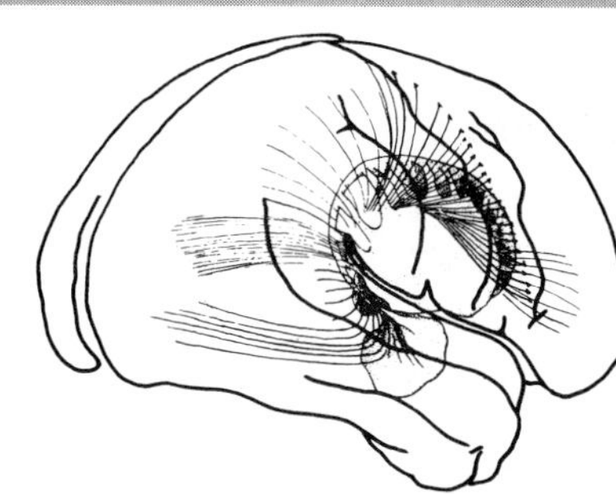

10.21. Label the specific parts indicated on the diagram.

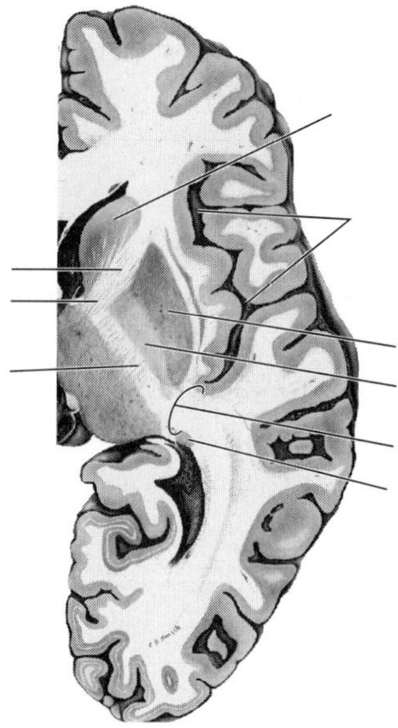

10.22. On the diagram, indicate and label the following: putamen, globus pallidus, head of caudate, tail of caudate, corona radiata, three divisions of internal capsule with names, and corticospinal fibers in internal capsule.

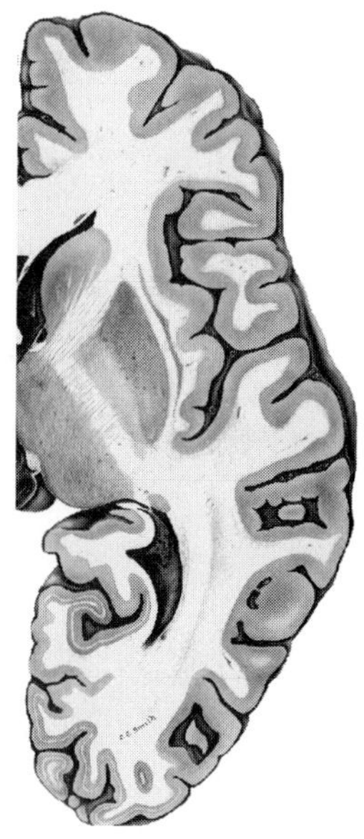

10.23. The corticospinal tract originates primarily in the gray matter of the ____________________ gyrus and passes from the cortical surface in a ____________ direction successively through the ____________ ____________ before turning inferiorly over the ____________________ nucleus as part of the ____________ limb of the ____________ ____________.

10.20A. internal capsule; transverse (cross)

10.21A.

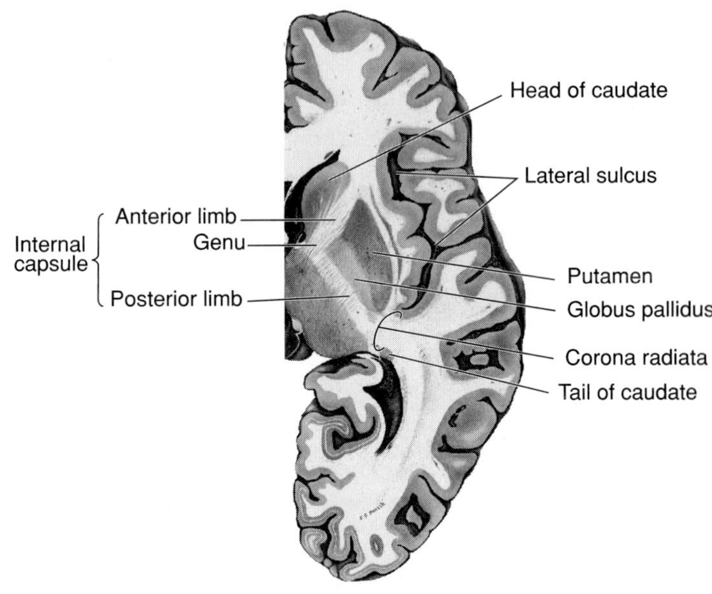

10.22A.

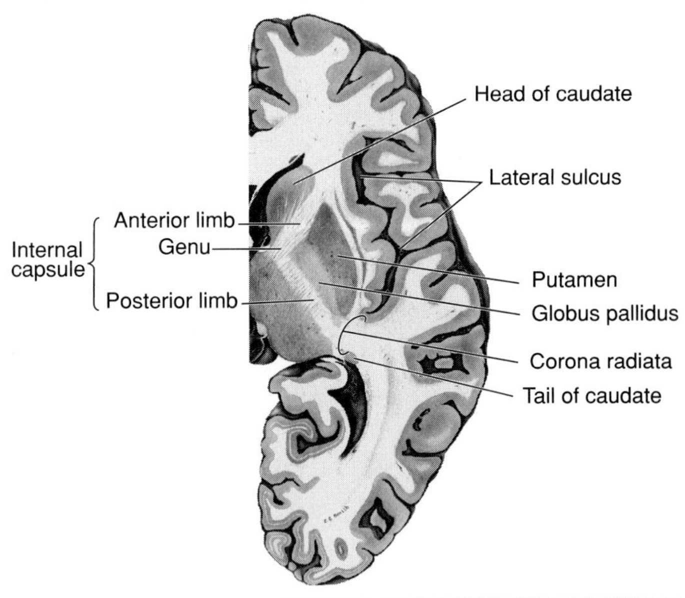

10.23A. precentral; medial (or inferior); corona radiata; lenticular; posterior; internal capsule

11 The Corticospinal System: Additional Relations to Deeper Structures

11.1. This section has been stained by a method that colors myelin black and leaves cell bodies relatively unstained. In the illustration, the white matter looks ______ er than the cell bodies.

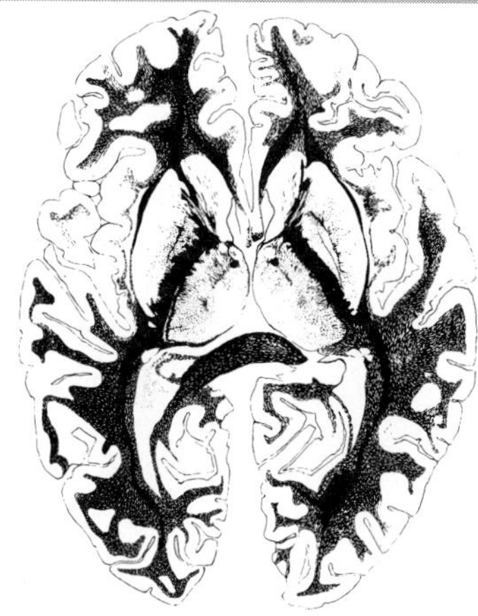

11.2. Indicate which section has the myelin stain and which has the cell stain.

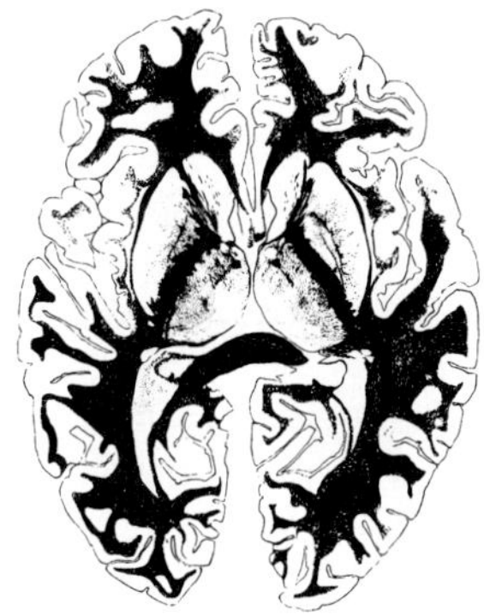

______ stain

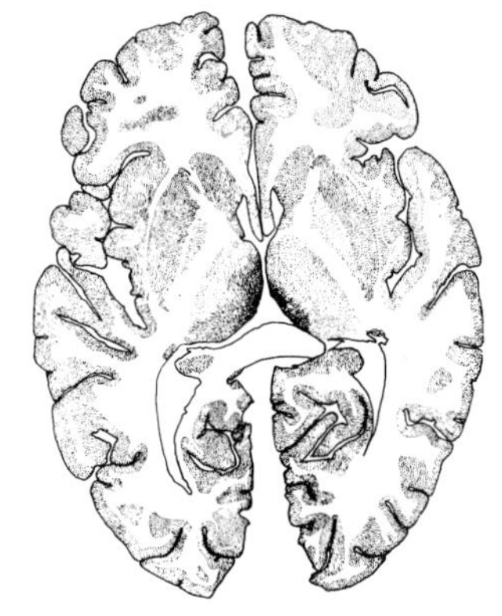

______ stain

11.3. On each section, label the anterior (A) and posterior (P) limbs of the internal capsule.

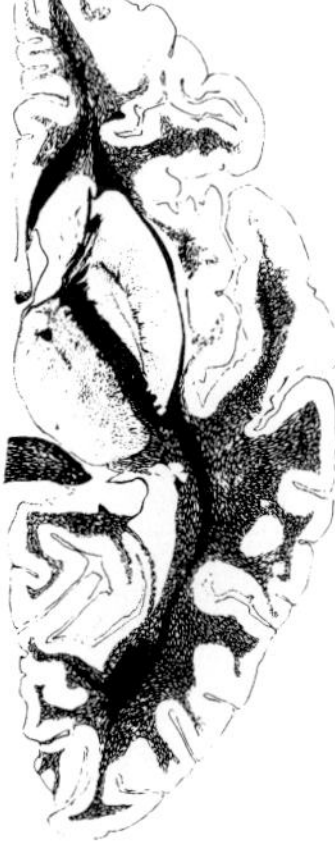

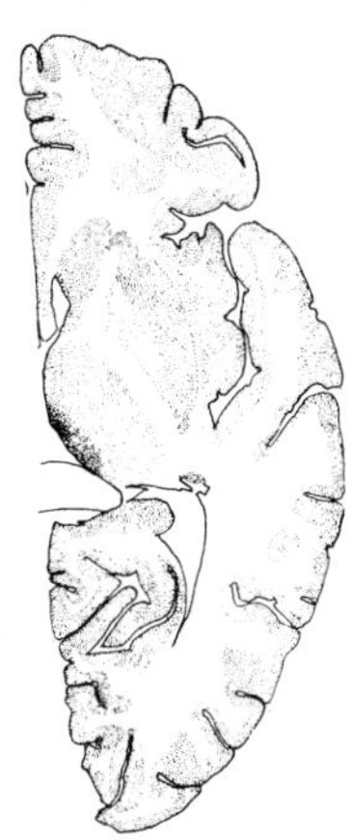

11.1A. darker

11.2A.

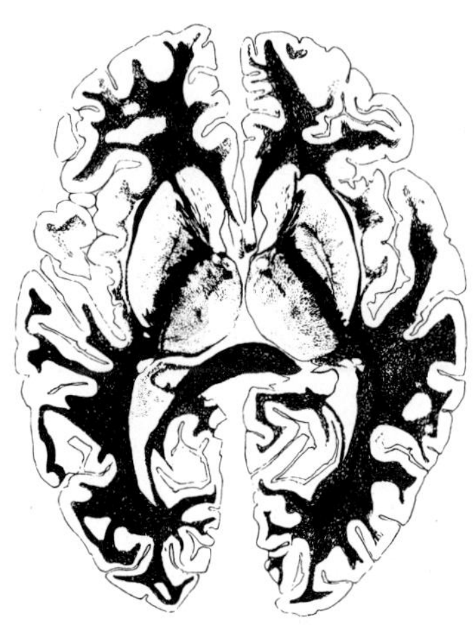

Myelin stain

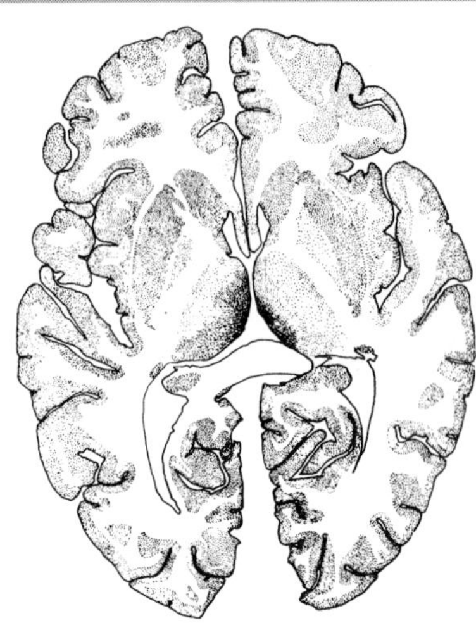

Cell stain

11.3A.

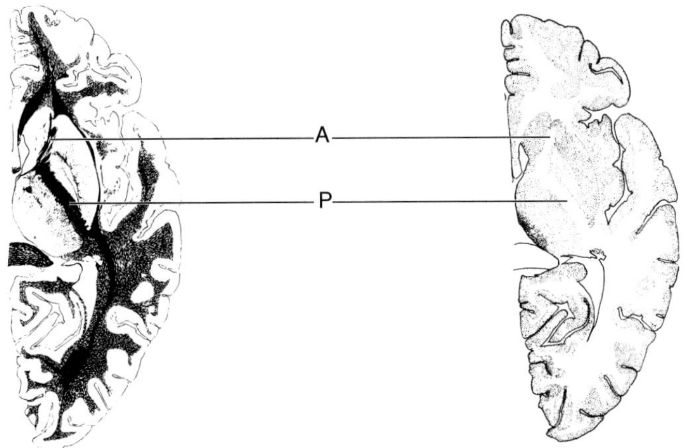

11.4. What color is the globus pallidus in this stain? ___________

Draw a line to the globus pallidus on the right side of the figure.

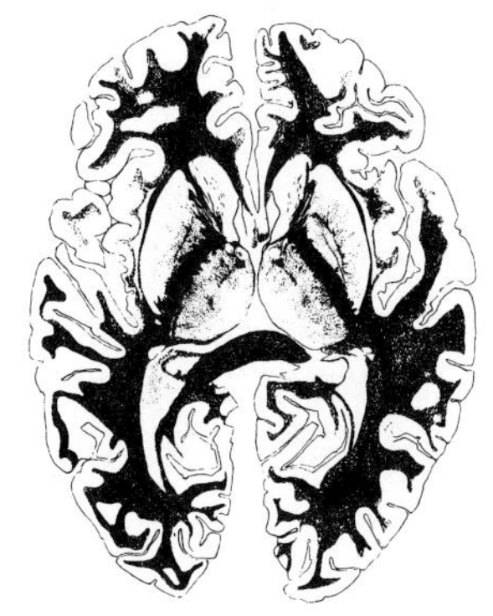

11.5. Draw lines to the appropriate structures.

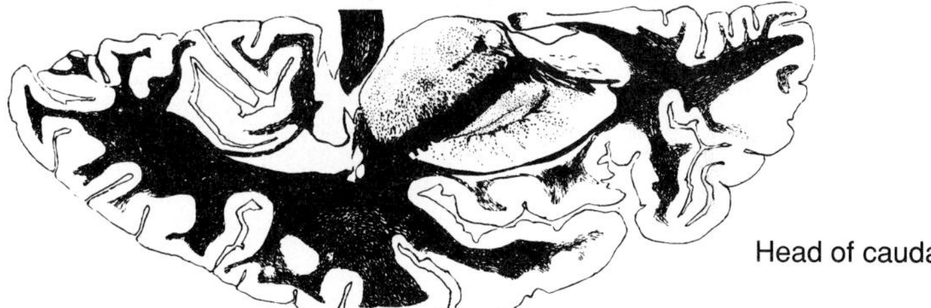

11.6. The head of the caudate typically lies antero-___________ to the internal capsule; the lenticular nucleus always lies ___________ to the internal capsule.

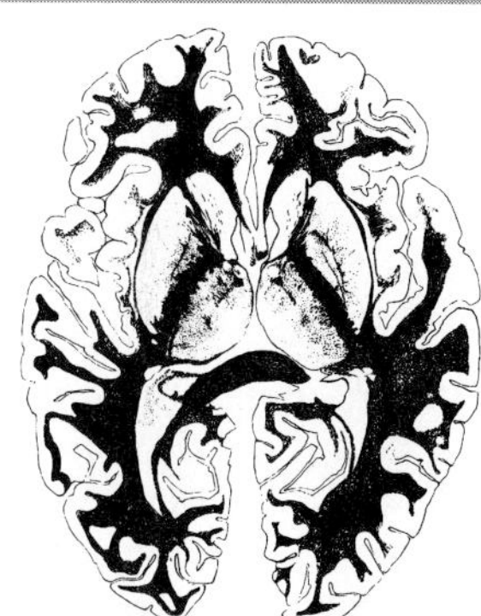

11.7. The anterior limb of the internal capsule is crossed by cell bridges that connect the putamen and the ___________ nucleus. At the level of this section, the putamen is also contiguous with another gray matter structure, the ___________ ___________.

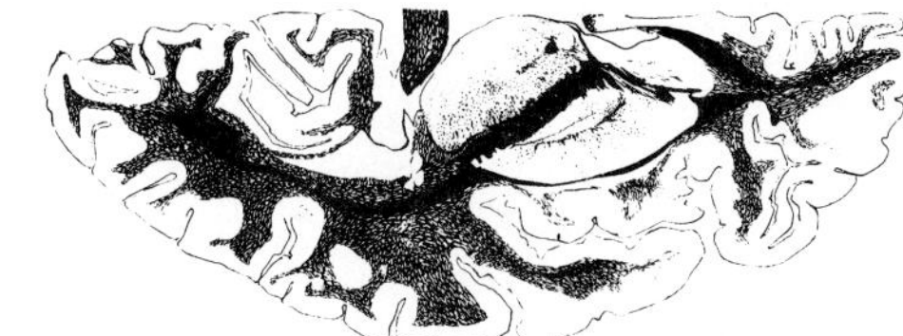

11.4A. White

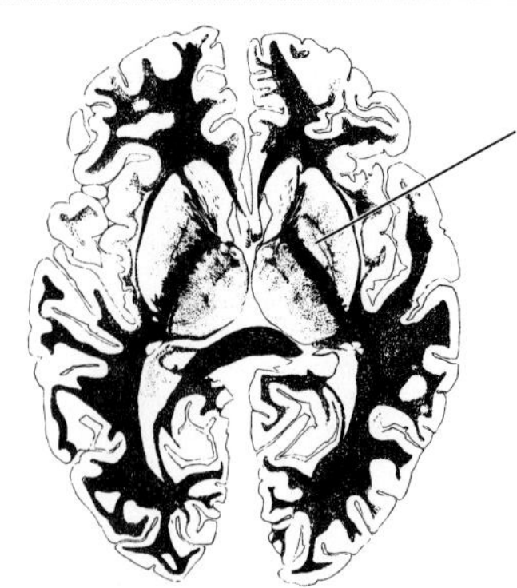

11.5A.

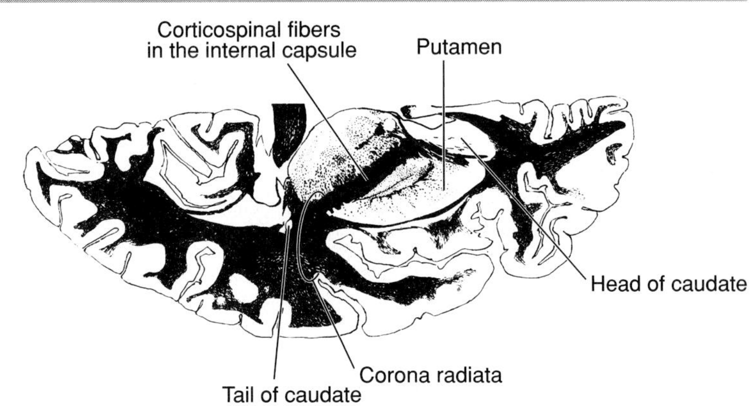

11.6A. antero-medial; lateral

11.7A. caudate; globus pallidus

11.8. The putamen is readily distinguishable histologically and functionally from the other part of the lenticular nucleus, the ___________ ___________. The putamen is more closely related to the nucleus from which it is partially separated by the internal capsule, the ___________ nucleus. Because of their structural resemblance, a single term, striatum, is often used to designate the head, body, and tail of the ___________ plus the ___________

11.9. Draw lines to relate the proper items in the middle column to the terms in the other two columns:

	Caudate	
Striatum	Putamen	Lenticular nucleus
	Globus pallidus	

11.10. The lateral sulcus partially separates the frontal and parietal lobes superiorly from the ___________ lobe inferiorly.

11.11. The tail differs from the rest of the caudate in position. It has swung around to a position inferior and lateral to the head, entering the medial part of the ___________ lobe.

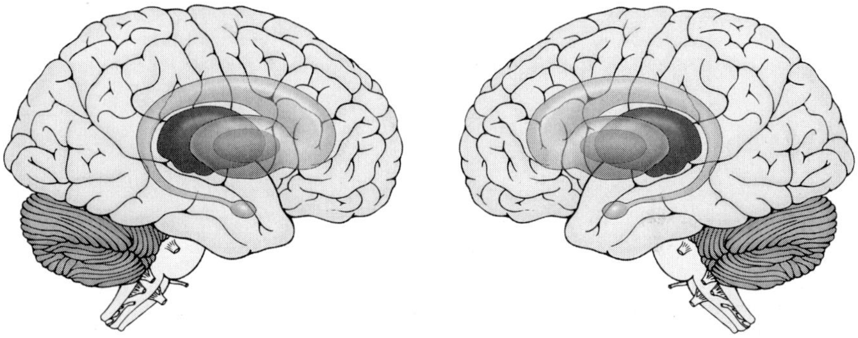

11.12. The head of the caudate (indicated by the "X") is in the ___________ lobe. "Y", which represents the ___________, is in the ___________ lobe.

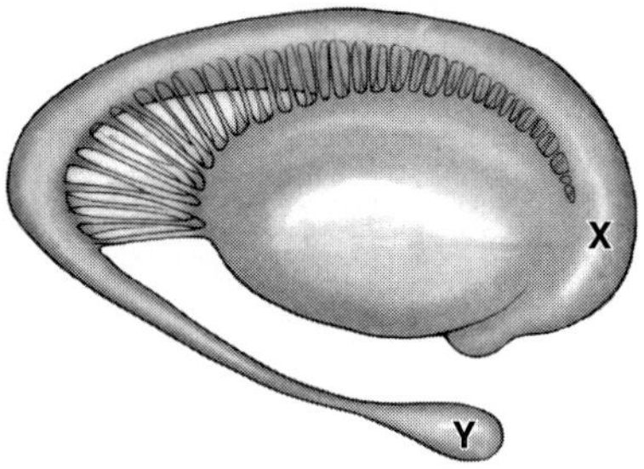

X

Y

11.13. In a section stained for myelin, the head and tail of the caudate appear ______ in color.

11.8A. globus pallidus; caudate; caudate; putamen

11.9A.

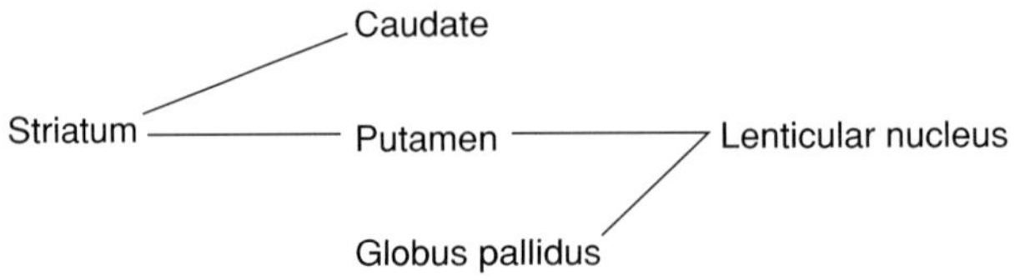

Caudate
Striatum — Putamen — Lenticular nucleus
Globus pallidus

11.10A. temporal

11.11A. temporal

11.12A. frontal; amygdala; temporal

11.13A. light

11.14. On the figure, label the indicated structures appropriately as:

Putamen

Cell bridges

Head of caudate

Tail of caudate

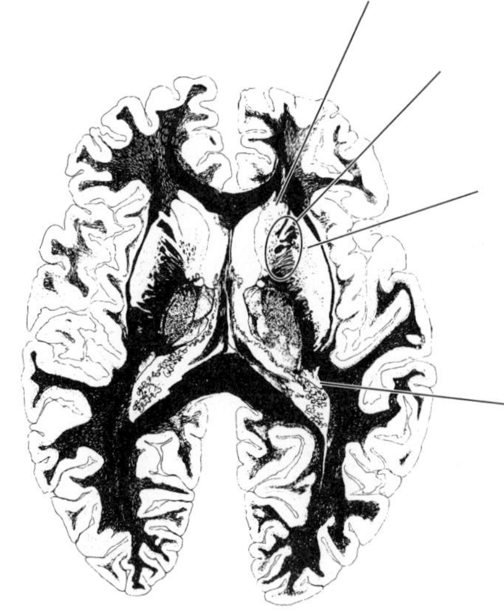

11.15. The head and tail of the caudate lie ______ al to the white matter of the internal capsule and corona ____________.

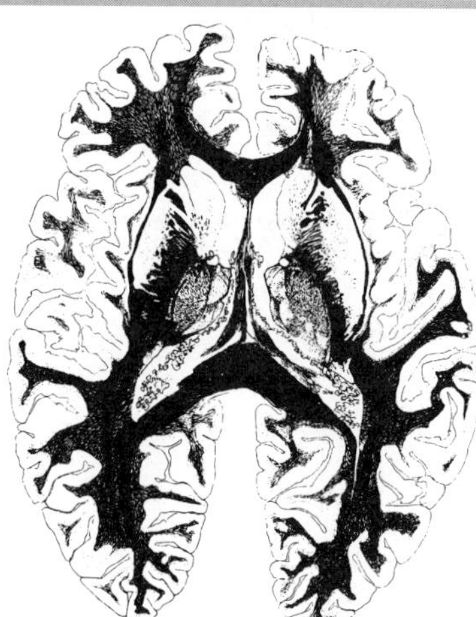

11.16. A horizontal section along the line indicated would cut across the corpus callosum in ______ places.

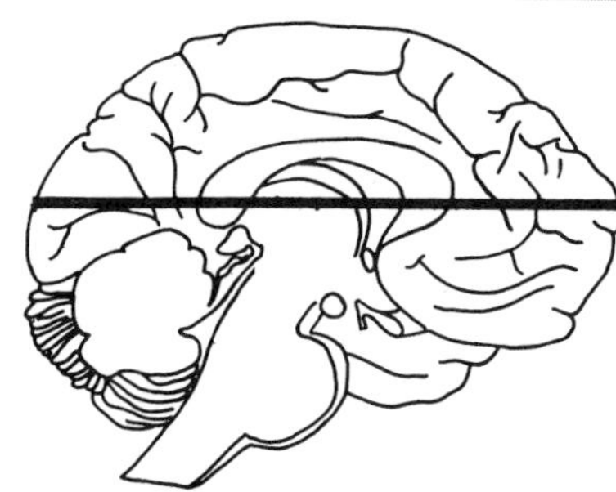

11.17. On the right hand picture, place an "A" and "P" on the structures so labeled on the left hand image.

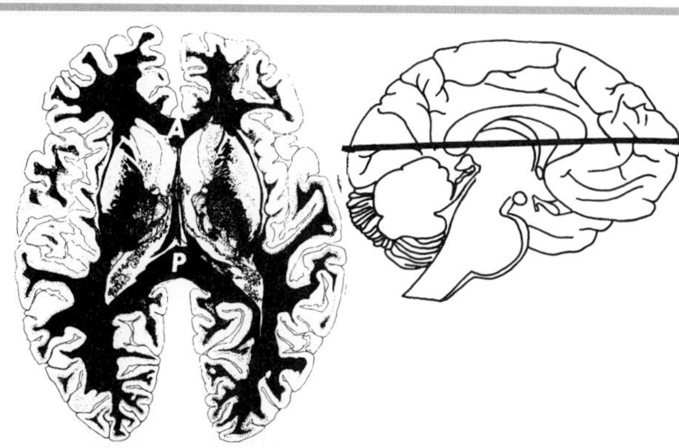

11.14A.

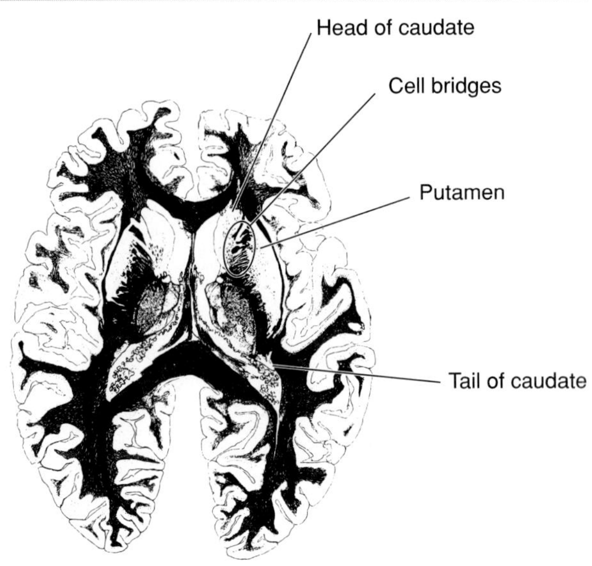

11.15A. <u>medi</u>al; <u>radiata</u>

11.16A. <u>two</u>

11.17A.

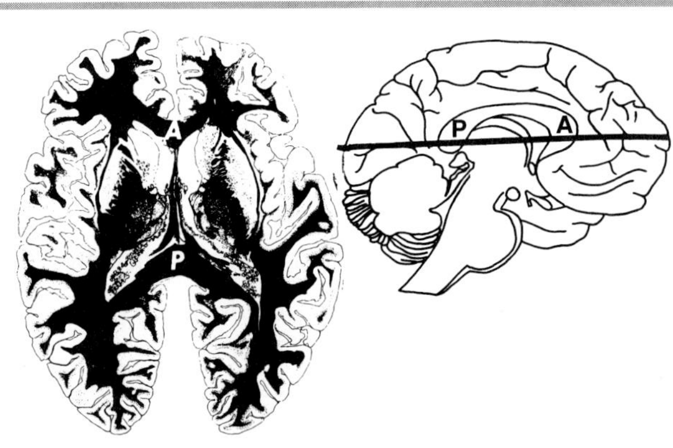

11.18. Label the head (H) and tail (T) of the caudate at the corresponding points on both pictures. The lateral ventricle (labeled "V" on the left hand image) occupies the interior of each cerebral hemisphere. The caudate nucleus forms the ______ al wall of the ventricle.

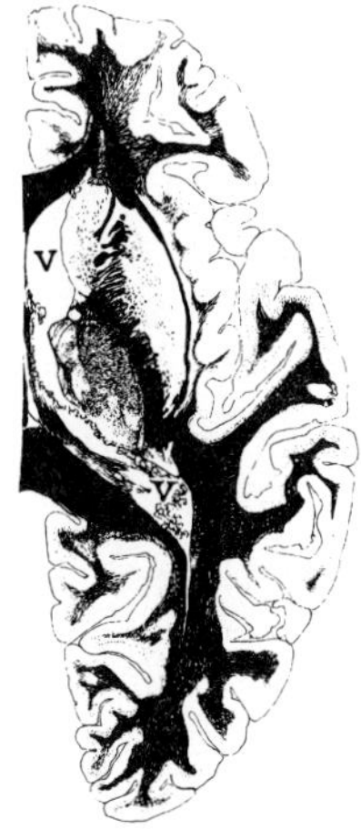

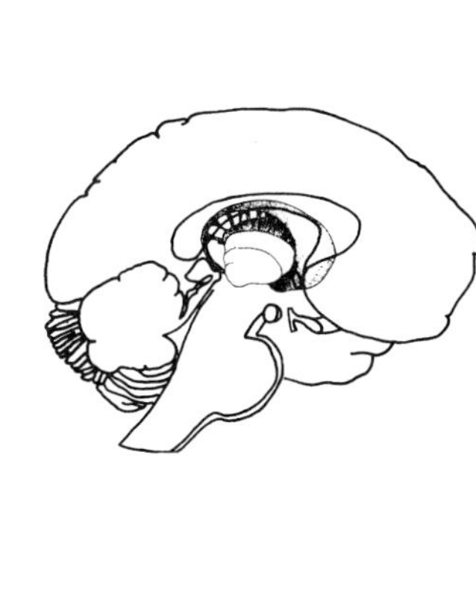

11.19. Label the head (H) and tail (T) of the caudate on both sides of each horizontal section. On the right hand image, each "V" lies in a lateral __________.

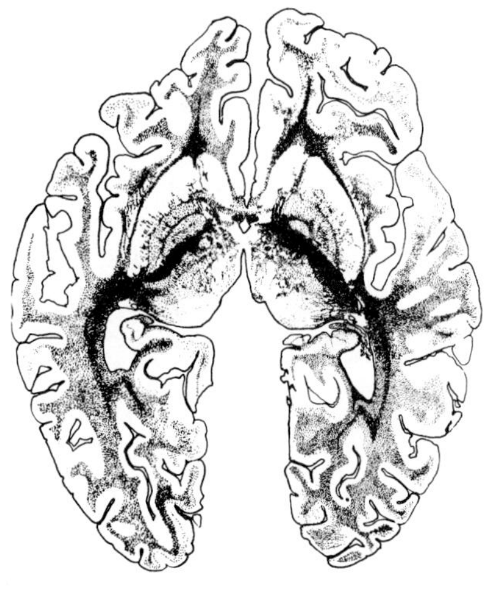

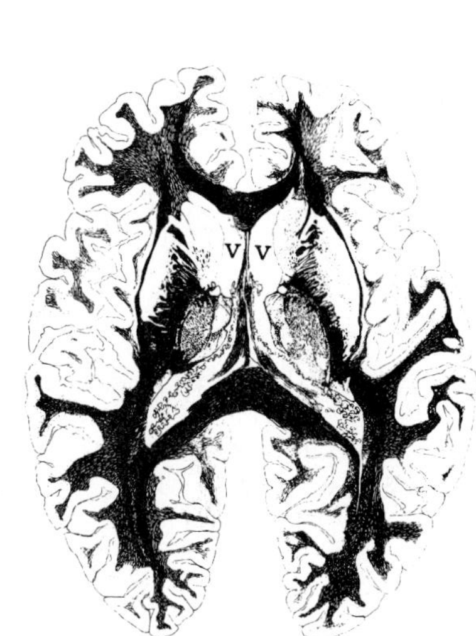

11.20. In the temporal lobe, the slender tail of the caudate is continuous with a thicker mass of gray matter, the __________.

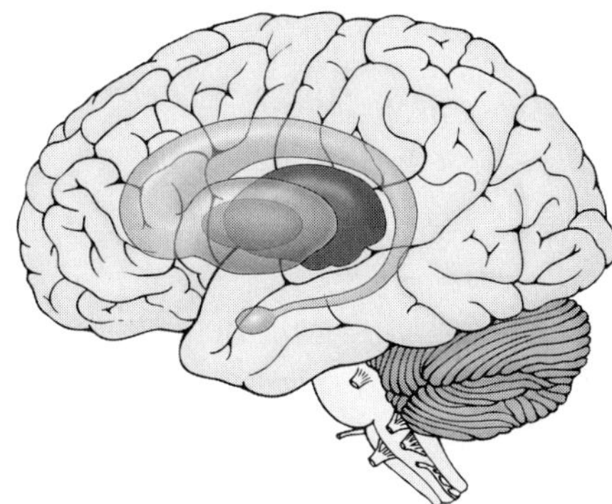

11.21. The masses of cells that lie deep within the lobes of the cerebral cortex in a basal position are the putamen, __________ __________, and __________ nucleus. They make up most of the cell masses collectively named the ______ __________.

11.18A. lateral

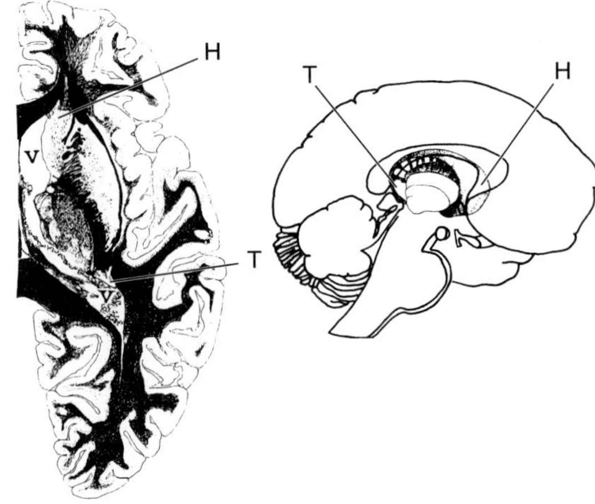

11.19A. ventricle

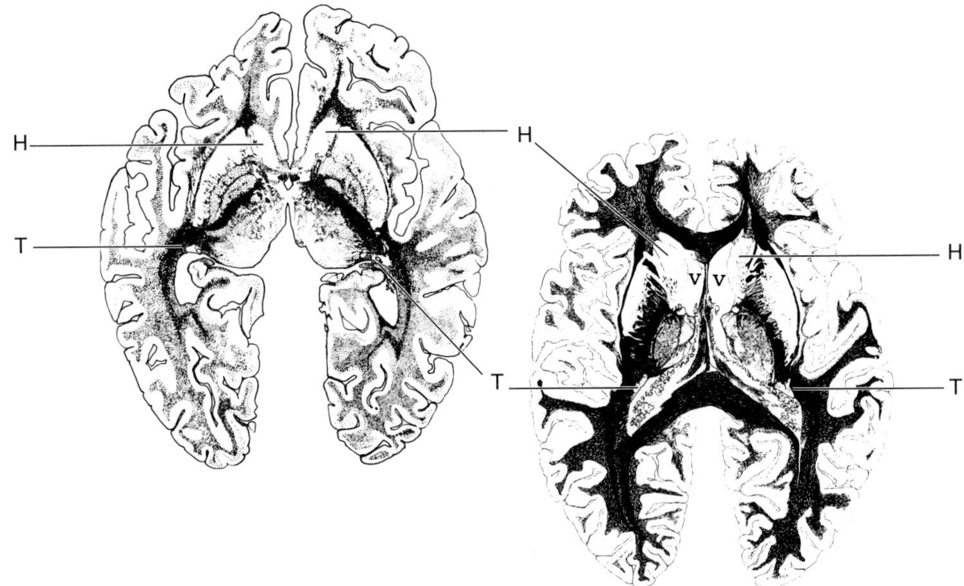

11.20A. amygdala

11.21A. globus pallidus; caudate; basal nuclei

11.22. Basal nuclei are continuous with or adjacent to one another. Name the specific structures that are continuous at the junctions indicated as "A," "B," "C," and "D."

A ______________________________

B ______________________________

C ______________________________

D ______________________________

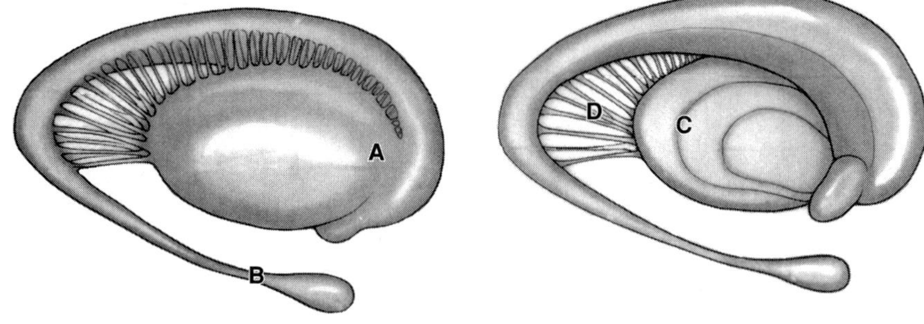

11.23. Which of the basal nuclei are included in the striatum? ____________ and ____________

11.24. On the horizontal section, are any basal nuclei visible? ______ Draw a line across the left diagram to indicate the approximate level of the horizontal section. Label the precentral gyrus on the horizontal section.

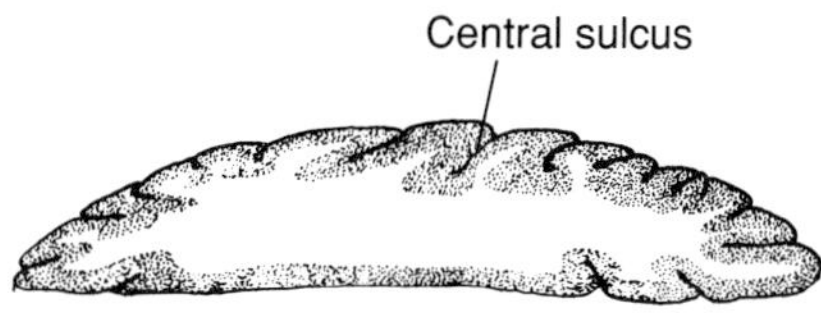

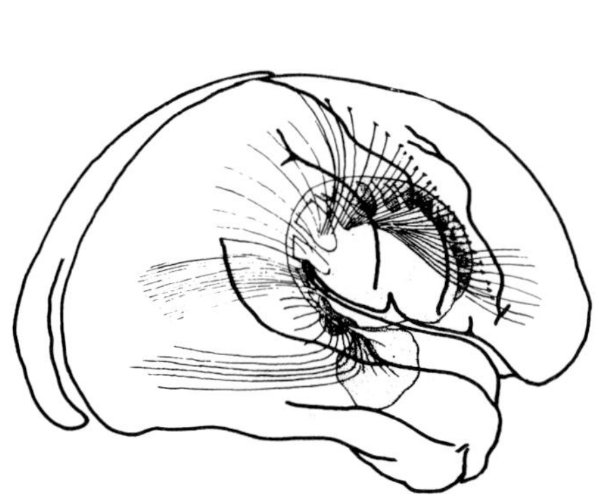

11.25. Label the two structures indicated on the diagram.

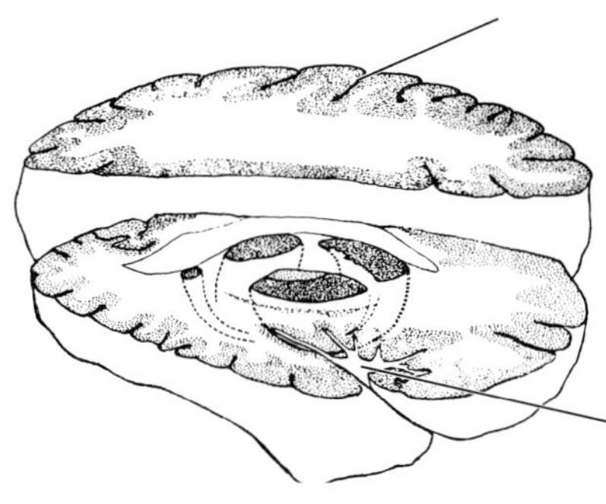

11.22A.

A Head of caudate and putamen

B Tail of caudate and amygdala

C Putamen and globus pallidus

D Putamen and body of caudate

11.23A. Putamen; caudate

11.24A. No

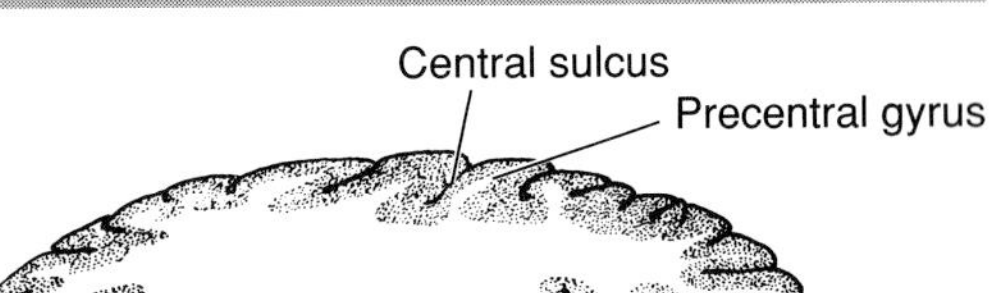

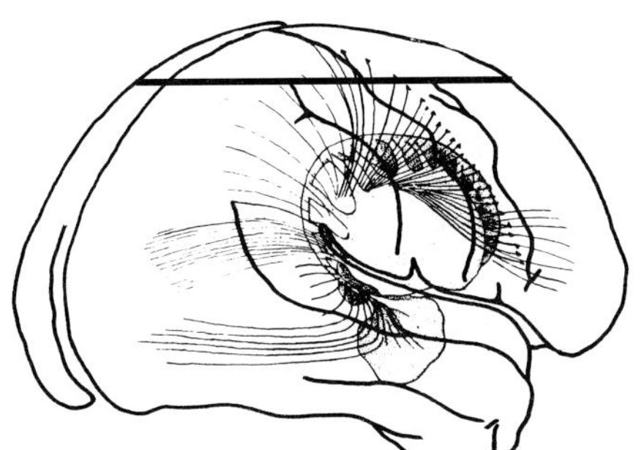

11.25A.

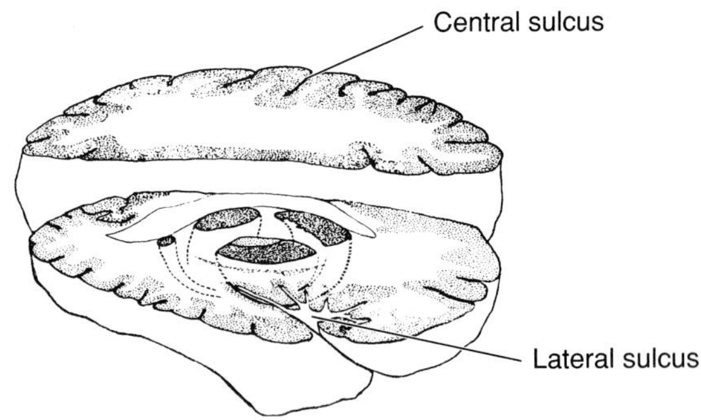

11.26. The head of the caudate and most of the lenticular nucleus are in the ______ al lobe.

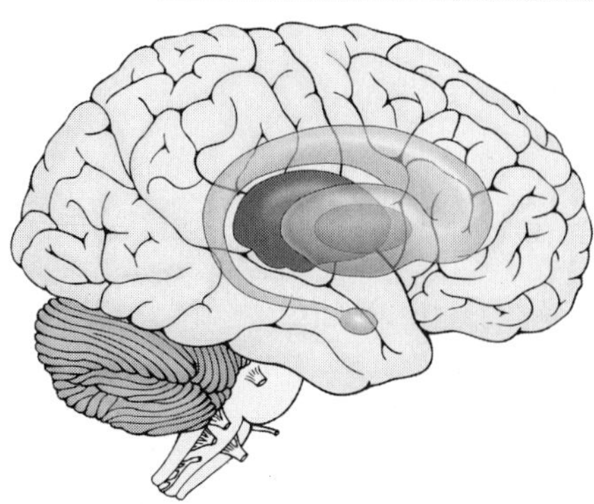

11.27. The deep lateral sulcus partially separates the frontal lobe from the __________ lobe.

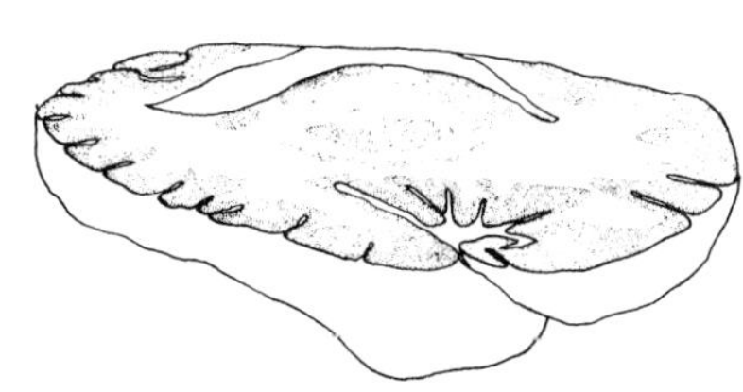

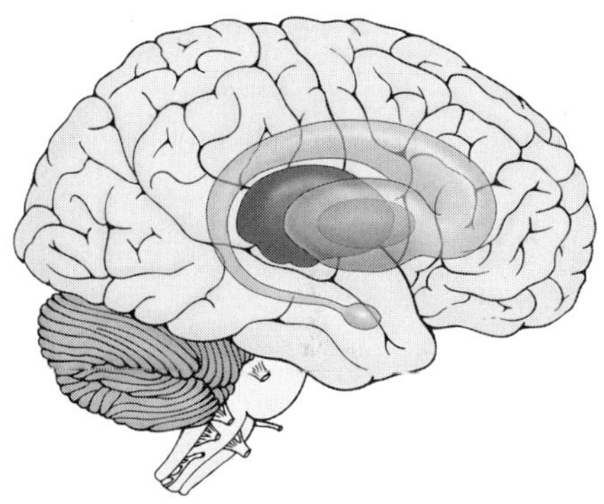

11.28. The arrows point to the ______ matter in the base of the ______ al lobe.

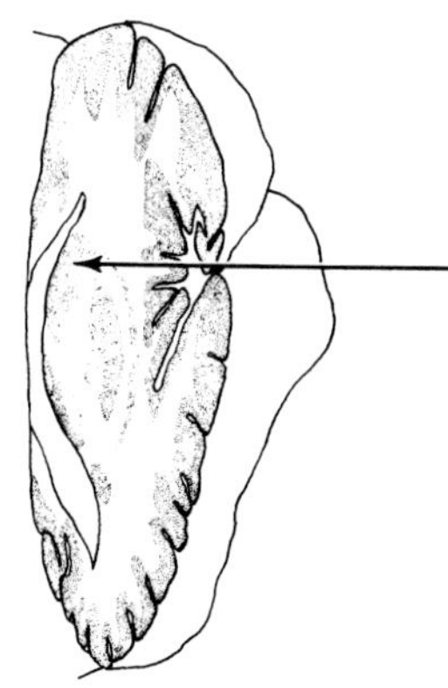

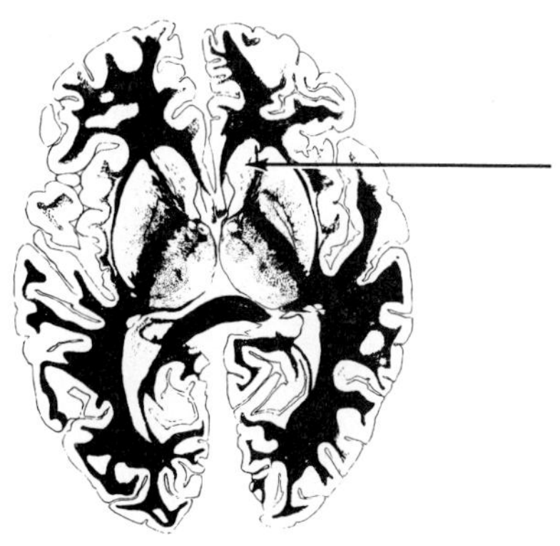

11.29. The horizontal section cuts across the basal nuclei in the plane indicated. Place a "T" on the cut surface of the tail of the caudate in both pictures.

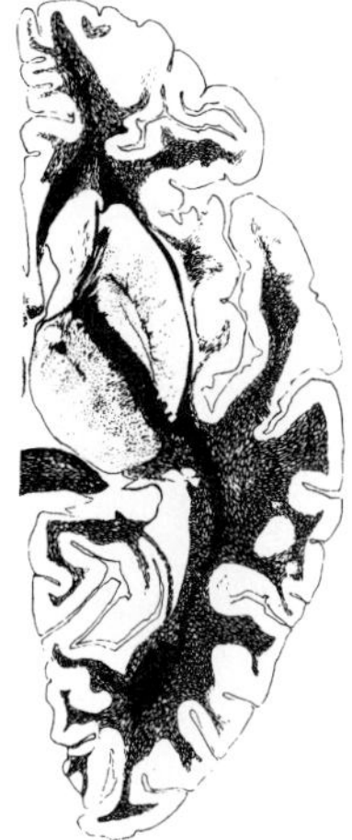

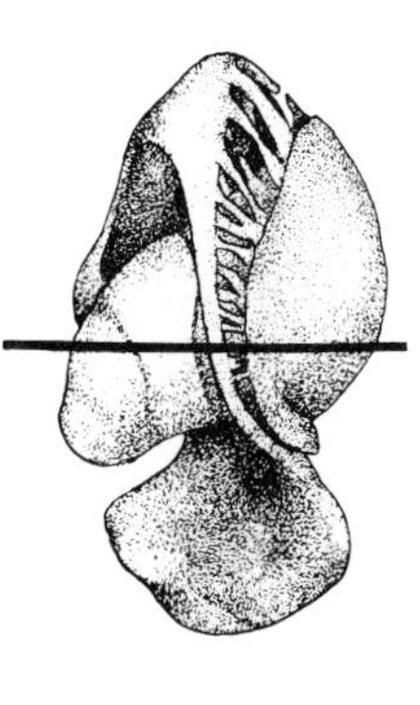

11.26A. <u>front</u>al

11.27A. <u>temporal</u>

11.28A. <u>gray</u>; <u>front</u>al

11.29A.

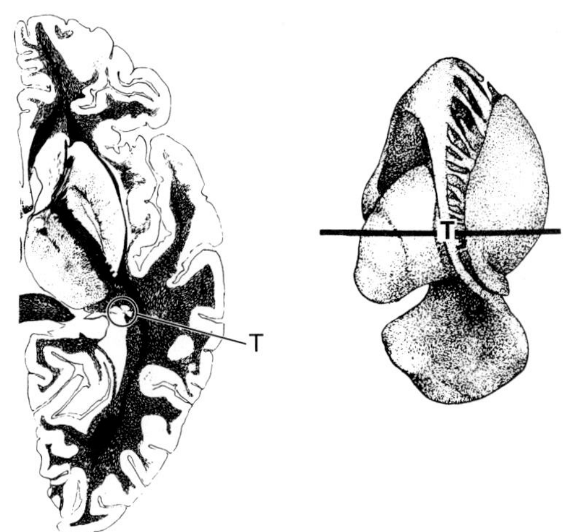

11.30. A vertical (sagittal) section in the indicated position would cut across a mass of gray matter inferior to the putamen and therefore would not appear in the horizontal section—the ____________. The latter structure is in the medial part of the ____________.

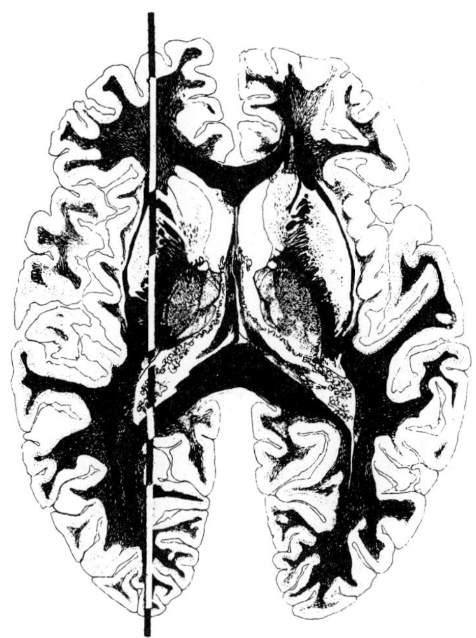

11.30A. amygdala; temporal lobe

12 The Corticospinal System: Relations Among the Insula, Claustrum, and White Matter Structures

12.1. The lateral sulcus is lined with surface ______ matter. The cortex hidden in the depths of the sulcus is called the *insula*. Label the indicated structures.

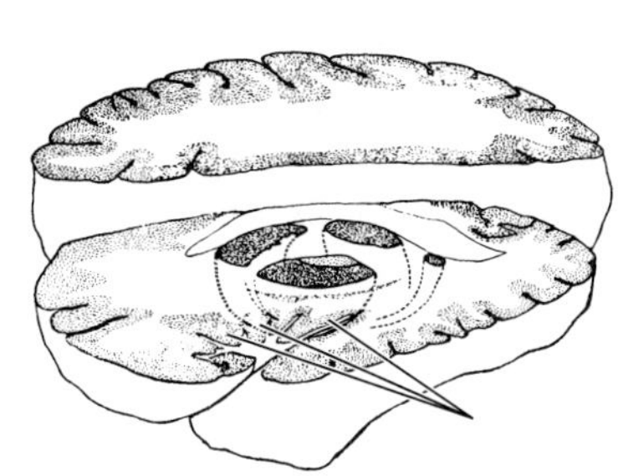

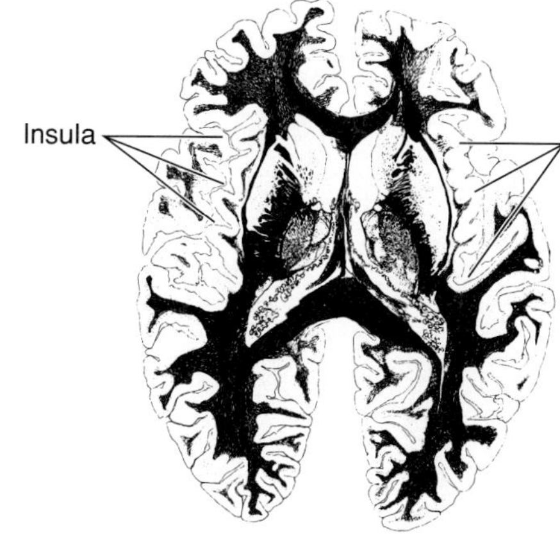

12.2. The lateral sulcus can be pulled open to expose the __________.

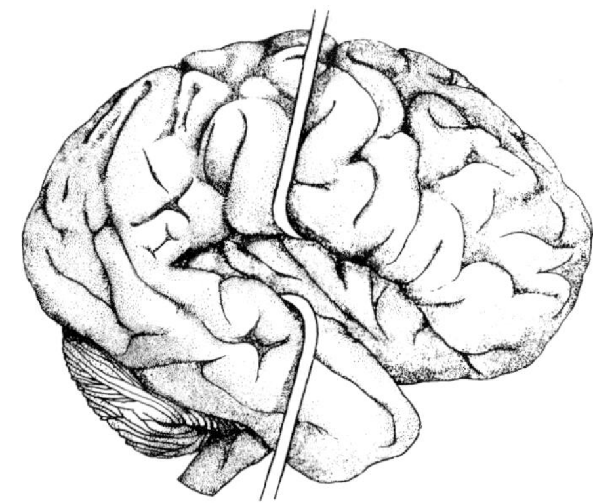

12.3. The surface of the insula is ______ matter. On both diagrams, draw lines to indicate the insula.

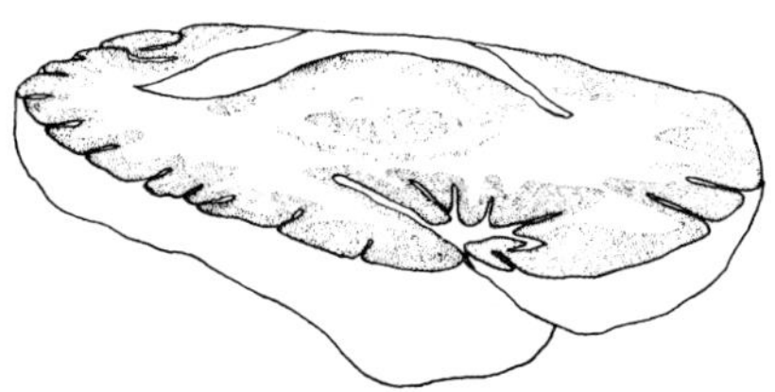

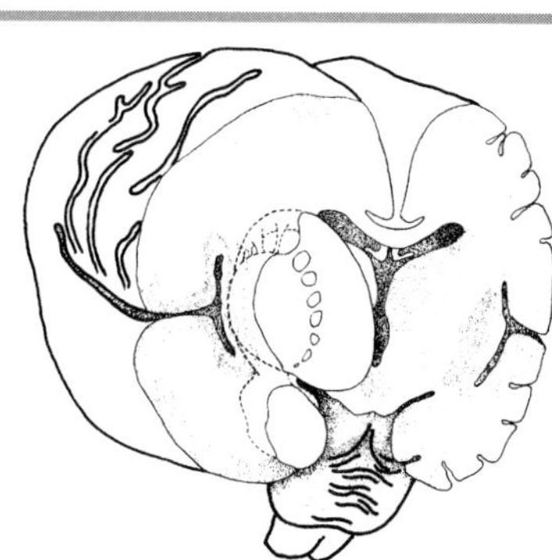

12.1A. gray

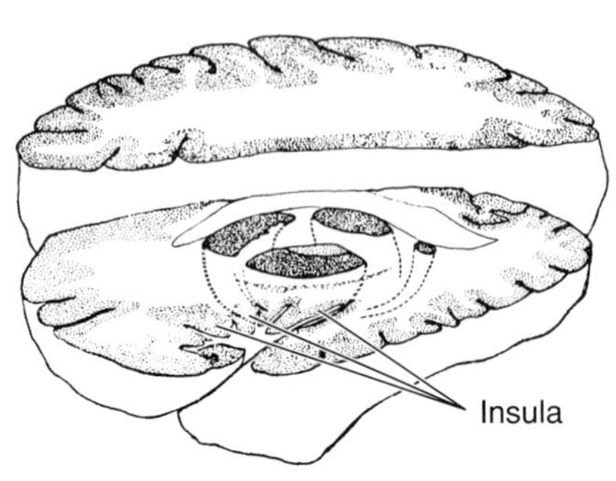

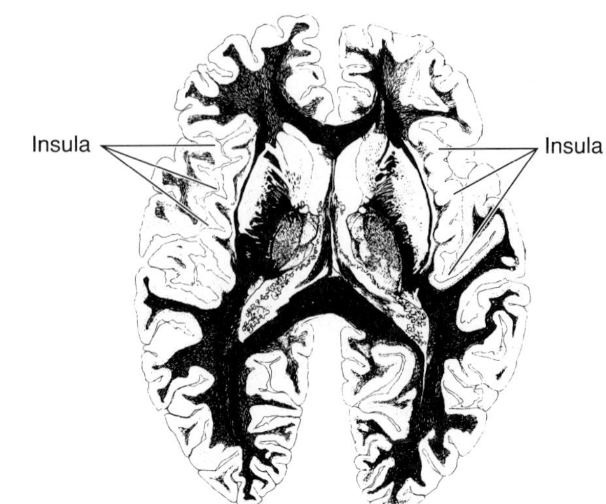

12.2A. insula

12.3A. gray

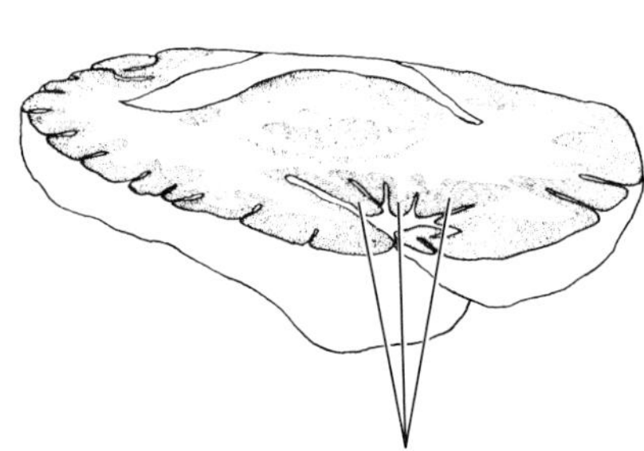

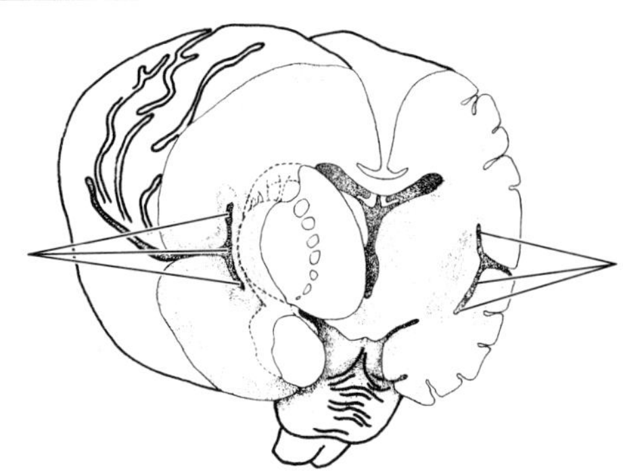

12.4. Deep to the surface of the insula, extending into its convolutions, is a thin zone of _____ matter.

12.5. While passing from the insula inward to the putamen, one crosses (in succession) the surface gray matter of the insula, thin zones of _____ matter, _____ matter, and _____ matter, and then putamen.

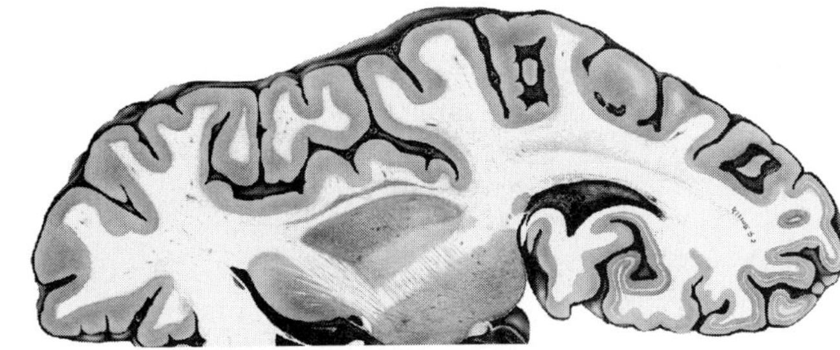

12.6. Just medial to the lenticular nucleus is the __________ capsule; just lateral to the lenticular nucleus is the __________ capsule.

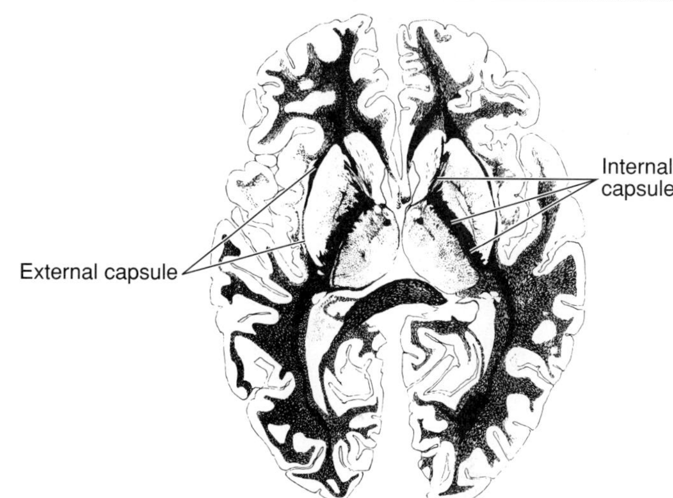

12.7. The internal and external capsules are _____ matter.

12.4A. white

12.5A. white; gray; white

12.6A. internal; external

12.7A. white

12.8. While passing from the putamen laterally, one crosses (in succession) the __________ __________, __________, __________ __________, and the surface gray matter of the __________.

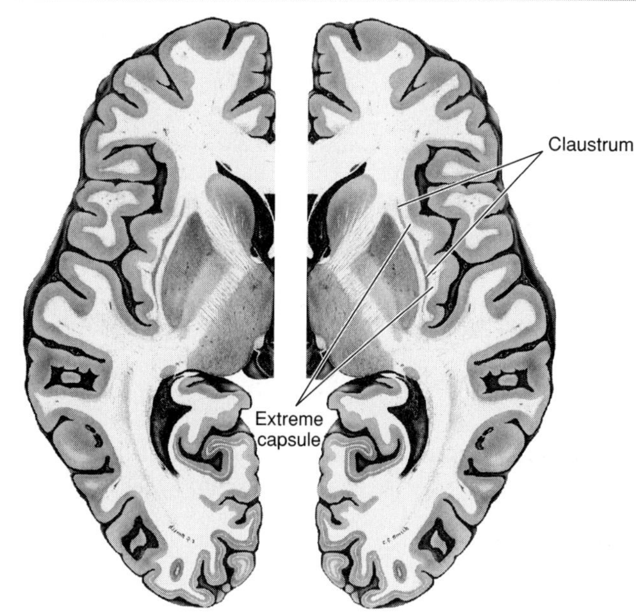

12.9. The pronunciation of the last two letters in "wow" is given to the "au" in cl______strum.

12.10. The cl______strum is ______ matter. It is usually classified (like caudate, putamen, and globus pallidus) as one of the ______ nuclei.

12.11. The claustrum has a very similar appearance in all horizontal sections. Draw an arrow to it on both sides of both figures.

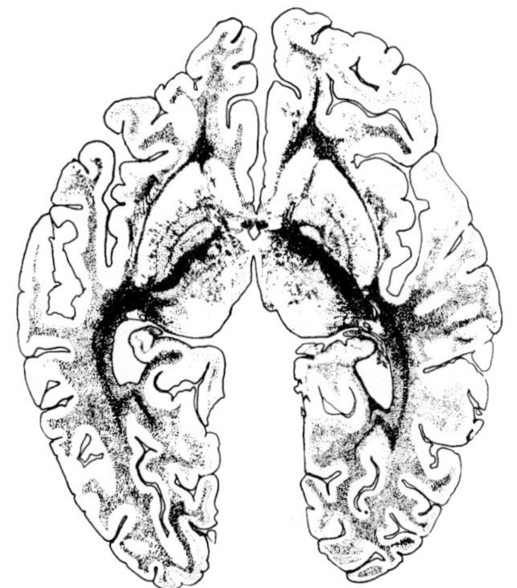

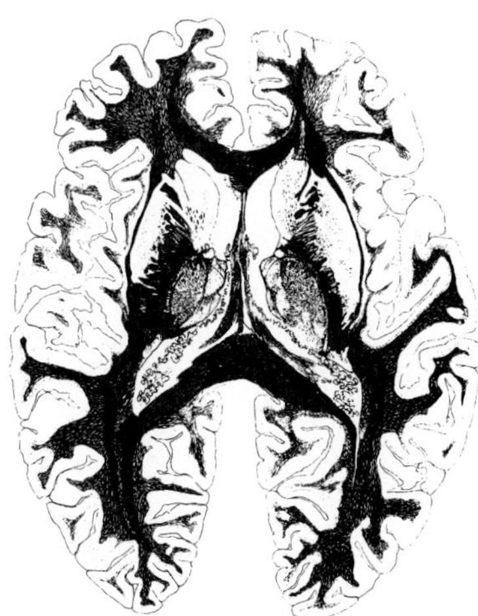

12.8A. external capsule; claustrum; extreme capsule; insula

12.9A. claustrum

12.10A. claustrum; gray; basal

12.11A.

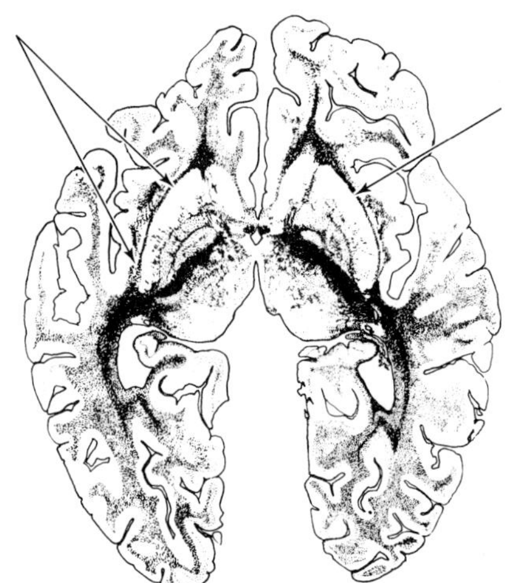

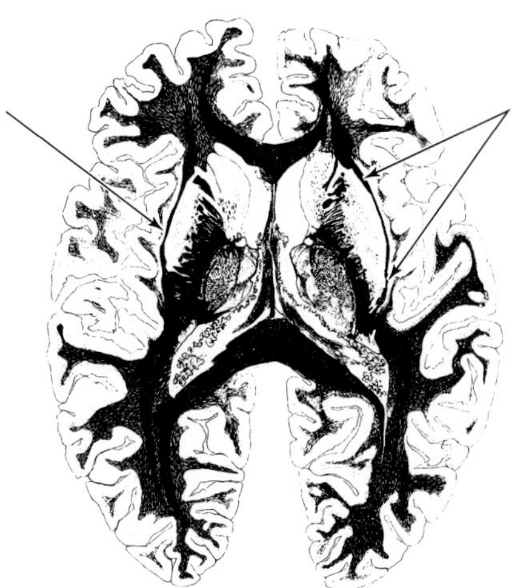

12.12. Even in sections cut at right angles to the previous ones, the claustrum looks about the same. Indicate it bilaterally with arrows.

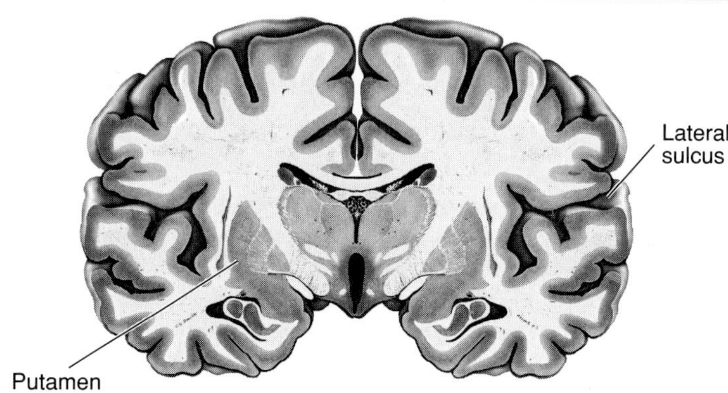

12.13. In this three-dimensional picture, the ____________ is a thin, somewhat crumpled sheet of gray matter separated from the putamen by the ____________ capsule.

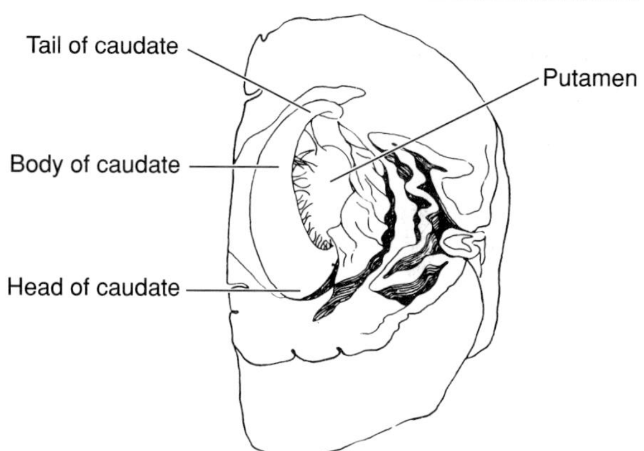

12.14. Label the internal capsule, external capsule, claustrum, and extreme capsule.

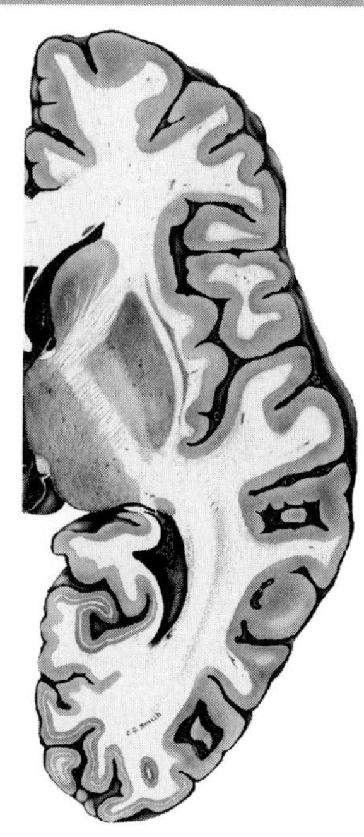

12.12A.

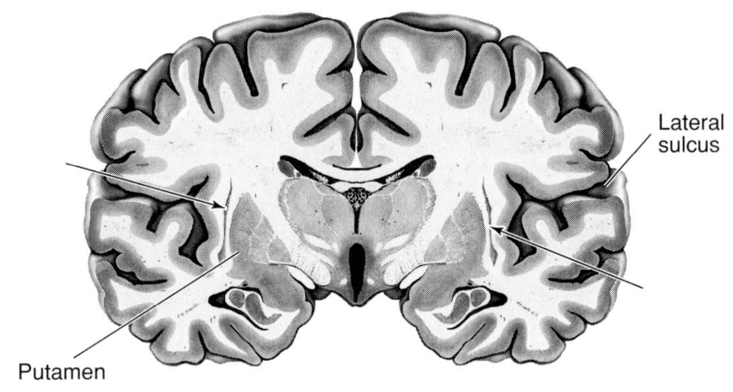

12.13A. claustrum; external

12.14A.

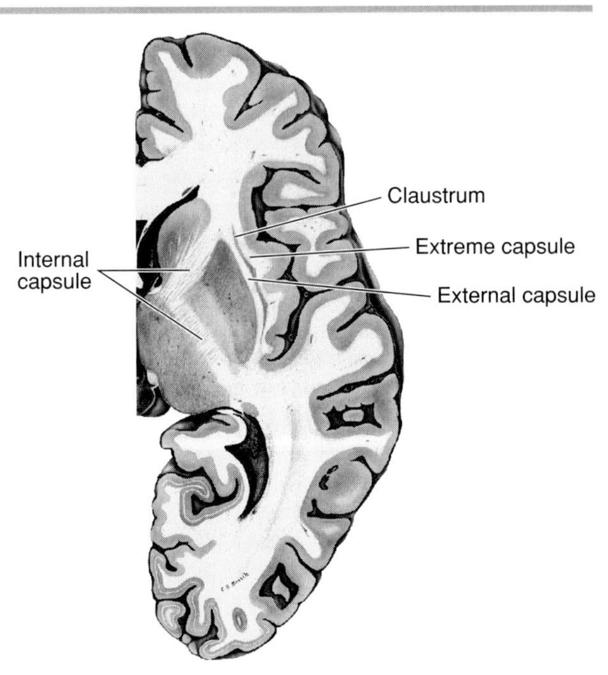

12.15. Indicate and name the white matter that separates the claustrum from the surface gray matter of the insula.

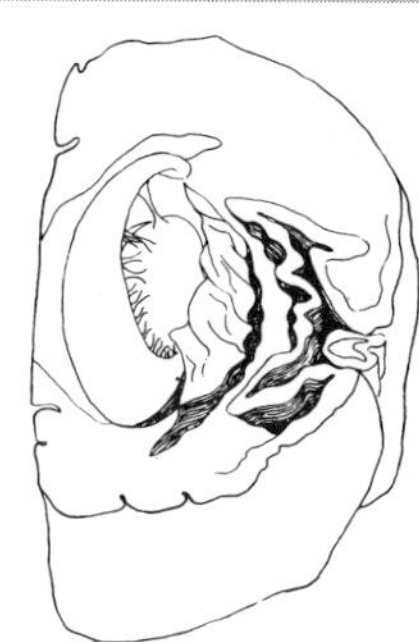

12.16. The extreme capsule is simply the white matter of a buried cortical surface region, the ____________.

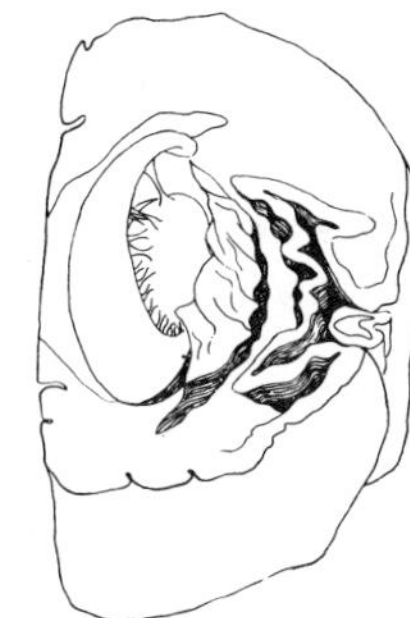

12.17. A section cut along the line drawn on the figure would cut across (beginning inferiorly) the ____________ in the temporal lobe and then the ____________________ nucleus and the junction of the ______ and ______ of the caudate.

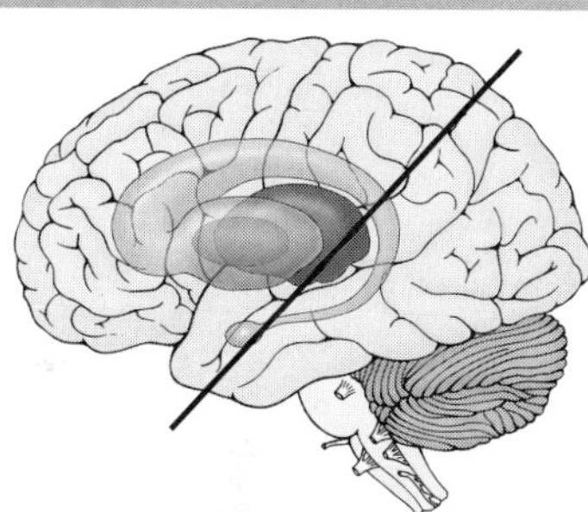

12.18. Basal nuclei are found in frontal, ____________, and ____________ lobes. List the four basal nuclei. Place checks beside the two basal nuclei that form the lenticular nucleus; place "X"s beside the two that form the striatum.

12.15A.

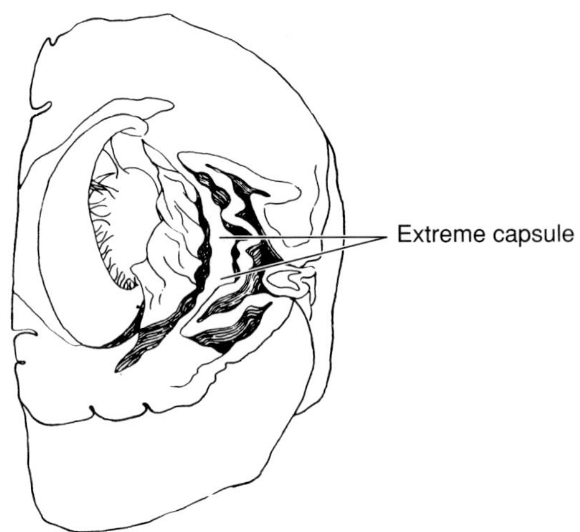

12.16A. insula

12.17A. amygdala; lenticular; tail; body

12.18A. parietal; temporal

Caudate ×

Putamen ✓ ×

Globus pallidus ✓

Amygdale

12.19. From the following list, select all of the white matter components and label them on the section:

Globus pallidus
External capsule
Extreme capsule
Corona radiata
Claustrum
Tail of caudate
Amygdala
Anterior limb of internal capsule
Corticospinal tract (show position in internal capsule)

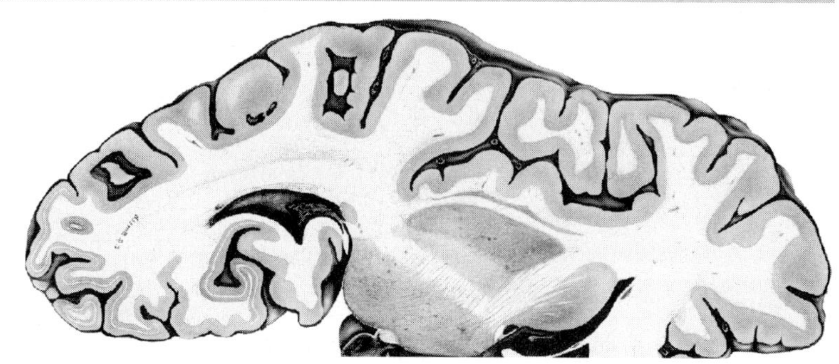

12.20. Label the extreme capsule, tail of caudate, head of caudate, globus pallidus, putamen, claustrum, and insula.

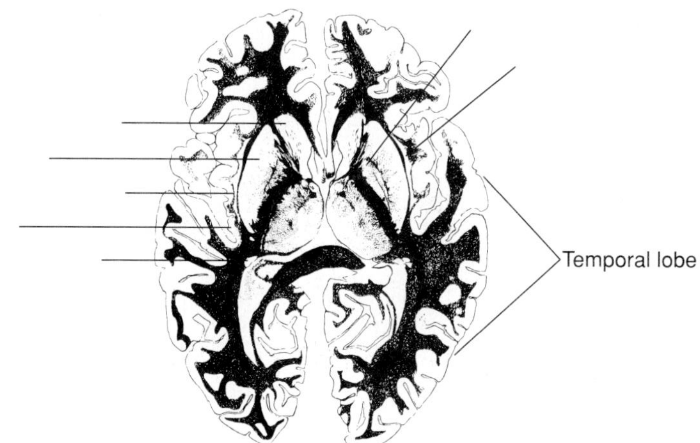

12.19A.

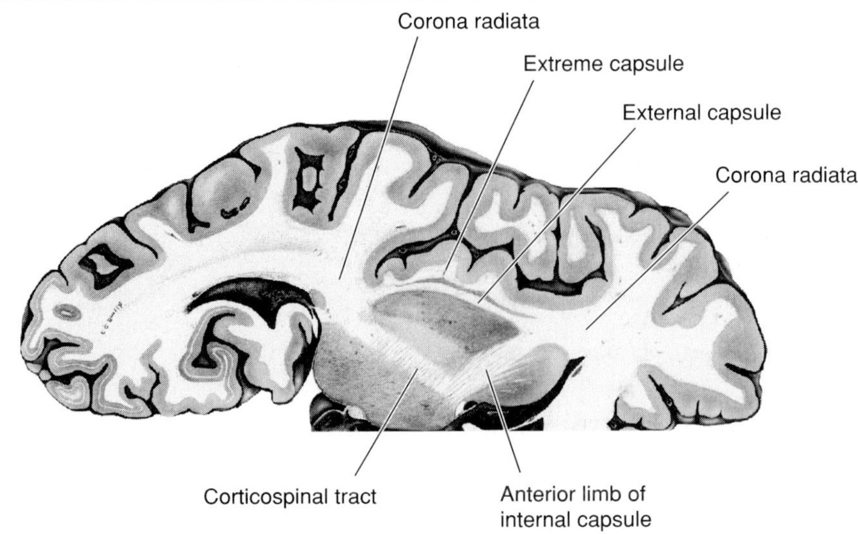
Corona radiata
Extreme capsule
External capsule
Corona radiata
Corticospinal tract
Anterior limb of internal capsule

12.20A.

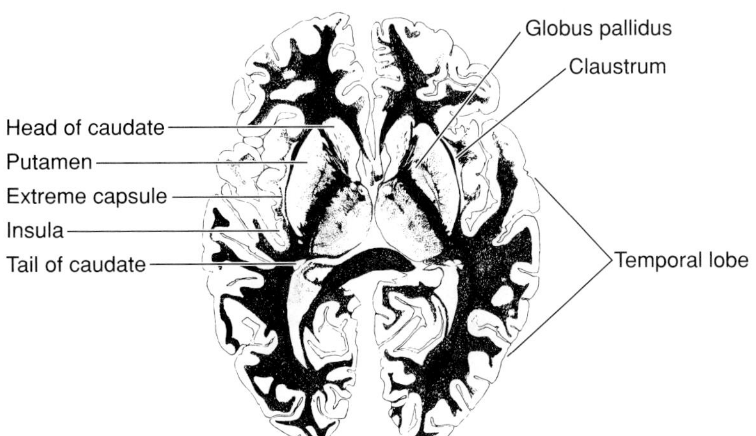
Globus pallidus
Claustrum
Head of caudate
Putamen
Extreme capsule
Insula
Tail of caudate
Temporal lobe

13 The Corticospinal System: Relations of Basal Nuclei to Thalamus

13.1. The name "thalamus" comes from the Greek word "thalamos" for couch, or bed. The cerebral hemispheres lie on the thalamus. Label the thalamus on the diagram.

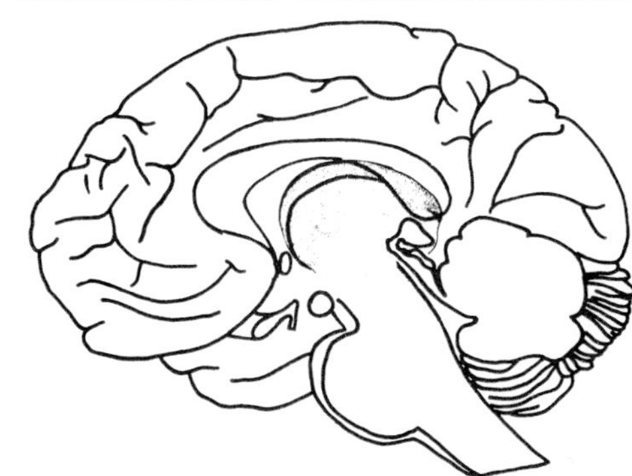

13.2. The thalamus has no distinct inferior border; it merges with the superior end of the ____________ region of the brainstem. The arrows point to the anterior- ______ ior border of the thalamus.

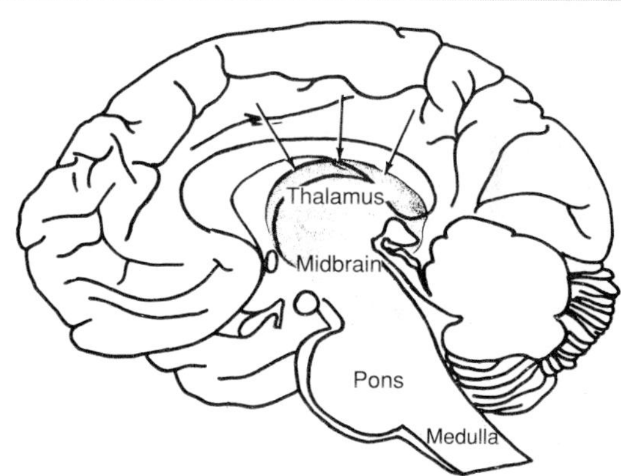

13.3. The arrows point to a thin groove that separates the ____________ below from the ____________ nucleus.

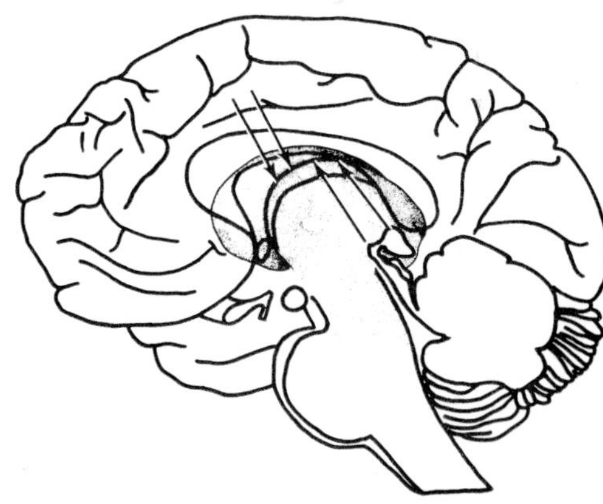

13.4. The "X" lies on the ____________ ior part of the corpus ____________, cut sagittally at midline. The dark tissue partially covered by the "X" is the posterolateral part of the ____________.

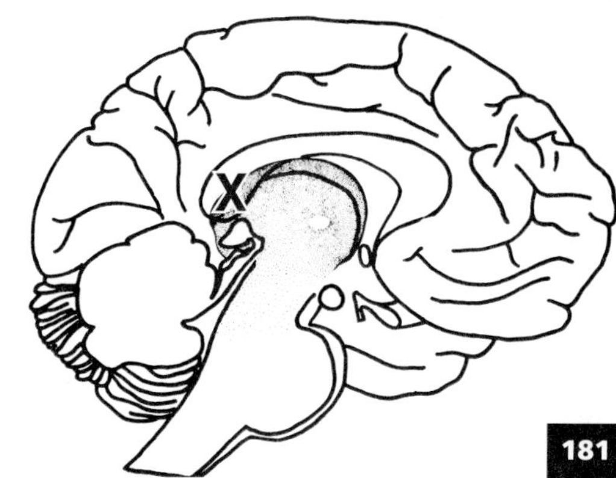

13.1A.

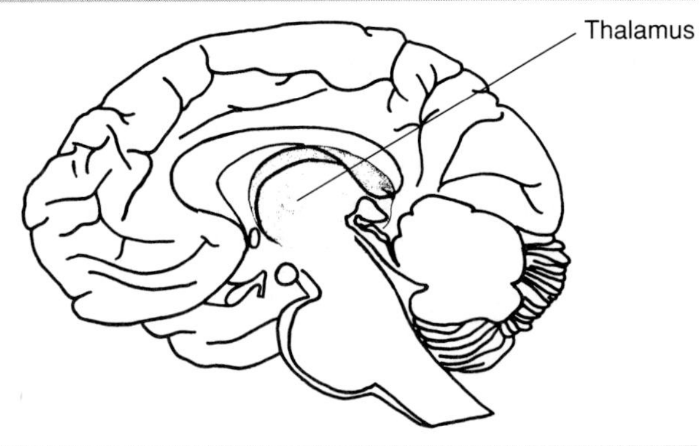

13.2A. midbrain; anterior-superior

13.3A. thalamus; caudate

13.4A. posterior; callosum; thalamus

13.5. In the left hand picture, the thalamus is opaque; in the right hand picture, it is transparent. The body of the caudate disappears from view at the arrow because it lies ______al to the thalamus.

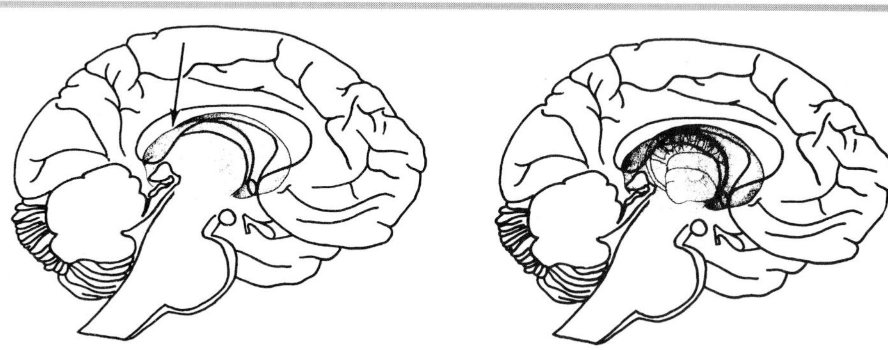

13.6. The arrows in each picture point to the groove between the __________ and __________.

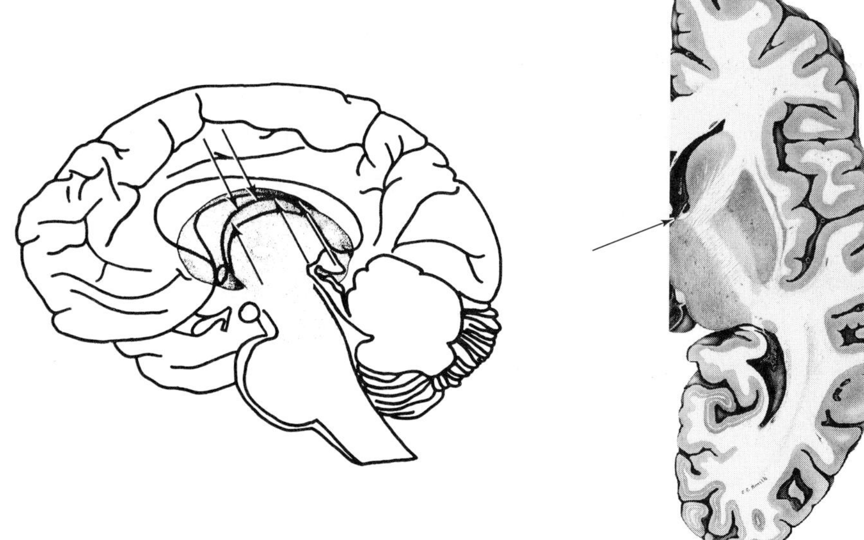

13.7. The line indicates the approximate plane of the horizontal section. Place an "H" on the line where it passes through the head of caudate, a "TH" where it passes through the thalamus, and a "T" where it passes through the tail of caudate. Label these three structures the same way on the horizontal section.

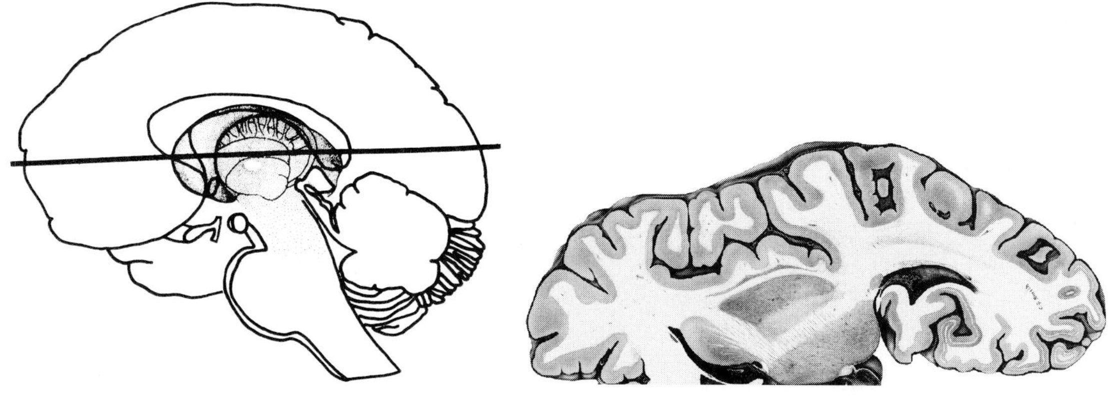

13.5A. lateral

13.6A. thalamus; caudate

13.7A.

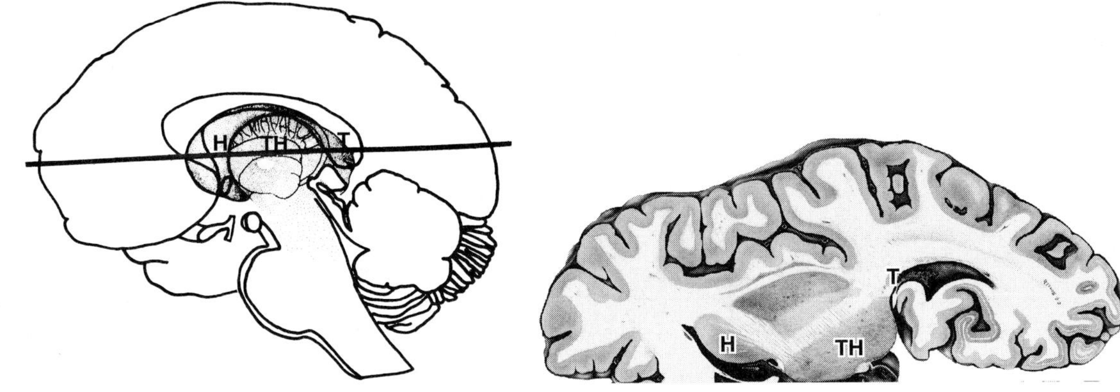

13.8. On the left hand picture, label with an "X" the gray matter structure that rises above the plane of the right hand section and is represented on that section by broken lines.

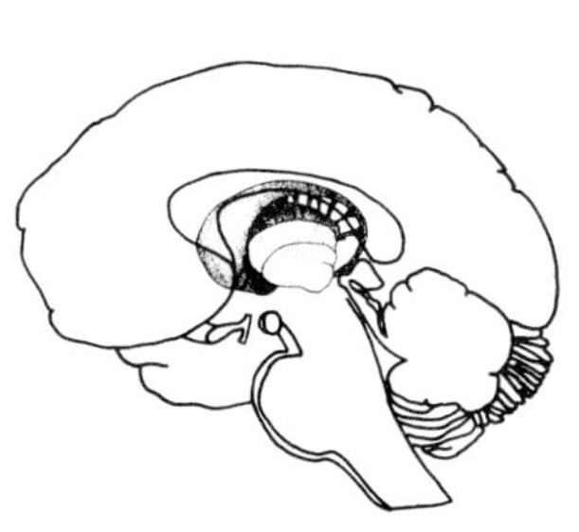

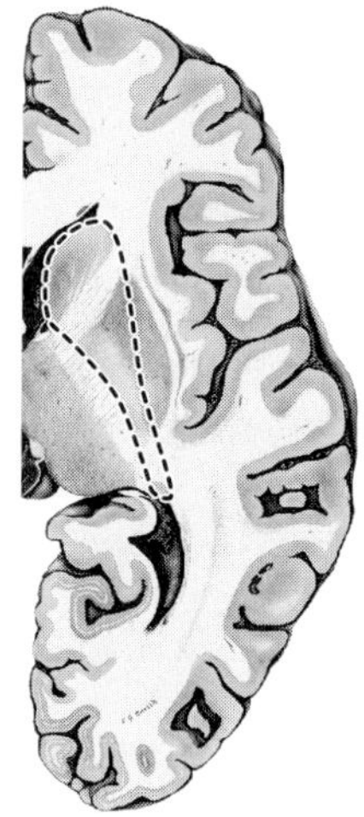

13.9. The head of the caudate lies close to the midline. It does not get in the way of the thalamus because it lies ____________ to the thalamus. Label the head of the caudate (H) and thalamus (TH) on the left side.

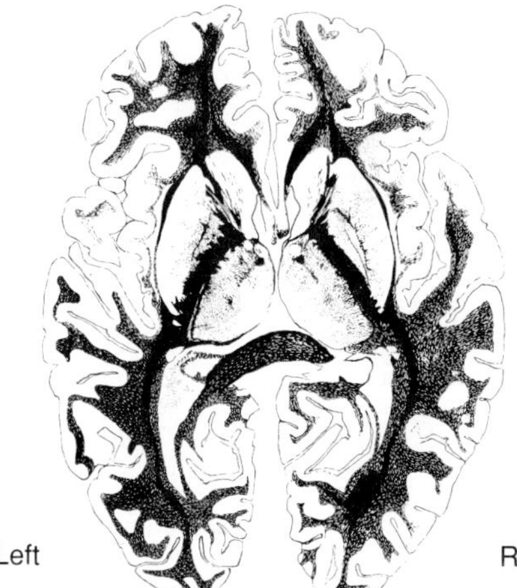

13.10. The brain contains two caudate nuclei, two lateral sulci, and ______ precentral gyri. The thalamus is also a paired structure, with the left and right sides joined by an ______ thalamic adhesion.

13.11. From the head of the caudate, one passes in a ____________ direction to reach the thalamus.

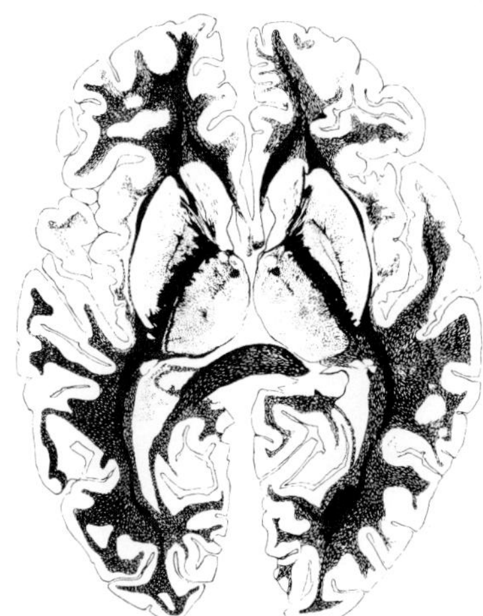

13.8A.

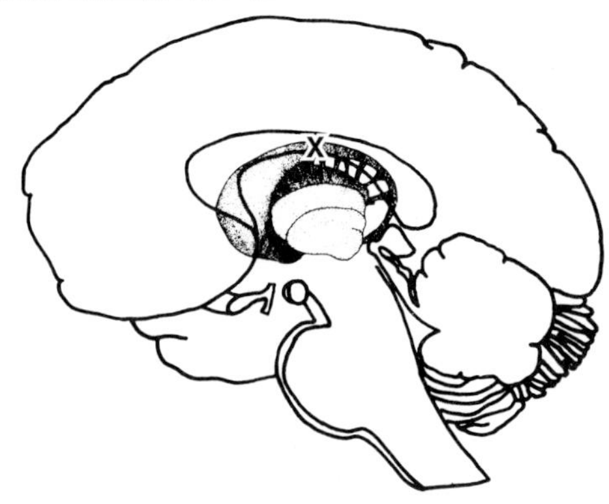

13.9A. rostral

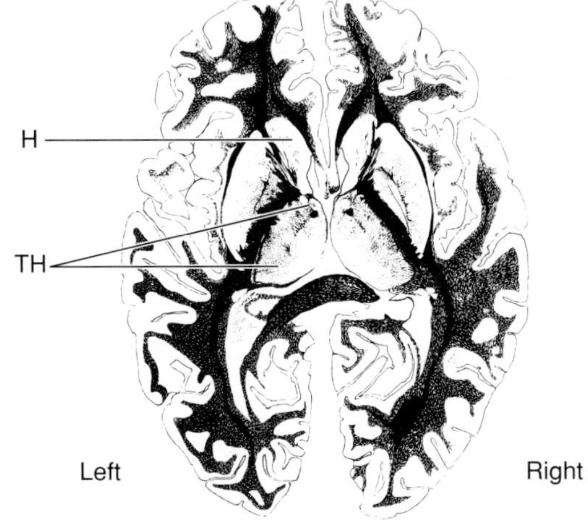

13.10A. two; interthalamic

13.11A. posterior

13.12. The tail of the caudate lies __________ ior and __________ to the head of the caudate.

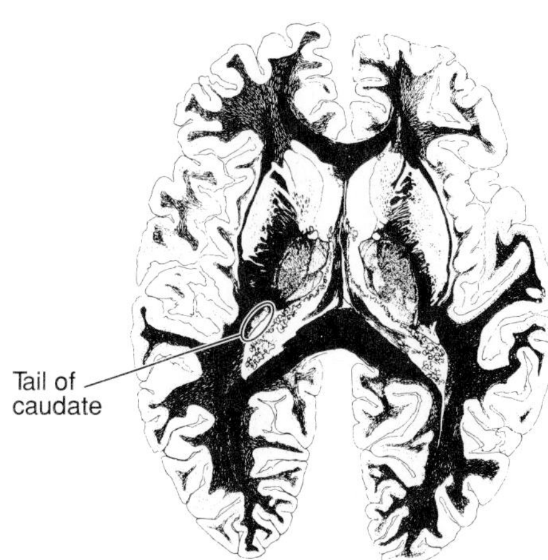

13.13. If the body of the caudate did not move laterally as it moves in a posterior direction, it would bump into the __________.

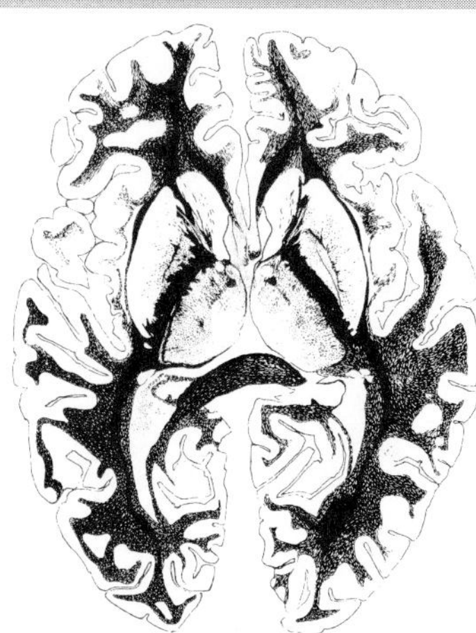

13.14. As the body of the caudate passes posteriorly from the head toward the tail, it gradually turns also in an inferior and __________ direction. The end of the tail is in the __________ lobe. In the bottom picture, encircle the tail of the caudate and place a "V" in the adjacent part of the lateral ventricle.

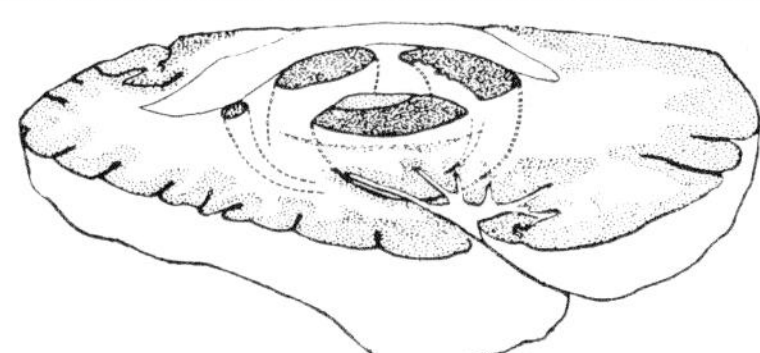

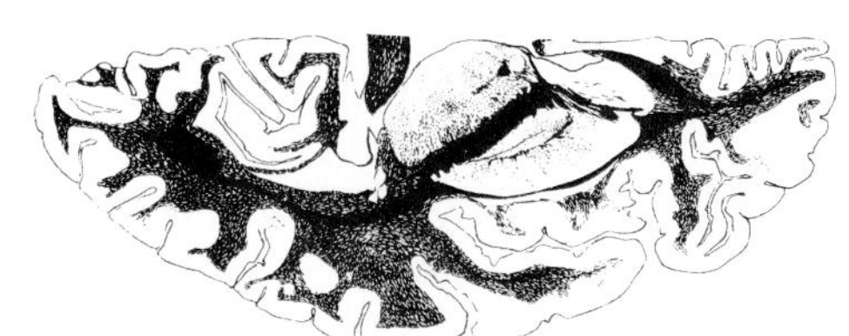

13.15. The tail of the caudate lies slightly posterior and __________ to the thalamus.

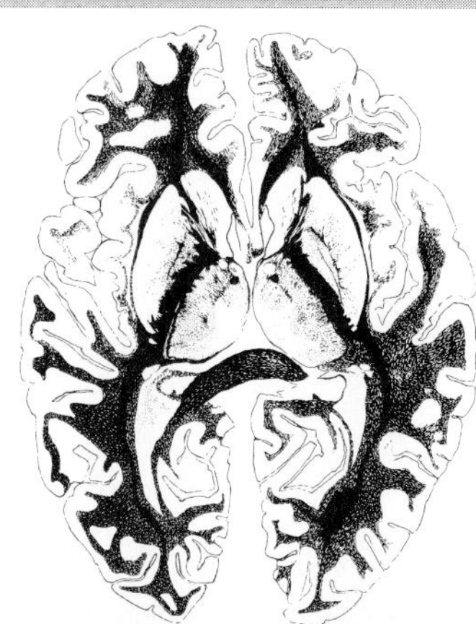

13.12A. posterior; lateral

13.13A. thalamus

13.14A. lateral; temporal

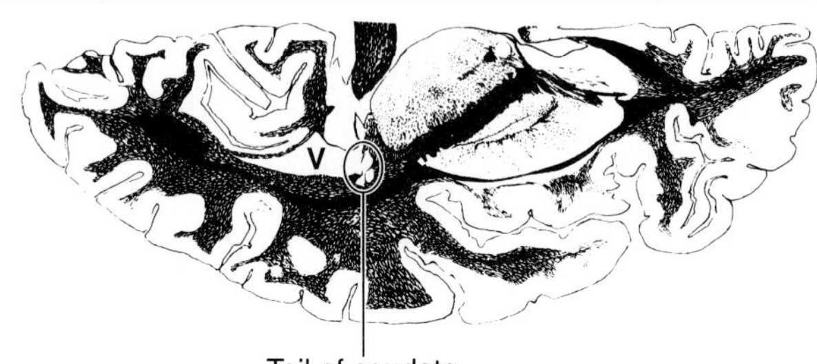

13.15A. lateral

13.16. The anterior limb of the internal capsule separates the lenticular nucleus from the ___________. The posterior limb of the internal capsule separates the lenticular nucleus from the ___________.

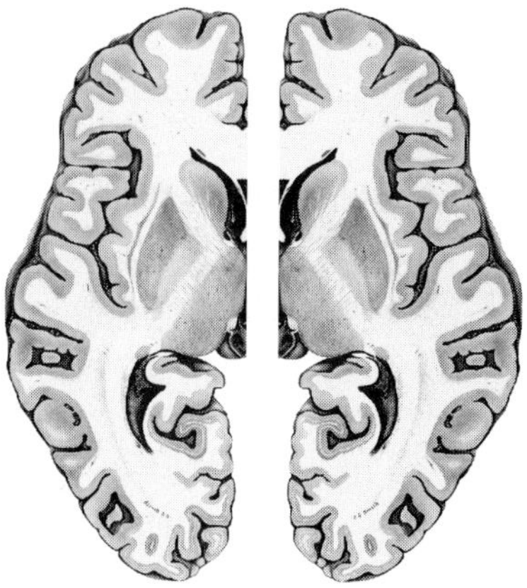

13.17. In *all* planes of section, the internal capsule lies ___________ to the thalamus and medial (internal) to the _________________ nucleus.

13.18. The thalamus is a large collection of cell bodies with many internal subdivisions. Like the basal nuclei, it is composed of _____ matter; unlike the basal nuclei, it is continuous with the brain _____.

13.19. The brainstem is joined to the cerebral hemispheres by a wall of white matter, the ___________ limb of the ___________ ___________. Encircle this white matter structure on both sides.

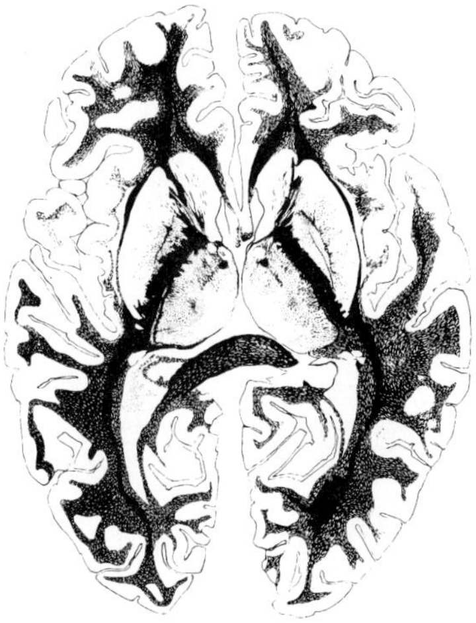

13.20. The thalamus lies ___________ to the posterior limb of the internal capsule.

13.21. The internal capsule is a part of the cerebral hemisphere and encapsulates (is the "internal capsule" of) the _________________ nucleus.

13.22. Information from sense organs often reaches the thalamus. The thalamus may then relay impulses to the cerebral cortex. With respect to the cortex, such impulses are _____ fferent.

13.16A. caudate; thalamus

13.17A. lateral (external); lenticular

13.18A. gray; brainstem

13.19A. posterior; internal capsule

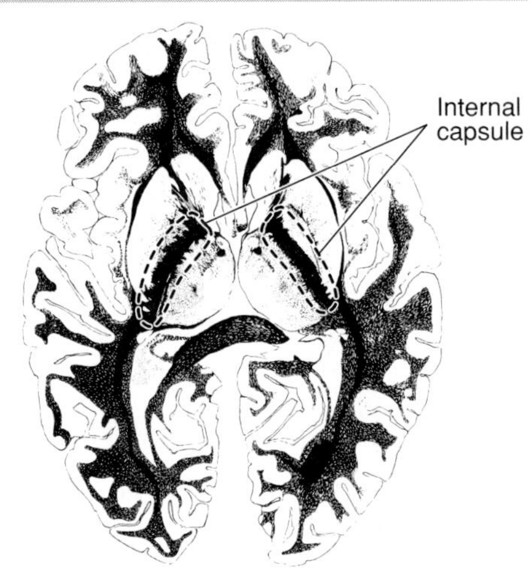

13.20A. medial

13.21A. lenticular

13.22A. afferent

14 The Corticospinal System, Basal Nuclei, and Thalamus

14.1. Sections cut at right angles to the horizontal plane, as illustrated and labeled, are in the __________ plane.

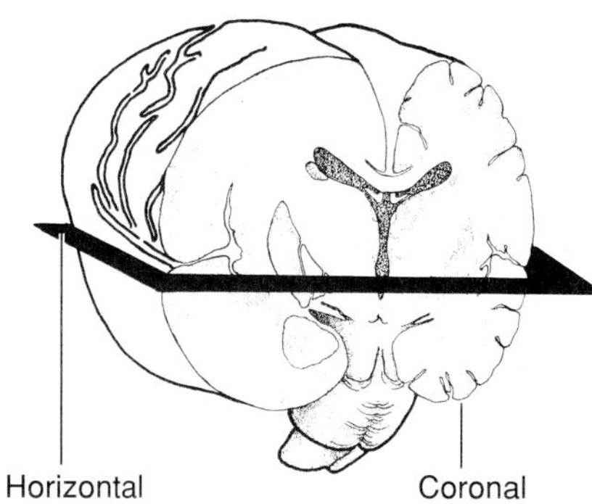

14.2. Look at the caudate and putamen. You are _____ ior to the brain. On the _____ side of the picture, a schematic representation of the __________ __________ is superimposed on the section, which is cut in the __________ plane.

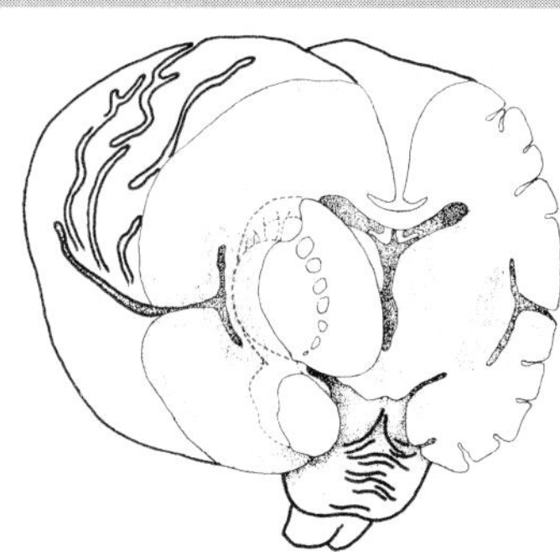

14.3. Label the indicated structures.

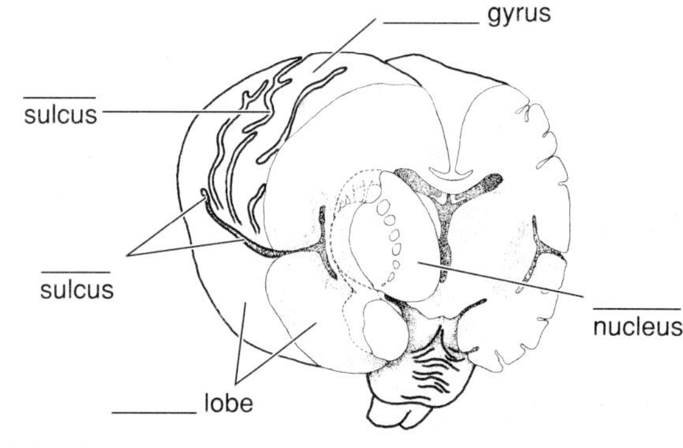

14.4. Place an "A" and a "B" on the putamen and head of caudate, respectively, where they project anteriorly from the cut surface.

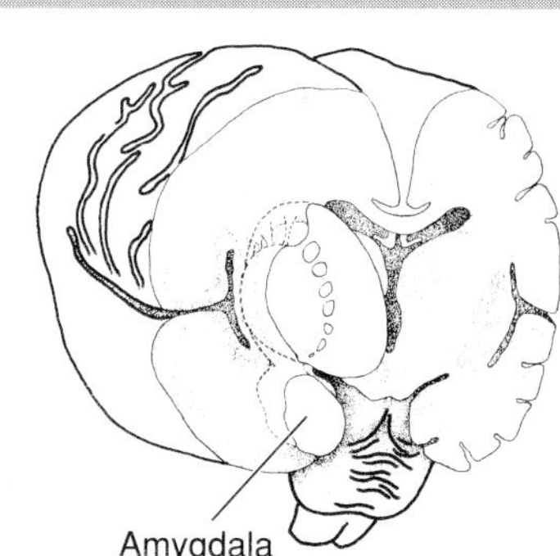

14.1A. coronal

14.2A. anterior; right; caudate nucleus; coronal

14.3A.

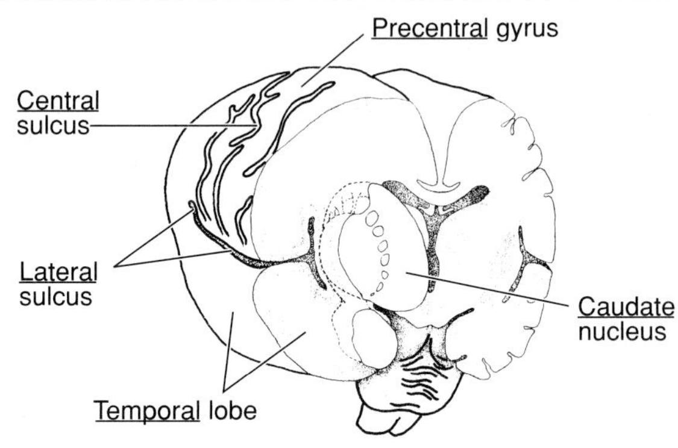

14.4A.

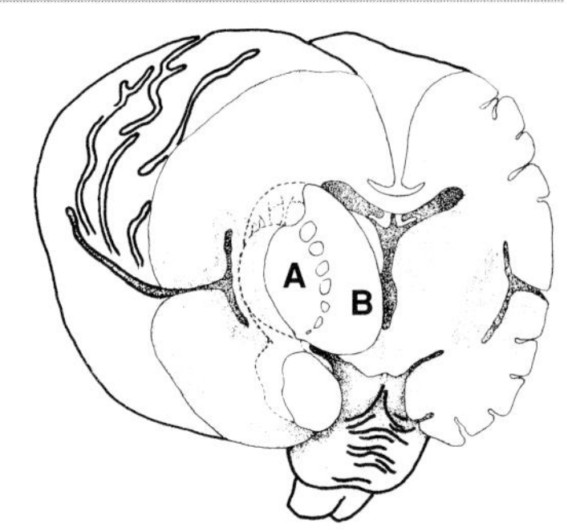

14.5. Place an "X" on the lateral surface of the lenticular nucleus where it is shown posterior to the plane of section. Indicate with an arrow where the body of the caudate emerges from the cut surface.

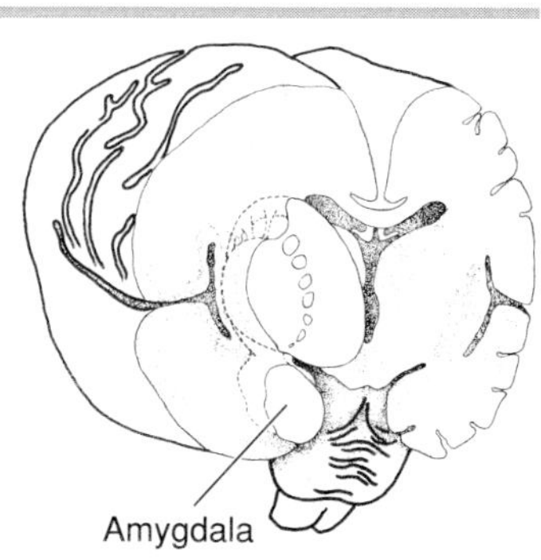

14.6. On the *cut* surface of the right hand diagram, label the amygdala, lenticular nucleus, and body of caudate.

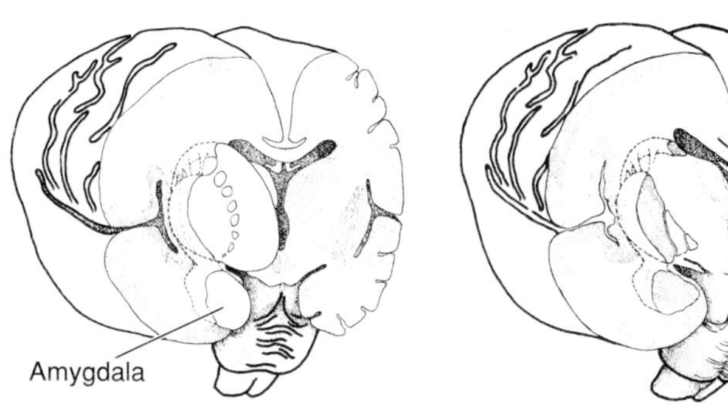

14.7. In a coronal section cut along plane "A," the thalamus lies mainly ______ al to the lenticular nucleus. The thalamus lies ____________ ior to the head of the caudate.

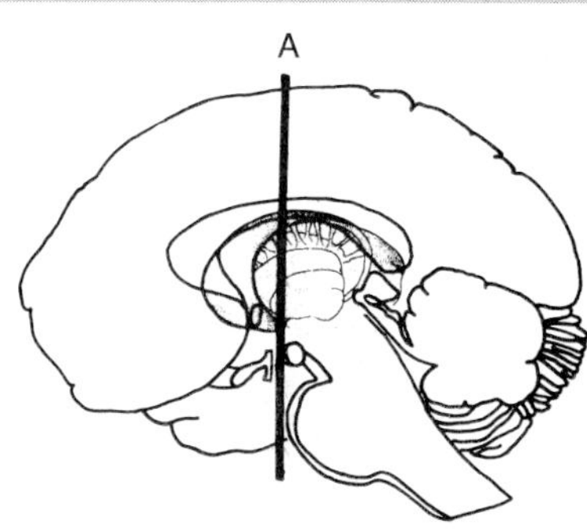

14.8. On the *cut surface* of *both* sides of the diagram, label the lenticular nucleus (L), body of caudate (C), amygdala (A), thalamus (T), and internal capsule (IC). In the indicated space above and below the picture, place the appropriate labels: superior (S) and inferior (I).

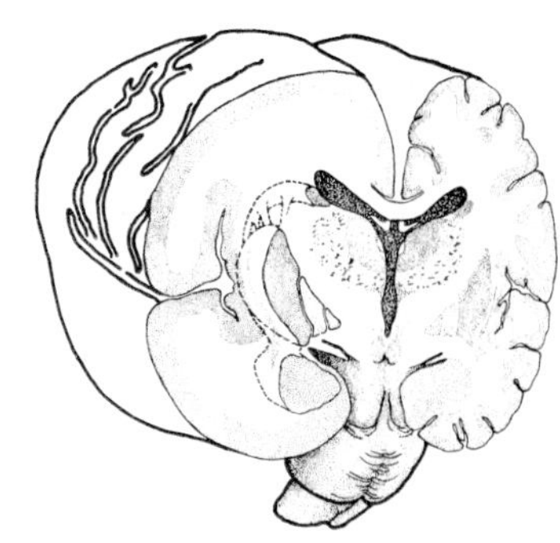

14.5A.

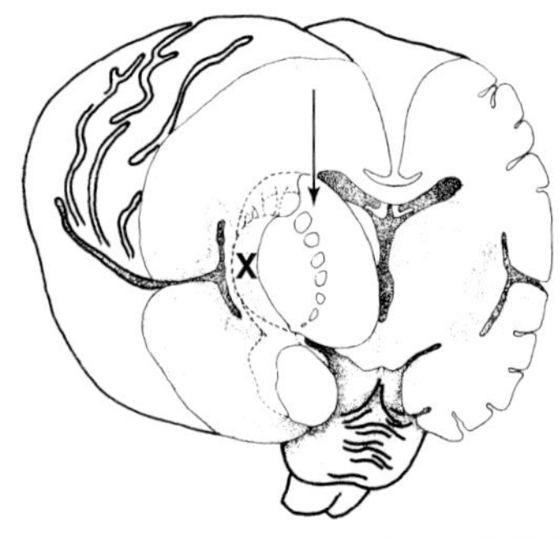

14.6A.

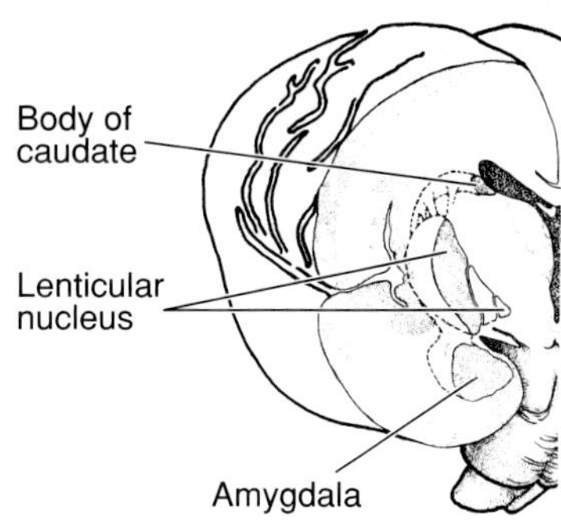

14.7A. medial; posterior

14.8A.

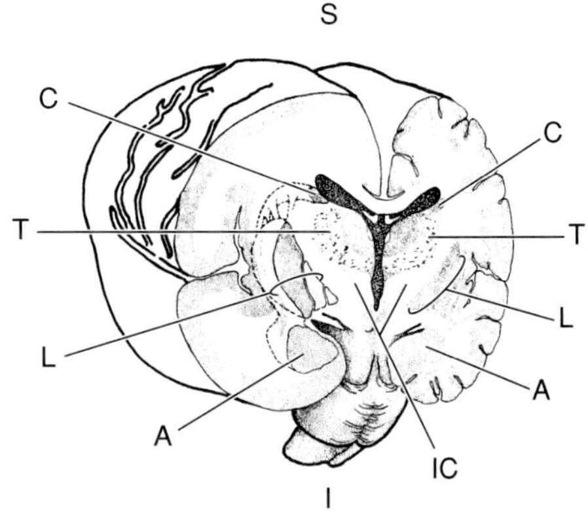

14.9. The left hand coronal section has been stained for ____________. Draw lines between the two diagrams to connect the following structures and label each appropriately: lenticular nucleus (L), internal capsule (IC), thalamus (T), body of caudate (C), and amygdala (A).

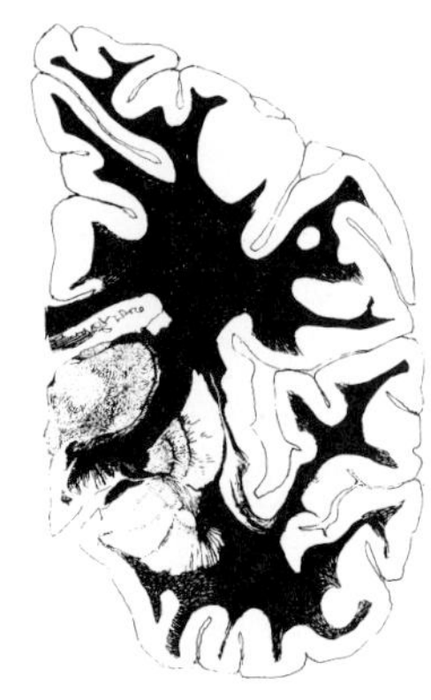

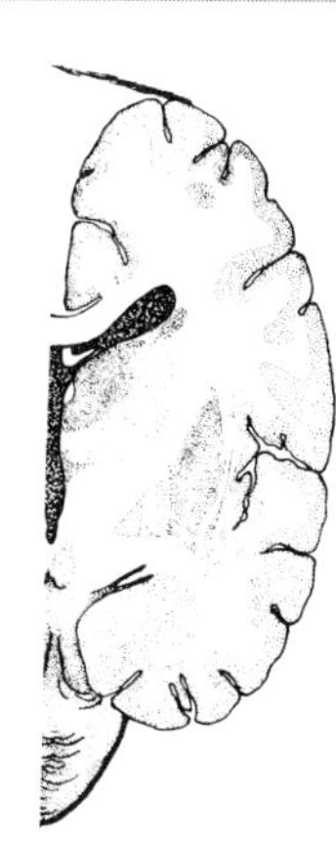

14.10. In the indicated space above and below each section, place the appropriate labels: anterior (A), posterior (P), superior (S), and inferior (I).

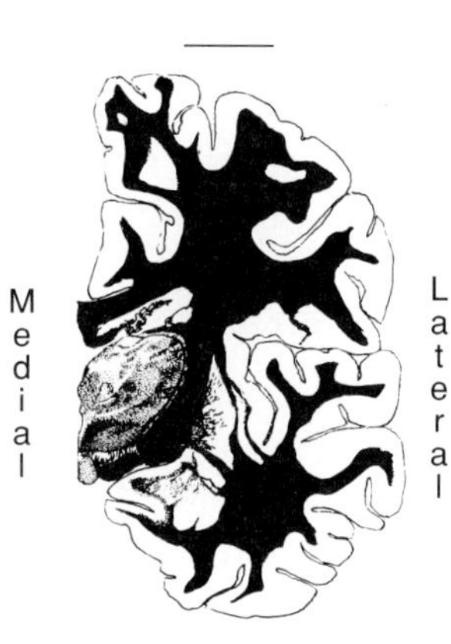

Coronal section

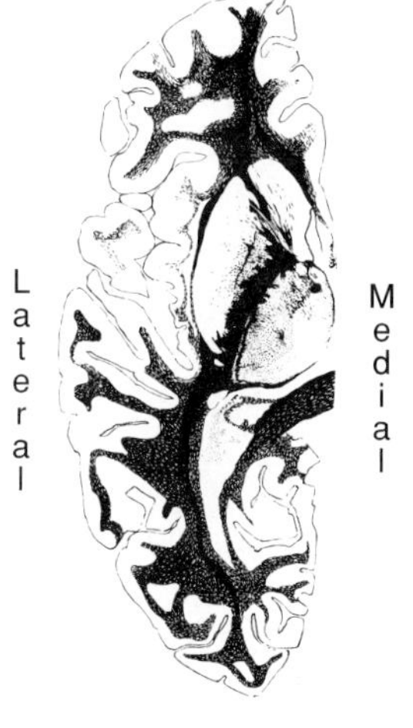

Horizontal section

14.11. In coronal sections at the levels marked "A," "B," and "C," section "A" passes through the ______ of the caudate but not through the thalamus; starting laterally, section "B" passes through the lenticular nucleus and then through myelinated fibers of the ________________ tract in the ____________ limb of the internal capsule; section "C" just catches the lenticular nucleus, then the internal capsule, and then passes through the broad part of the ____________.

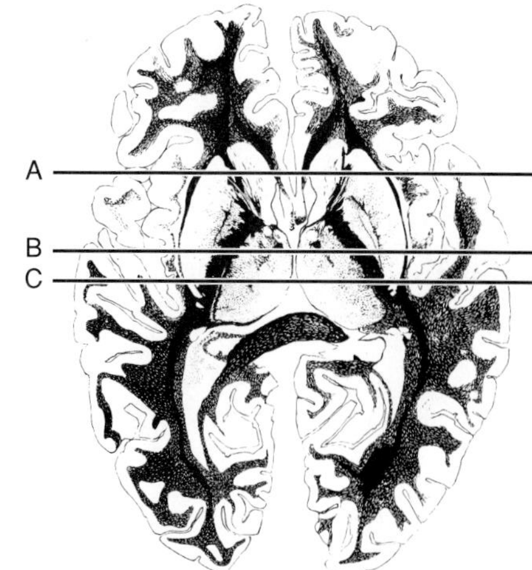

14.9A. myelin

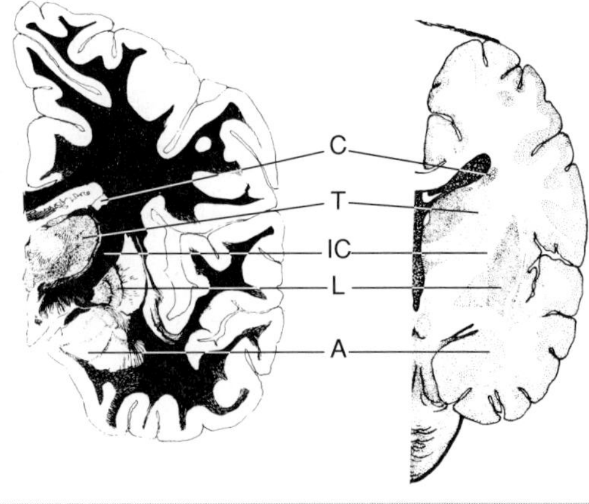

14.10A.

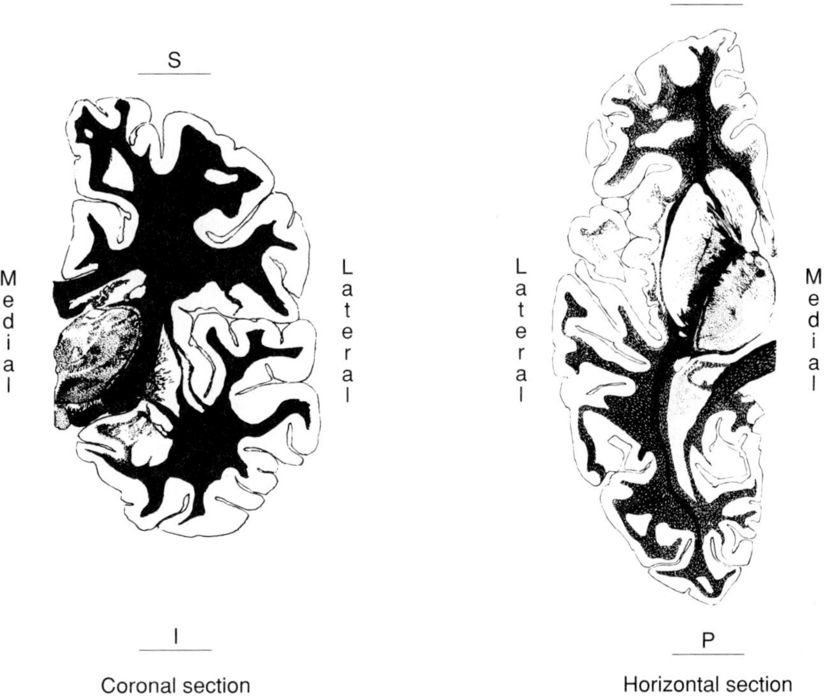

14.11A. head; corticospinal; posterior; thalamus

14.12. Does the coronal section show the globus pallidus? ______ The level of the coronal section is indicated at ______ on the horizontal section.

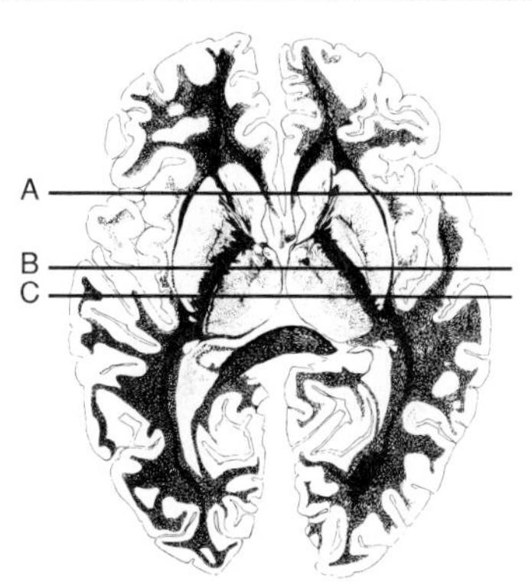

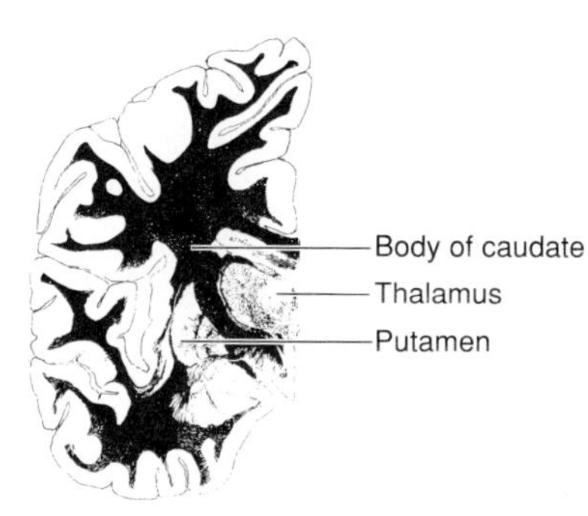

14.13. The thalamus lies ____________ ior to the *head* of the caudate.

14.14. Check the names of four structures that could be cut across in one coronal section:

______ Head of caudate

______ Body of caudate

______ Posterior limb of internal capsule

______ Lenticular nucleus

______ Calcarine fissure

______ Thalamus

14.15. Does the right hand section show the globus pallidus? ______ The thalamus? ______ The level of the right hand section is indicated at ______ on the section to the left. Beneath each section, indicate its plane.

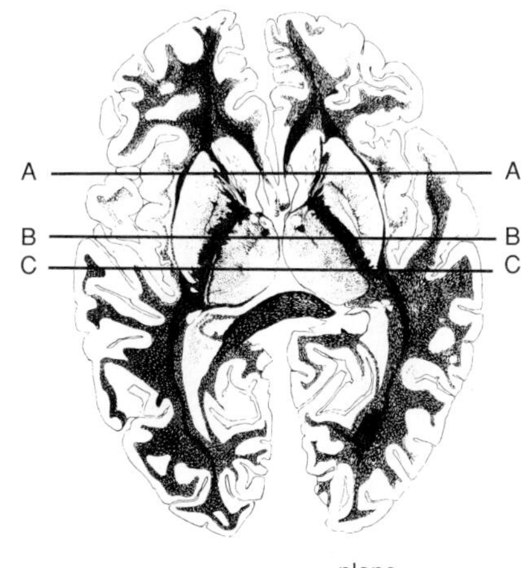

______ plane

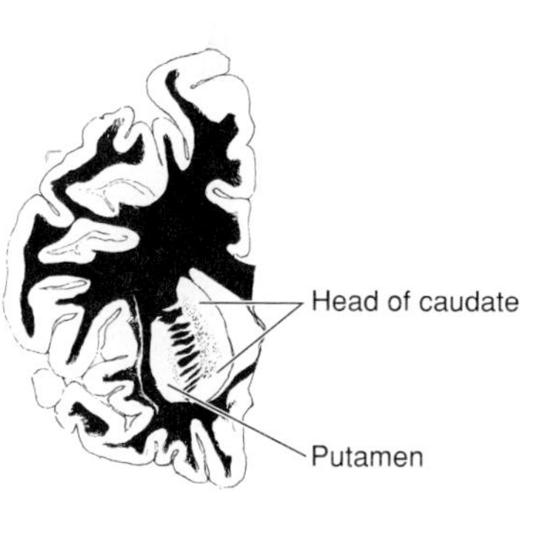

______ plane

14.16. This coronal section shows putamen connected to the head of the caudate by cell bridges. Label the putamen (P), head of the caudate (H), and lateral ventricle (LV).

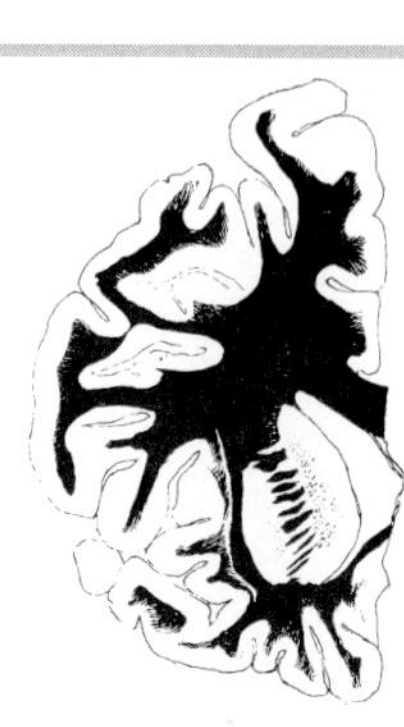

14.12A. Yes; B

14.13A. posterior

14.14A.

______ Head of caudate
__√__ Body of caudate
__√__ Posterior limb of internal capsule
__√__ Lenticular nucleus
______ Calcarine fissure
__√__ Thalamus

14.15A. No; No; A

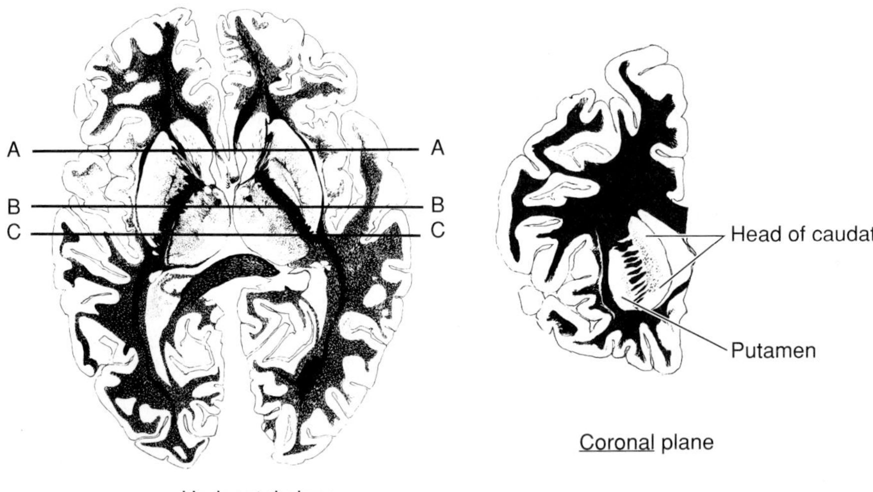

14.16A.

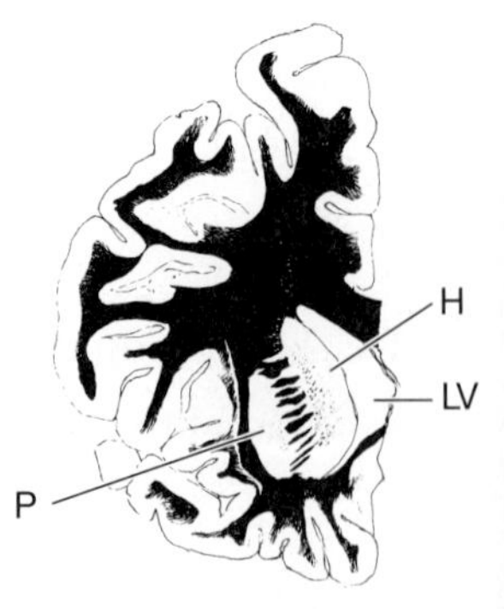

14.17. In this coronal section, the body of the caudate is separated from the lenticular nucleus by the junction of the corona radiata and internal capsule. Label the body of caudate, thalamus, and putamen.

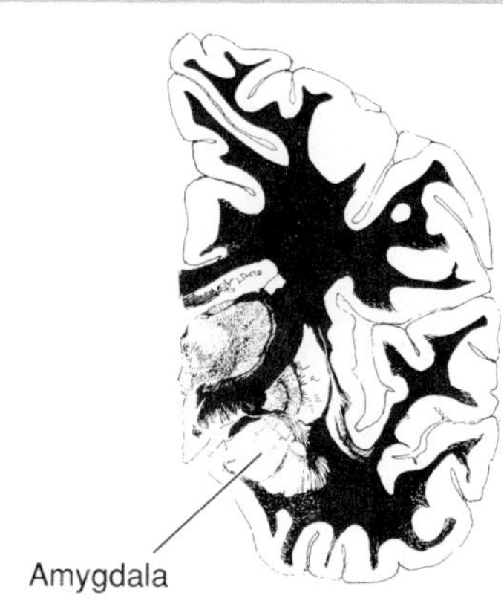

14.18. Indicate with a check the more anterior of the two coronal sections.

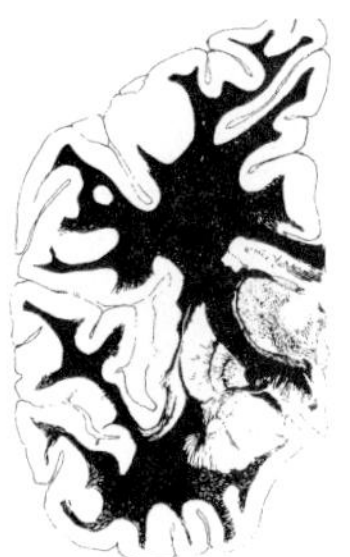

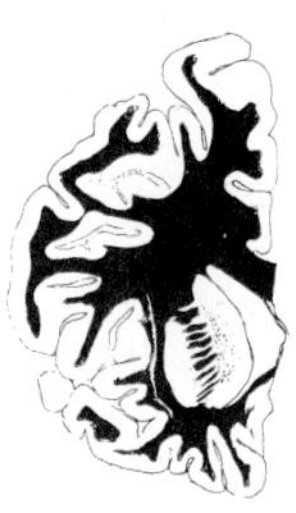

14.19. Vertical sections cut through the same level in left and right cerebral hemispheres are called ____________ sections. Sections cut roughly parallel to the ground are called ____________________ sections. Sagittal sections are a third type that are also vertical but are cut through the midline or through one hemisphere from ____________ to ____________.

14.20. Label the indicated structures.

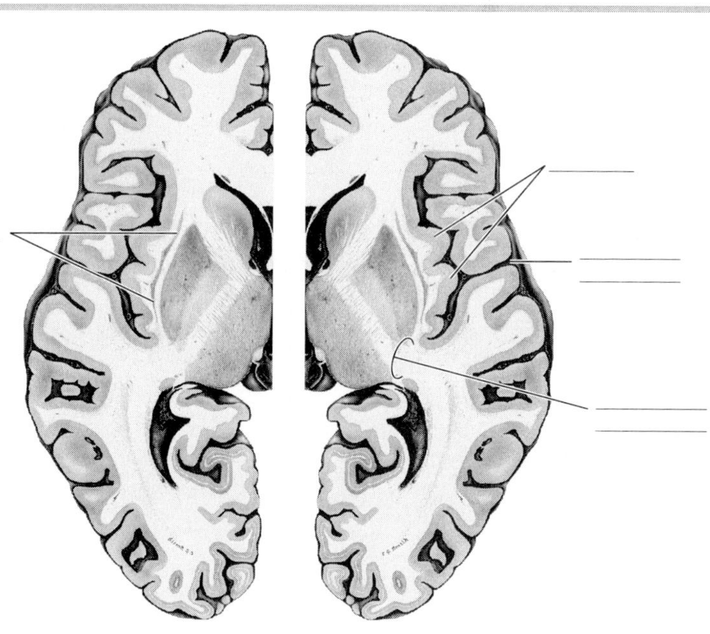

14.17A.

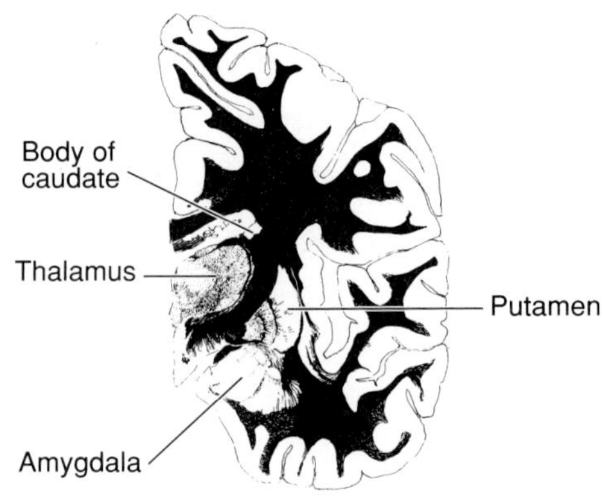

14.18A.

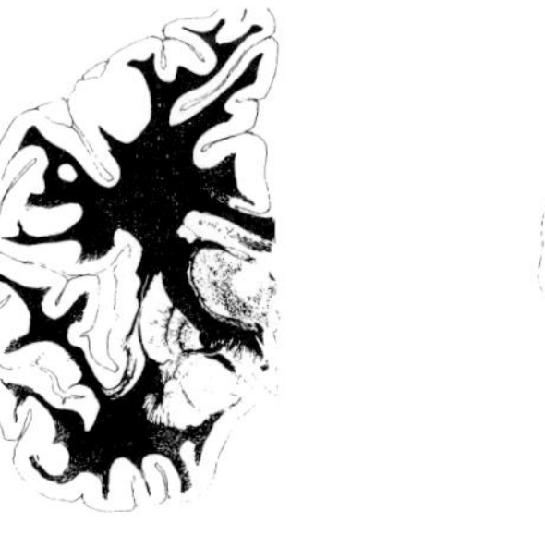

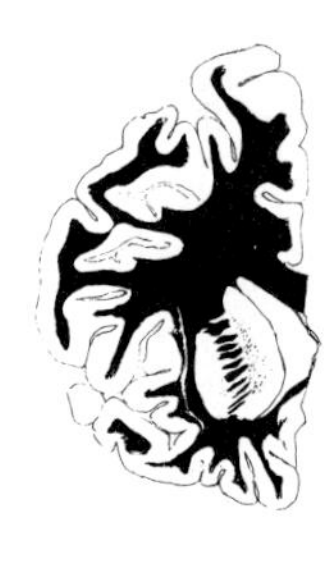

14.19A. coronal; horizontal; anterior; posterior

14.20A.

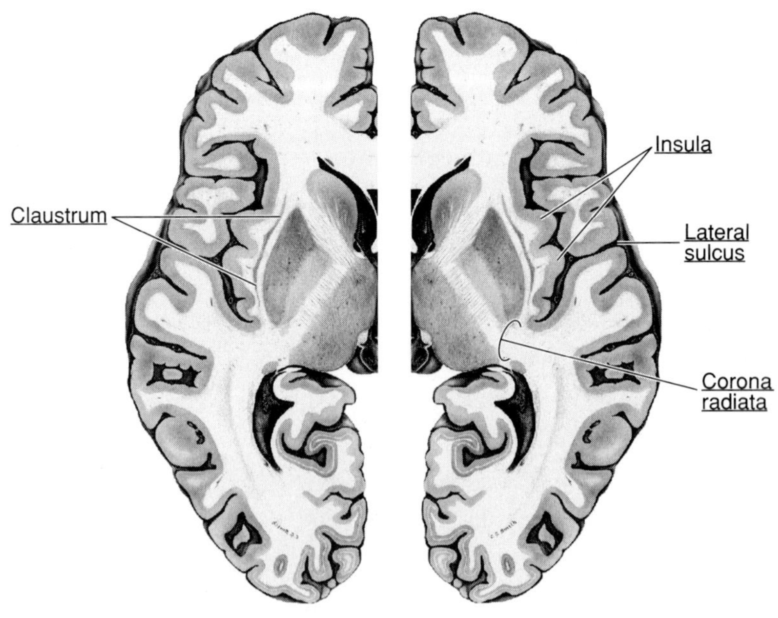

14.21. Label the indicated structures.

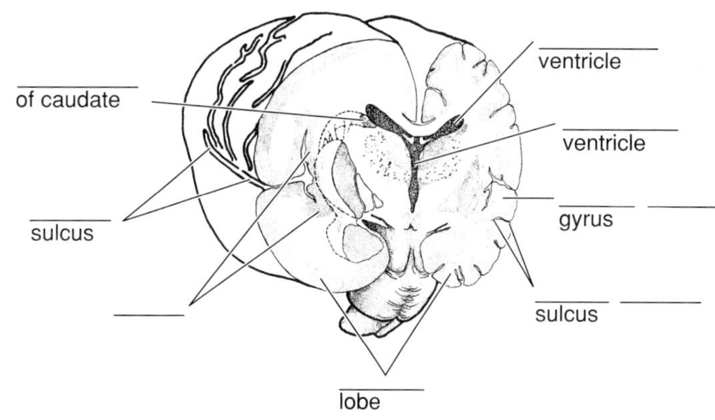

14.22. Draw lines to the appropriate structures.

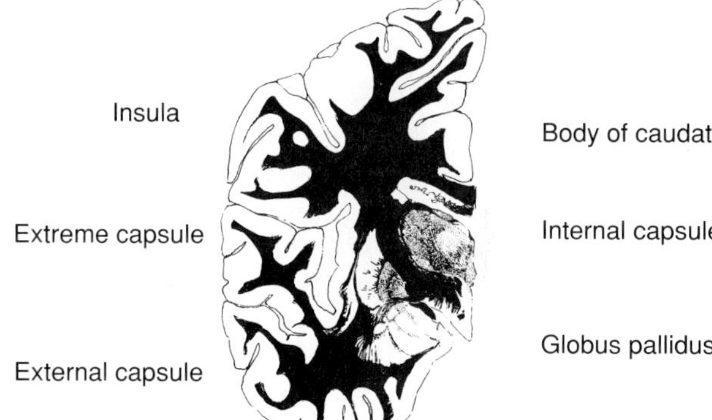

14.23. Draw a line through the left hand diagram to indicate the plane of the right hand section.

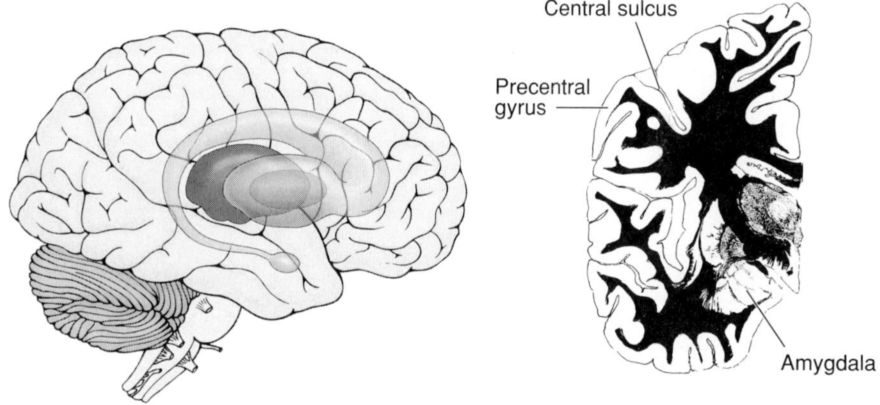

14.24. In this diagram, is the frontal pole at your left or your right? ______ The broadest part of the thalamus lies at a level that is posterior and __________ to the broadest part of the lenticular nucleus.

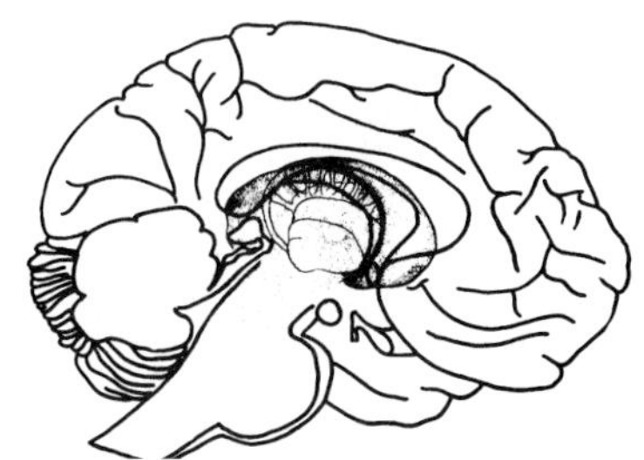

14.21A.

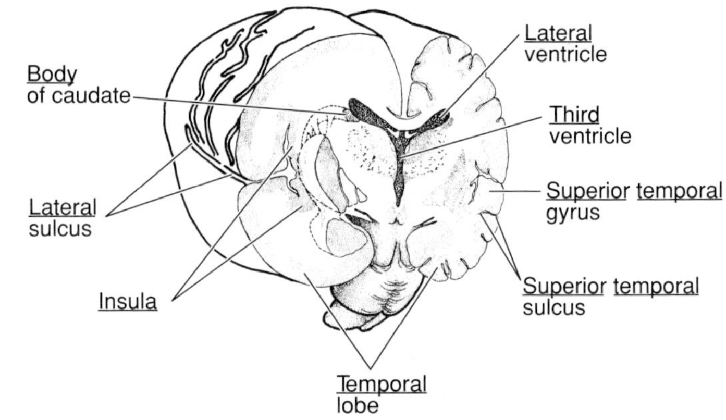

14.22A.

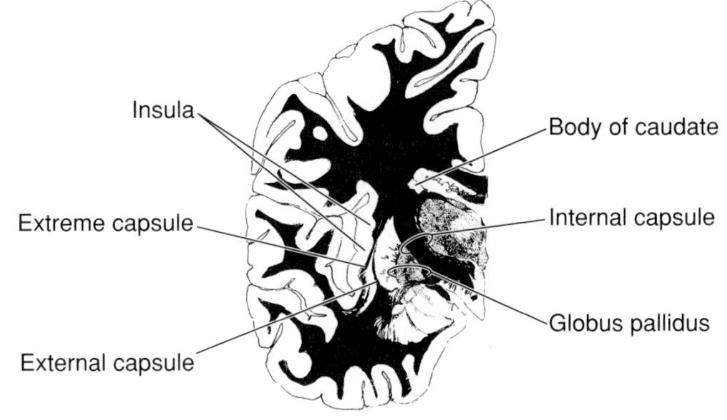

14.23A.

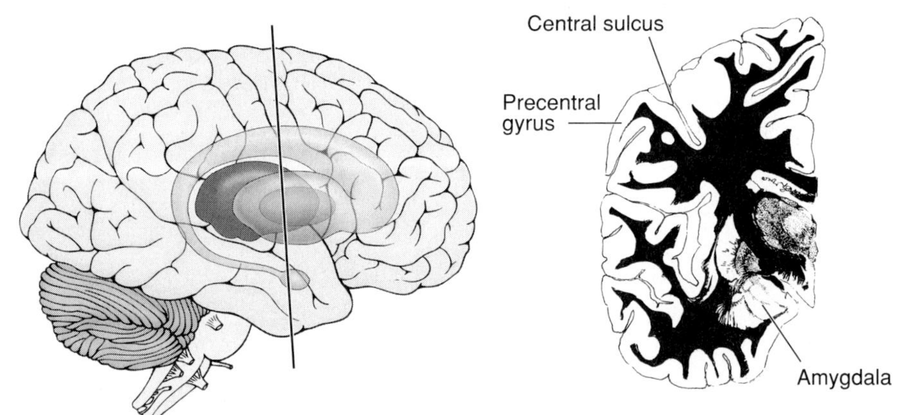

14.24A. Right; medial

14.25. The more posterior the coronal section is, the larger the thalamus and the smaller the lenticular nucleus. The section on the ______ side is cut at a slightly more posterior level.

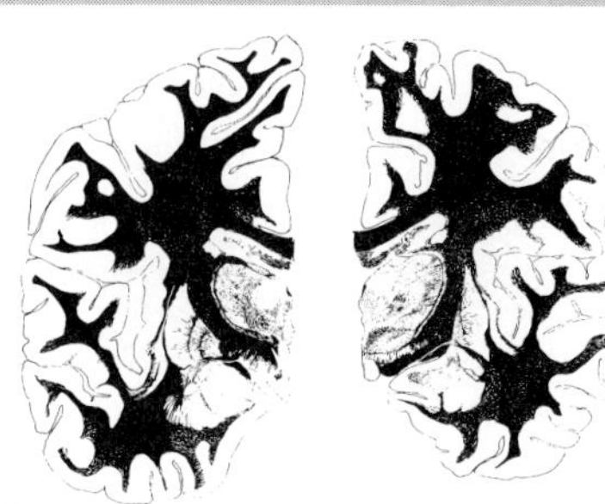

14.26. The sequence of numbered sections from the most anterior to the most posterior section is: ______, ______, ______, and ______.

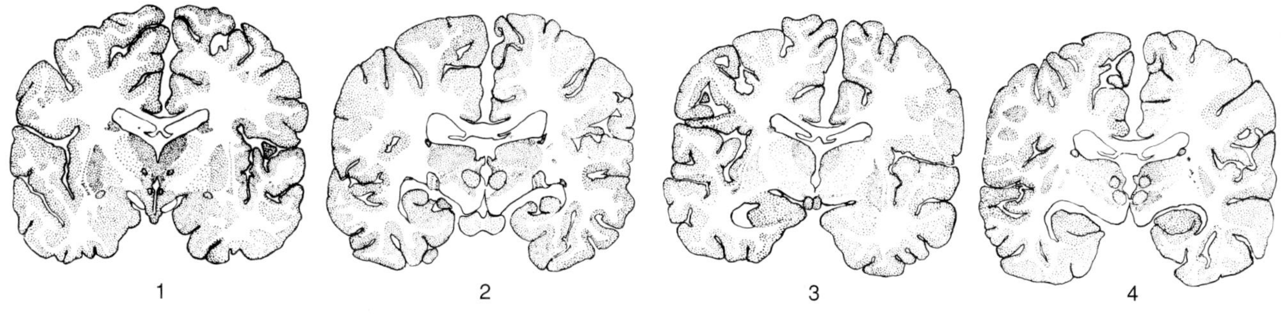

14.27. Number the following structures in the correct anterior to posterior sequence, beginning with number 1:

______ Globus pallidus

______ Head of caudate

______ Calcarine fissure

______ Frontal pole

14.28. In both pictures, the lateral ventricle (indicated by "LV") lies immediately ______ al to the __________ nucleus.

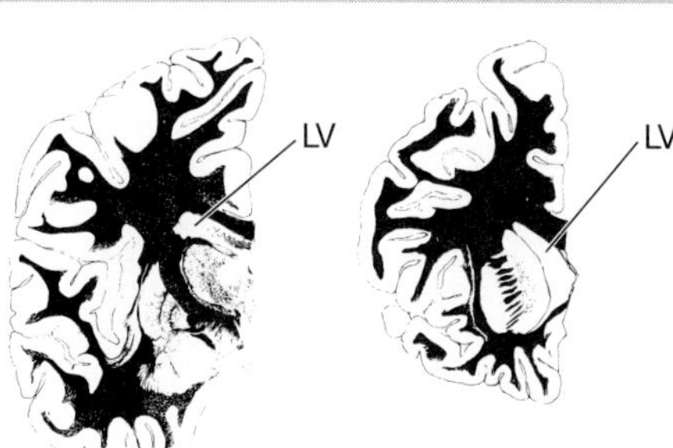

14.29. In both horizontal and coronal sections, the head and body of the caudate nucleus lie immediately medial to the __________ capsule and immediately __________ to the ventricle.

14.25A. right

14.26A. 1; 3; 4; 2

14.27A.

3 Globus pallidus
2 Head of caudate
4 Calcarine fissure
1 Frontal pole

14.28A. medial; caudate

14.29A. internal; lateral

14.30. List all *gray matter* structures encountered in passing along the line drawn from "X" on the surface gray matter of the insula to the midline.

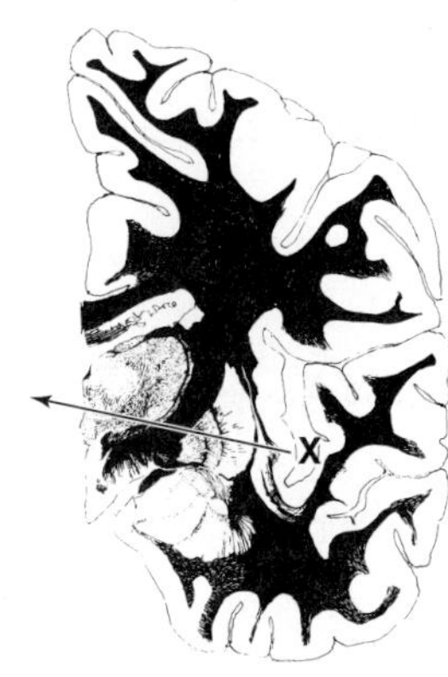

14.31. Draw lines to the structures indicated.

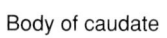

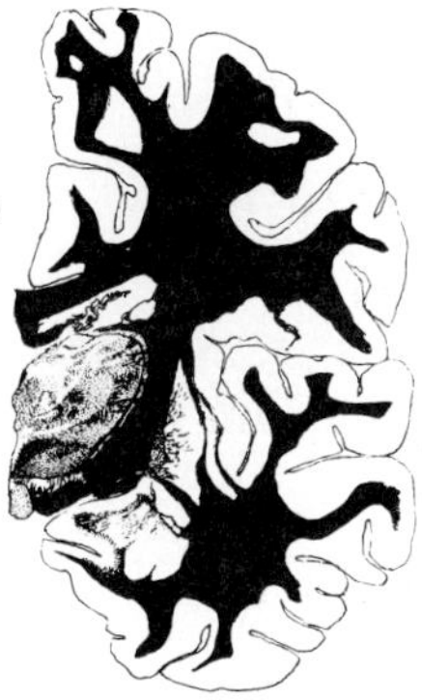

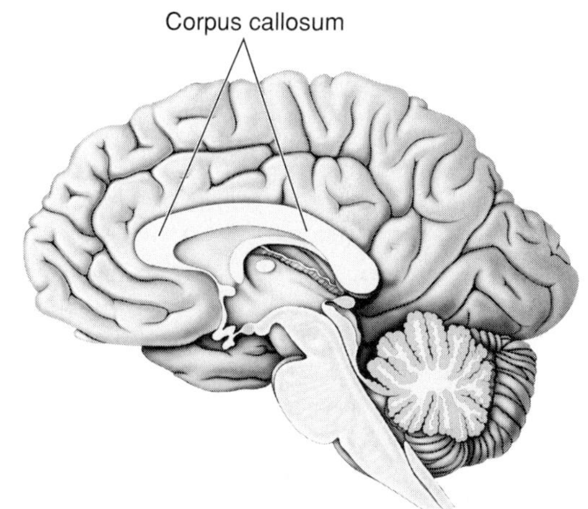

14.32. In this picture, one sees midsagittal (midline) structures, but one does not see into the right cerebral hemisphere. One of the few cerebral structures cut at the midline is the massive white matter tract that passes between the hemispheres, the ____________ ____________.

14.33. Label the corpus callosum. It is composed of ______ matter. As its fibers run *laterally*, they pass ______ ior to the basal nuclei.

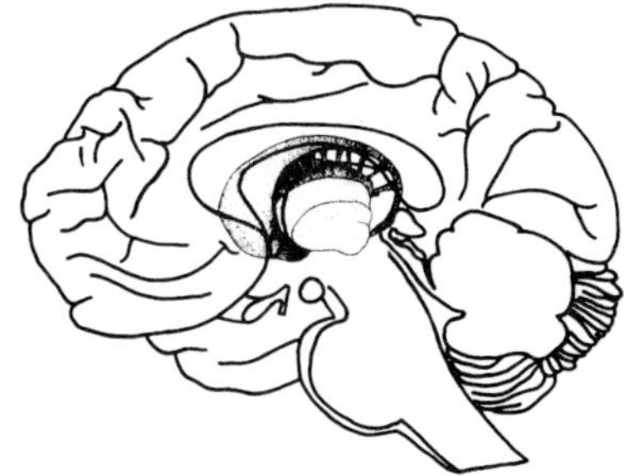

14.30A. Claustrum; putamen; globus pallidus; thalamus

14.31A.

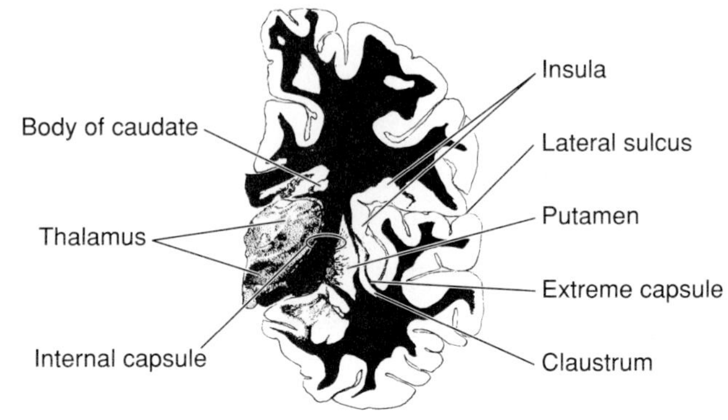

14.32A. corpus callosum

14.33A. white; superior

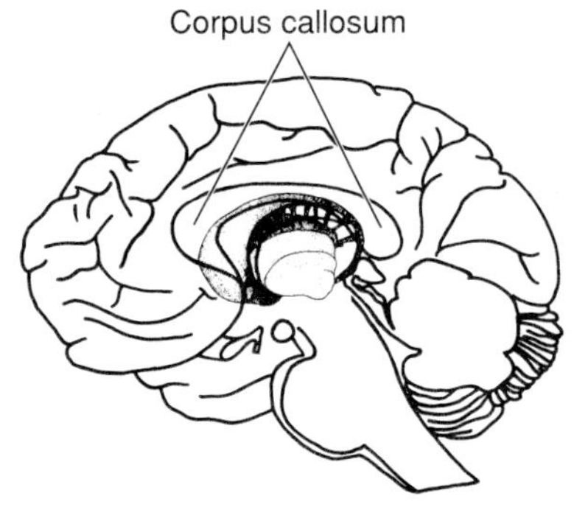

14.34. The corpus callosum is composed of ______ matter. Indicate it with an arrow at the midline.

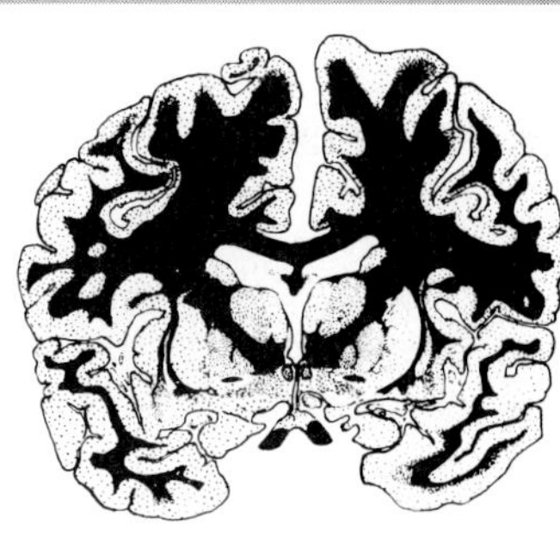

14.35. Some cell bodies of the corticospinal system lie in gyri anterior to the precentral gyrus. Three such cell bodies are drawn on the left side of the figure. Draw efferent fibers from these cell bodies across the corona radiata into the internal capsule.

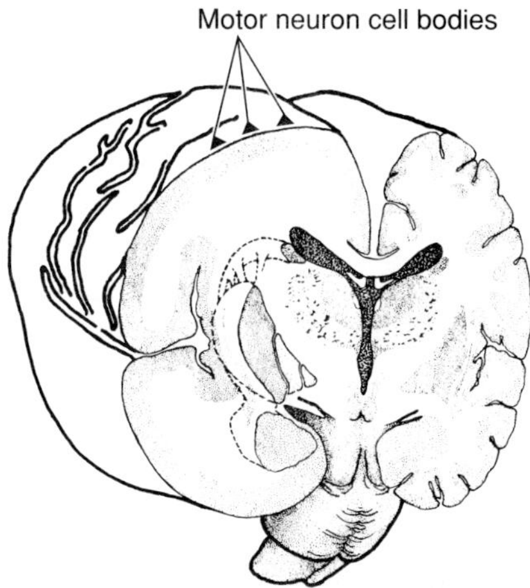

14.36. On the cut surface of the left side of the picture (right side of the brain), place an "X" accurately on the site where the corticospinal fibers pass between the putamen and the body of caudate.

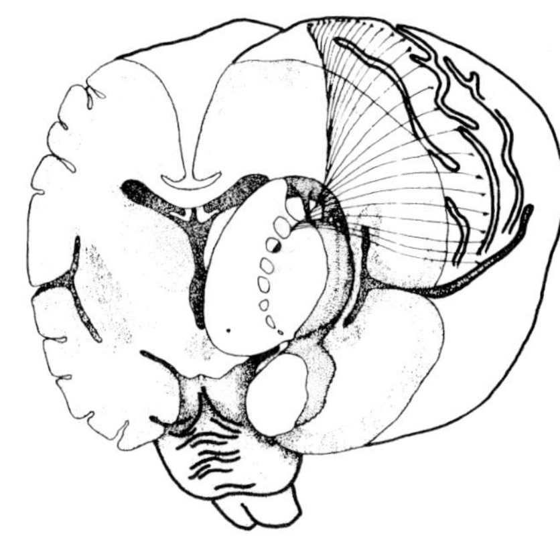

14.34A. <u>white</u>

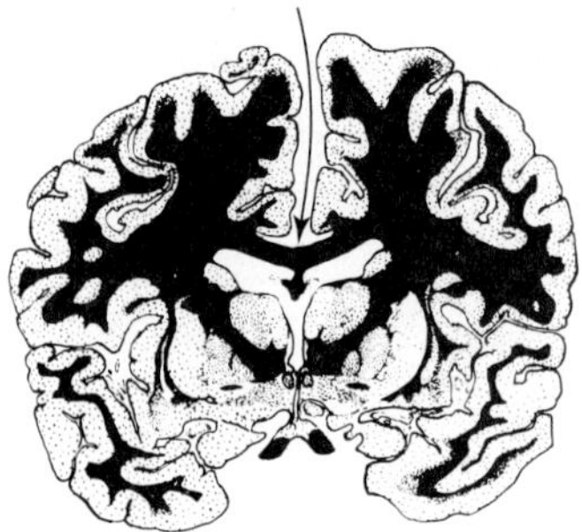

14.35A.

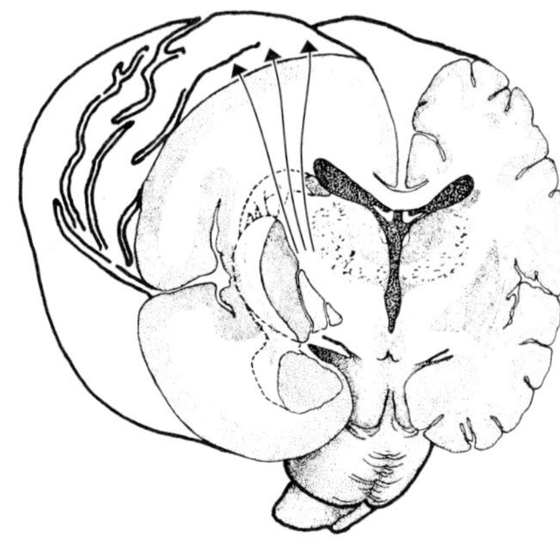

14.36A.

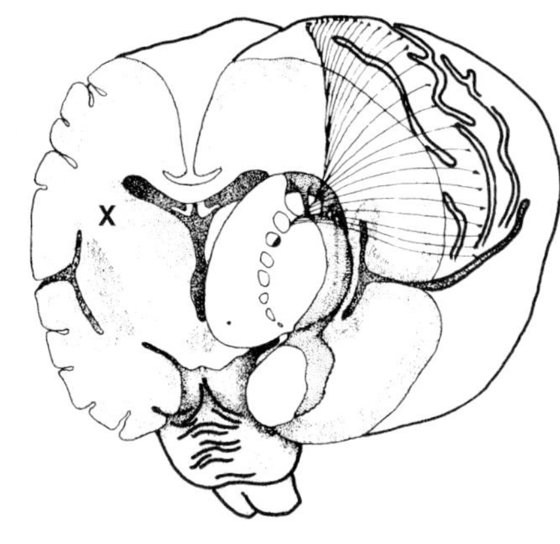

14.37. Encircle the corticospinal fibers where they pass through the corona radiata.

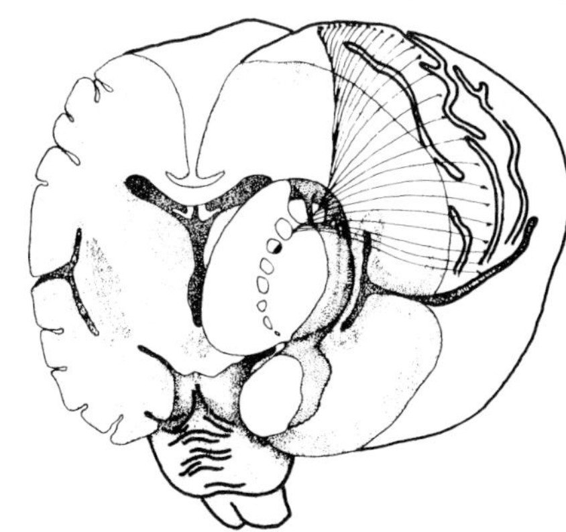

14.38. The fibers on the left side of the figure form part of the ____________ tract. They contribute to the following regions: at 1, the ________ ________; at 2, the ________ ________.

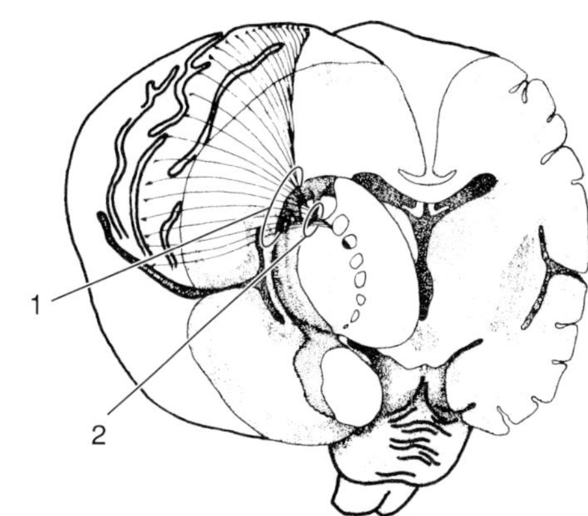

14.39. On both sides of this section, draw fibers of corpus callosum crossing the midline and intersecting with other fibers of the corona radiata.

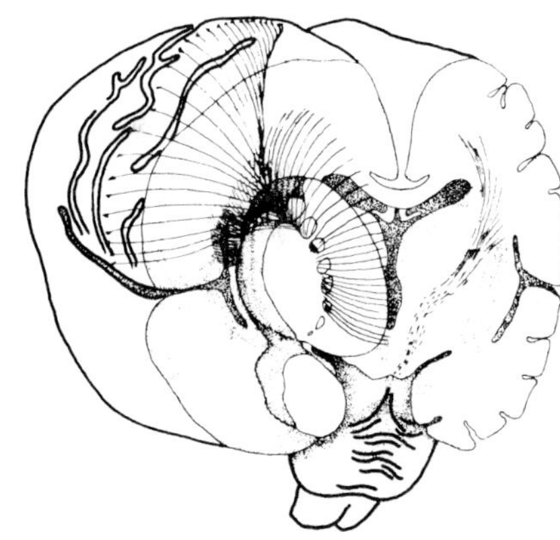

14.37A.

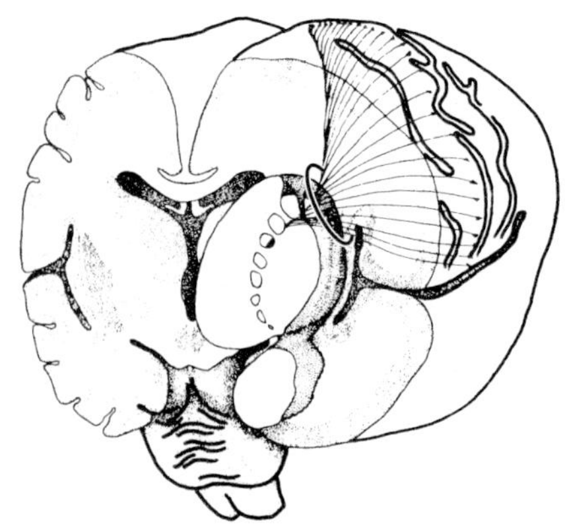

14.38A. corticospinal; corona radiata; internal capsule

14.39A.

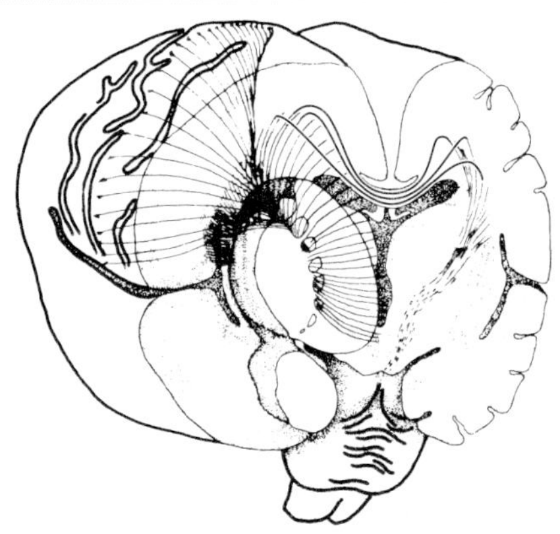

15 Relations Between the Thalamus and Cortex: Location of the Hypothalamus

15.1. The arrows represent the corticospinal fibers passing lateral to the ____________ nucleus. Further down, as part of the ____________ limb of the internal capsule, the corticospinal fibers pass just medial to the globus pallidus and lateral to the ____________.

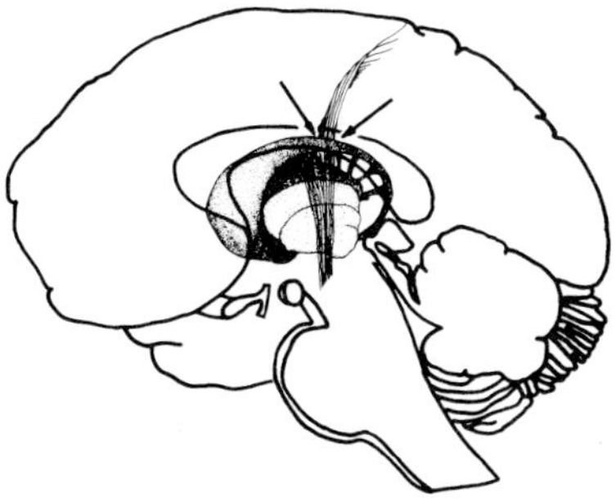

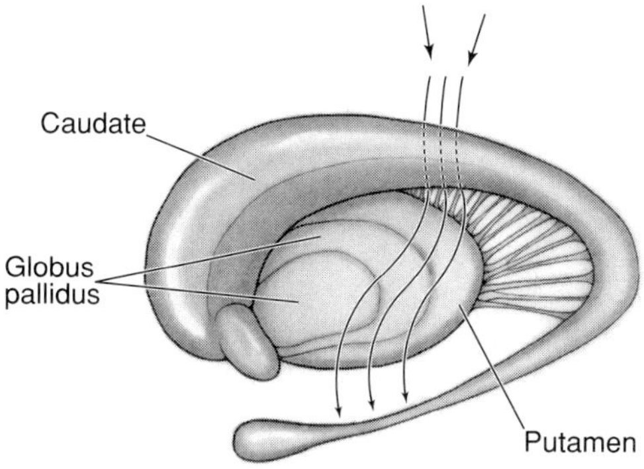

Caudate
Globus pallidus
Putamen

15.2. The medial wall of the cerebral hemisphere separates the basal nuclei from the brainstem. The medial wall of the cerebral hemisphere is formed by the ____________ ____________. Medial to this wall, at the level illustrated, is the ____________.

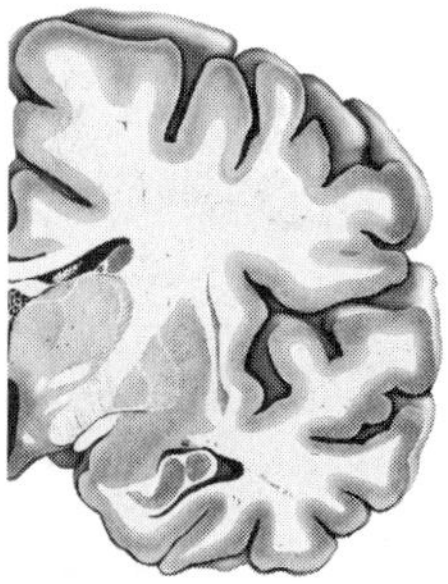

15.3. The thalamus receives information generated in sense organs. The thalamus is a relay and integration station in ____________ pathways to the cerebral cortex.

15.4. Many of the encircled fibers passing through the region of the ____________ ____________ are afferent. These fibers arise from nerve cell bodies in the ____________.

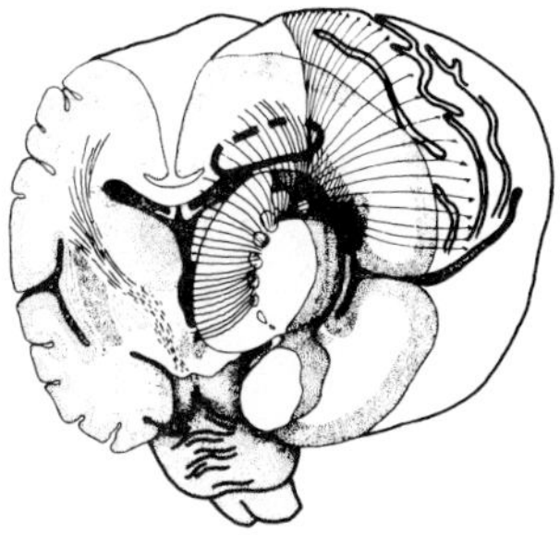

15.1A. caudate; posterior; thalamus

15.2A. internal capsule; thalamus

15.3A. sensory

15.4A. corona radiata; thalamus

15.5. Sensory fibers pass from the thalamus to the cortex via the ____________ ____________ and the corona radiata. Motor fibers of the corticospinal tract enter the same white matter regions but bypass the ____________.

15.6. Except for corticospinal fibers, most fibers in the posterior limb of the internal capsule are ____________ fibers.

15.7. Draw a line from "E" to "H." You have drawn an approximately transverse plane across the brainstem, from epithalamus (E), through ____________, to hypothalamus (H).

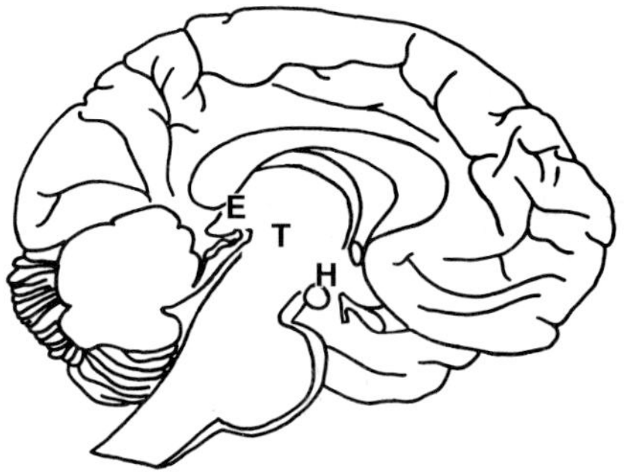

15.8. Look at the plane transverse to the brainstem. The small region above the thalamus *in the transverse plane* is called the epithalamus. The region below the thalamus is called the hypothalamus. Label the three zones indicated in the picture with their names. Look at the midsagittal plane. When the brain as a whole is considered, the hypothalamus is the most anterior and ______ ior of the three structures, and the most posterior structure is the ____________.

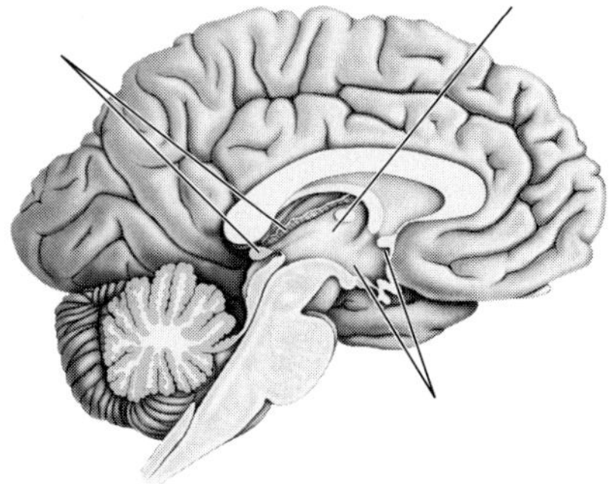

15.9. A section indicated by the line, in the ____________ plane, would cut through all but one of the following: lenticular nucleus, thalamus, hypothalamus, and epithalamus. The missing one would be the ____________.

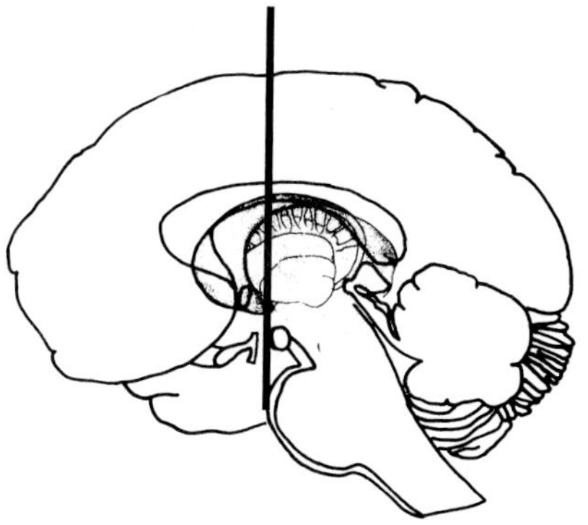

15.5A. internal capsule; thalamus

15.6A. afferent

15.7A. thalamus

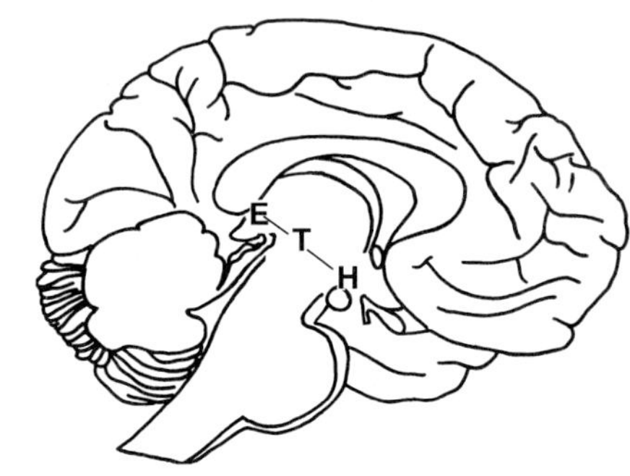

15.8A. inferior; epithalamus

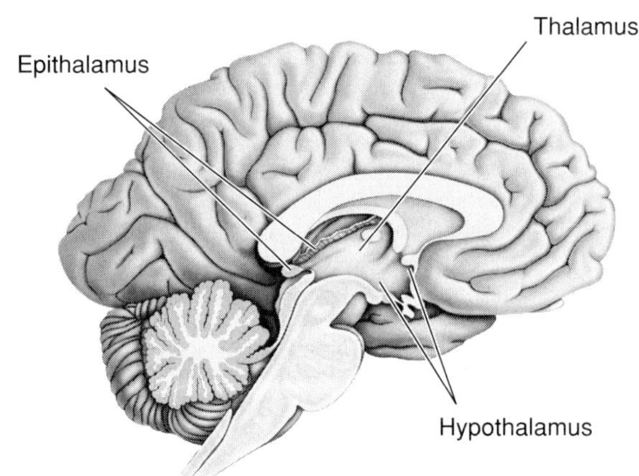

15.9A. coronal; epithalamus

15.10. On this coronal section, the encircled area indicated by the arrow is the ________________.

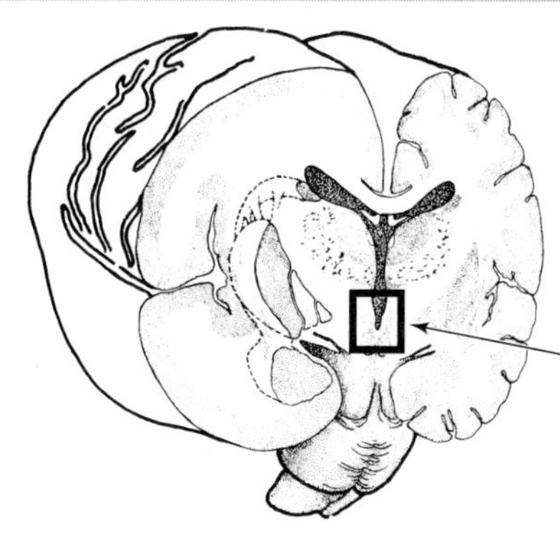

15.11. On each coronal section, label the two enclosed areas with their names.

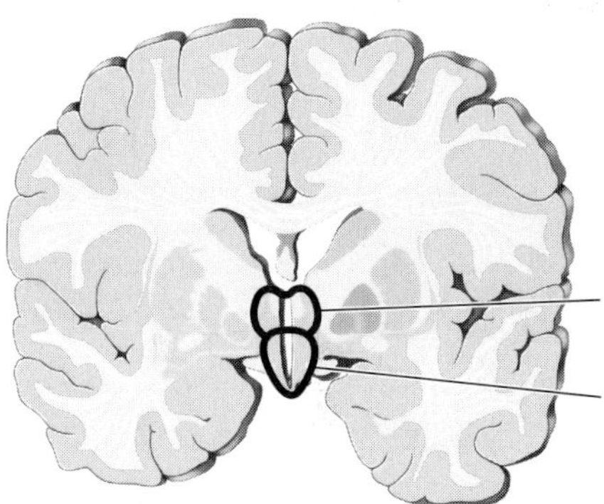

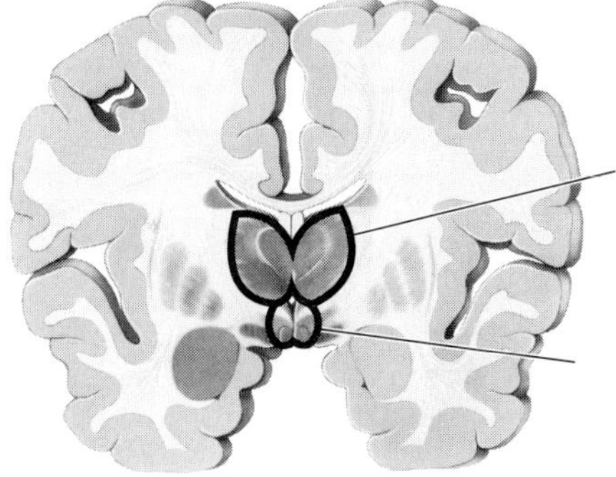

15.10A. hypothalamus

15.11A.

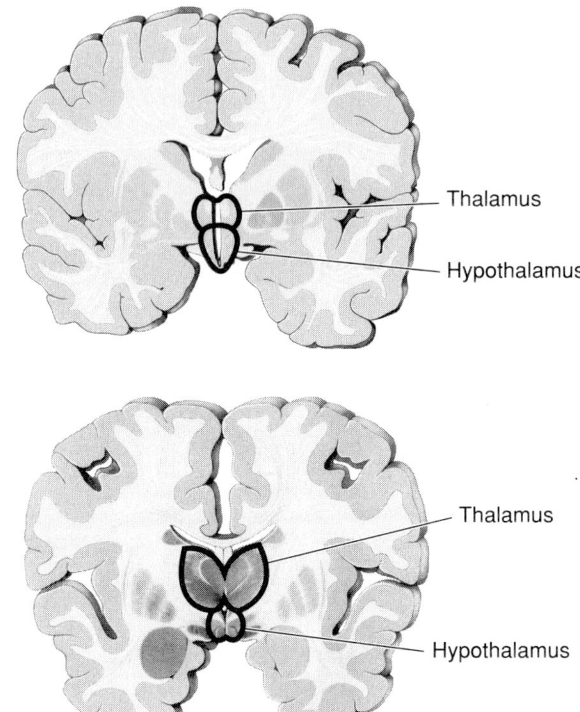

16 Relations Between Cortex and Upper Brainstem: Sagittal Views

16.1. The right side of the lower brainstem has been added in the ______ hand picture.

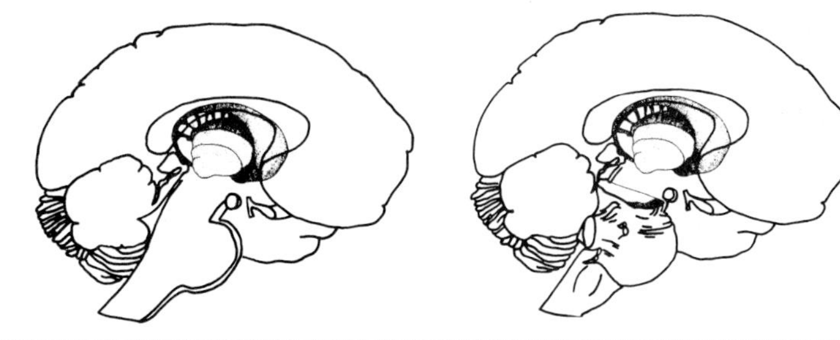

16.2. On the right hand picture, label those structures that are already labeled on the left hand picture.

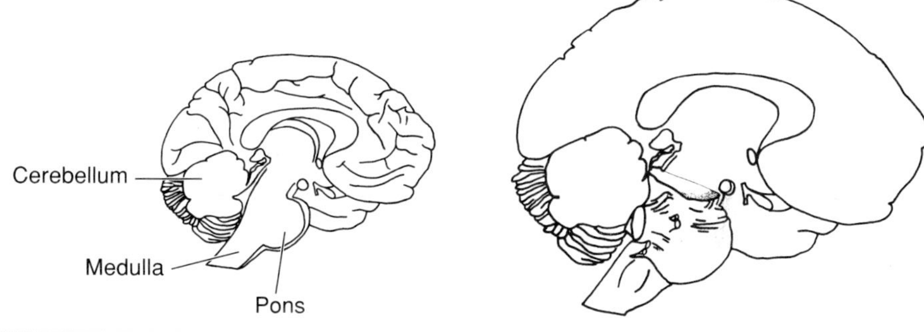

16.3. Label the indicated regions of the brainstem with their names.

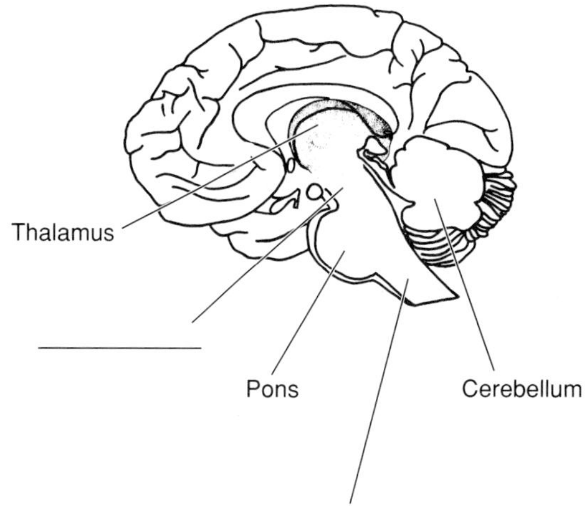

16.1A. right

16.2A.

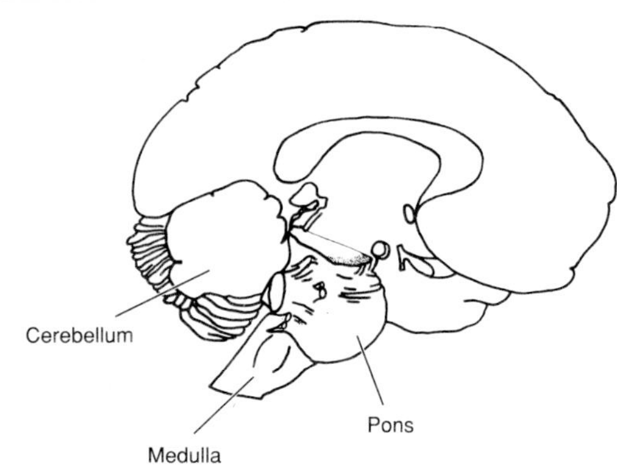

16.3A.

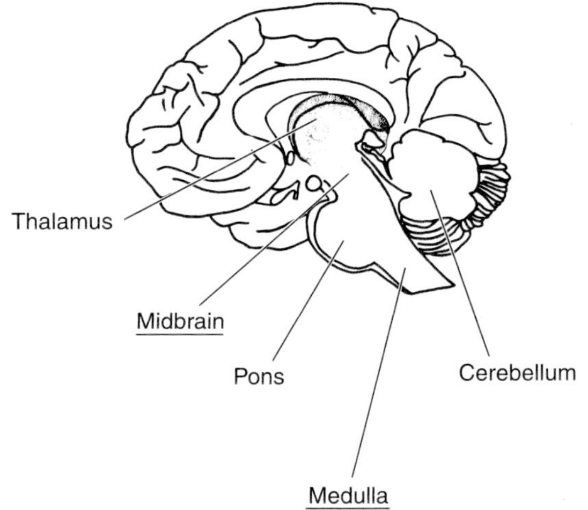

16.4. In the indicated spaces, label anterior (A) and posterior (P). "M" is the transected surface of the ______ hand side of the ____________ region of the brainstem.

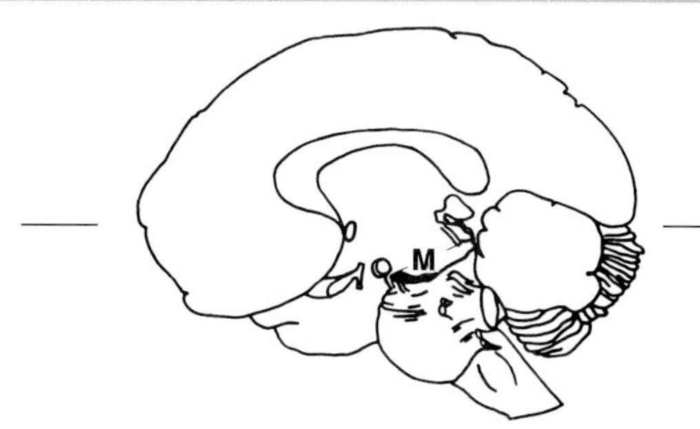

16.5. The right hand picture shows basal nuclei in the ______ side of the brain and lateral surfaces of the medulla and ______ on the ______ side. The corticospinal tract illustrated arises in the ____________________ gyrus of the hemisphere on the ______ side. On the right hand picture, draw an arrow to the just visible central sulcus.

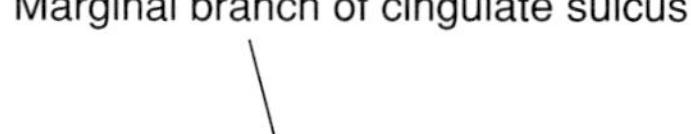

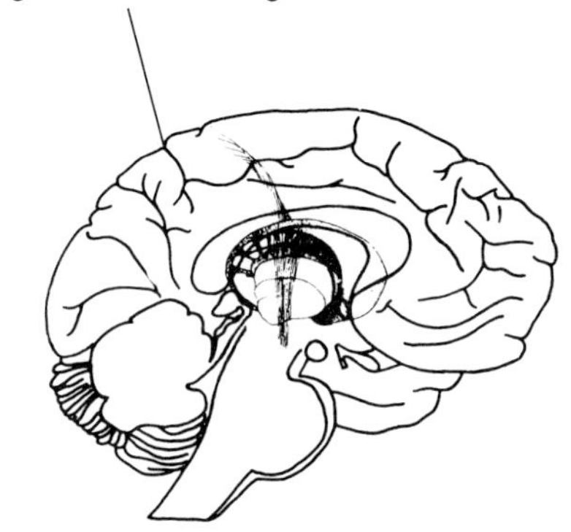

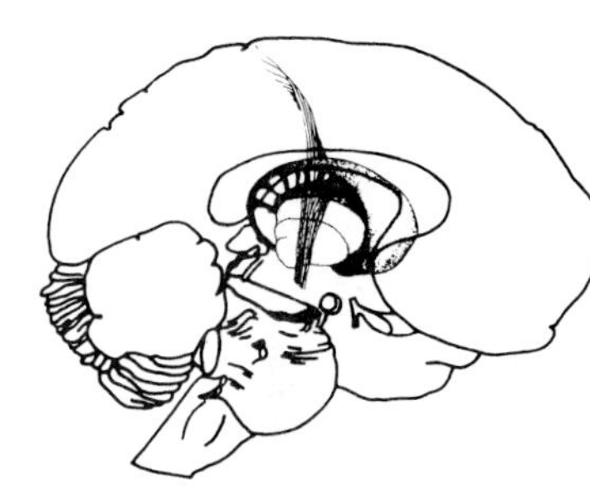

16.6. Here the transection at "M" has been carried across *both* sides of the ____________. The dark areas on the cut surface of the midbrain represent transverse sections of nerve fibers, including fibers of the ____________________ tract. The corticospinal tract illustrated disappears, without crossing the midline, into the ______ side of the midbrain.

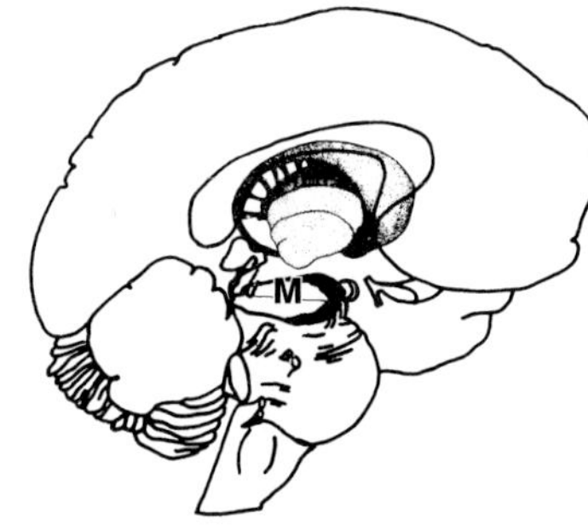

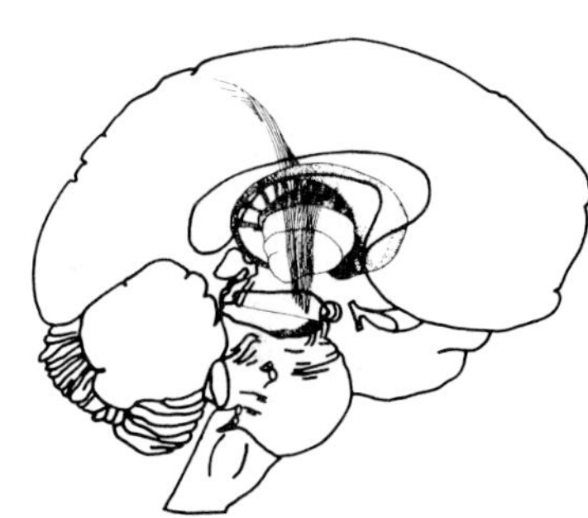

16.4A. left; midbrain

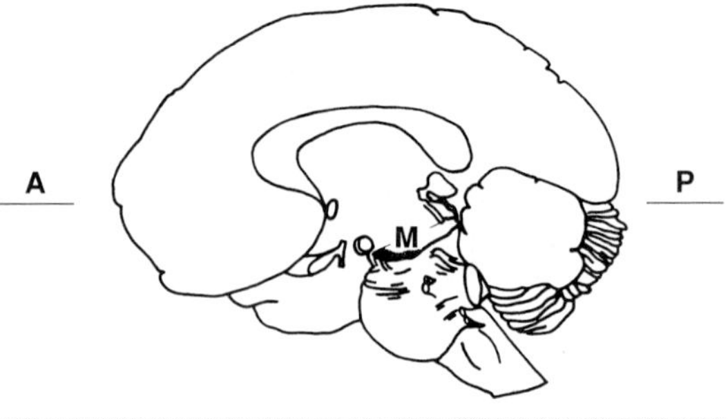

16.5A. left; pons; right; precentral; left

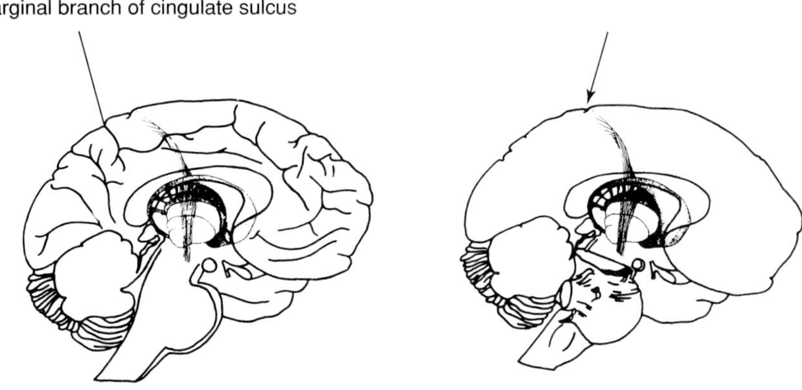

16.6A. midbrain; corticospinal; left

16.7. The occipital pole is posterior, while the frontal pole is anterior. In the midbrain, the dark area is ______ior. All efferent tracts from cortex to brainstem enter the ______ior part of the midbrain.

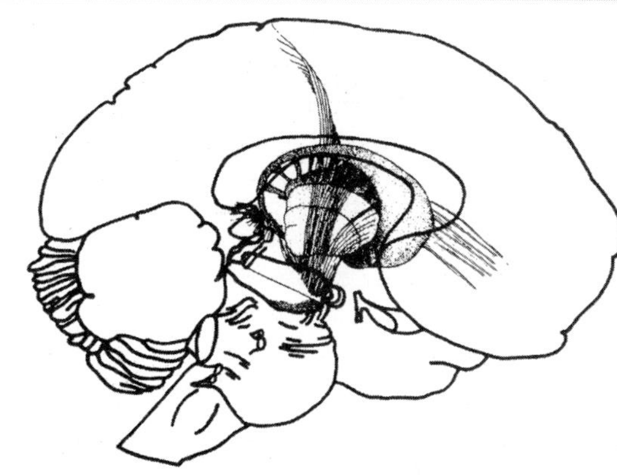

16.8. Before entering the brainstem, efferent fibers run in the internal capsule, along the lateral surface of the __________.

16.9. Efferent fibers from the cortex pass lateral to the thalamus and medial to the __________ __________ in the __________ __________ and then emerge on the basal, or ______ior, surface of the midbrain.

16.10. As the name states, the corticospinal fibers are destined to terminate in the __________ ______. From the midbrain, they must pass in sequence through the ______ and __________ of the brainstem.

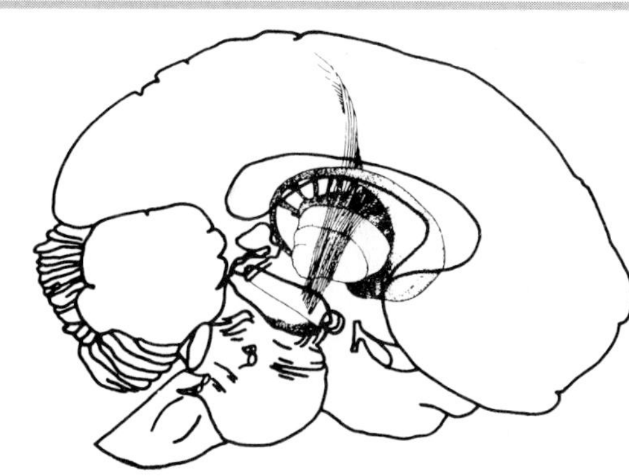

16.11. The three main regions of the brainstem in direct sequence are the __________, ______, and __________. Fiber bundles "A," "B," and "C" pass through the internal capsule lateral to the __________ and immediately enter the anterior surface of the __________ region of the brainstem.

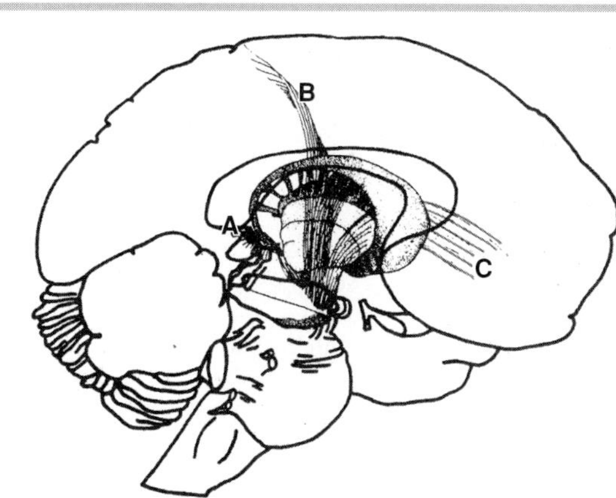

16.7A. anterior; anterior

16.8A. thalamus

16.9A. globus pallidus (or lenticular nucleus); internal capsule; anterior

16.10A. spinal cord; pons; medulla

16.11A. midbrain; pons; medulla; thalamus; midbrain

16.12. The frontopontine tract originates in the frontal lobe and terminates in the region of the brainstem called the ______. Label it with a "C" where it lies in the internal capsule.

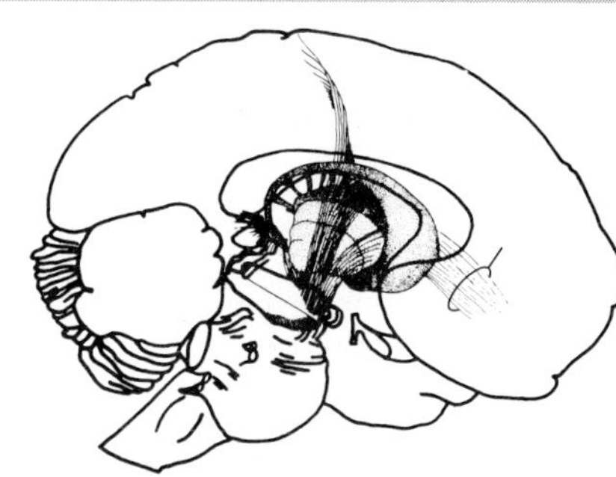

16.13. The fiber bundle labeled "A" originates in the parietal, temporal, and occipital lobes. It will terminate in the pons, after (as seen at the arrow) it passes through the ____________ region of the brainstem.

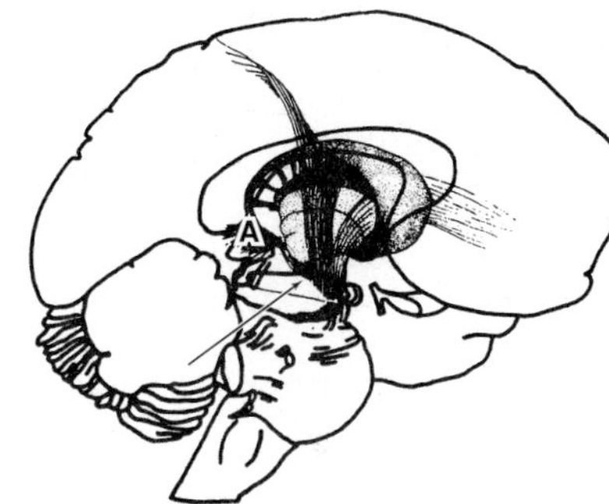

16.14. Two major efferent tracts from the cortex terminate in the pons. They are the ____________pontine tract and the cortico____________ tract. Label them as "A" and "C," respectively, on the diagram.

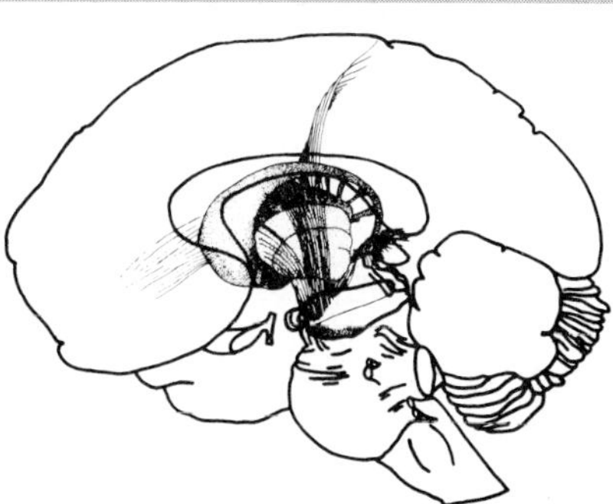

16.15. Tracts "A" and "C" terminate in the ______; "B" terminates in the ____________ ______.

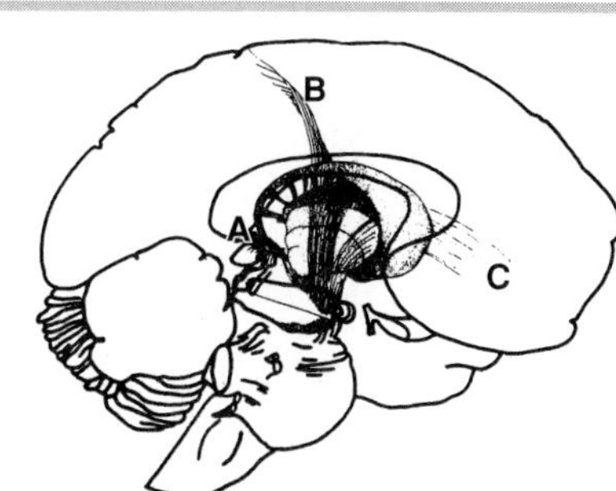

16.12A. pons

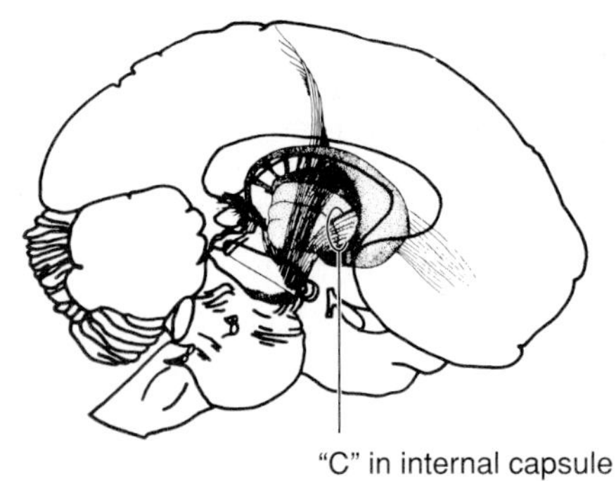

16.13A. midbrain

16.14A. frontopontine; corticopontine

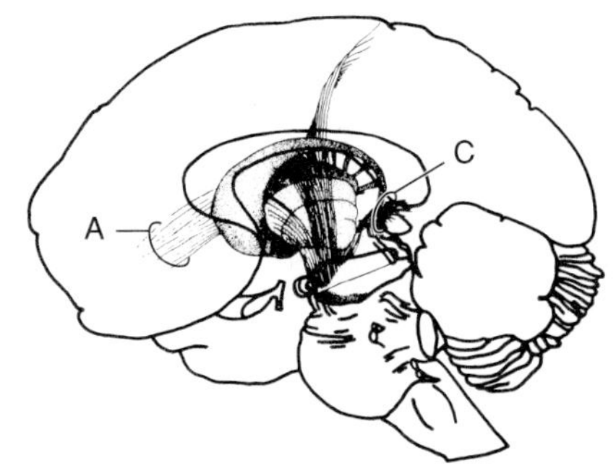

16.15A. pons; spinal cord

16.16. All efferent tracts from cortex to brainstem pass between the caudate and lenticular nucleus. The corticopontine tract passes between the ______ of the caudate and the part of the lenticular nucleus called the __________ __________.

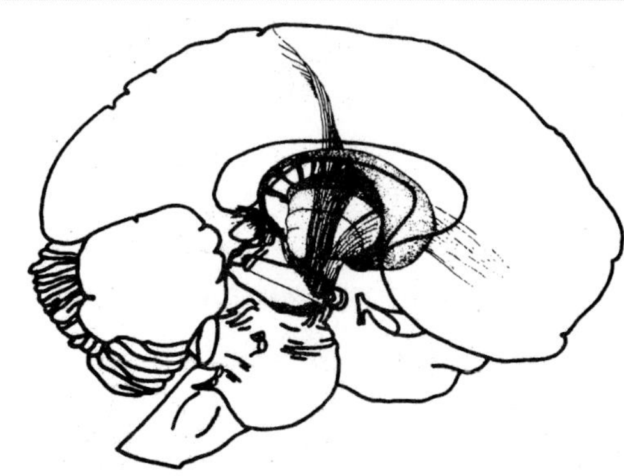

16.17. Some efferent fibers from the surface of the cortex terminate in the basal nuclei. Others pass down into the brainstem, mainly in the __________spinal, fronto__________, and __________pontine tracts.

16.18. At the level of the internal capsule, encircle and label the three main tracts that reach the brainstem from the cortex.

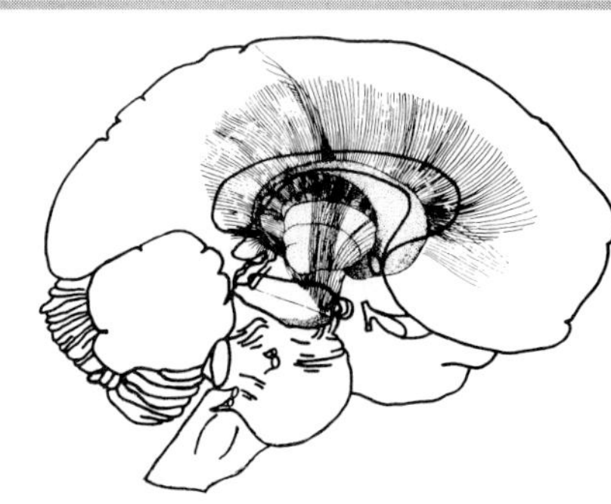

16.19. Some efferent tracts pass from cortex to basal nuclei. However, the only *direct* efferent pathways from cortex to brainstem are the cortico__________, fronto__________, and cortico__________ tracts.

16.20. Apart from the tracts from cortex to cord, brainstem, and basal nuclei, the large number of other fibers in the internal capsule are ______ferent with respect to cortex. These fibers arise from cell bodies in the __________.

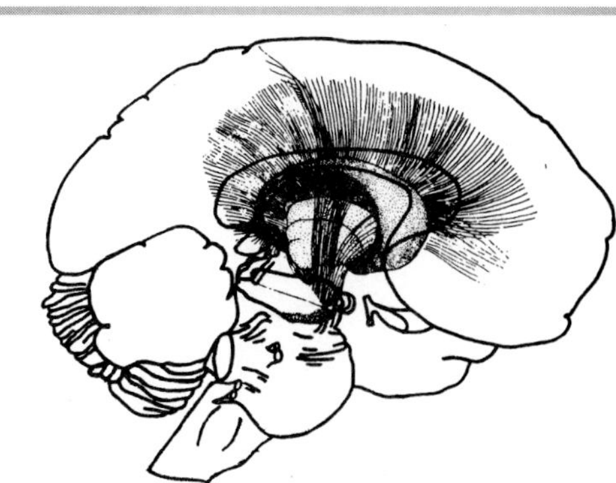

16.16A. tail; globus pallidus

16.17A. corticospinal; frontopontine; corticopontine

16.18A.

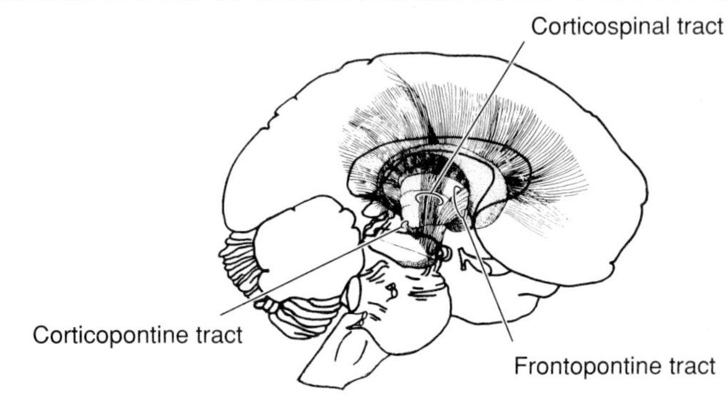

16.19A. corticospinal; frontopontine; corticopontine

16.20A. afferent; thalamus

16.21. Primary sensory information comes from the thalamus predominantly to the ____________, ____________, and ____________ lobes. The arrow in the left picture points to a sulcus that marks the boundary between the ____________ and ____________ lobes. With arrows, point to the same sulcus in the right picture.

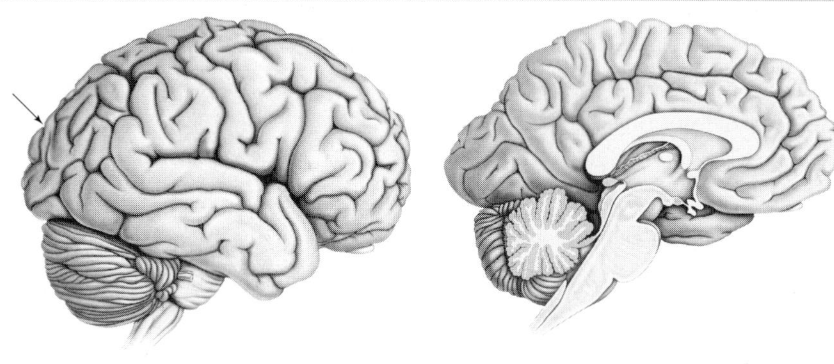

16.22. Although all cortical lobes may send some efferent fibers to lower centers, one lobe is not known to send any major motor tract to the brainstem or cord. Draw the boundaries of this lobe on both diagrams.

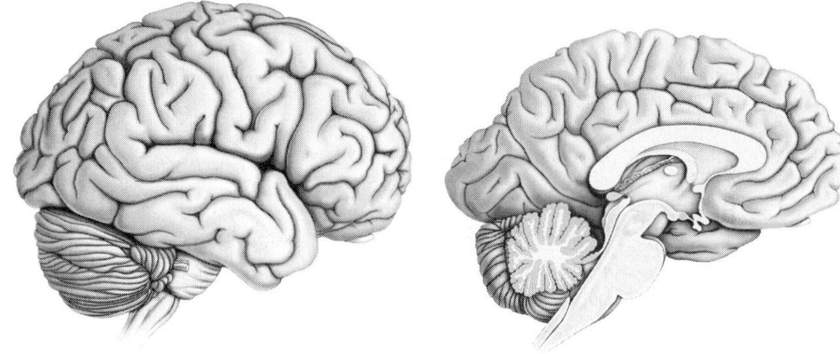

16.23. Lesions affecting the internal capsule and corona radiata are very common. A lesion at "X" will impair both motor and sensory functions because fibers pass through the internal capsule and corona radiata in ______ directions.

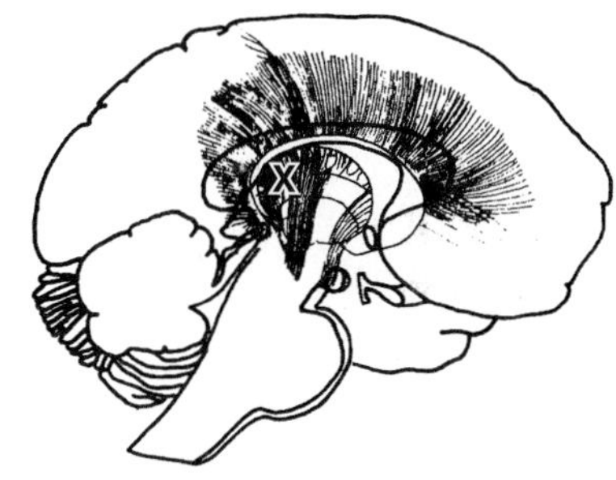

16.21A. parietal; temporal; occipital (in any order); parietal; occipital (in either order)

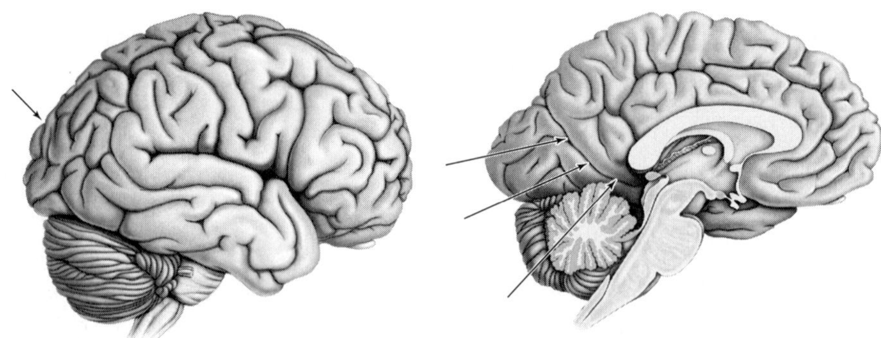

16.22A.

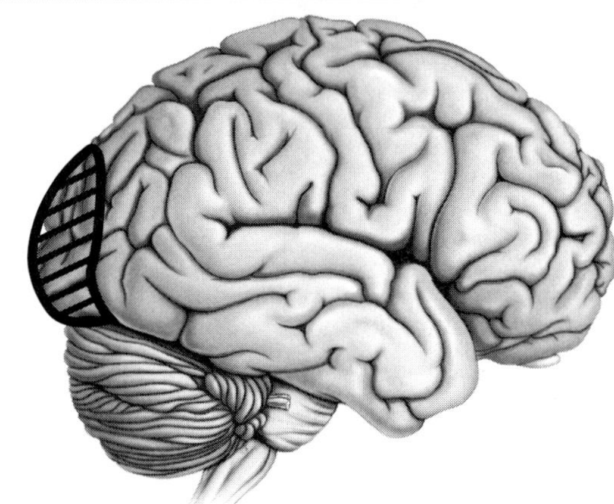

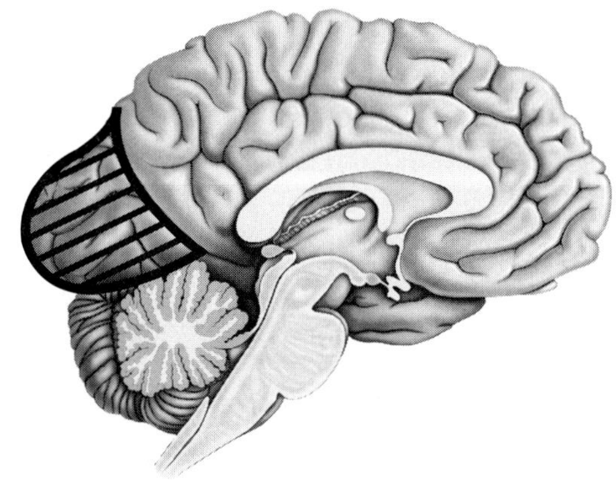

16.23A. both

17 The Corticospinal System and Brainstem Structures: Midbrain

17.1. The "little hills" on the midbrain are called, according to their longitudinal position, the superior and __________ colliculi.

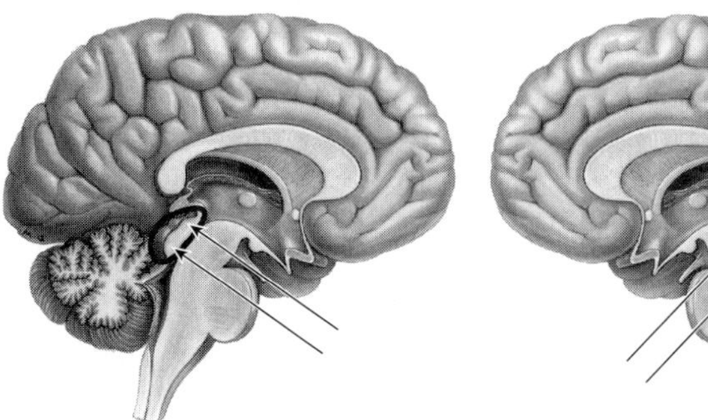

17.2. Uppermost are the left and right ______ior colliculi and below them are the left and right __________ __________. The total number of "little hills" in the midbrain is ______.

17.3. The superior and inferior colliculi lie in the __________ region of the brainstem.

17.4. Label the structure indicated on this midsagittal view; include the side of the brain in which it is located.

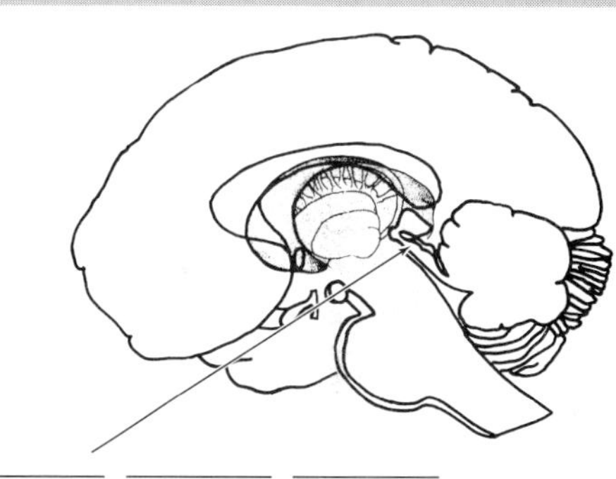

17.5. In referring to the cerebral hemispheres, we have indicated "front" with the directional term __________; "rear" with the term __________; "above" with the term __________; and "below" with the term __________.

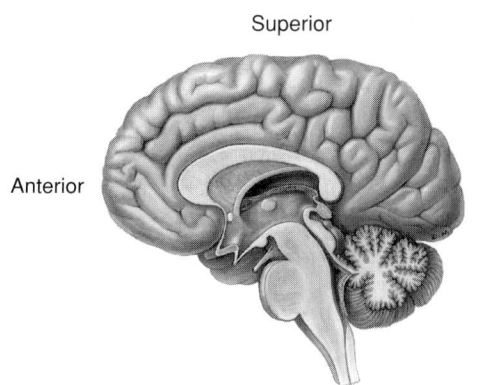

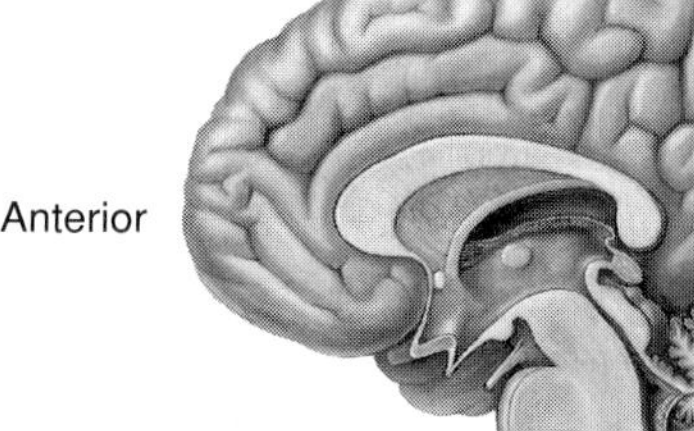

17.1A. inferior

17.2A. superior; inferior colliculi; four

17.3A. midbrain

17.4A.

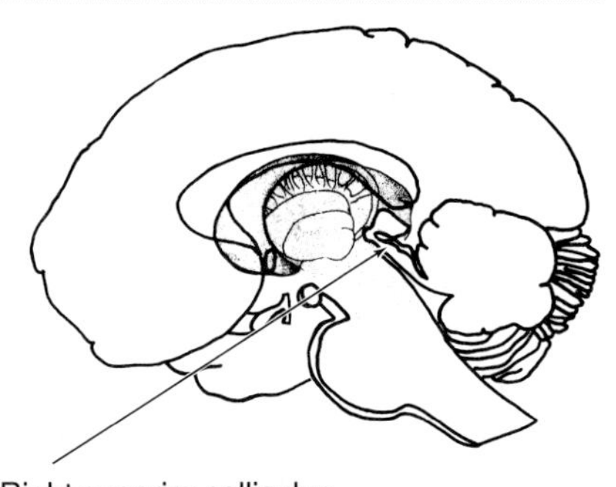

17.5A. anterior; posterior; superior; inferior

17.6. The cerebellum lies ____________ior to the medulla, ______, and midbrain portions of the brainstem.

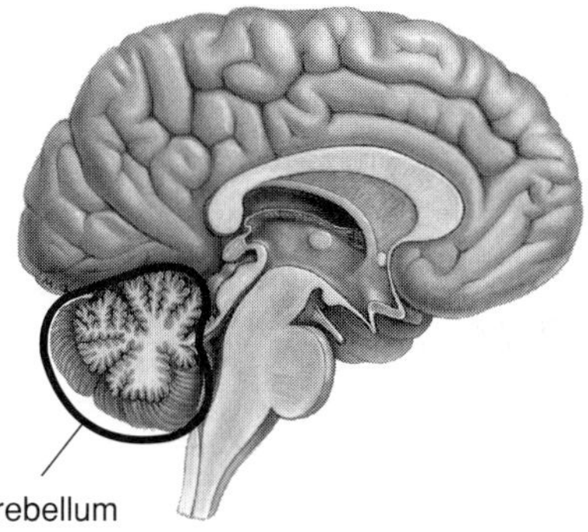

Cerebellum

17.7. The two indicated structures are visible on the ____________ior surface of the midbrain. Label these two structures.

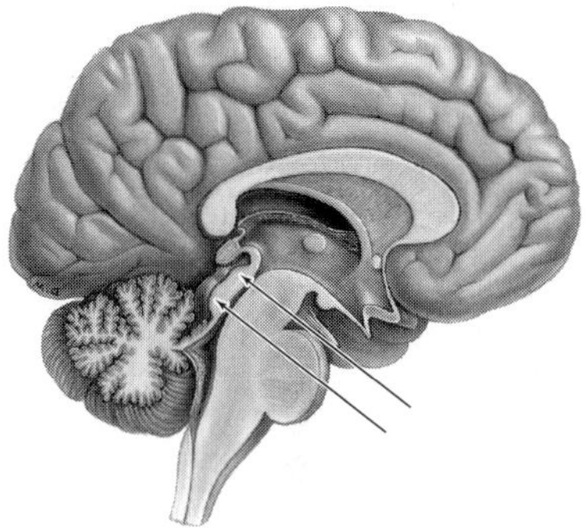

17.8. At the base of each side of the midbrain, ______ior to the colliculi, is a massive white matter structure, the ______ ____________.

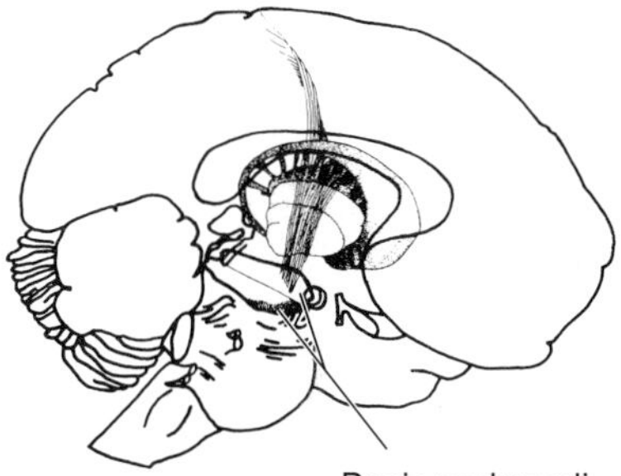

Basis pedunculi

17.9. Corticospinal fibers pass from the internal capsule to the midbrain and pass through the base of the midbrain in the ______ pedunculi.

17.10. Label the outlined region just below the thalamus.

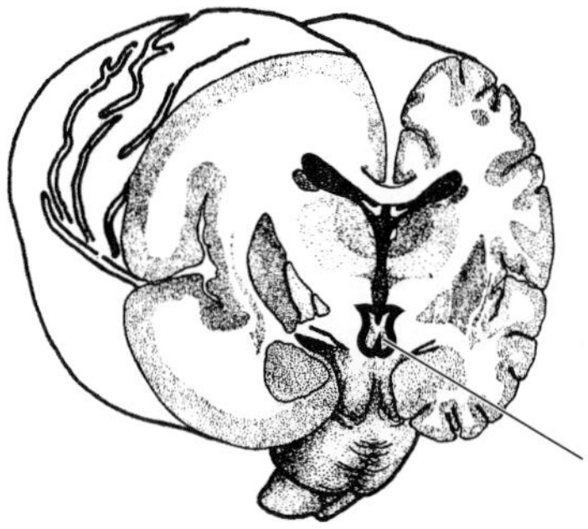

17.6A. posterior; pons

17.7A. posterior

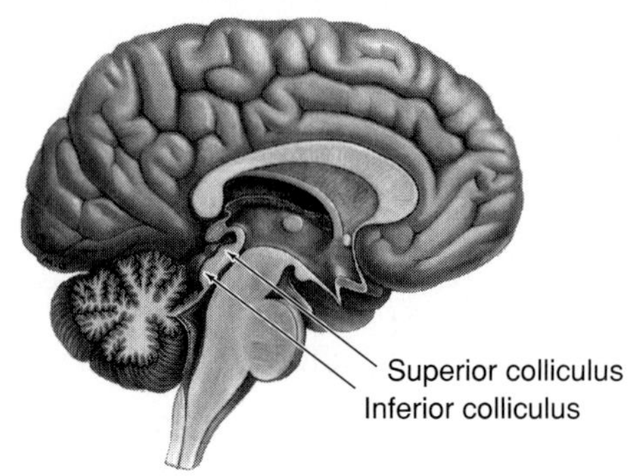

17.8A. anterior; basis pedunculi

17.9A. basis

17.10A.

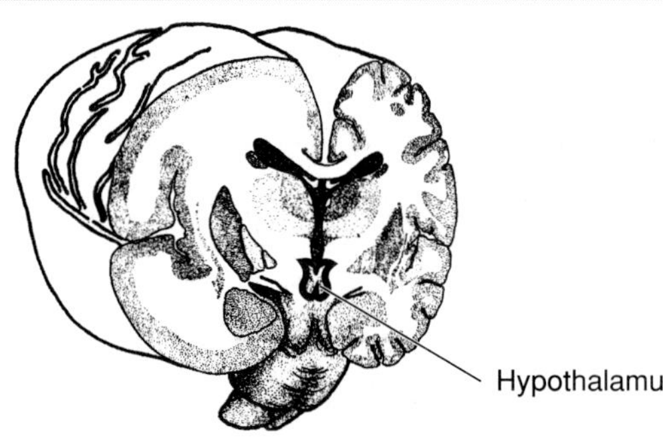

17.11. The internal capsule runs along the ______al boundary of the thalamus and ____________________us.

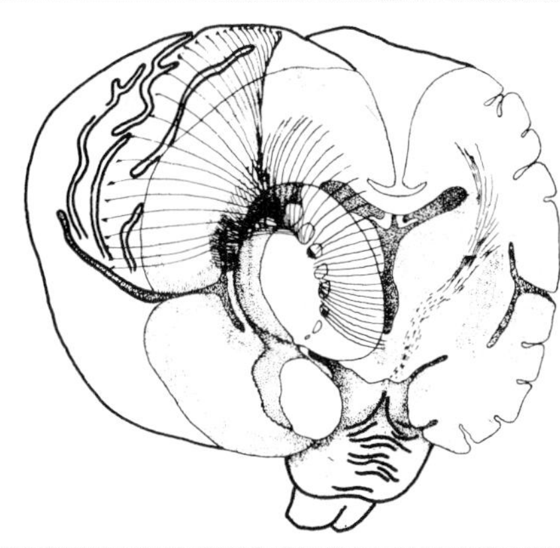

17.12. The midbrain (encircled) lies between the ______ (label it on figure) inferiorly and the thalamus and ____________________ (label it on figure) superiorly.

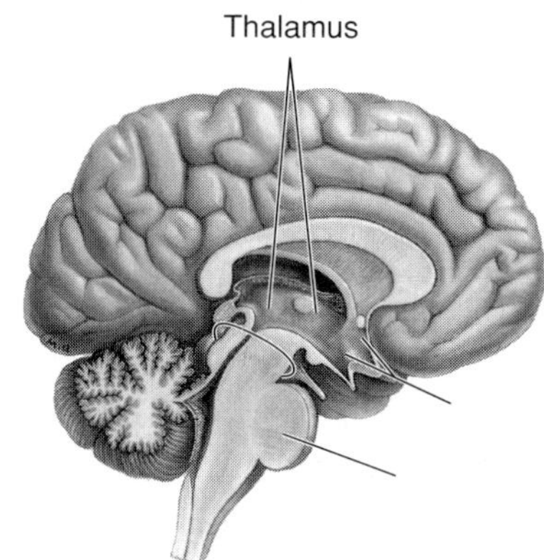

17.13. A coronal section at the level indicated would be difficult to use for study of brainstem anatomy because it passes obliquely through the midbrain, ______, and medulla.

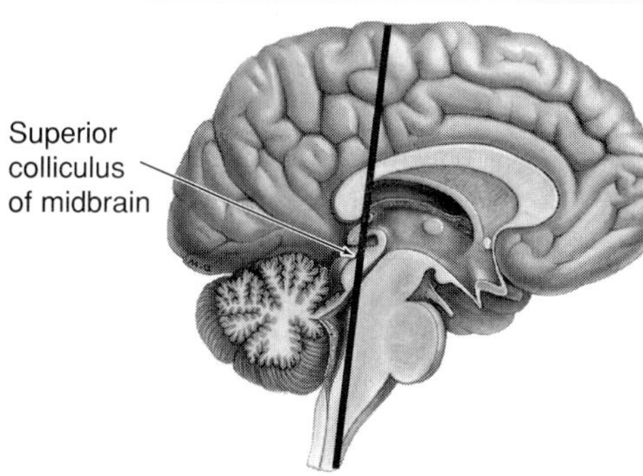

17.14. Does the *cut surface* on the right hand figure show the thalamus? ______ Hypothalamus? ______ Midbrain? ______ Pons? ______. Draw a line on the left hand figure to indicate the position of the cut surface of the right hand figure.

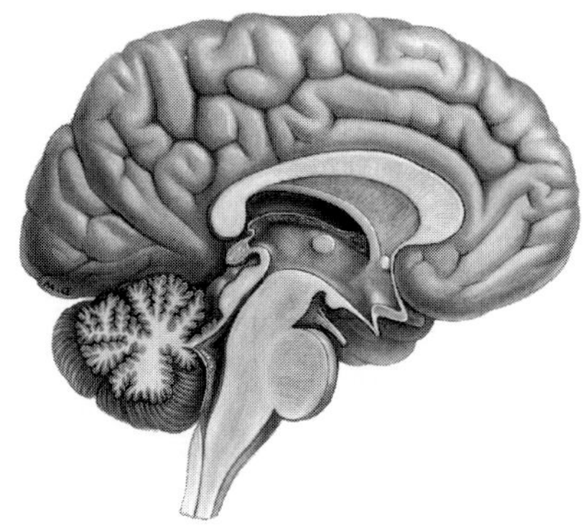

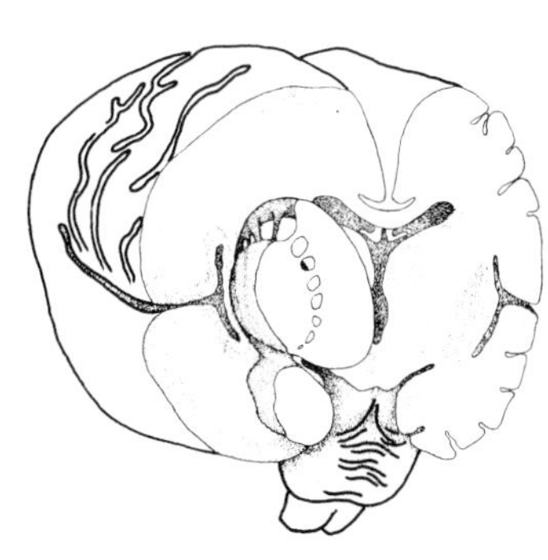

17.11A. lateral; hypothalamus

17.12A.

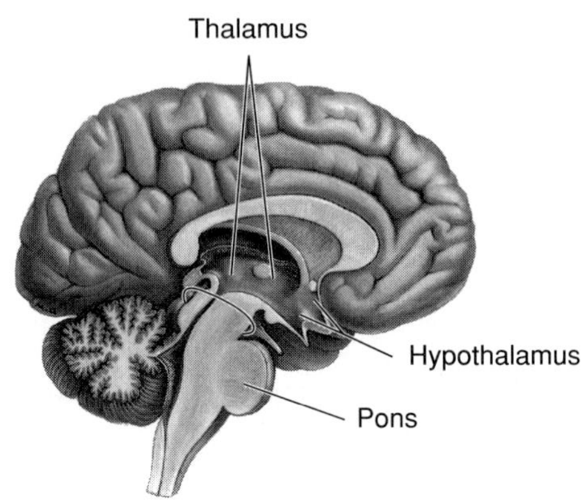

17.13A. pons

17.14A. Yes; Yes; Yes; No

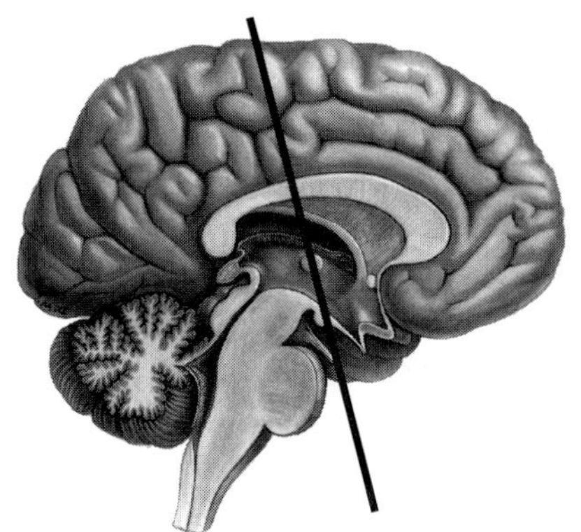

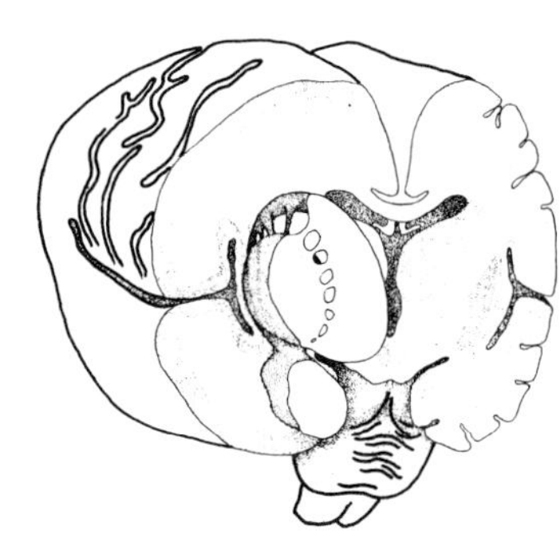

17.15. The passage of fibers from the internal capsule to the base of the __________ would be shown well on a myelin-stained coronal section at this level and in sections __________ior to this level.

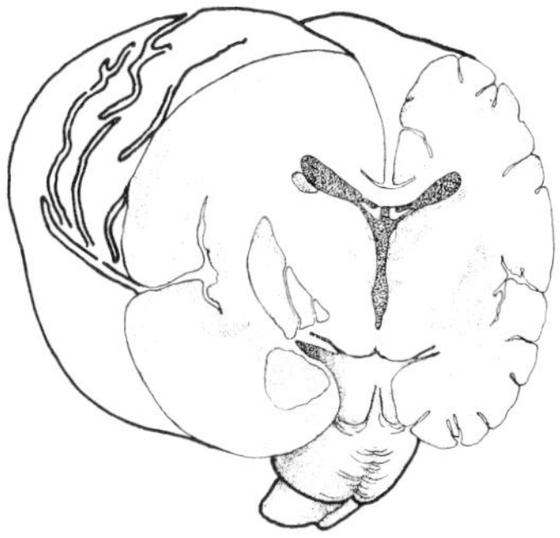

17.16. This section, cut in a plane indicated by the broken line, passes through the thalamus superiorly and through a small portion of the hypothalamus and __________ inferiorly. The white matter indicated by the arrow on the section is just below the internal capsule and barely into the __________ region of the brainstem.

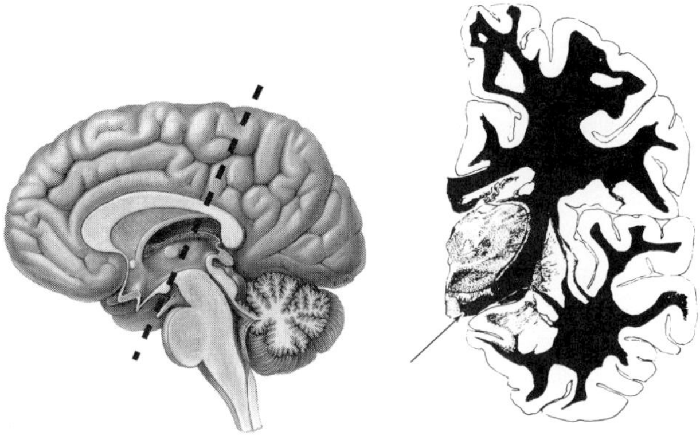

17.17. The corticospinal fibers leave the cerebral hemisphere by passing without interruption from the internal capsule to the basis __________, on the base of the __________. Place an "X" on the basis pedunculi.

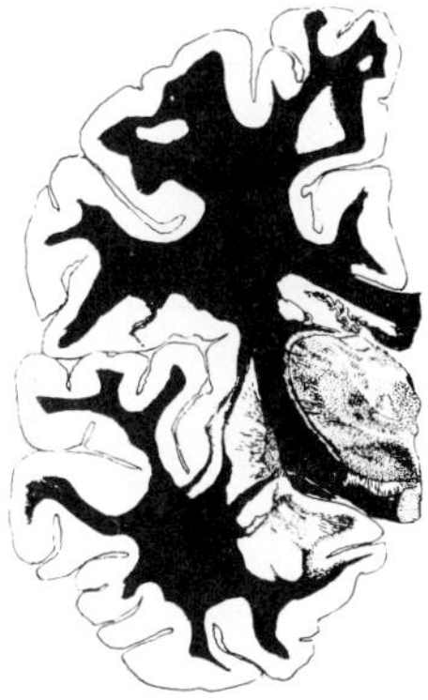

17.18. In the midbrain, the superior and inferior __________ are gray matter, and the basis pedunculi is ______ matter.

17.19. The two planes of section intersect in the ______ nucleus. Both planes also pass through the ______ __________ of the midbrain, but only the plane transverse to the brainstem passes, at the posterior side of the midbrain, through the __________ ______________.

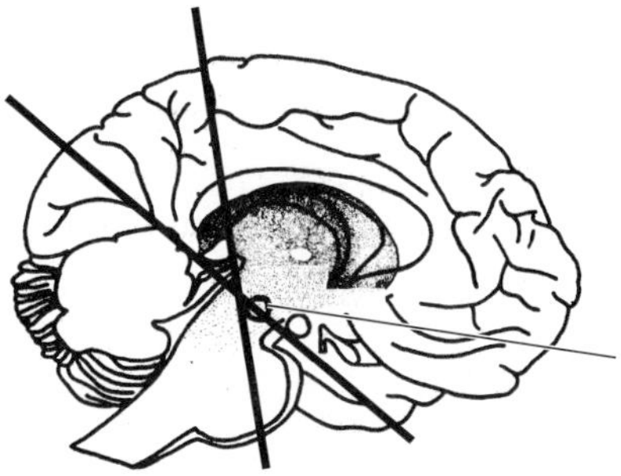

Red nucleus

17.15A. midbrain; posterior

17.16A. midbrain; midbrain

17.17A. pedunculi; midbrain

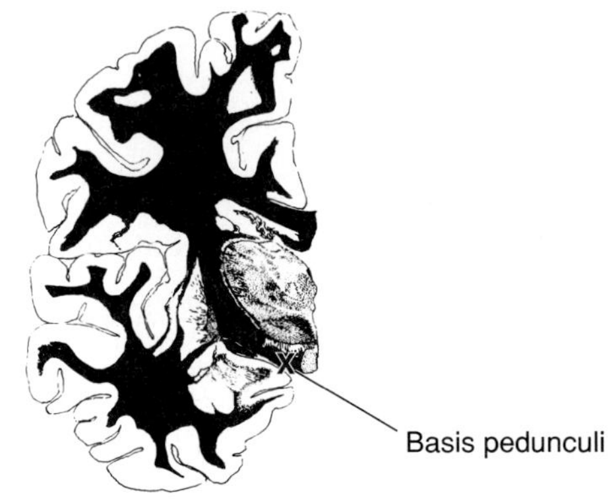

17.18A. colliculi; white

17.19A. red; basis pedunculi; superior colliculus

17.20. The basis pedunculi lies ___________ to the colliculi of the midbrain and both anterior and lateral to the ______ nucleus. Encircle the region of the basis pedunculi.

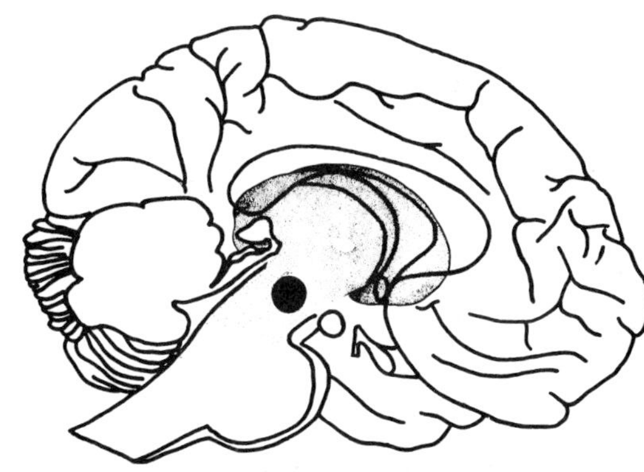

17.21. In the midbrain, the corticospinal tract passes anterior to the four ___________ and to the ______ nucleus.

17.22. Encircle the midbrain region of the brainstem. A line has been drawn on the diagram to indicate a coronal section. Draw an intersecting line to indicate a section *transverse* to the *midbrain*, with the intersection in the left superior colliculus.

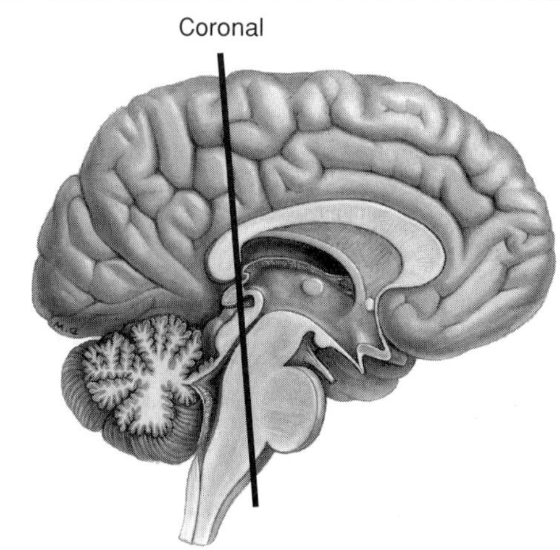

17.23. Note the labeled structures on the transverse section. Draw a line through the left hand picture to show the level of the section.

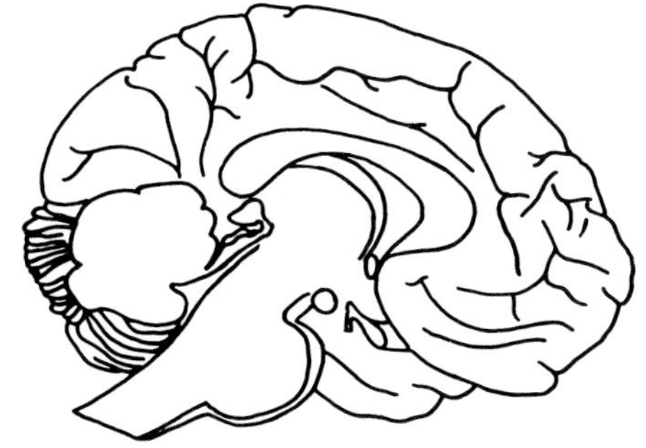

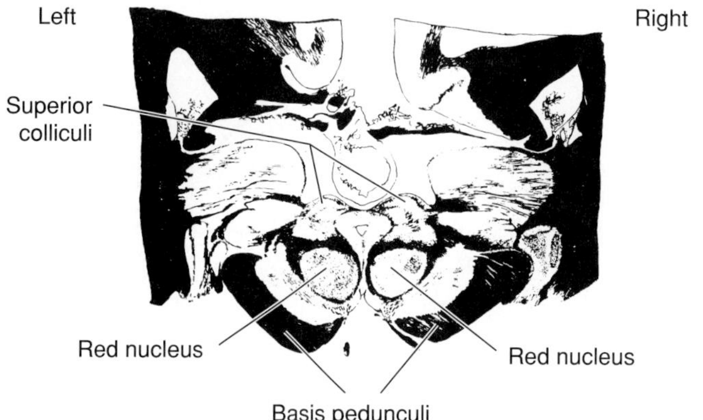

17.20A. anterior; red

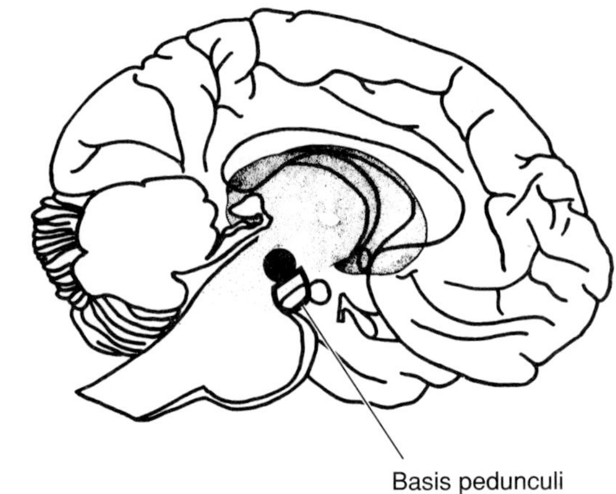

17.21A. colliculi; red

17.22A.

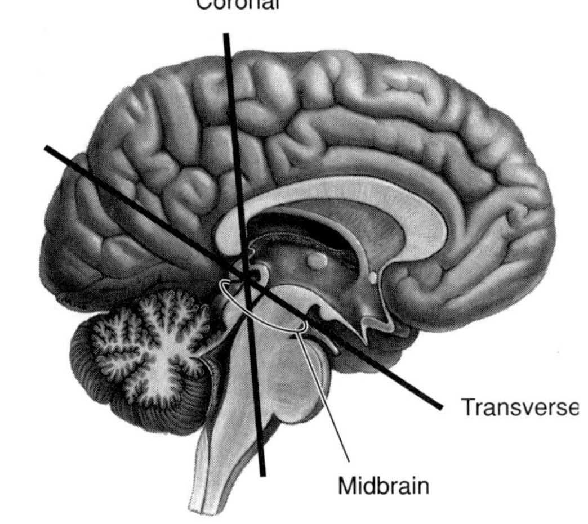

17.23A.

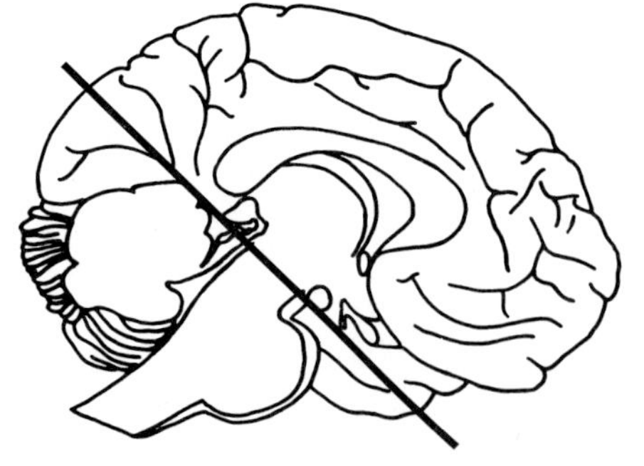

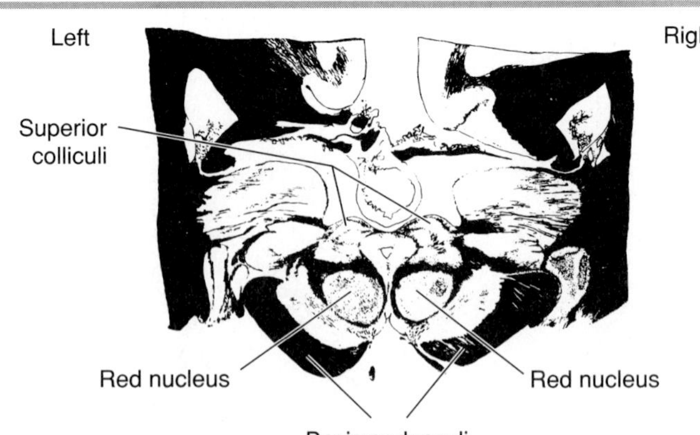

17.24. Label the three indicated structures. Encircle the labels of the two most anterior structures.

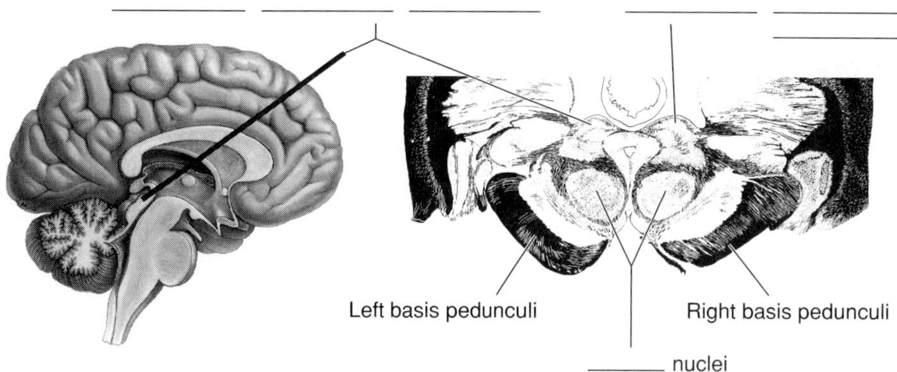

17.25. The red nuclei lie _______ior to the colliculi. On both sides of the section, label the red nuclei and superior colliculi.

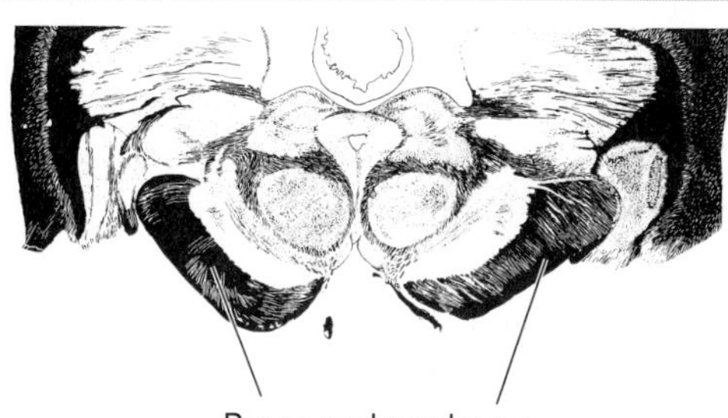

17.26. Look at the diagram. The basis pedunculi is part of a larger structure, the _____________ _____________.

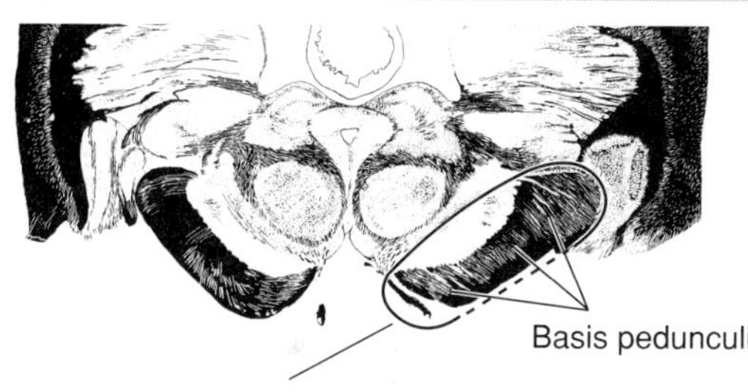

17.27. A *ped*uncle is a foot piece (pillar or column) that supports another structure. The _______ uncle on each side of the midbrain "holds up" the cerebral hemisphere, which lies in a position _______ior to the midbrain.

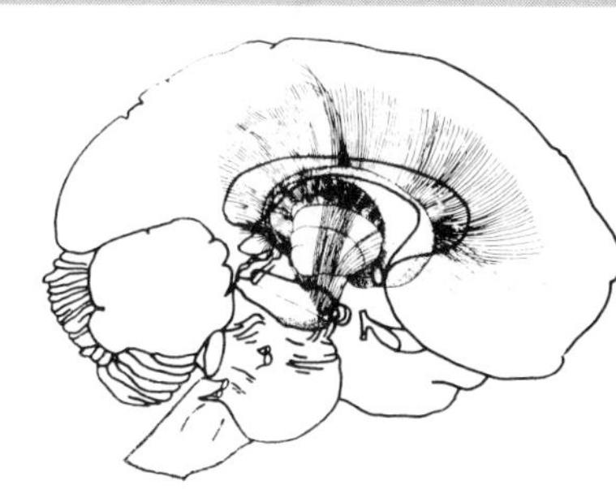

17.24A.

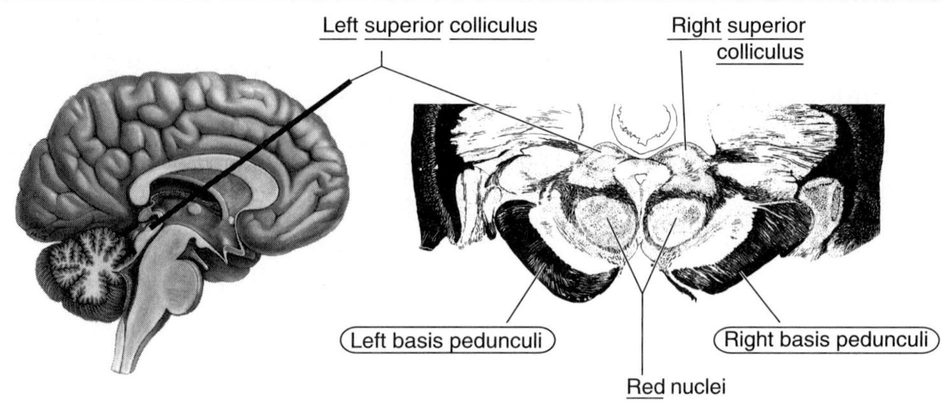

17.25A. anterior

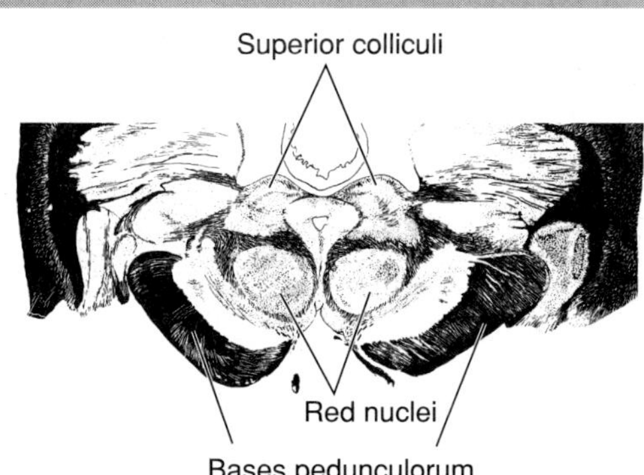

17.26A. cerebral peduncle

17.27A. peduncle; superior

17.28. The portion of the midbrain that holds up the cerebral hemisphere is called the ____________ ____________ (label it on the figure). The white matter that forms the *base of the peduncle* is called, in direct Latin translation, the ______ ____________ (label it on the figure).

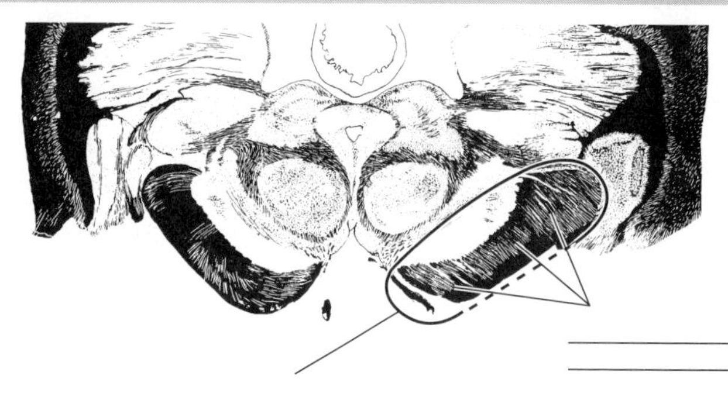

17.29. The basis pedunculi is composed of ______ matter. The whole cerebral peduncle is composed of both ______ and ______ matter. At the posterior side of the section are two "little hills," the ____________ ____________.

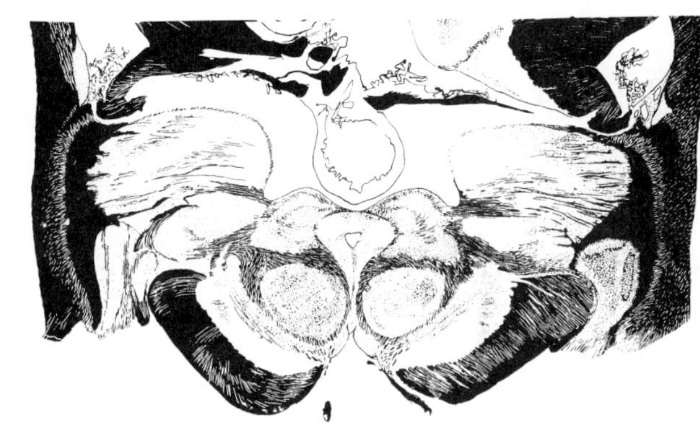

17.30. Label the indicated structures.

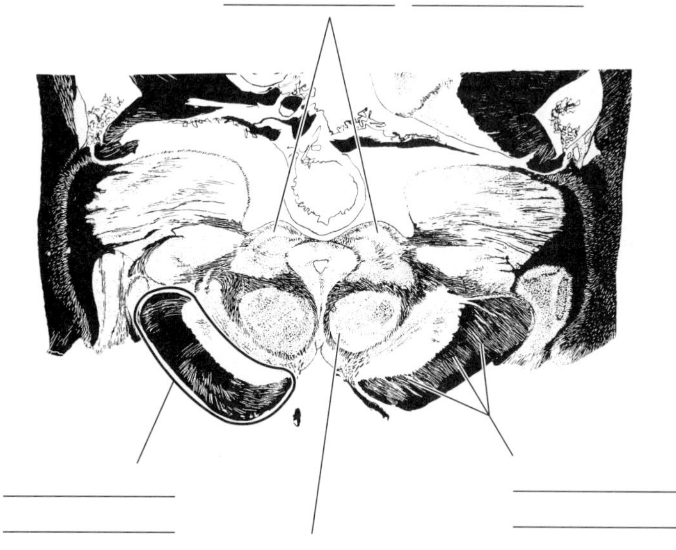

17.28A.

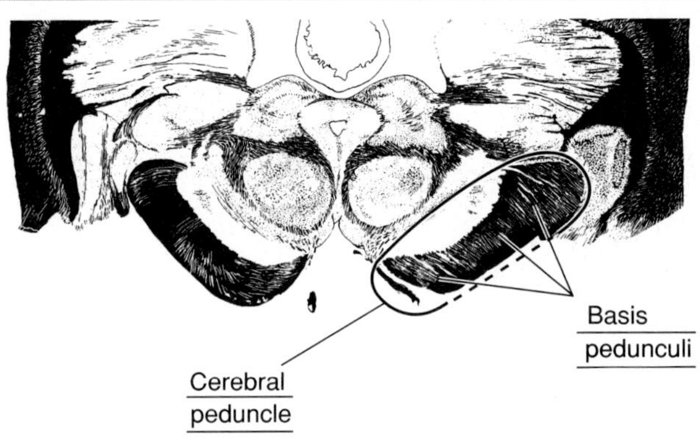

17.29A. <u>white</u>; <u>gray</u>; <u>white</u>; <u>superior</u> <u>colliculi</u>

17.30A.

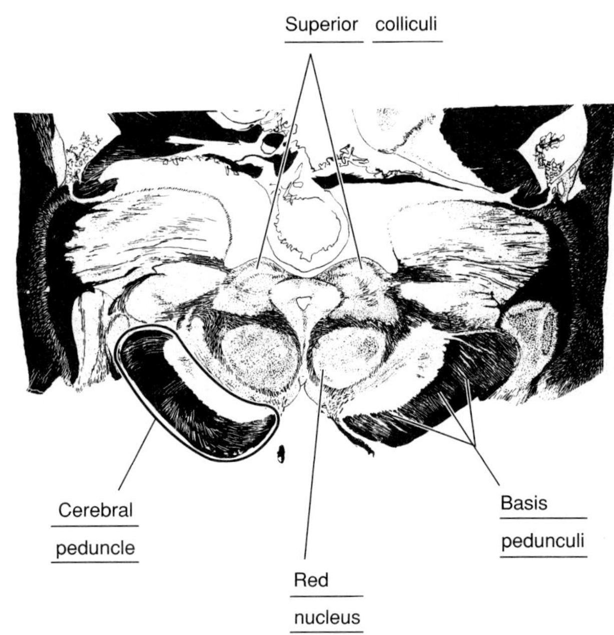

18 The Corticospinal System and Brainstem Structures: Pons and Medulla

18.1. Before it enters the pons, the corticospinal tract traverses the ______ __________ of the midbrain.

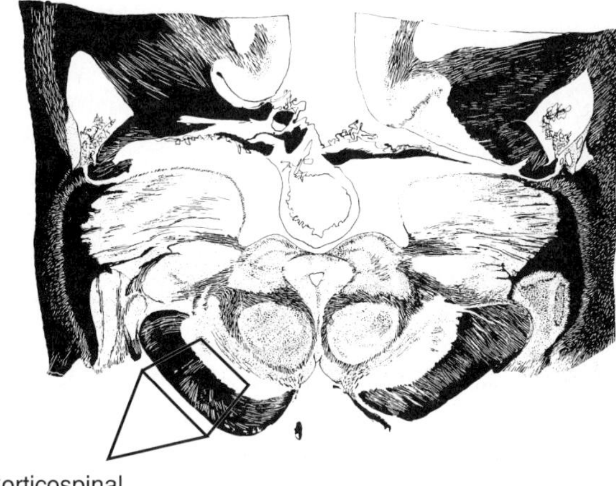

18.2. In the coronal section, the corticospinal fibers in the internal capsule are cut lengthwise (longitudinally); in a section transverse to the midbrain, the same fibers are cut in ________________ section.

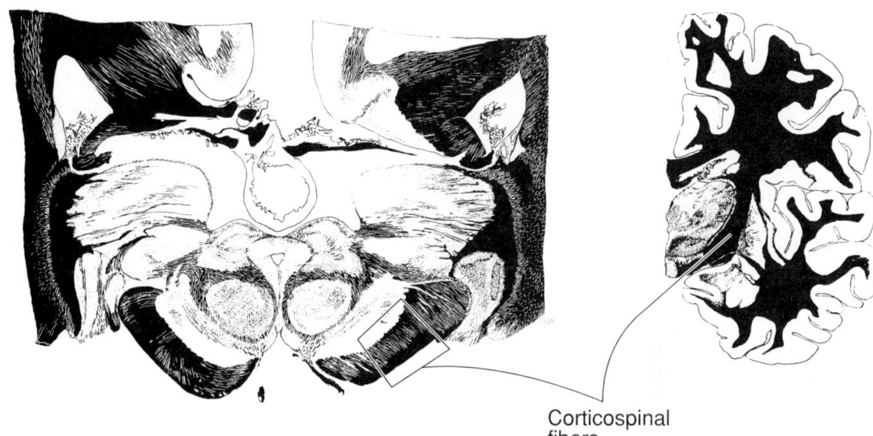

18.3. The pons appears rounded and bulging on its __________ side.

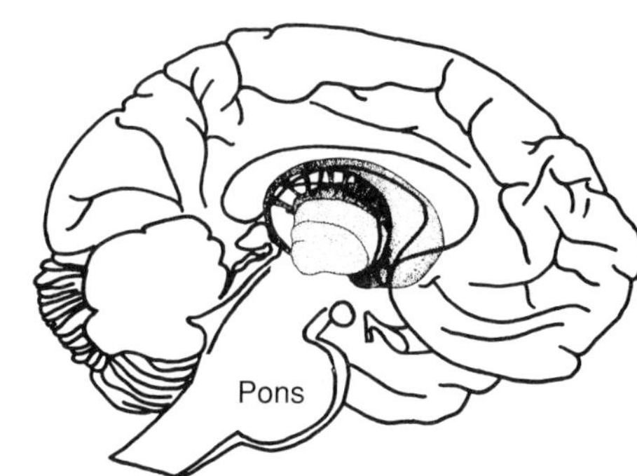

18.1A. basis pedunculi

18.2A. transverse (or cross)

18.3A. anterior

18.4. Note the fourth ventricle (IV) in the transverse section through the pons. The section is at the level marked ______ on the left hand diagram.

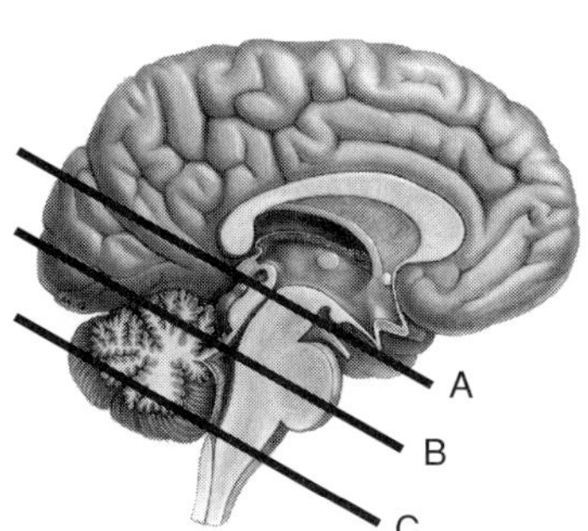

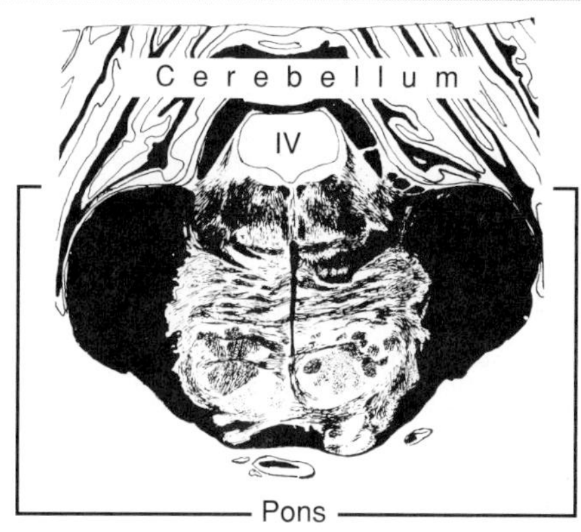

18.5. Label the pons (P) and medulla (M). A distinctive structural feature of the pons is the pattern made by the interlacing bundles of white matter fibers in its anterior, bulging part. The arrow lies along fibers running to the cerebellum. Most of the other fibers are heading for the medulla and belong to the ________________ tract.

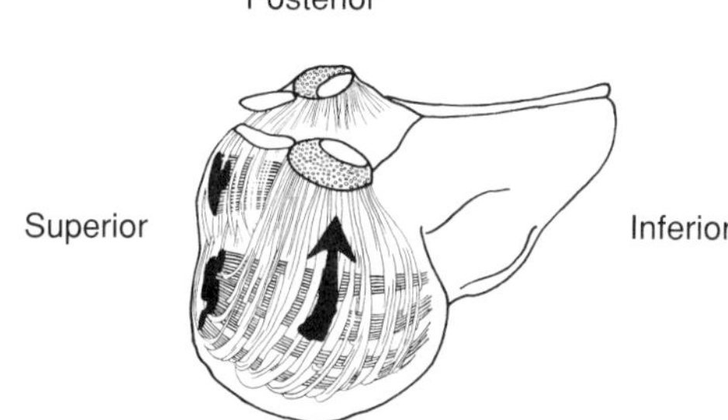

18.6. Draw lines to bundles of corticospinal fibers and label them "CS." Draw arrows on the laterally placed masses of white matter to indicate the direction of impulse conduction in them.

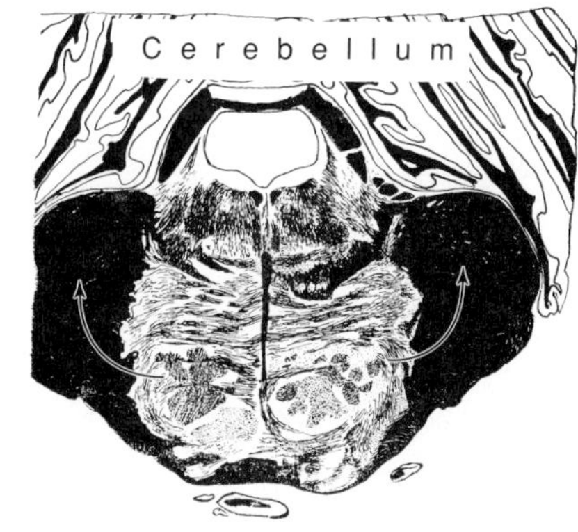

18.7. The region of the brainstem represented by the left section is the ____________; the region represented by the right section is the ______. The area encircled on the two pictures contains the fibers of the ________________ tract.

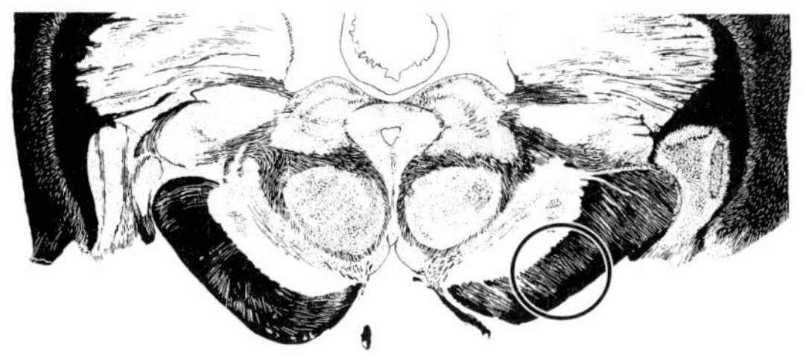

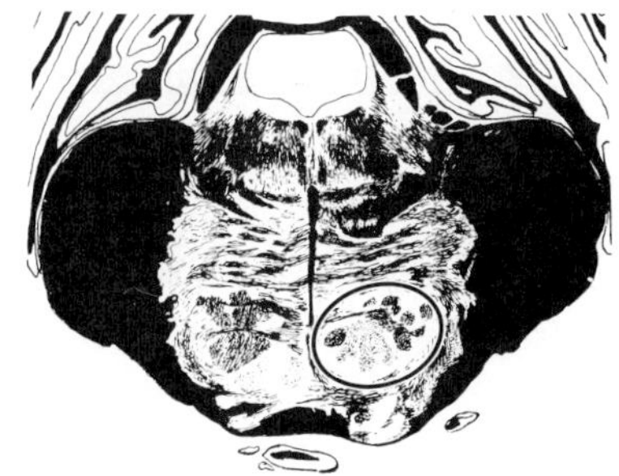

18.4A. B

18.5A. corticospinal

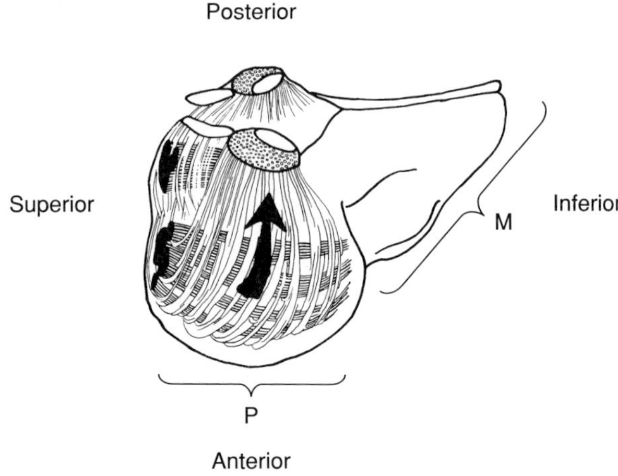

18.6A.

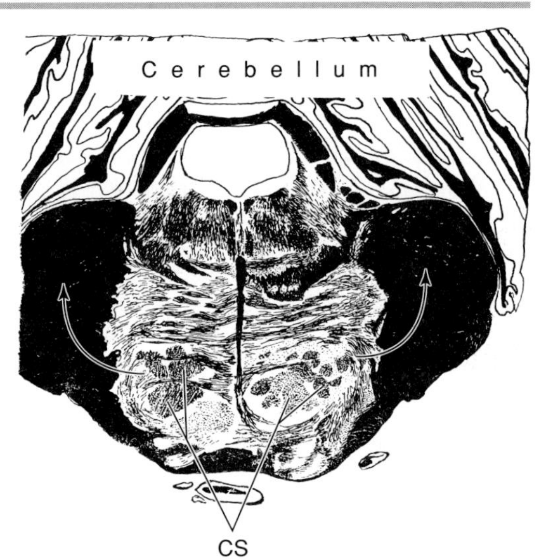

18.7A. midbrain; pons; corticospinal

18.8. The parietal, temporal, and occipital lobes send efferent fibers to the pons. This __________ pontine tract follows the expected white matter route through the posterior limb of the __________ __________ and then through the ______ __________ of the midbrain.

18.9. Another efferent tract from the frontal lobe to the pons follows a similar route, except that it passes through the __________ limb of the internal capsule. It is named the __________ pontine tract.

18.10. Encircle and label the corticopontine tract and the frontopontine tract at the level of the internal capsule. In the basis pedunculi, the ________________ tract is closest to midline.

18.11. Number the following tracts as 1 to 3 in sequence, with *1* being most lateral and *3* being most medial in the basis pedunculi:

_____ Frontopontine

_____ Corticopontine

_____ Corticospinal

18.12. Label tracts 1 to 3 on the figure with their names.

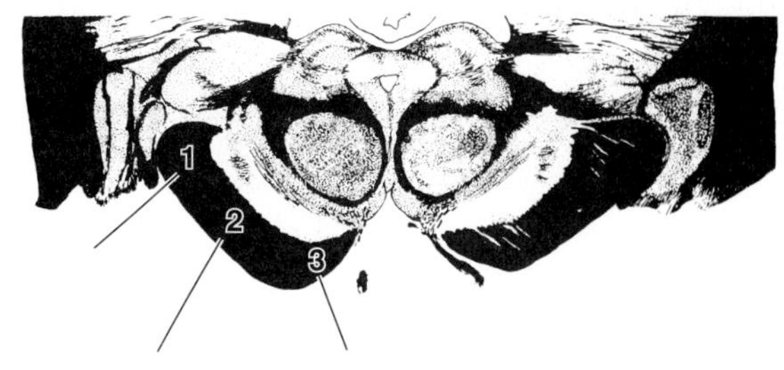

18.8A. corticopontine; internal capsule; basis pedunculi

18.9A. anterior; frontopontine

18.10A. corticospinal

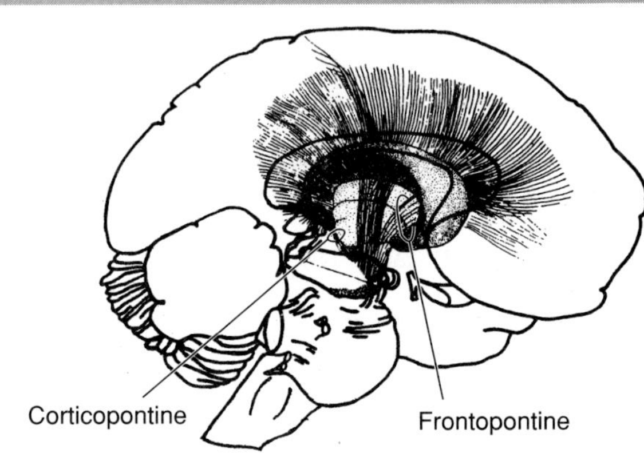

18.11A.

3 Frontopontine

1 Corticopontine

2 Corticospinal

18.12A.

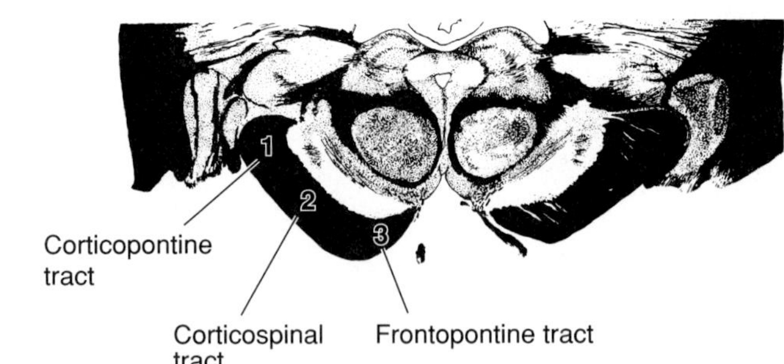

18.13. Fibers of tract "A" terminate in the ______. Fibers of tract "B" pass downward from the level of this section, successively through the ______ and ____________ and into the ____________ ______ .

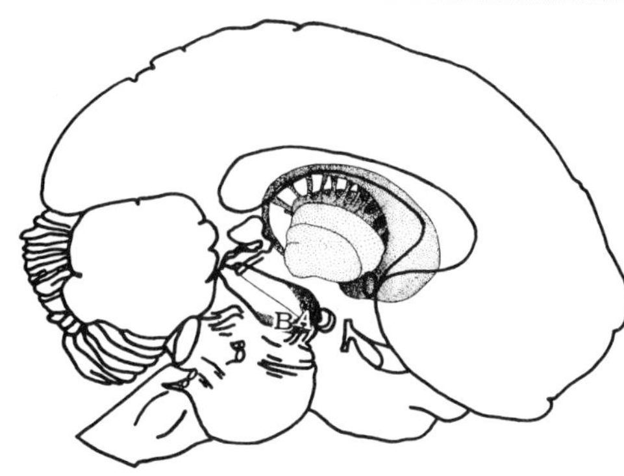

18.14. The line through the left hand diagram indicates the level of the section. From which region of the *brainstem* is the transverse section cut? ____________

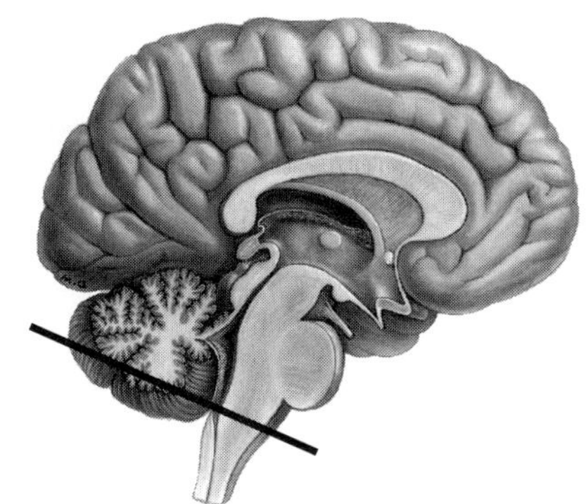

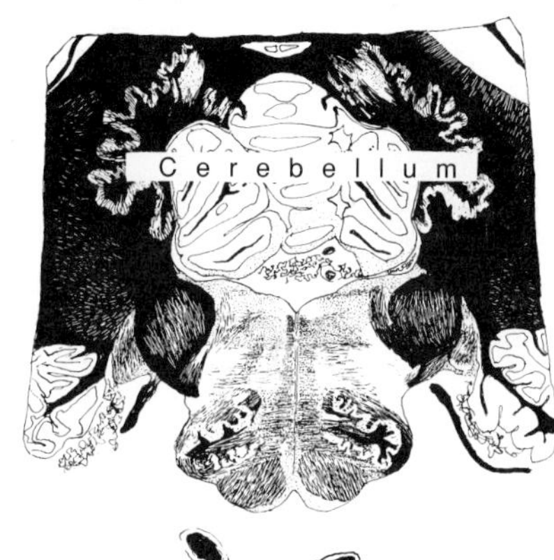

18.15. The corticospinal fibers again form a compact bundle along the ____________ surface of the medulla. At some levels of the medulla, the corticospinal fibers form a compact bundle with a *pyramidal* shape. Because of this shape, the portion of the corticospinal system that lies in the medulla is called the ____________ al tract.

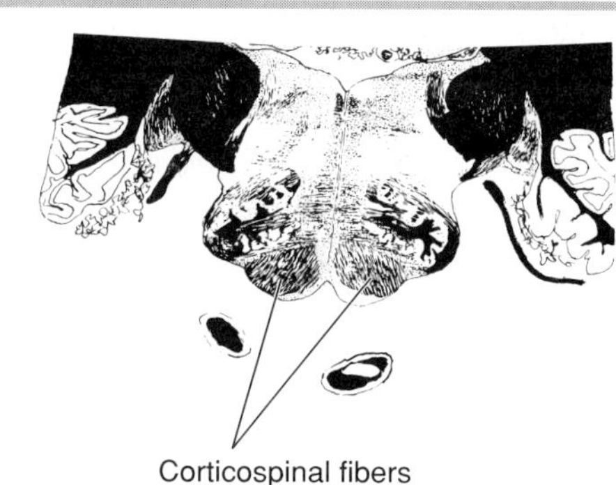

18.16. The pyramidal tract is ______ matter. The stain applied to the right side of this diagram colors the ______ matter (cranial nerve XII was drawn in on this diagram; it would not be stained in this way). On the right side, label the inferior olive, cranial nerve XII, and pyramidal tract.

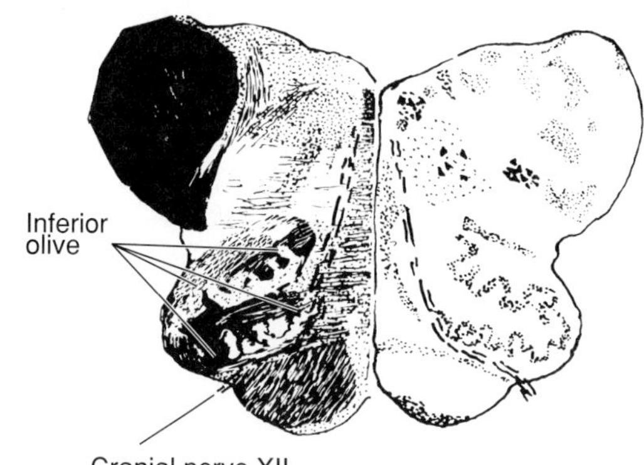

18.13A. pons; pons; medulla; spinal cord

18.14A. medulla

18.15A. anterior; pyramidal

18.16A. white; gray

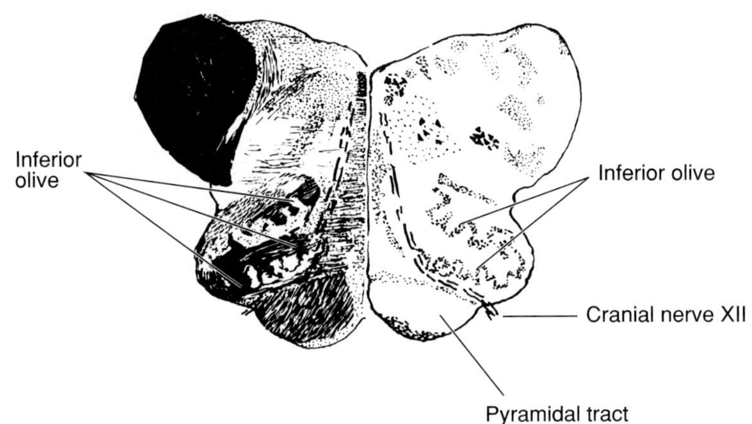

18.17. Cranial nerve XII emerges from the brainstem between the inferior olive and the pyramidal tract. On both sides of the diagram, indicate its point of emergence with arrows. Cranial nerve XII, the inferior olive, and the pyramid all help to identify a transverse section across the ___________.

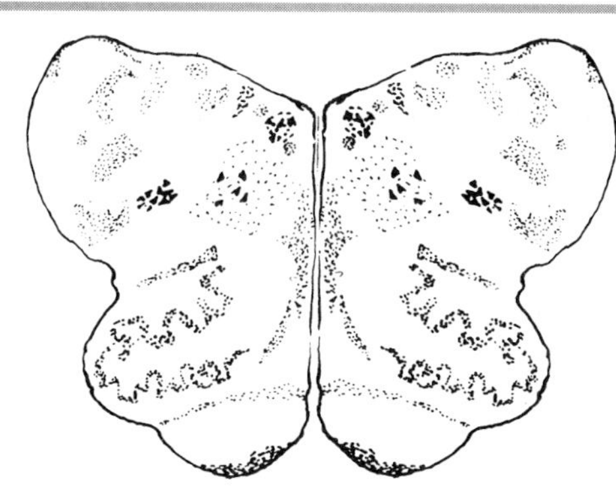

18.18. The pons is in the section numbered _____; the medulla is in the section numbered _____.

In the following list, place a "P" beside the structures found in the section through the pons and an "M" beside the structures found in the section through the medulla. Place both letters if the structure is common to both sections and neither letter if neither section shows the structure.

_____ Inferior olive
_____ Corticopontine tract
_____ Cranial nerve XII
_____ Internal capsule
_____ Corticospinal fibers
_____ Pyramidal tract
_____ Cerebellum
_____ Fourth ventricle

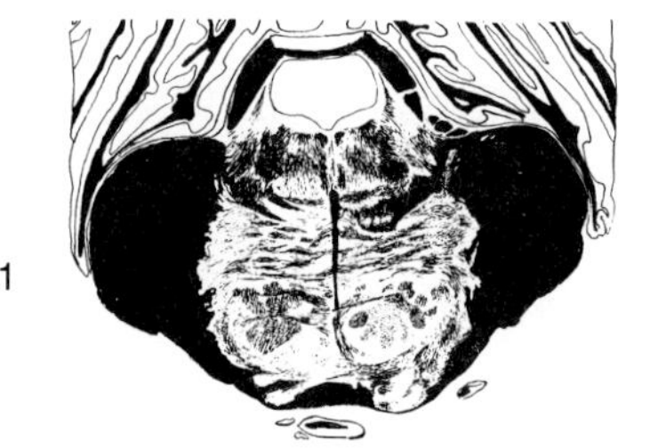

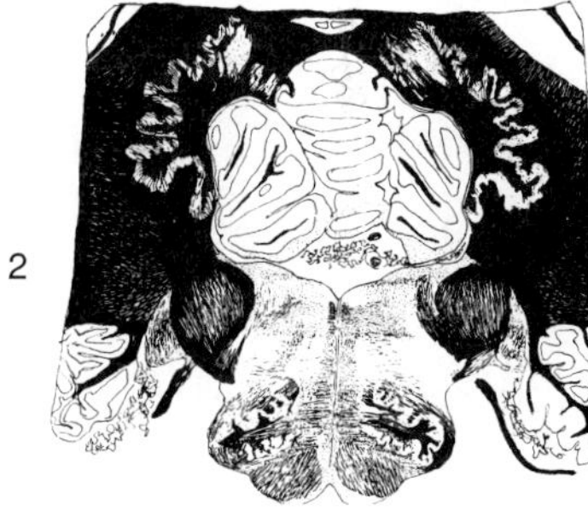

18.19. Label each section with its brainstem level. On the right side of each figure, place an "X" in the region that contains corticospinal fibers.

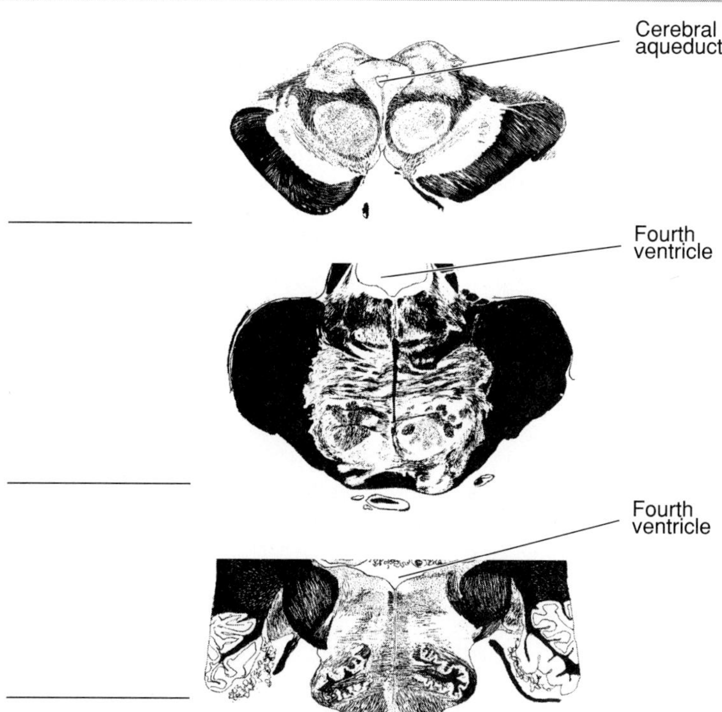

18.17A. medulla

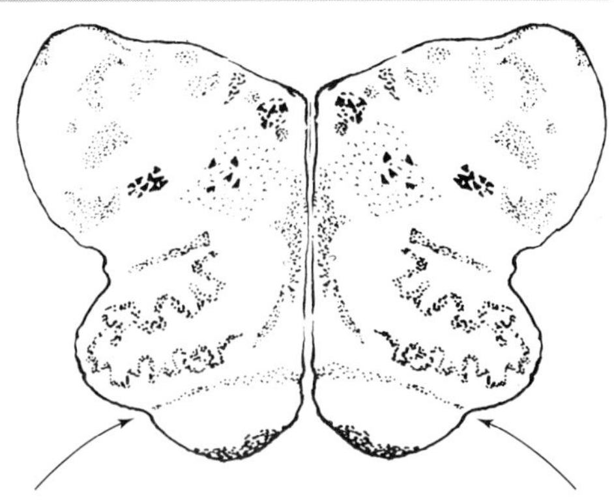

18.18A. 1; 2

__M__ Inferior olive

__P__ Corticopontine tract

__M__ Cranial nerve XII

______ Internal capsule

__PM__ Corticospinal fibers

__M__ Pyramidal tract

__PM__ Cerebellum

__PM__ Fourth ventricle

18.19A.

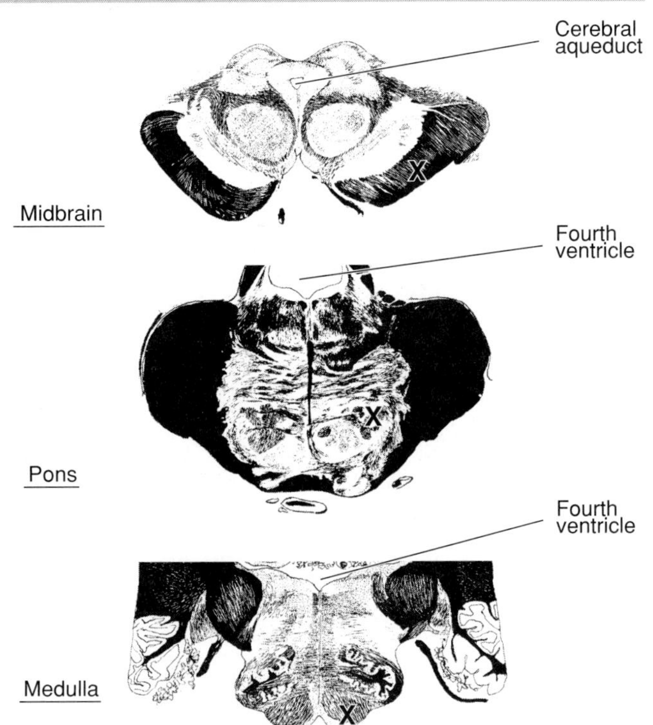

18.20. Corticospinal fibers, notable for their length, pass without ________________ from cerebral cortex to spinal cord. Depending on their location, corticospinal fibers may be referred to in several ways. For example, just before reaching the basal nuclei, they are part of the fan-shaped ___________ ___________; passing around the lenticular nucleus, they join the other fibers of the ___________ ___________; within the medulla, they become part of the ___________ _____.

18.21. Corticospinal fibers, plus the other components of the internal capsule, form the _____al wall of the thalamus.

18.22. This schematic view of the brainstem shows three efferent nerve fibers, A through C, from the cerebral cortex. At the level where they are lettered, they are in the ___________ ___________, and just medial to them is a large mass of gray matter, the ___________. At the cut surface indicated by the arrow, the fibers are entering the ___________ region. Look also at the pons. The corticospinal fiber is labeled with the letter _____.

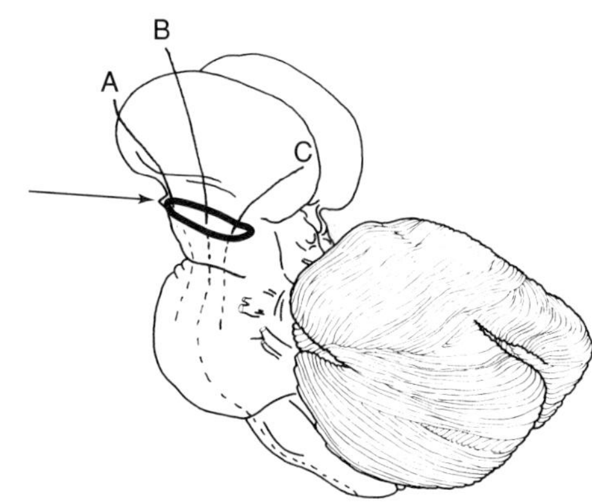

18.23. When an axon is interrupted, the functional loss is likely to be the same regardless of where the interruption occurs along the length of the axon. *Some* of the effects of a lesion in the internal capsule are identical to the effects of a lesion that involves the ___________ tract in the medulla. The most obvious consequence of damage to corticospinal fibers is ___________ of movement.

18.24. The destructive lesion marked with a cross in the midbrain causes loss of motor function in an arm and leg. Place crosses on the *sections* through the pons and medulla to indicate lesions that would cause the same motor loss in this arm and leg.

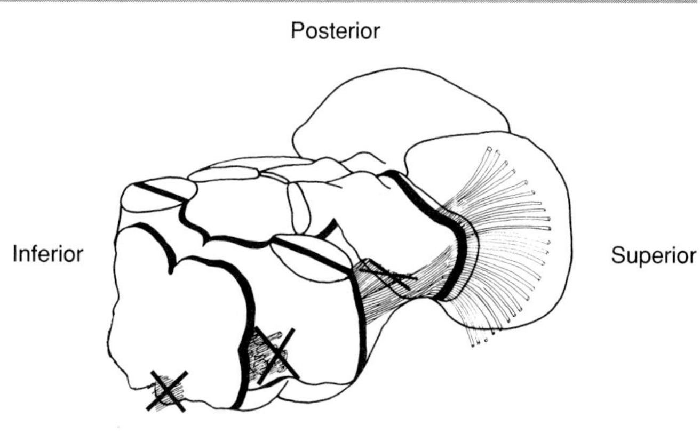

18.20A. interruption; corona radiata; internal capsule; pyramidal tract

18.21A. lateral

18.22A. internal capsule; thalamus; midbrain; B

18.23A. pyramidal; paralysis

18.24A.

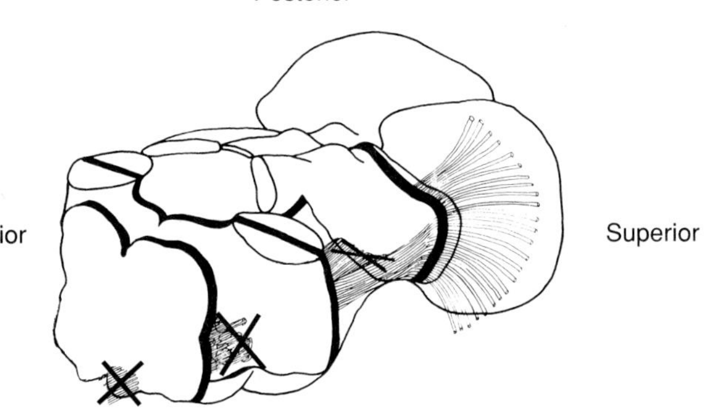

19 The Decussation of the Pyramids

19.1. The term *pyramidal tract* refers to fibers in the pyramids on the anterior surface of the ____________ of the brainstem

19.2. In this schematic diagram, parts of the brainstem and spinal cord are seen from an *anterior* view. At the most superior level of the pons, encircle the group of fibers that originates in the *left* cerebral *hemisphere*. The corticospinal system is bilaterally symmetrical.

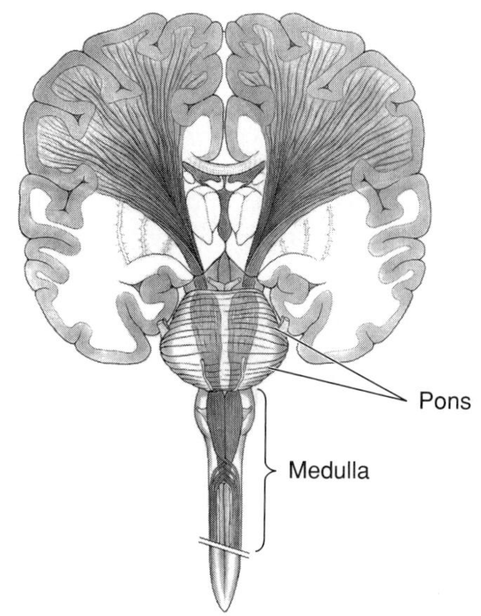

19.3. As the fibers of the left pyramidal tract descend, most of them ______ the midline in the lower medulla and enter the ____________ ____________________ tract on the ____________ side.

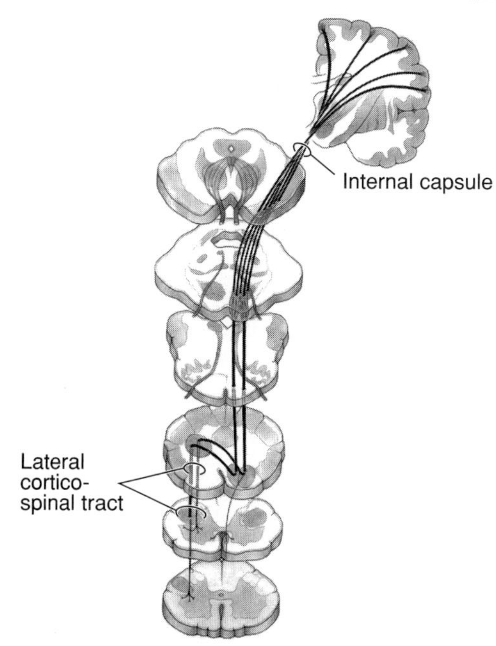

19.1A. medulla

19.2A.

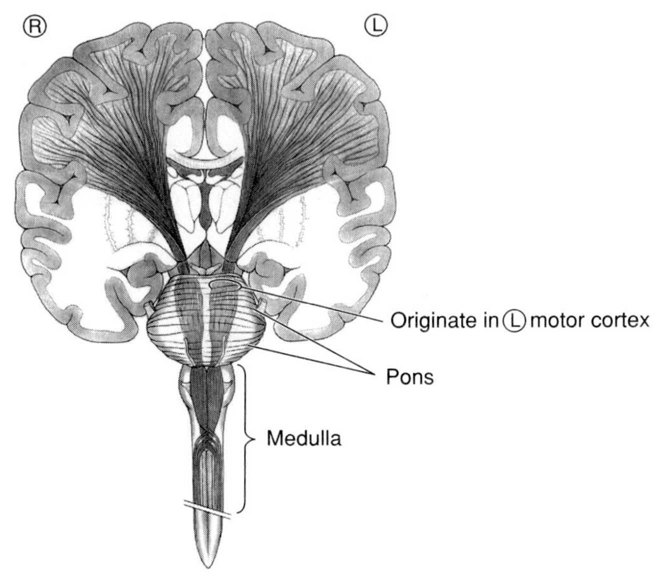

19.3A. cross (decussate); lateral corticospinal; opposite (contralateral)

19.4. As labeled, about 10 to 30% of the pyramidal fibers enter the spinal cord *uncrossed* as the ___________ corticospinal tract. Fibers of the *right lateral* corticospinal and *left anterior* corticospinal tracts arise from cell bodies in the cerebral cortex on the ______ side.

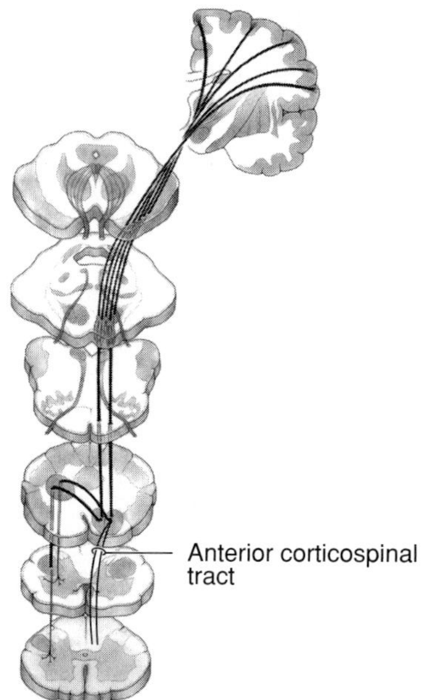

19.5. In the gradual transition zone between the medulla and spinal cord, 70 to 90% of the corticospinal fibers cross the midline from one side to the other. At the lowest level shown on the diagram, encircle the fibers from the *left hemisphere* that have crossed the midline.

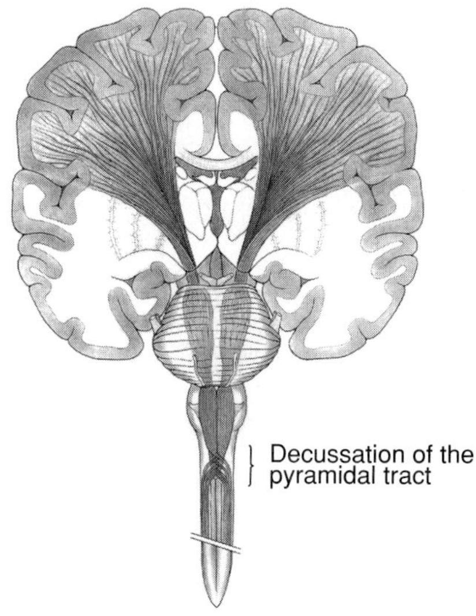

19.6. Darken the nerve fibers labeled as "A" over their whole visible length on the diagram. Do all of the diagrammed fibers cross the midline within the territory included in the diagram? ______

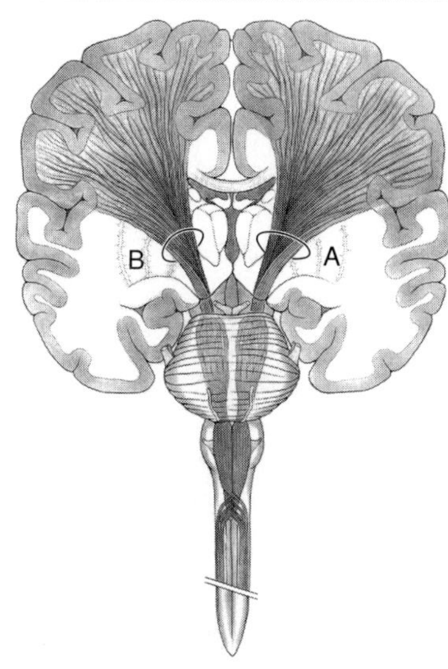

19.4A. anterior; left

19.5A.

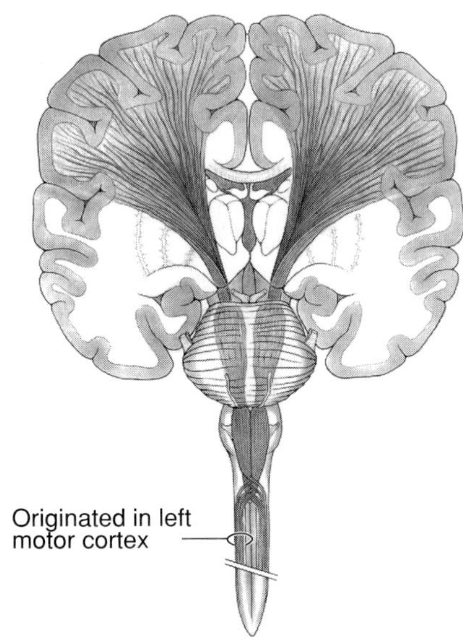

19.6A. No

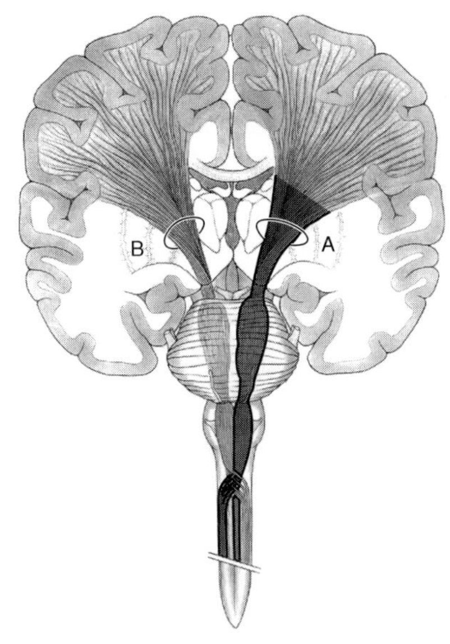

19.7. The decussation of the pyramidal tract extends over several millimeters of the junction area between the ___________ region of the brainstem and the ___________ ______. On the diagram, indicate with an arrow the level at which the decussation begins.

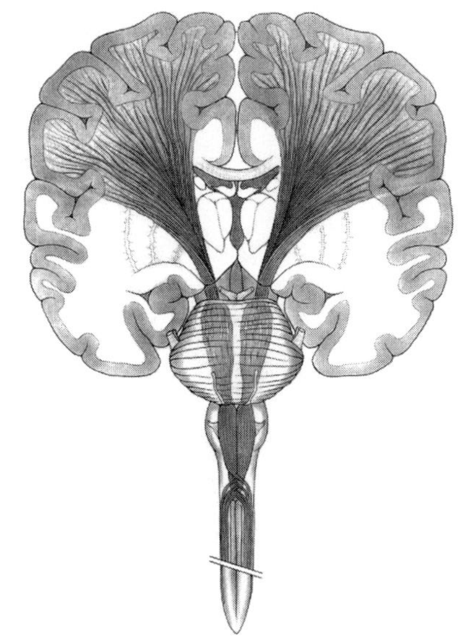

19.8. The descending corticospinal fibers of the right motor cortex appear stained on the transverse sections. At the lowest level of the diagram, encircle the transverse section of the *fibers* that arose in the left hemisphere and have crossed the midline.

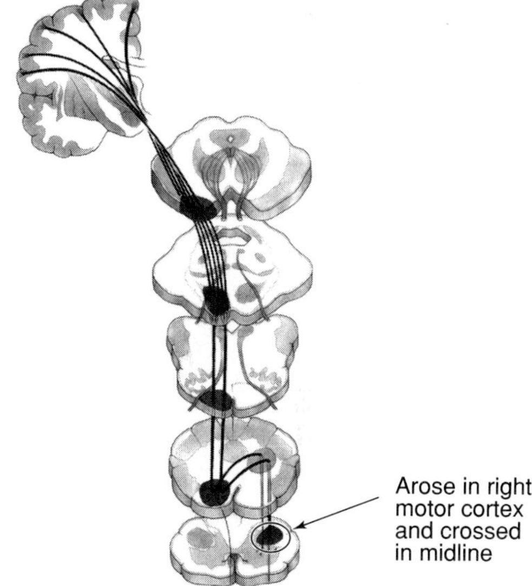

19.9. The descending fibers marked "X" are beginning to cross from the ______ side to the ______ side of the medulla. In the left hand diagram, encircle the cross section of these same fibers, both where they begin to cross and where they are completely crossed.

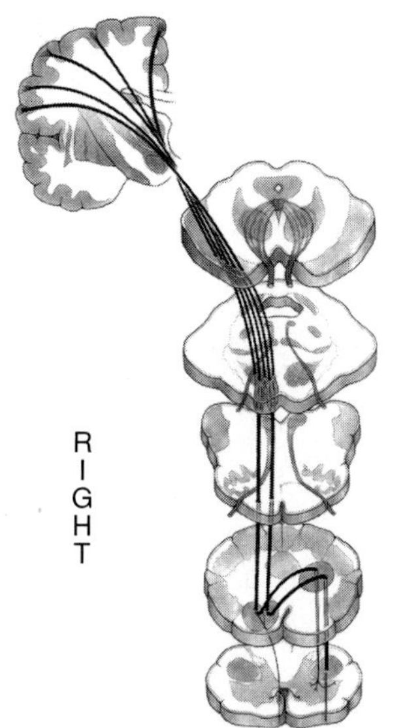

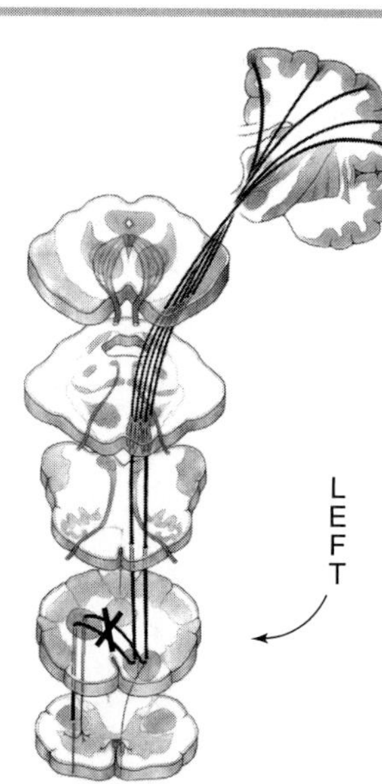

19.7A. medulla; spinal cord

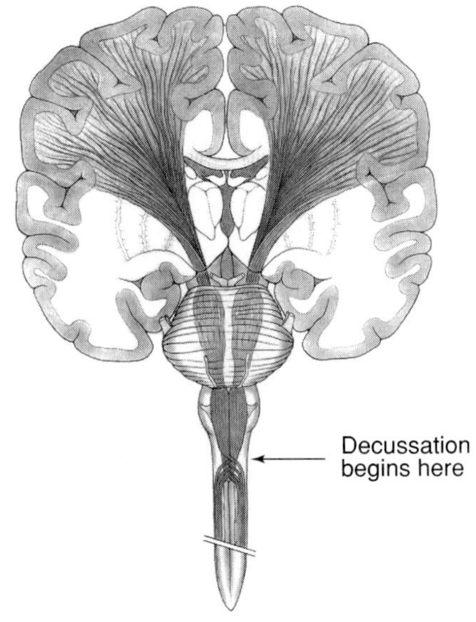

19.8A.

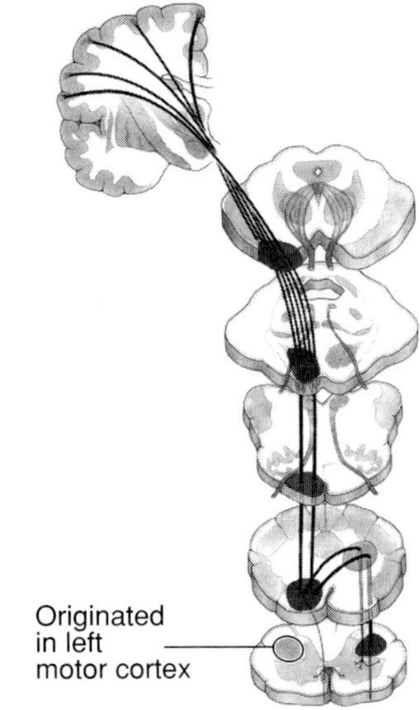

19.9A. left; right

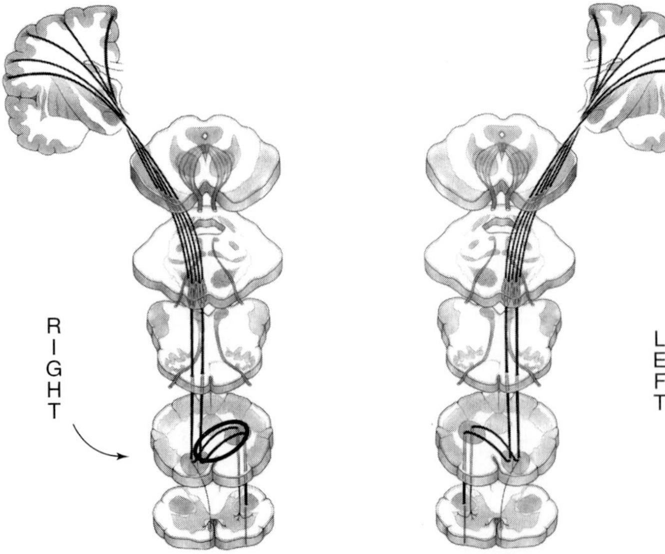

19.10. The lines on the *left* diagram represent segments of the corticospinal tract. The arrows indicate the direction of impulse conduction. Draw arrows on the right hand diagram to indicate the direction of impulse conduction.

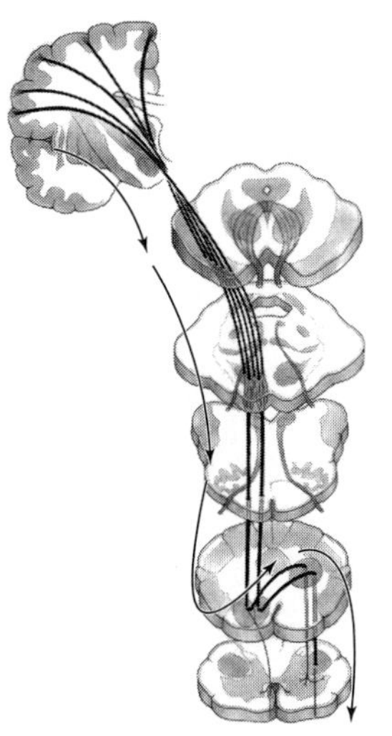

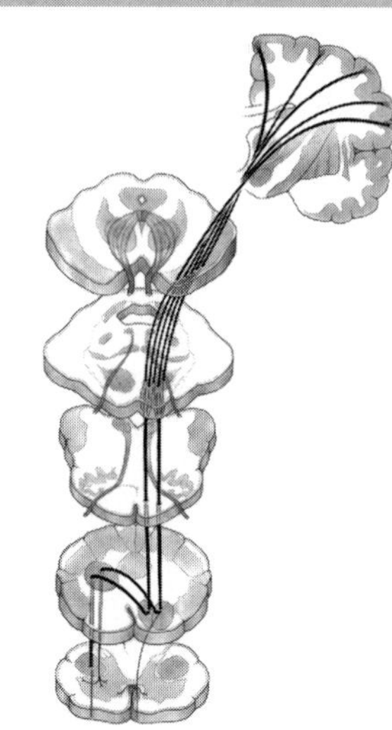

19.11. Draw arrows to indicate the direction of impulse conduction at the sites marked as "A," "B," "C," and "D" on the diagram.

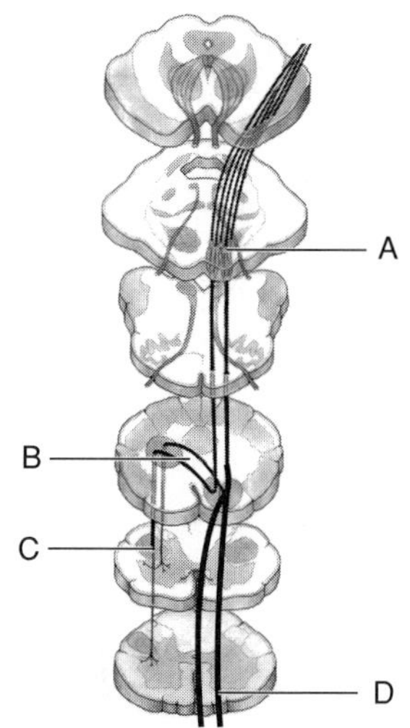

19.12. The pyramidal fibers in level "A" occupy an anterior position in the medulla. By "D," in the lower medulla and upper spinal cord, most of the fibers reach a posterior and lateral position. Between "B" and "C" in the pyramidal decussation, the fibers pass from an ____________ position on one side across the midline in a ____________ and ____________ direction. Draw a decussating fiber originating in the right pyramid from "B" to "C."

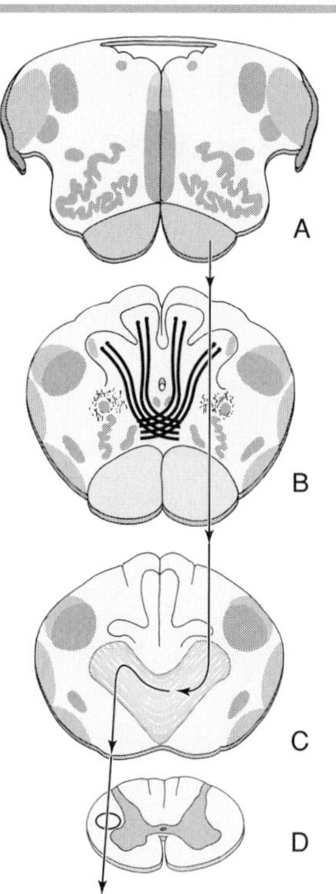

19.10A.

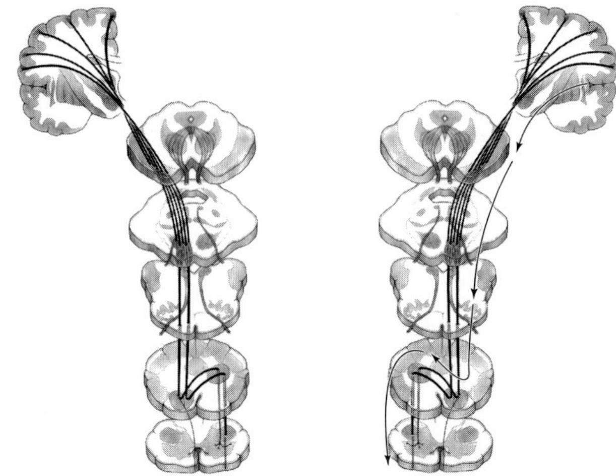

19.11A.

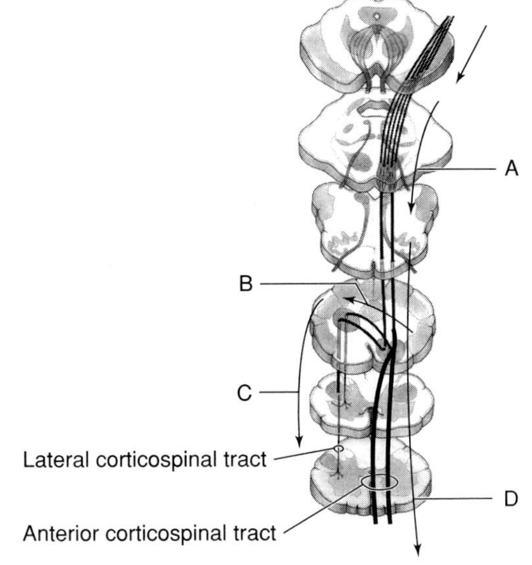

19.12A. anterior; lateral; posterior

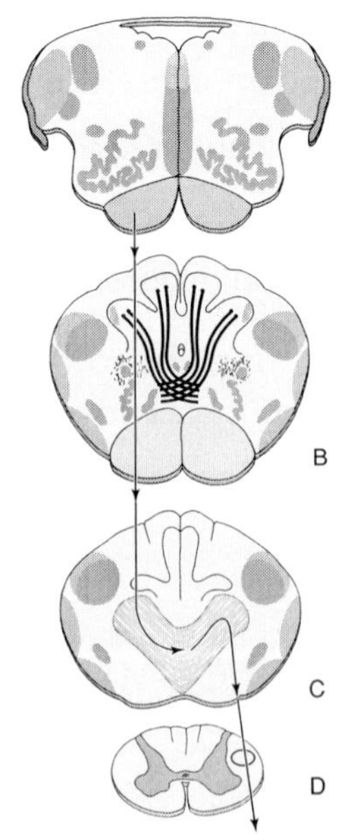

19.13. If you look at a transverse section of the medulla from an inferior view (looking up from the spinal cord), the *left* side of the picture represents the *left* side of the medulla. If you view the same section of the medulla from a superior view (looking down from the midbrain), the left side of the picture represents the ______ side of the medulla.

19.14. Label each picture "L" or "R" to indicate, respectively, the left and right sides of the brain.

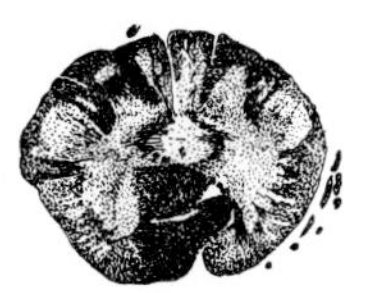

Viewed from spinal cord

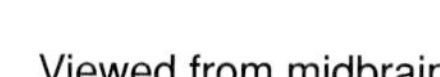

Viewed from midbrain

19.15. Of the three sections labeled "A," "B," and "C," which one shows fibers of the pyramidal tract decussating from the left to the right side of the medulla? ______ Decussating from the right to left side of the medulla? ______ At a level above the pyramidal decussation? ______

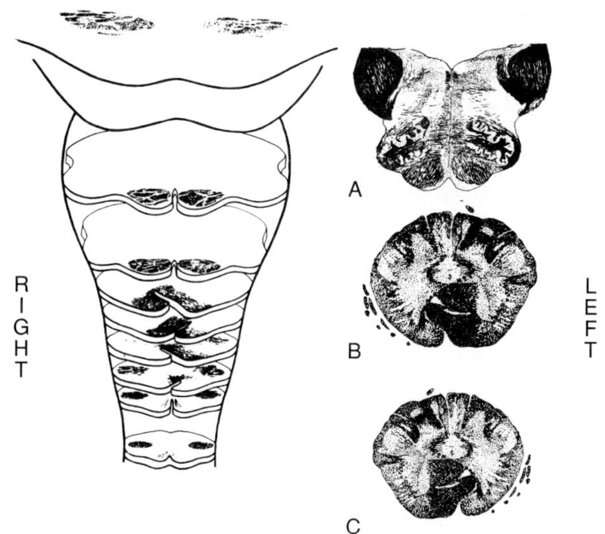

19.16. On each picture, draw an arrow on the decussating fibers to show the direction of impulse conduction from one side of the medulla to the other.

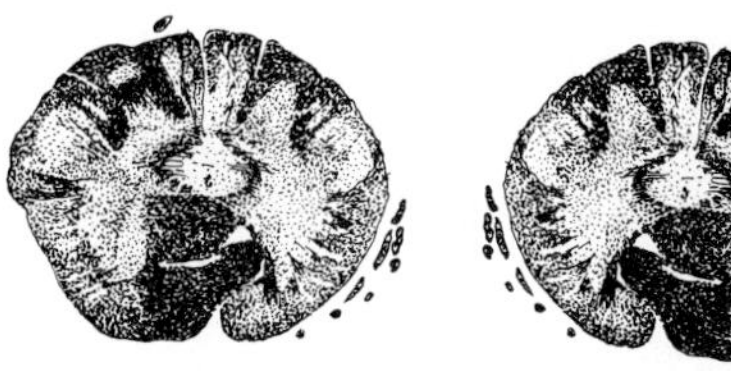

19.17. Extend the fiber labeled as "1" inferiorly to the spinal cord. Let it decussate (cross) in the section indicated by the arrow.

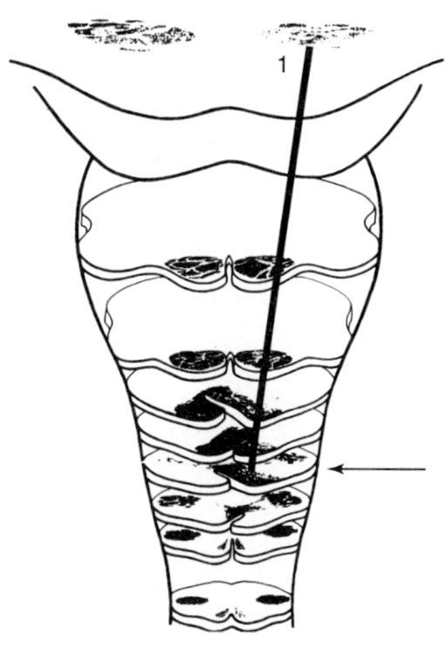

19.13A. right

19.14A.

L 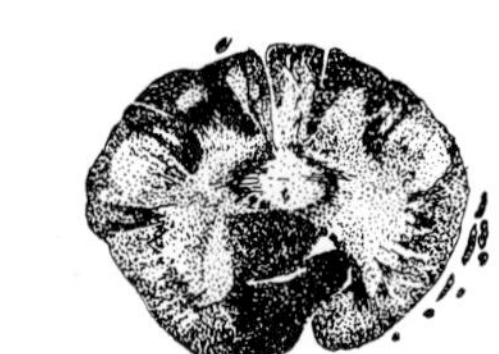 R

Viewed from spinal cord

R L

Viewed from midbrain

19.15A. B; C; A

19.16A.

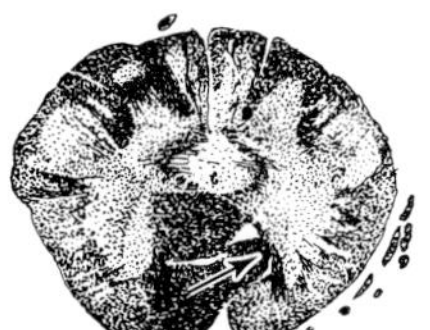

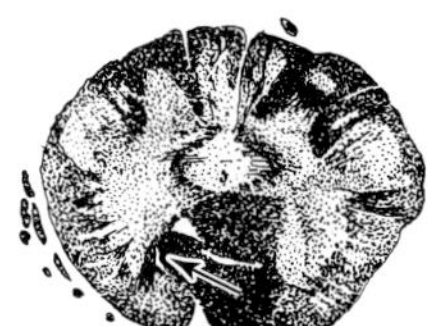

19.17A.

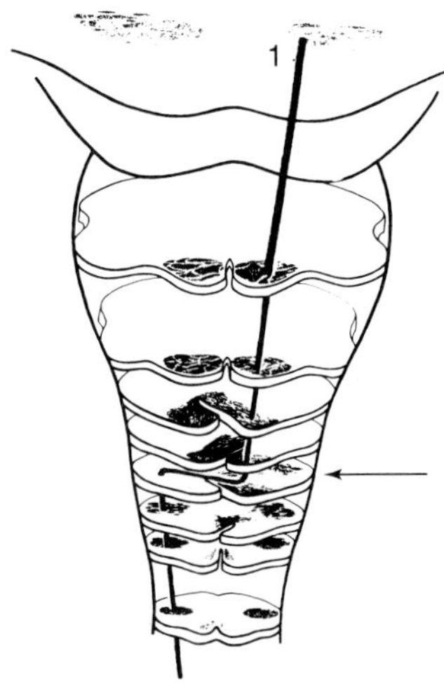

19.18. Draw the decussating fibers "1" and "2" inferiorly to the spinal cord.

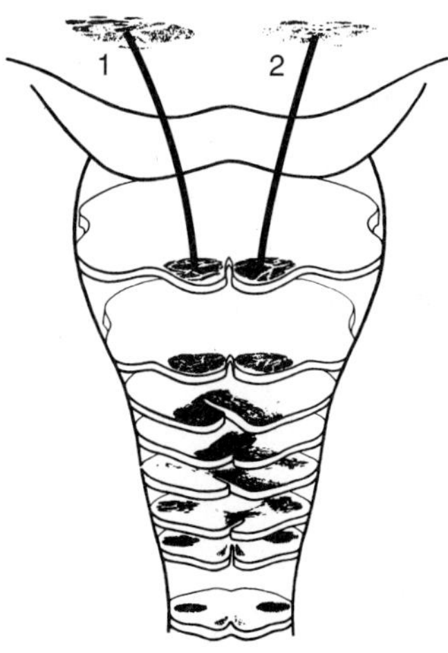

19.19. The fibers shown decussating in section "A" arise mainly in the ______ cerebral hemisphere and end in the ______ side of the spinal cord.

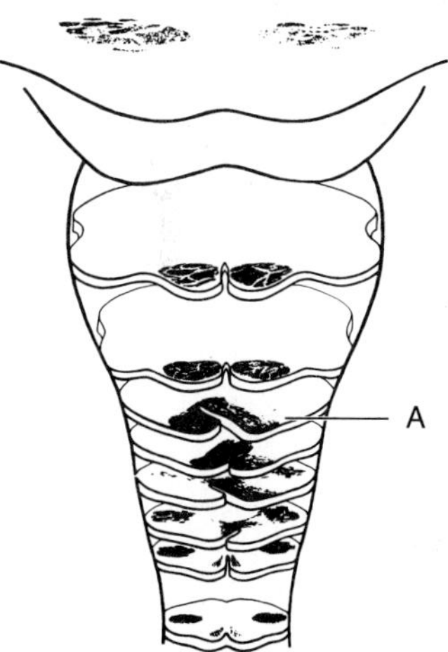

19.20. Look at these two sections of the medulla. The more rostral of the sections is ______ Explain your answer:

____.

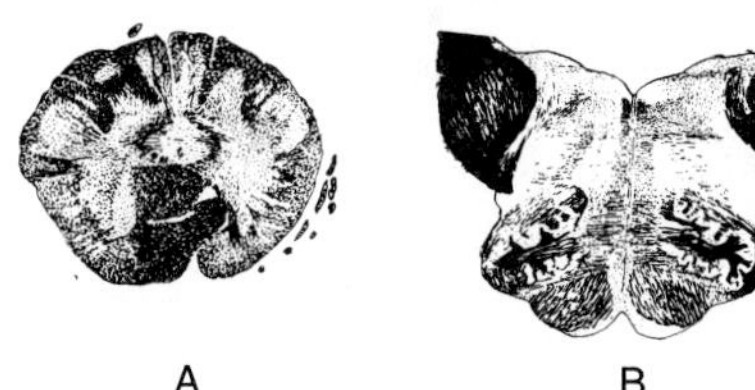

19.21. Place an "X" at the midline on two sections that show pyramidal fibers decussating from the left to the right side of the specimen.

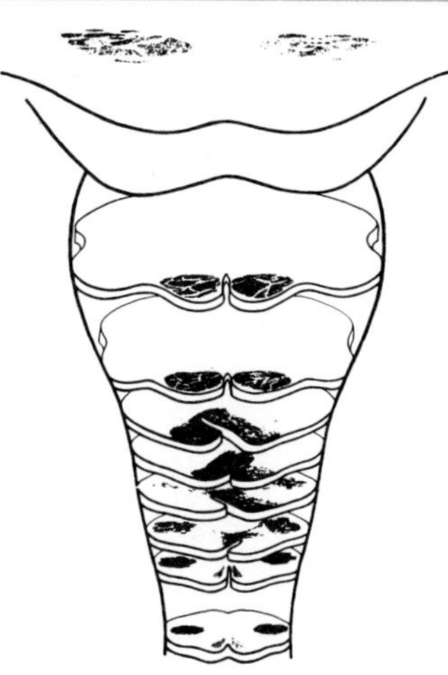

19.18A.

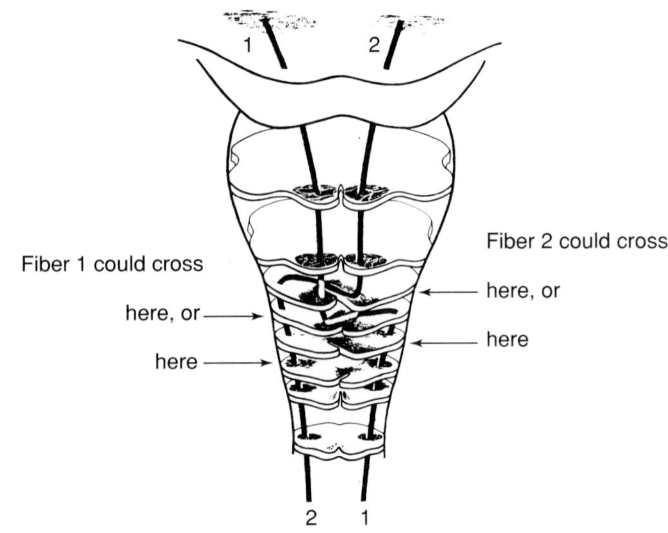

19.19A. <u>left</u>; <u>right</u>

19.20A. <u>B</u>; <u>Section "B" does not show the decussation of the pyramidal tract.</u>

19.21A.

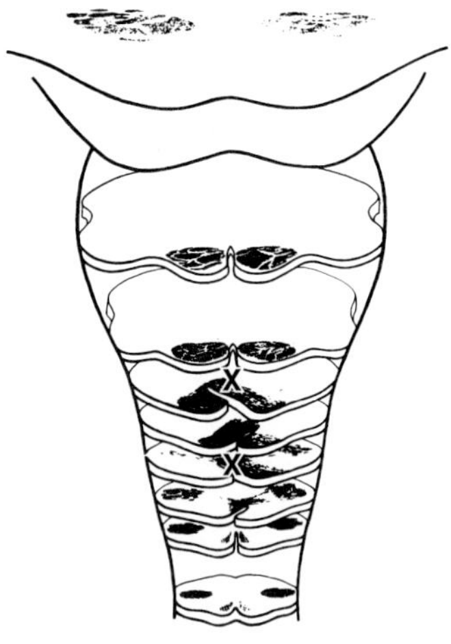

19.22. As corticospinal fibers descend, bundles of fibers from one side cross the midline alternately with bundles from the other side, so that a given transverse section is likely to show the decussation mainly from one side. On the diagram, fibers crossing the medulla from left to right are shown in levels numbered ______ and ______. Fibers crossing the medulla from right to left are shown in levels numbered ______ and ______.

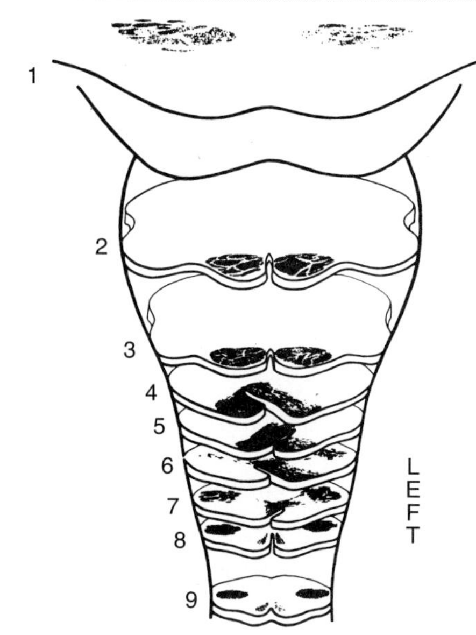

19.23. The alternating pyramidal decussations from left to right and right to left give a braided appearance to the ______ior surface of the lower medulla.

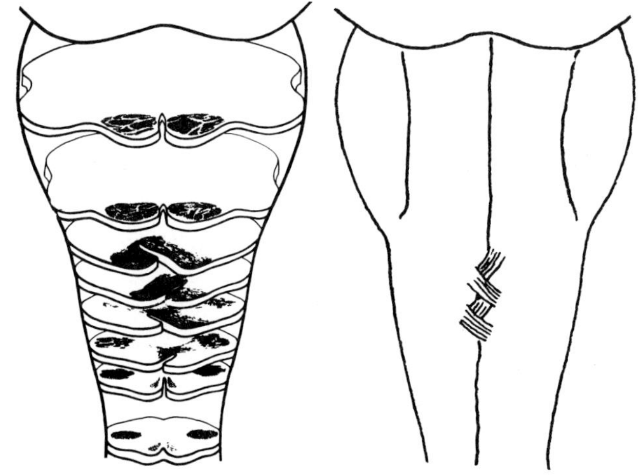

19.24. In passing from medulla to spinal cord, corticospinal fibers cross the midline in the __________ation of the __________ tract.

19.25. Corticospinal fibers cross in the pyramidal decussation from the ______ior surface of the medulla to a postero ______al position in the spinal cord.

19.22A. 4; 6; 5; 7

19.23A. anterior

19.24A. decussation; pyramidal

19.25A. anterior; posterolateral

19.26. Label the transition area between the medulla and spinal cord. In the spinal cord, the decussated fibers take up a postero ____________ position.

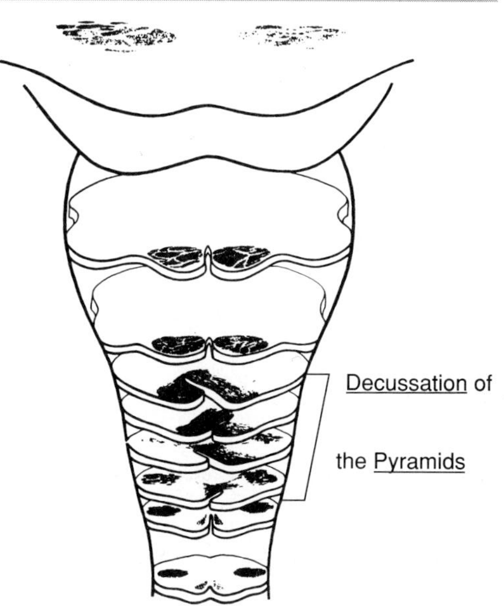

19.27. Corticospinal fibers arise from cells in the surface gray matter of the cortex, pass into the depths of the cortex, and emerge on the anterior surface of the ____________ region of the brainstem. They pass inferiorly through the pons and again move toward the anterior surface while in the medulla's ____________ tract. The fibers then decussate to a ______ero ____________ position inside the cord. Interruption of corticospinal fibers on one side of the brain at the level of the rostral medulla or above is likely to produce paralysis on the ____________ side of the body.

19.28. Corticospinal fibers on the right side of the top diagram are encircled. Identify the level of each section.

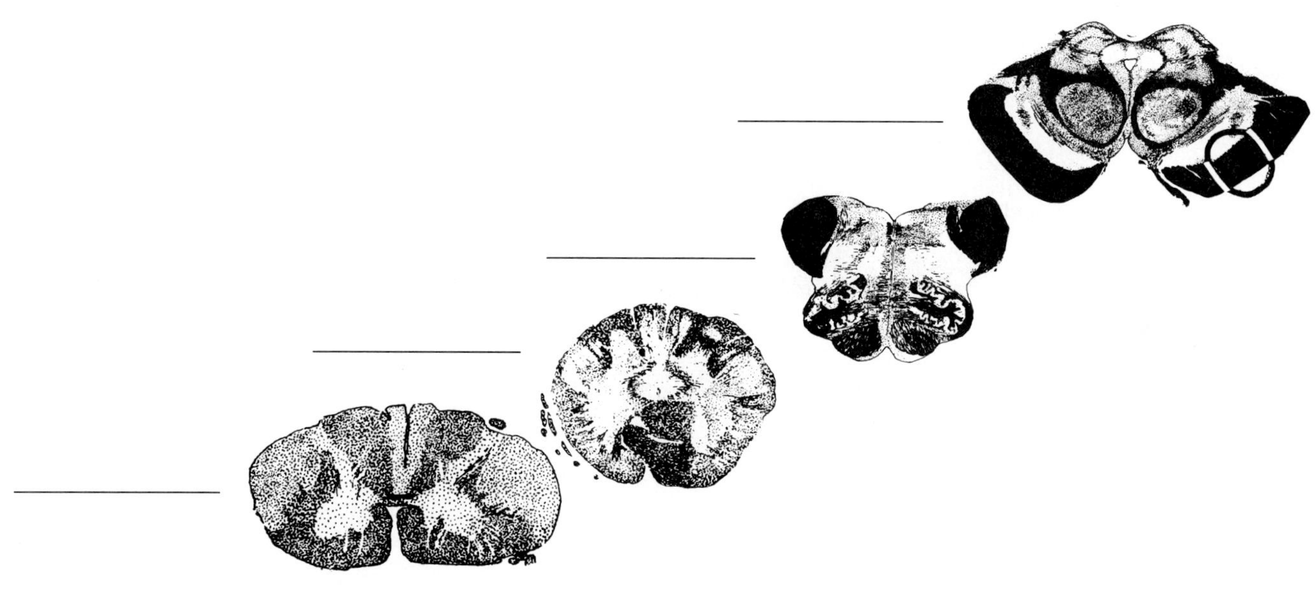

19.26A. posterolateral

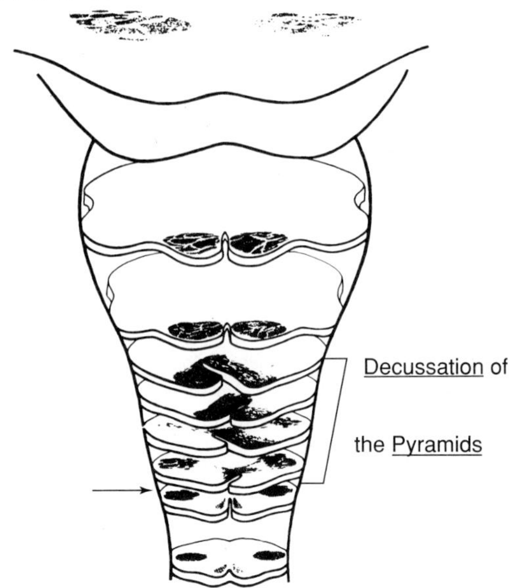

19.27A. midbrain; pyramidal; posterolateral; opposite

19.28A.

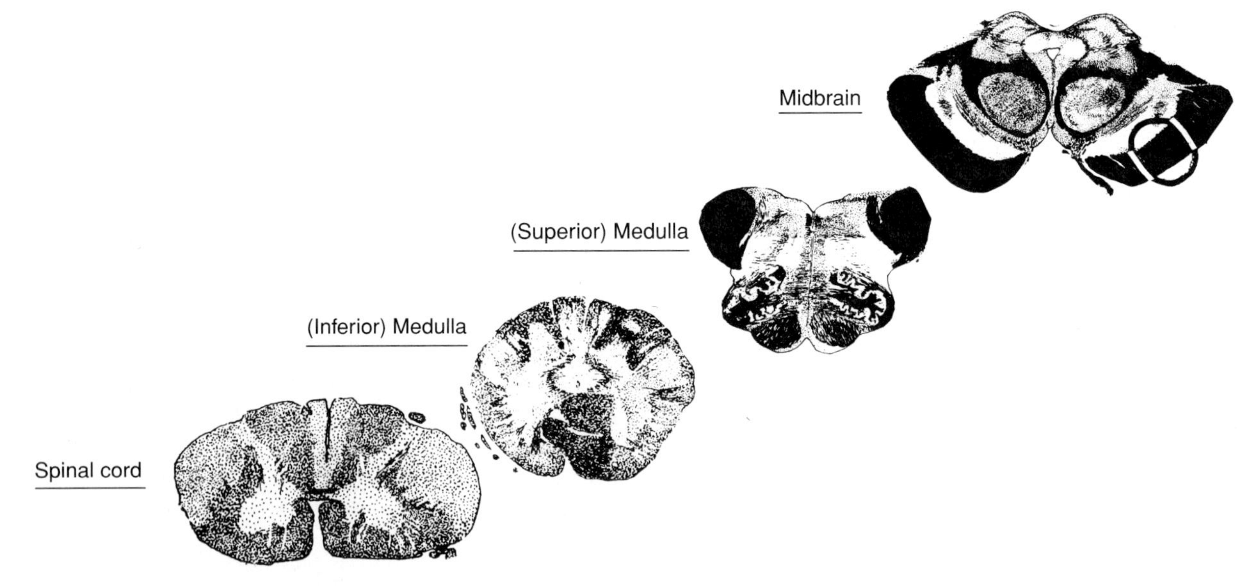

20 Representation of Body Parts in the Corticospinal System: Cortex and Brainstem

20.1. We have followed corticospinal fibers that originate in the ________________ gyrus. Many of the efferent fibers of the pyramidal tract actually arise from cells more widely distributed in the same lobe, the __________ lobe.

20.2. Most of the efferent fibers of the basal nuclei travel in paths outside the pyramidal route; hence, the term extra __________ motor system is often used for the basal nuclei and their connected structures.

20.3. The extrapyramidal system, like the pyramidal system, by definition is a _____ system.

20.4. Of the wide range of neurons contributing efferent fibers to the brainstem and spinal cord, much attention has been given to a relatively small population of giant neurons in the precentral gyrus. In honor of their discoverer, Betz (1874), these giant neurons are referred to as _____ cells.

20.5. The body is represented on the precentral gyrus as indicated on the diagram. Cells on the most inferior part of the lateral surface of the gyrus, closest to the __________ sulcus, influence the _____. Over the superior surface and onto the medial side of the precentral gyrus is the representation of the _____ limb.

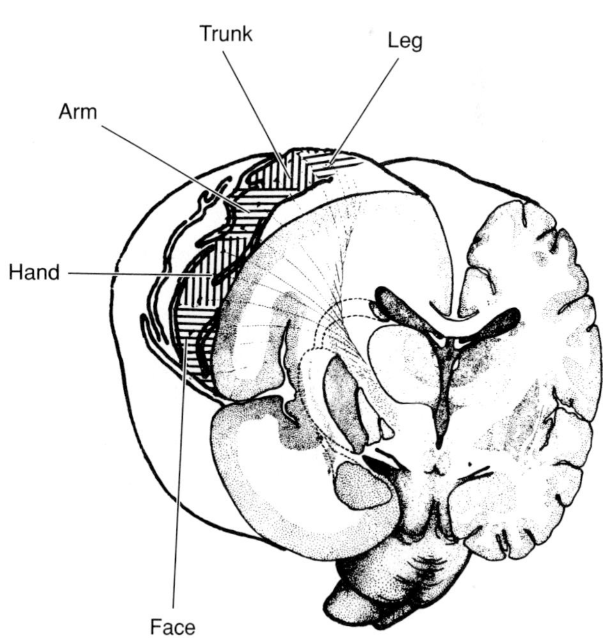

20.1A. <u>precentral</u>; <u>frontal</u>

20.2A. extra<u>pyramidal</u>

20.3A. <u>motor</u>

20.4A. <u>Betz</u>

20.5A. <u>lateral</u>; <u>face</u>; <u>lower</u>

20.6. Movements of the fingers on the opposite side are produced by stimulation of an area on the precentral gyrus __________ in size than the area representing the entire thorax plus abdomen.

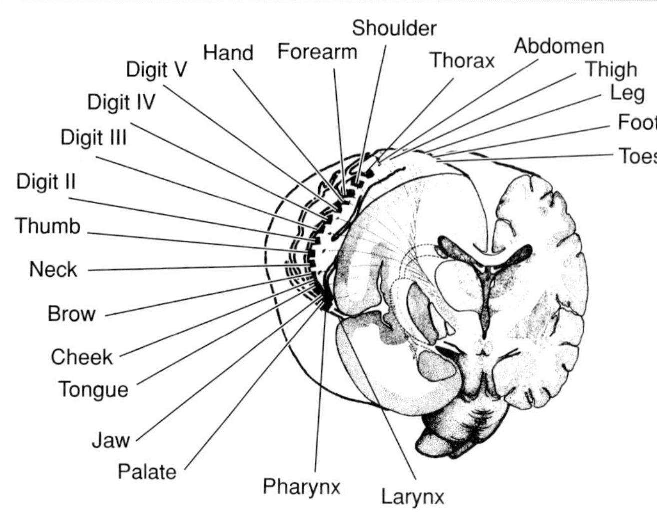

20.7. An important principle is that the complexity of motor control for a given body part is proportional to the ______ of precentral gyrus on which that body part is represented. The same principle applies to sensory representation of body parts on the ________________ gyrus.

20.8. In conformity with this principle, the ______ is represented by an area larger than that for the rest of the face. If the area of precentral gyrus influencing movements of the toes were as large as the area for the fingers, we might modify the piano and place a keyboard within reach of our ______.

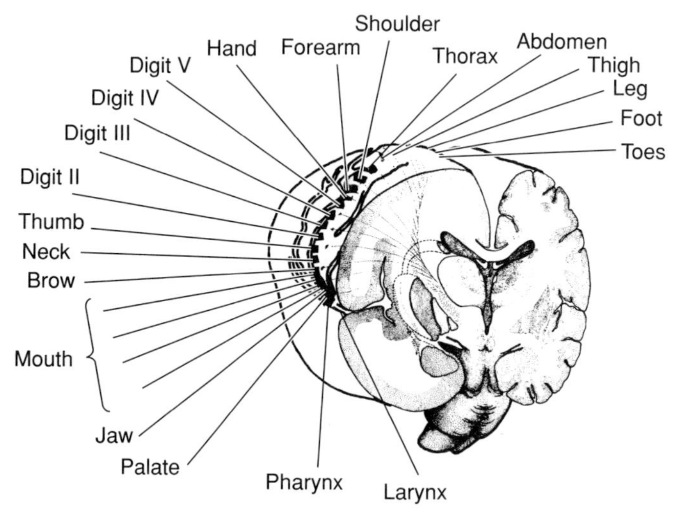

20.9. The cortex is insensitive to pain and can be stimulated directly in human beings. Dr. Harvey Cushing was among the first to describe that movements of different parts of the body are produced on stimulation of different parts of the ________________ gyrus.

20.10. Weak electrical stimulation of the superior postcentral gyrus usually leads a conscious human subject to report some sensation localized to the opposite ______er limb. Some motor responses may be obtained when the postcentral gyrus is stimulated, but responses are more consistently obtained on stimulation of the ________________ gyrus. Likewise, sensory responses may be obtained on both sides of the __________ sulcus.

20.6A. greater

20.7A. area; postcentral

20.8A. mouth; toes

20.9A. precentral

20.10A. lower; precentral; central

20.11. Penfield has drawn a homunculus as represented on the sides of the central sulcus of the human cortex. The distortions of the homunculus emphasize the principle that complexity of function is ________________ to the ______ of the cortex.

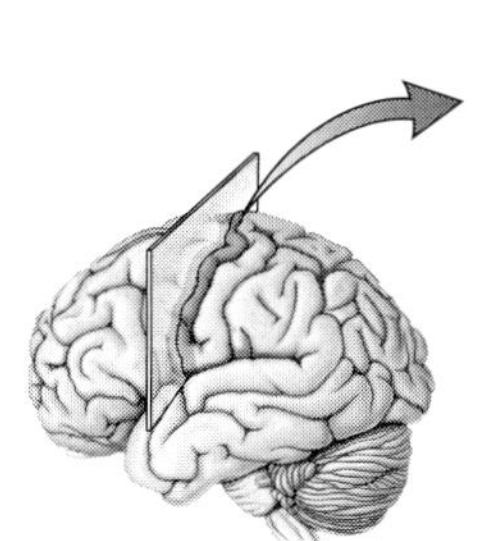

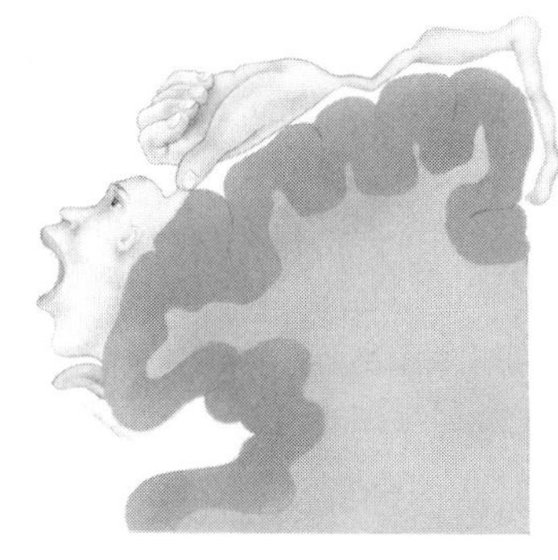

20.12. The position, as well as the relative size, of body parts is distorted on the homunculus. For example, that part of the face represented nearest the neck is not the chin, but the ___________. On the other side of the neck are cells that influence not the shoulders but the ___________.

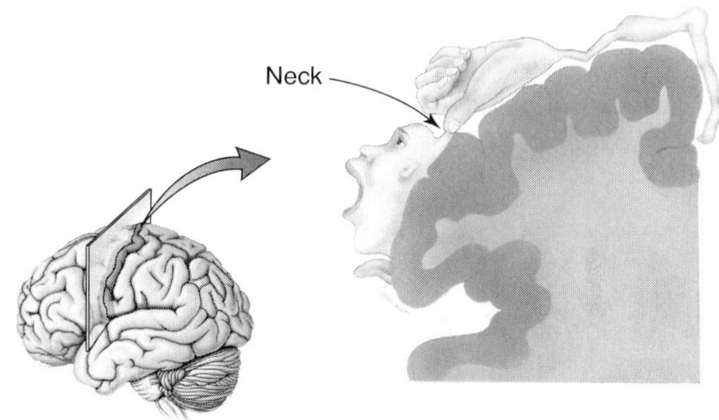

20.13. On stimulation of appropriate parts of the precentral gyrus, the opposite arm is raised, or the knee bends. Apparently, no individual muscles but, instead, coordinated ___________ of body parts are represented on the cerebral cortex.

20.14. The head is represented in the most inferior parts, the hands are represented more superiorly, and the ______ are represented over the superior surface and onto the medial surface of the two gyri bordering on the ___________ sulcus.

20.15. Fibers line up in topographic sequence as they descend from the cortex. Fibers representing the head lie in the most ______ior part of the precentral gyrus and in the most ______ior part of the internal capsule's posterior limb.

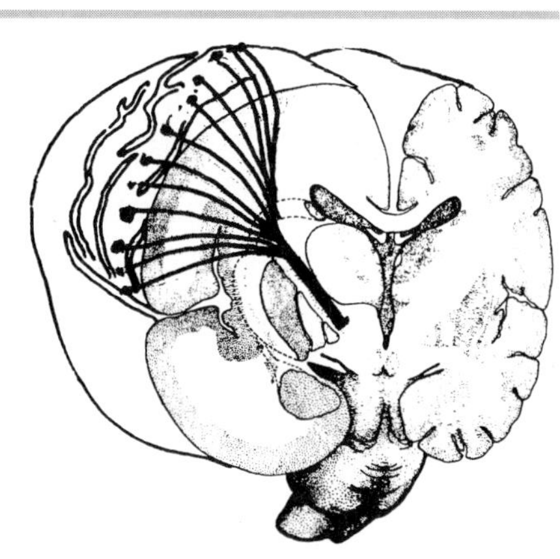

20.11A. proportional; area

20.12A. forehead; fingers

20.13A. movements

20.14A. feet; central

20.15A. inferior; anterior

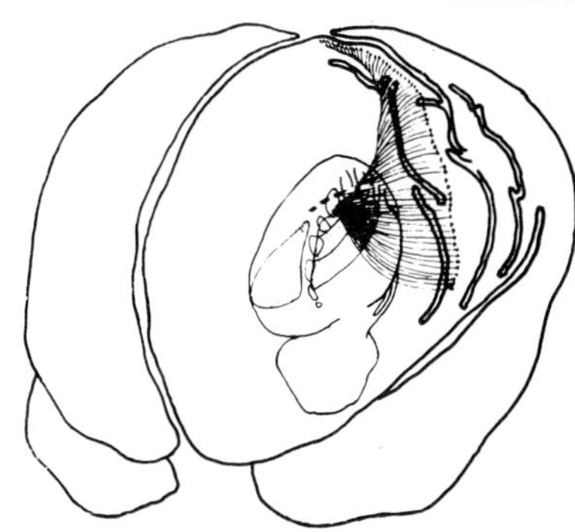

20.16. Encircle the leg area of the precentral gyrus. Compared to fibers from other parts of the precentral gyrus, fibers from the encircled cells pass through the internal capsule in the most ____________ior position.

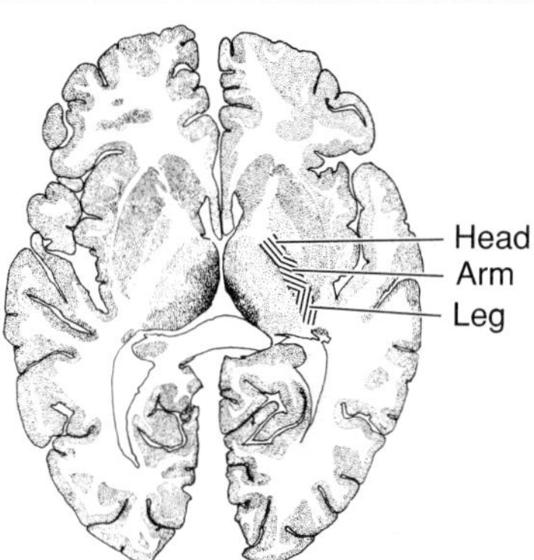

20.17. The linear arrangement of fibers from the precentral gyrus is shown on the diagram. Represented most anteriorly is the ______. All of these fibers are in the ____________ limb of the internal capsule.

20.18. Fibers influencing voluntary motor control of the head and face lie ____________ior to the ______ of the internal capsule. Considerable overlap is found in the topographic distribution of efferent fibers from the precentral gyrus. However, the predominant arrangement of these fibers in the internal capsule, from anterior to posterior, is ______, arm, and ______.

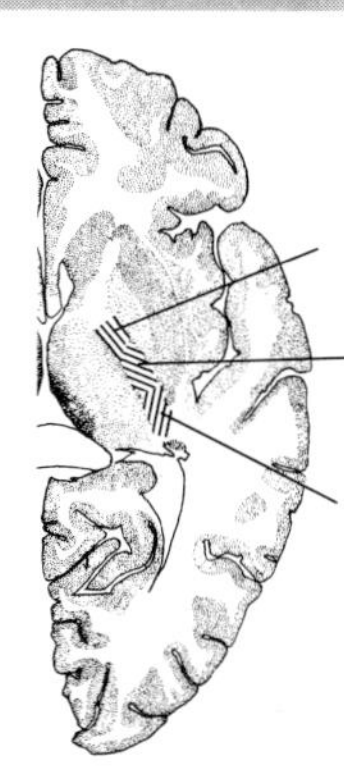

20.19. Label with an "S" those indicated fibers whose cell bodies lie mainly on the superior surface of the precentral gyrus; label with an "I" those indicated fibers whose cell bodies lie in the most inferior part of the precentral gyrus.

20.20. A patient has a stroke that leaves him severely paralyzed in the left leg, mildly weak in the left arm, and unaffected in the left side of the face. His lesion is in the internal capsule on the ______ side. The lesion involves primarily the ____________ part of the ____________ limb of the internal capsule.

20.16A. posterior

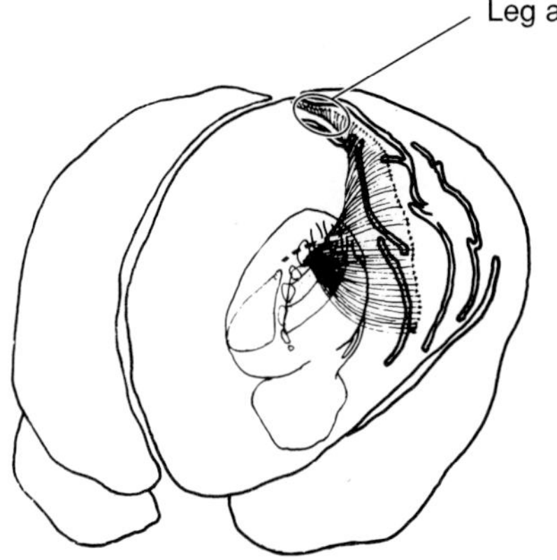

20.17A. head; posterior

20.18A. posterior; genu; head; leg

20.19A.

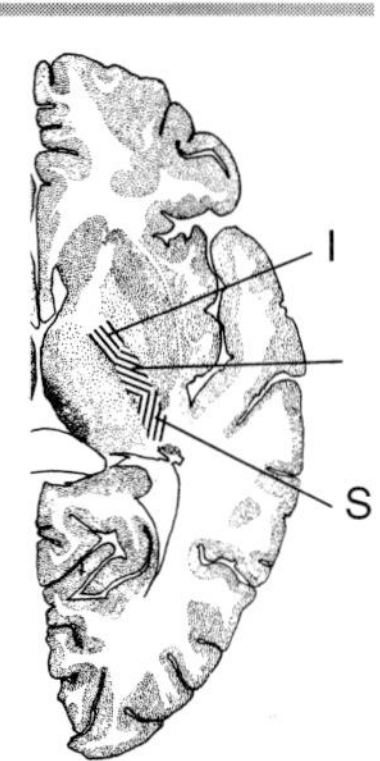

20.20A. right; posterior; posterior

20.21. This is a transverse section through the ____________. Label the structures indicated.

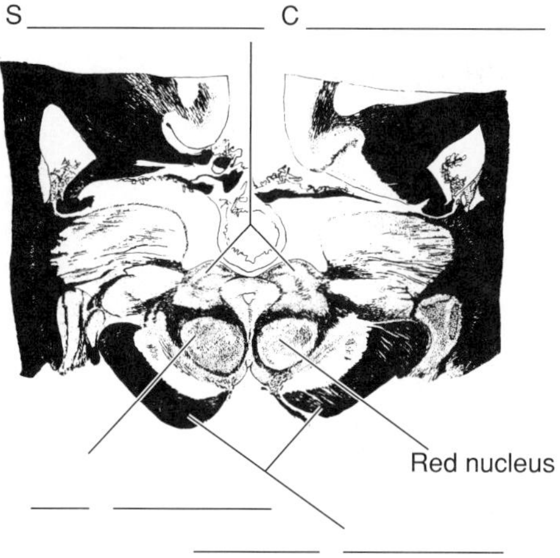

20.22. Neurons in the *left* precentral gyrus send axons in the ______ internal capsule and the ______ basis pedunculi. These fibers influence the ______ arm and leg because they decussate at the junction of the ____________ and ____________ ______.

20.23. Fibers from the precentral gyrus lie in the middle ______-fifths of the ______ ____________. The ______ is represented most medially, and the legs are represented most ____________.

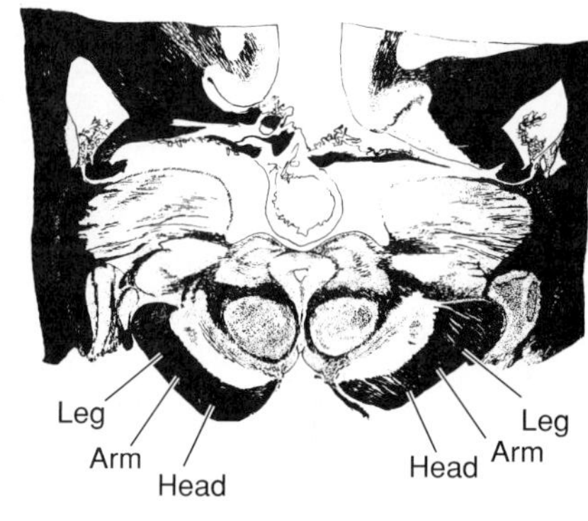

20.24. Indicate the head-arm-leg sequence in *each* basis pedunculi on the diagram.

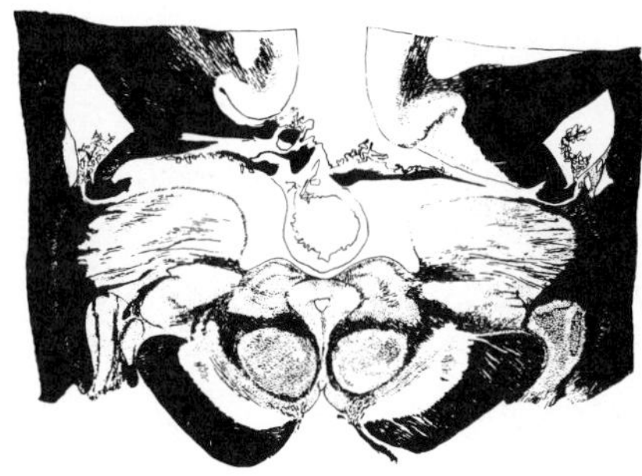

20.25. Corticospinal fibers labeled "A" originate in the ______ior part of the precentral gyrus and pass through the ____________ior part of the posterior limb of the internal capsule; fibers labeled ______ lie closest to the genu of the internal capsule.

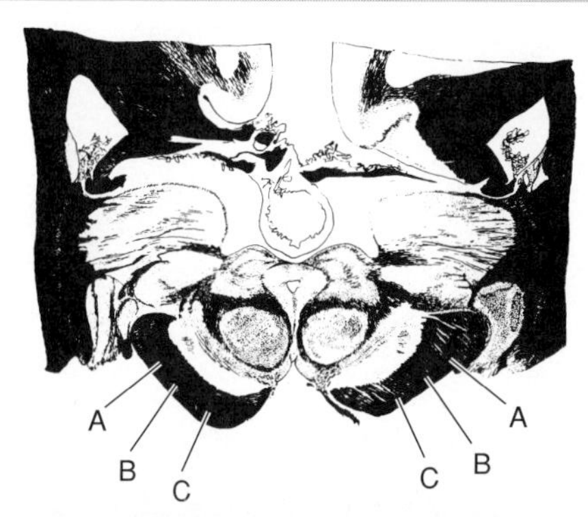

20.21A. midbrain

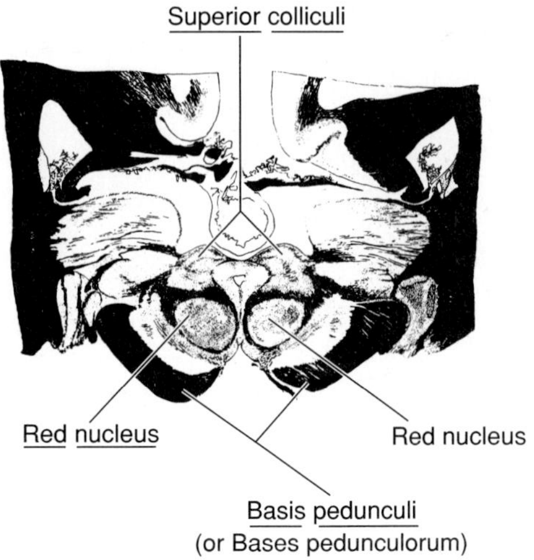

20.22A. left; left; right; medulla; spinal cord

20.23A. three-fifths; basis pedunculi; head; laterally

20.24A.

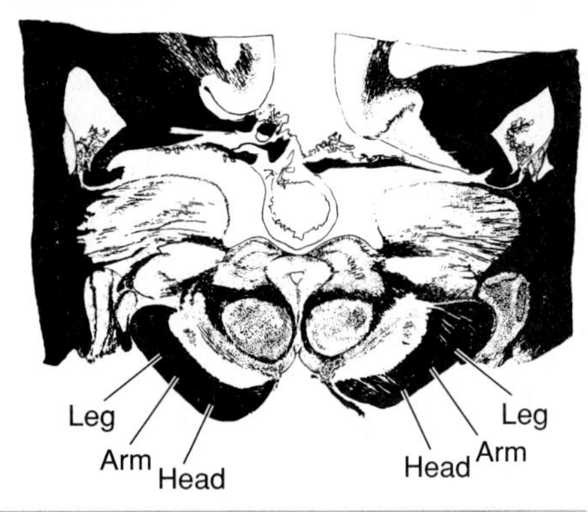

20.25A. superior; posterior; C

20.26. Fibers arising in the cortex and influencing motor control of the trunk and limbs terminate in the spinal cord (cortico___________ fibers). Fibers arising in cortex and influencing motor control of the head terminate in brainstem nuclei (cortico___________ fibers). An older term for these fibers is corticobulbar, referring to the fact that *bulb* is an old term for brainstem.

20.27. Within the middle three-fifths of each basis pedunculi, corticospinal fibers lie in a position ______al to fibers supplying the head (________________ fibers).

20.28. Indicate the two regions traversed by corticonuclear and corticospinal axons in the middle three-fifths of each basis pedunculi. Label the two regions on each side as "CN" or "CS."

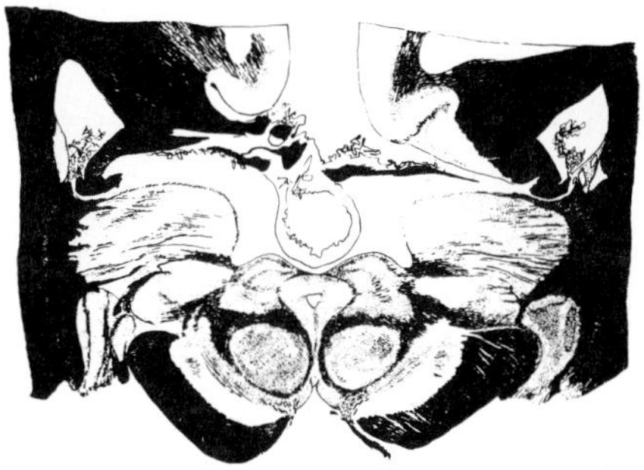

20.29. Since cortico___________ fibers influence face and head muscles, they do not pass to the spinal cord but instead terminate at various levels of the brainstem from midbrain inferiorly to ___________.

20.30. In the internal capsule, the predominant arrangement of efferent fibers, from anterior to posterior, is ______, arm, ______. In the internal capsule, the corticonuclear fibers lie ______erior to corticospinal fibers; in the basis pedunculi, the corticonuclear fibers lie ___________ to corticospinal fibers.

20.31. The other sectors of the basis pedunculi are occupied mainly by axons that terminate in the pons. The most lateral fibers arise mainly in cell bodies in the ___________ and ___________ lobes; the most medial ones arise in the ___________ lobe.

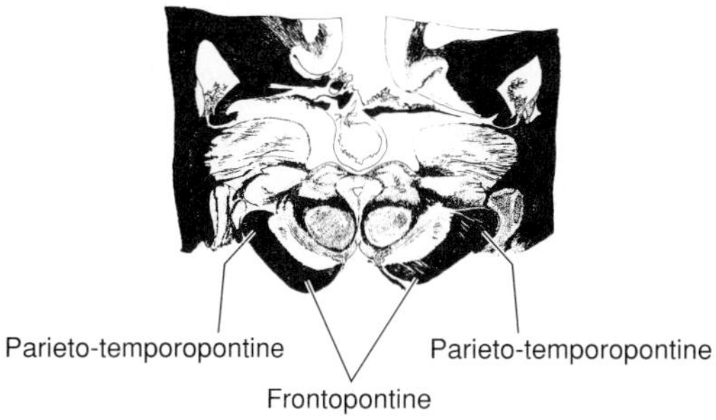

20.32. On both sides, encircle each label that indicates a tract with all fibers terminating superior to the level of the medulla.

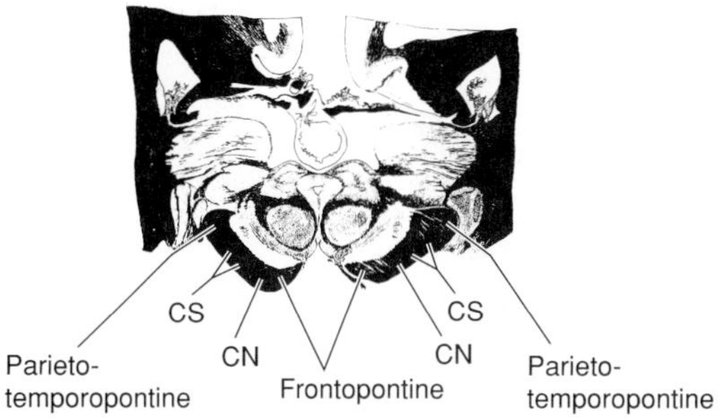

20.26A. corticospinal; corticonuclear

20.27A. lateral; corticonuclear

20.28A.

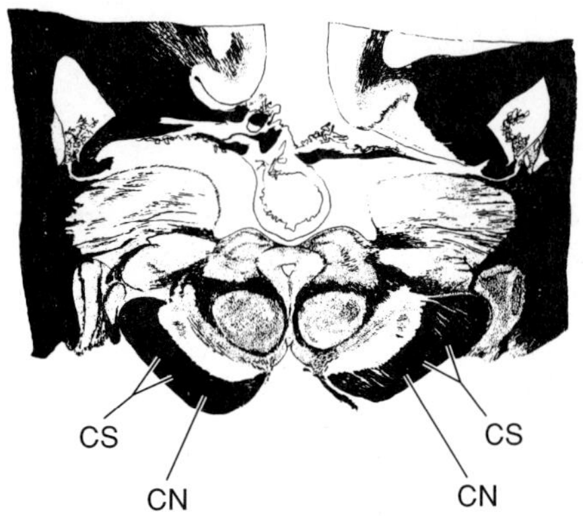

20.29A. corticonuclear; medulla

20.30A. head; leg; anterior; medial

20.31A. parietal; temporal; frontal

20.32A.

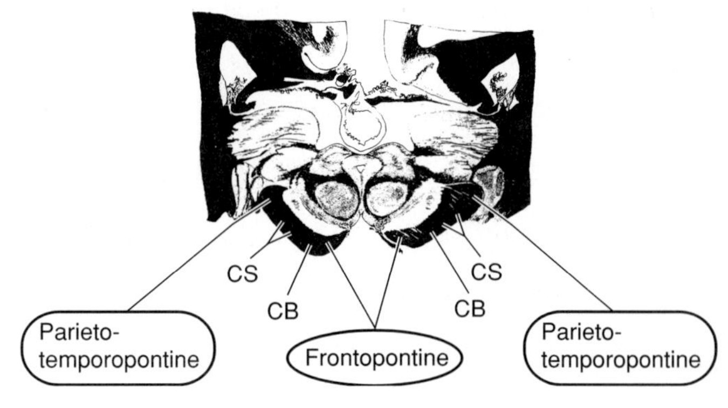

21 Lesions in the Corticospinal System

21.1. On this section drawn in the ____________ plane, draw a Betz cell axon as it courses through the white matter.

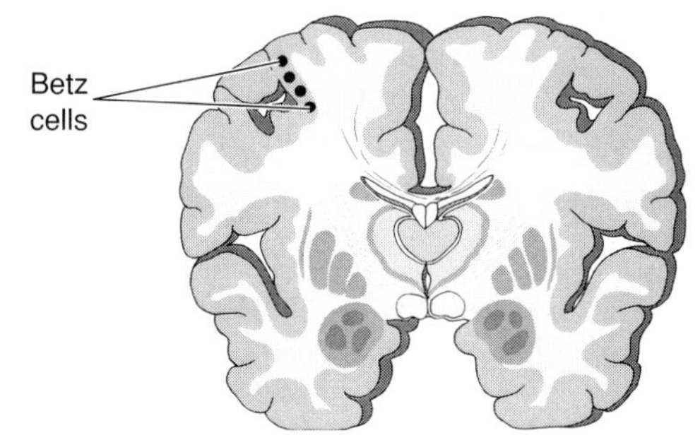

21.2. The medical term "stroke" is commonly used for an acute loss of some neurological function because of blood vessel disease. One manifestation of the stroke resulting from the lesion diagrammed is ____________ of voluntary movement of the face, arm, and leg on the ______ side.

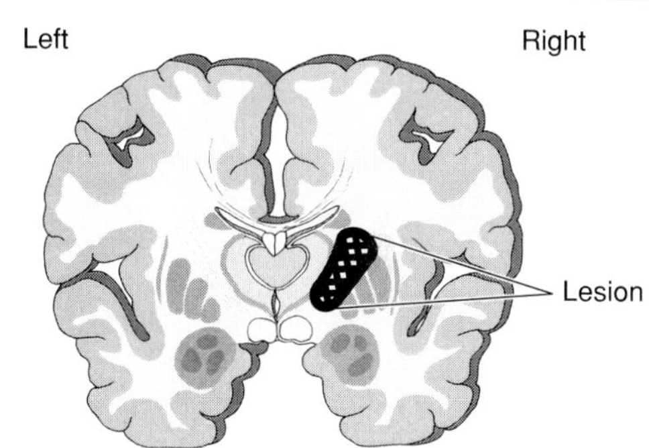

21.3. When the lesion, as diagrammed, is in the ____________ ____________, limb reflexes are still present but ____________ use of the limb is lost.

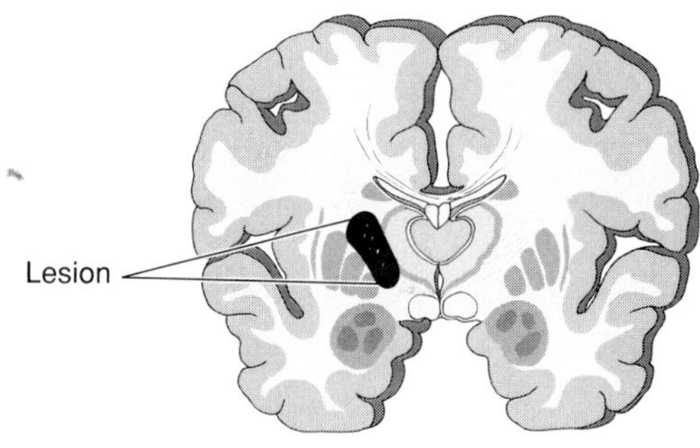

21.4. Lesions of corticospinal fibers above the level of the decussation of the pyramids cause paralysis on the __________________ side of the body; lesions below the decussation cause paralysis on the ____________ side. "Paralysis" is the term meaning inability to ______.

21.5. A lesion in this shaded area leads to paralysis of the arm and leg on the ______ side of the body. In addition, the axons of cranial nerve XII cease to function on the ______ side.

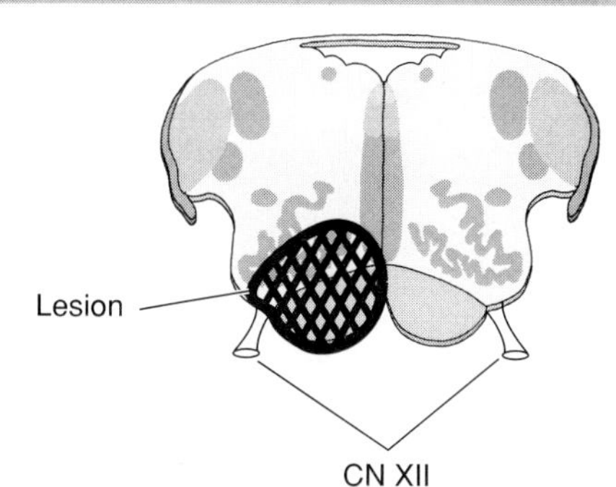

21.1A. coronal

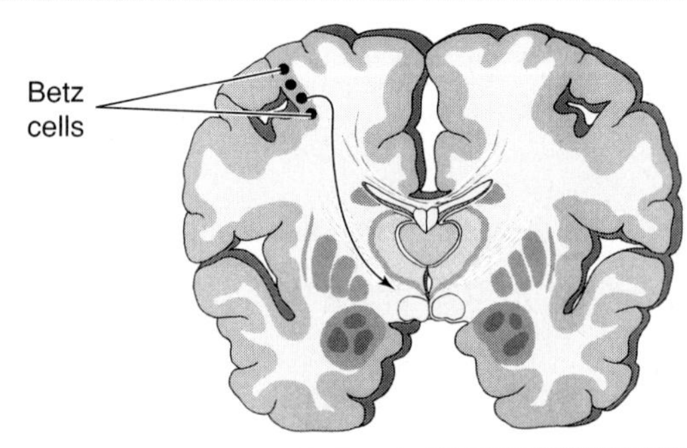

21.2A. paralysis; left

21.3A. internal capsule; voluntary

21.4A. contralateral (opposite); ipsilateral (same); move

21.5A. right (contralateral); left (ipsilateral)

21.6. In all three lesions, there is loss of ____________ movement of the left arm and ______. The only lesion that abolishes function in cranial nerve XII as well is the one in the section through the ____________.

Lesion 1

Lesion 2

Lesion 3

21.7. A lesion in the corona radiata that interrupts all corticospinal axons influencing the left arm and leg is much ____________ in size than a lesion in the medulla with the same consequences. Shade in the affected area on the section.

Left

Right

21.8. This lesion (shaded) in the internal capsule affects efferent corticospinal fibers as well as afferent fibers coming to the __________________ gyrus from cell bodies in the ____________. The resulting loss is in ______ function and in the __________________ class of sensory function.

21.9. A lesion may produce many effects if different types of axons all pass through the damaged area. On the diagram, shade in the smallest lesion that would concurrently affect voluntary motor, somesthetic sensory, and visual functions.

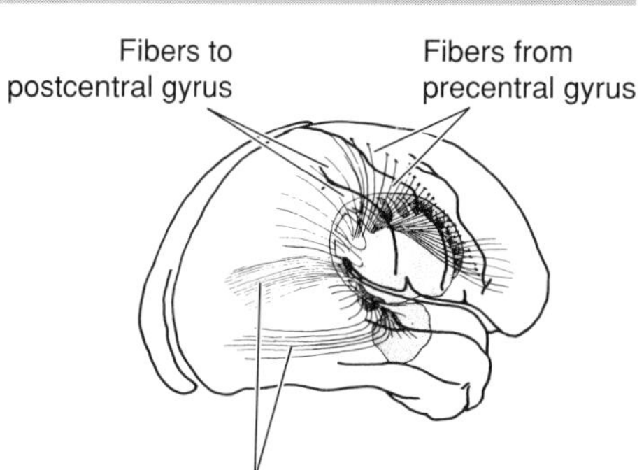

21.6A. voluntary; leg; medulla

21.7A. larger

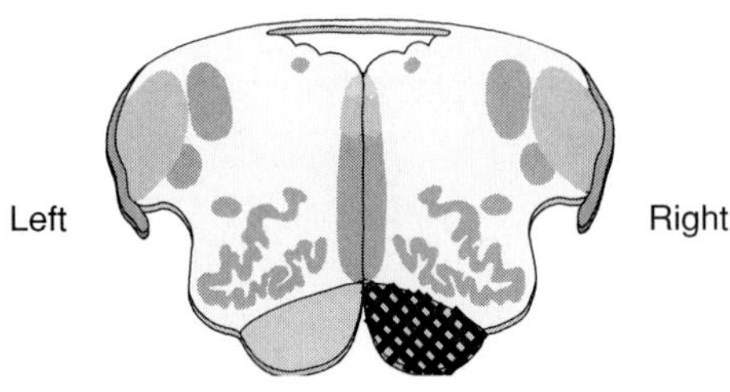

21.8A. postcentral; thalamus; motor; somesthetic

21.9A.

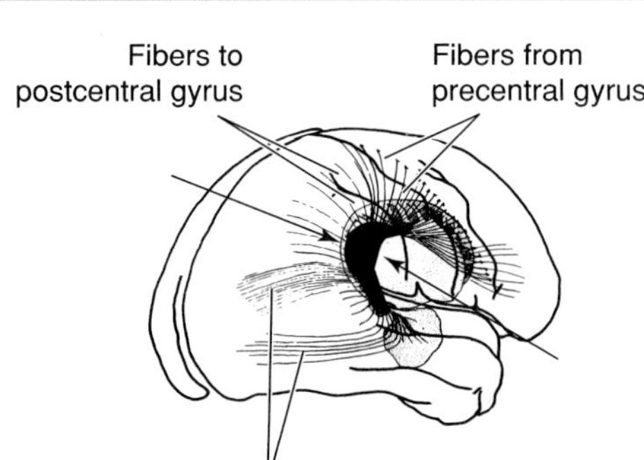

21.10. From the combinations of symptoms reported and signs detected by examination, the physician, knowing the kinds of axons that would have to be involved, deduces the anatomical ____________ and size of the lesion.

21.11. This patient had a stroke with occlusion of the artery supplying the corona radiata in the central part of his ______ cerebral hemisphere.

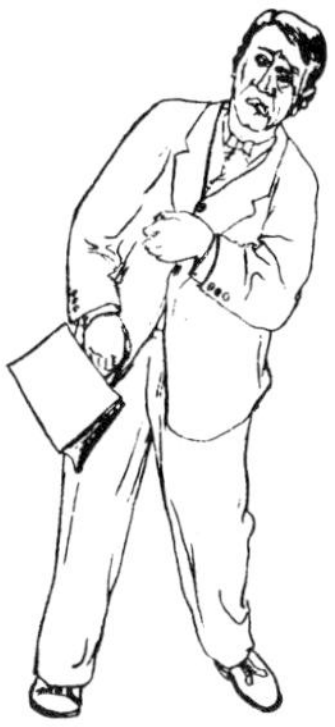

21.12. A lesion at "A" lies ____________ to the pyramidal decussation and affects voluntary control of the ______ leg. A lesion at "B" affects voluntary control of the ______ leg.

Left Right A B

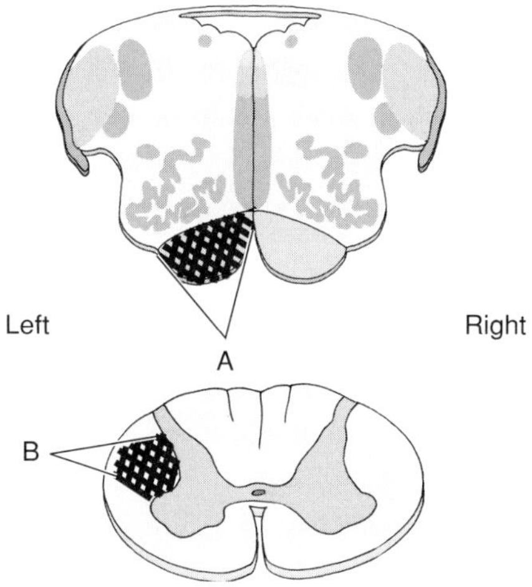

21.13. Since the right lower side of the face is paralyzed in a left cortical lesion, many cortico____________ fibers also must cross the midline.

21.14. Decussation of corticonuclear fibers is not easily demonstrated in stained sections, even though clinical data make it clear that such decussations must occur. Corticonuclear fibers must cross at many levels in groups of ____________ size.

21.10A. location

21.11A. right

21.12A. superior; right; left

21.13A. corticonuclear

21.14A. variable

21.15. If the shaded area were destroyed by sudden occlusion of the artery that nourishes it, the patient would likely be unable to move the lower ______ side of the face or the ______ arm and leg.

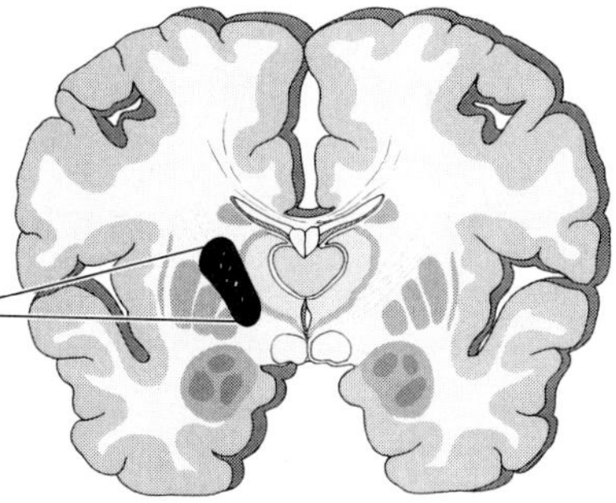

Left

Right

Lesion

21.16. Much of our knowledge of human neuroanatomy comes from the study of neurological disease. For example, since corticospinal lesions on one side do not paralyze breathing, we conclude that nerve cells that directly innervate intercostal muscles and the diaphragm are influenced by corticospinal fibers of ______ sides of the brain.

21.17. A unilateral lesion affecting corticonuclear fibers commonly has no effect on voluntary chewing, swallowing, or phonating. Also, upper facial muscles that control forehead and brow movement are spared. Presumably, the neuromuscular apparatus directly affecting these motor functions is influenced by corticonuclear fibers of ______ sides. Corticonuclear lesions that do affect these functions must be ____________.

21.18. The movements characteristically affected in unilateral corticonuclear and corticospinal lesions are movements of the tongue (transiently affected), lower face, arm, and leg on the ____________________ side from the lesion. Whether or not the anatomist can demonstrate it, most of these fibers must ____________.

21.15A. right (contralateral); right (contralateral)

21.16A. both

21.17A. both; bilateral

21.18A. contralateral; decussate

22 Clinical Signs of Corticospinal Damage

22.1. Between 70 and 90% of corticospinal fibers from the left cortex decussate and are found in the spinal cord in the ____________ corticospinal tract. Corticospinal fibers that do not cross the midline in the anterior commissure form the ____________ corticospinal tracts.

22.2. A lesion affecting corticospinal fibers in the left side of the pons impairs voluntary movement of the arm and leg on the ______ side.

22.3. Because its fibers have already decussated above the level of the limbs, lesions of the ____________ corticospinal tract affect limbs on the same side.

22.4. The indicated lesion has no effect on motor function noticeable by the usual clinical tests, since 70 to 90% of the axons affecting the same body parts are in the intact ____________ corticospinal tract on the ______ side.

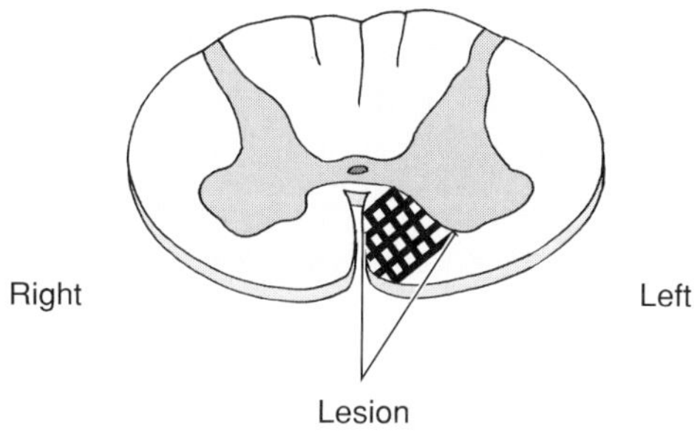

Right

Left

Lesion

22.5. Beginning laterally near the lateral sulcus and passing superiorly and medially, the cortical representation of movement in the face and extremities is, successively, ______, ______ limb, and ______ limb.

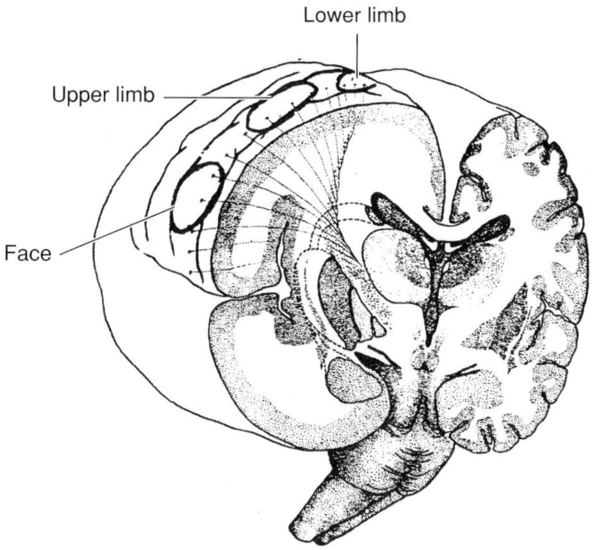

Lower limb

Upper limb

Face

22.1A. lateral; ventral

22.2A. right

22.3A. lateral

22.4A. lateral; right (contralateral)

22.5A. face; upper; lower

22.6. Mark with their appropriate initials (L, A, F) the approximate position of Betz cells that influence movement of the *right* leg, *right* arm, and *right* lower side of the face.

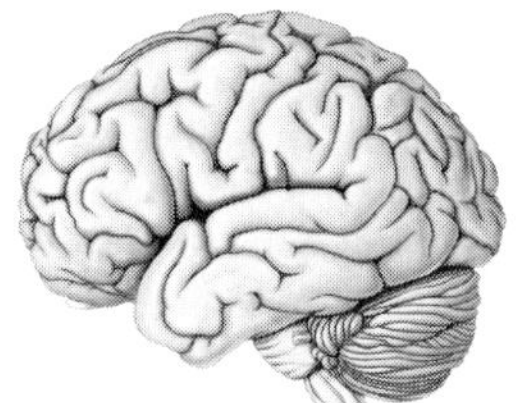

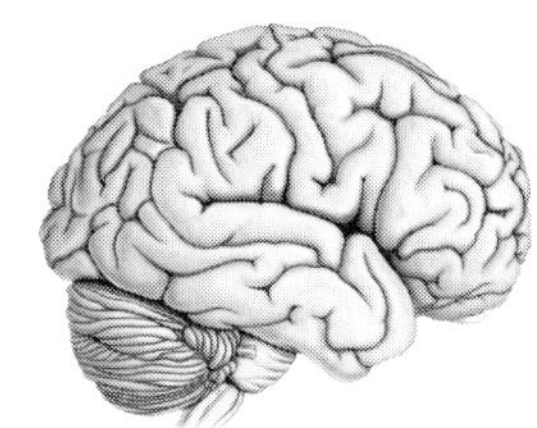

22.7. The representation of the face, arm, and leg is lateral to medial on the cortical surface and anterior to posterior in the internal capsule. Label the indicated regions as representing face (F), arm (A), and leg (L).

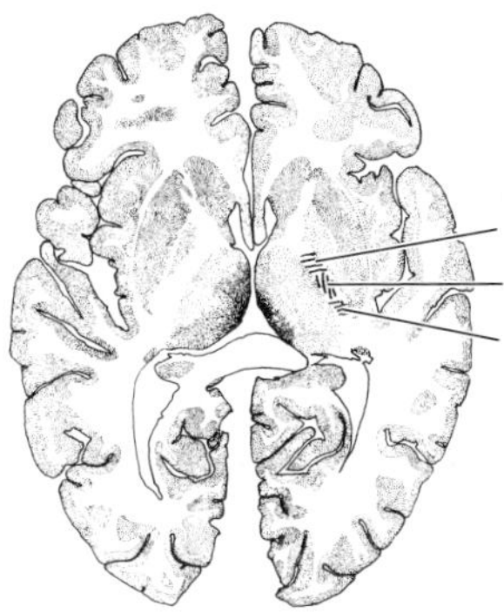

22.8. A lesion just posterior to the genu of the internal capsule on the *right* side causes loss of voluntary movement in muscles of the ______ on the ______ side.

22.9. Fibers from the precentral gyrus lie in the middle ______-fifths of the ______ __________. The lateral-to-medial representation in the midbrain is comparable to the posterior-to-anterior representation in the internal capsule. Label the indicated regions as representing face (F), arm (A), and leg (L).

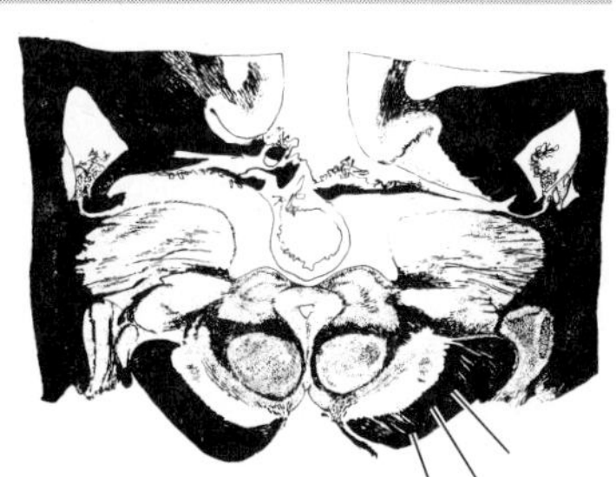

22.10. The indicated lesion in the basis pedunculi would cause voluntary paralysis in the ______er limb on the ______ side.

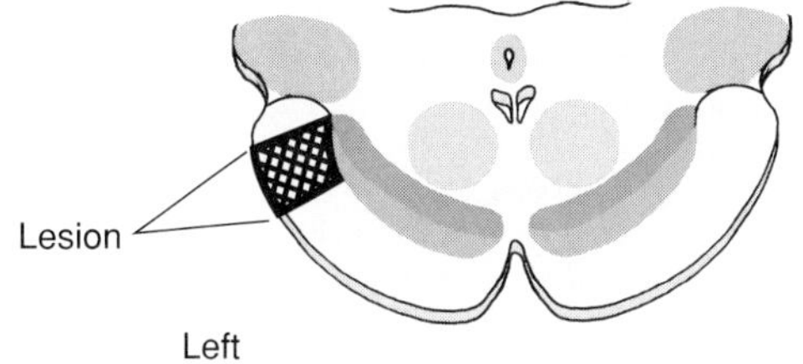

22.6A.

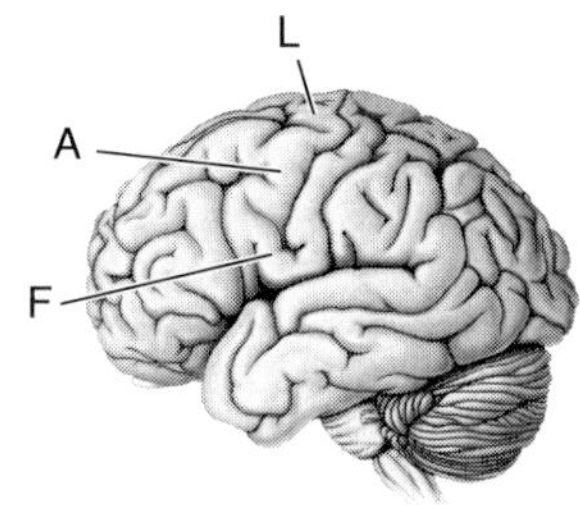

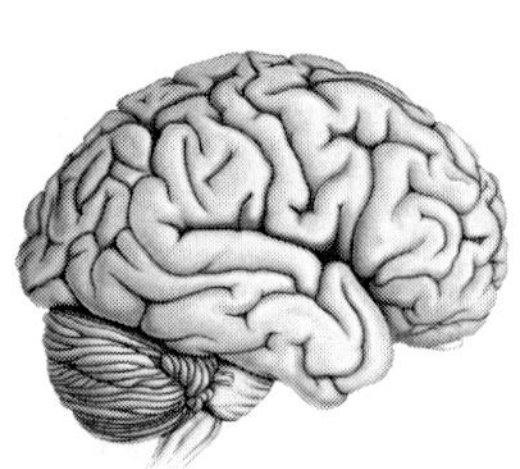

22.7A.

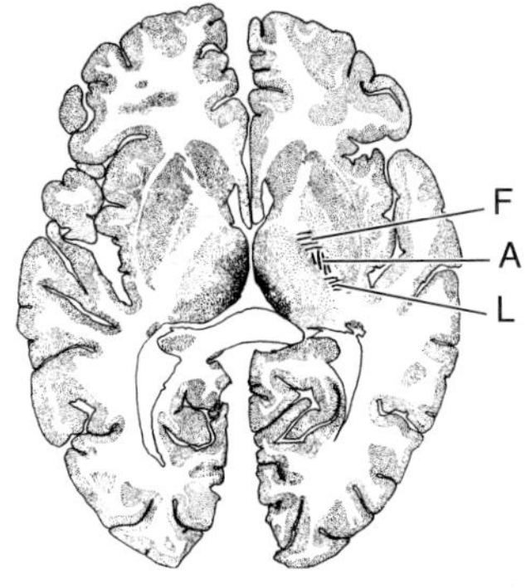

22.8A. face; left (contralateral)

22.9A. three-fifths; basis pedunculi

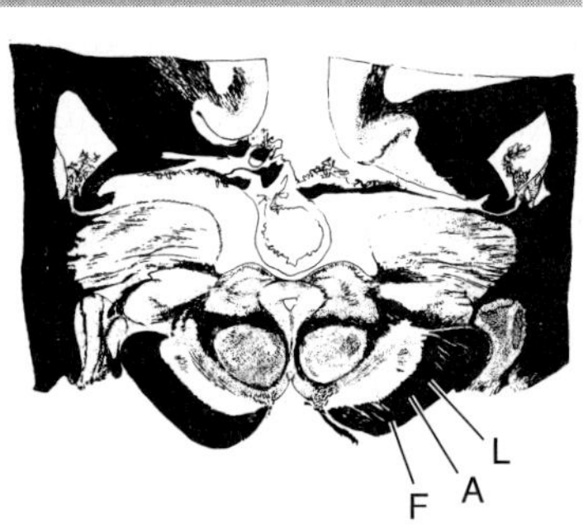

22.10A. lower; right

22.11. On each section, indicate with an arrow the approximate position of corticospinal axons carrying impulses that influence movement of the right arm.

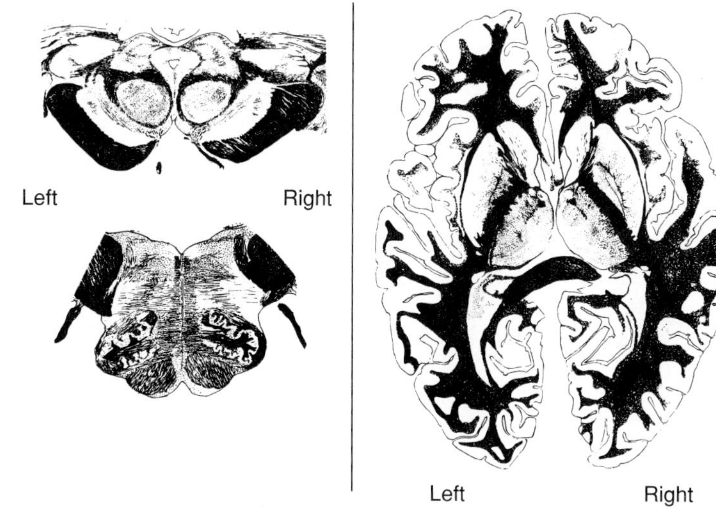

22.12. T1 and the lower *cervical* spinal nerves form a plexus that innervates the ______. A similar arrangement is seen in the innervation of the legs by S1 and several of the __________ spinal nerves.

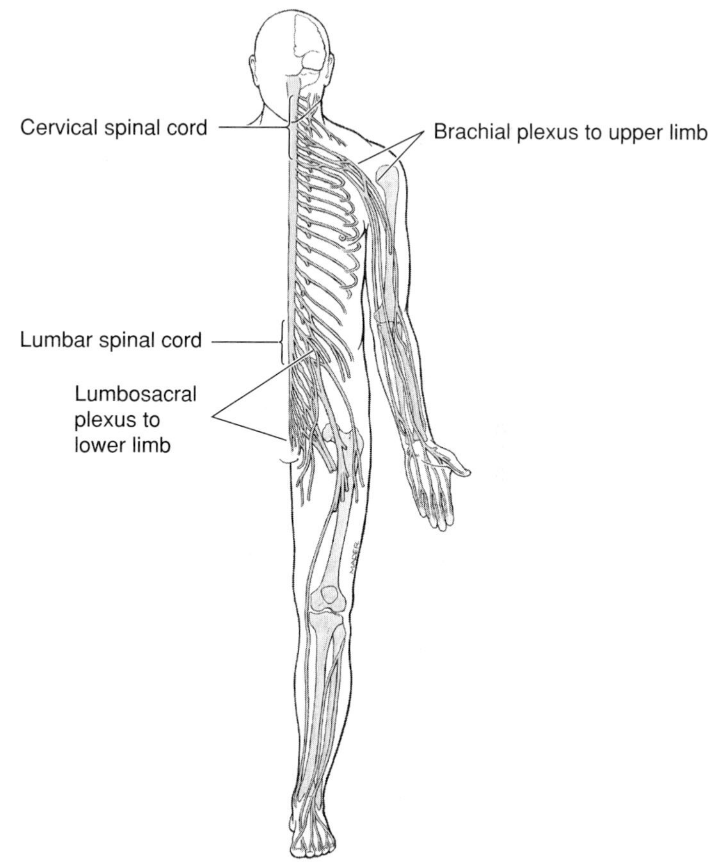

22.13. A complete transection of the spinal cord at a midthoracic level does not affect motor influences descending from the brain to the ______er limbs.

22.11A.

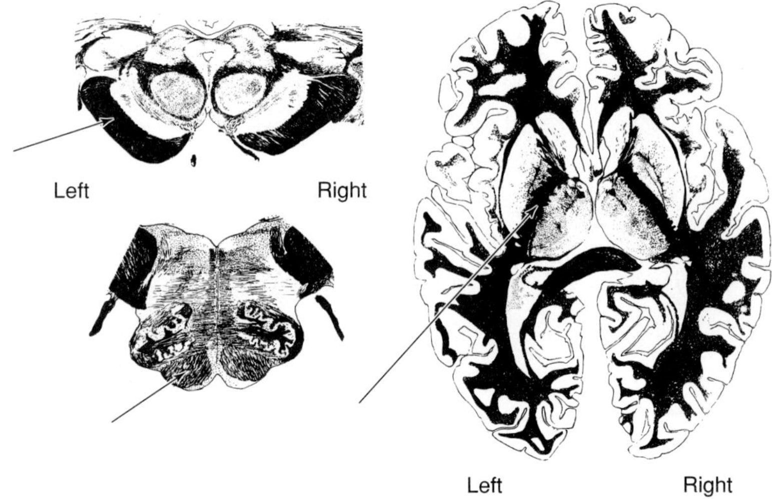

22.12A. arm; lumbar

22.13A. upper

22.14. This diagram shows a section through the T12 spinal cord level. A lesion at the site indicated would affect motor function in the arms because the relevant corticospinal fibers have already terminated at a ______er level.

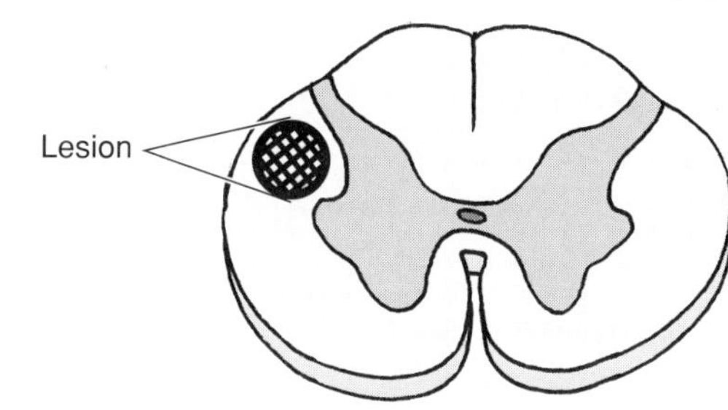

22.15. The neuron of the precentral gyrus is called the upper motor neuron. Correspondingly, the neuron of the anterior horn of the spinal cord is often called the ______ motor neuron. A lesion of the corticospinal fibers causes impairment of movement, not of particular muscles. Paralysis of voluntary movement results from lesions of the ______er motor neurons.

22.16. Within the anterior horn of the spinal cord, the most distal parts of the body are represented most ___________ly in position.

22.17. Place an "X" on cell bodies that might be damaged to produce paralysis solely of the flexor muscles associated with the right wrist.

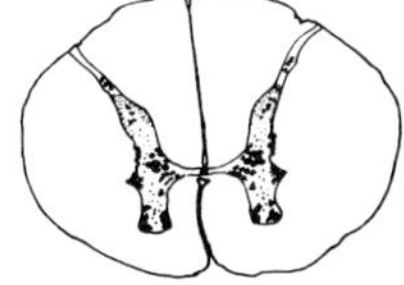
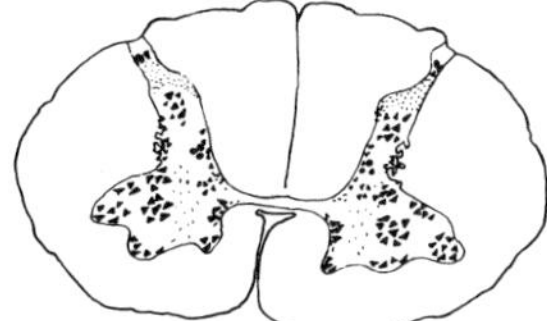
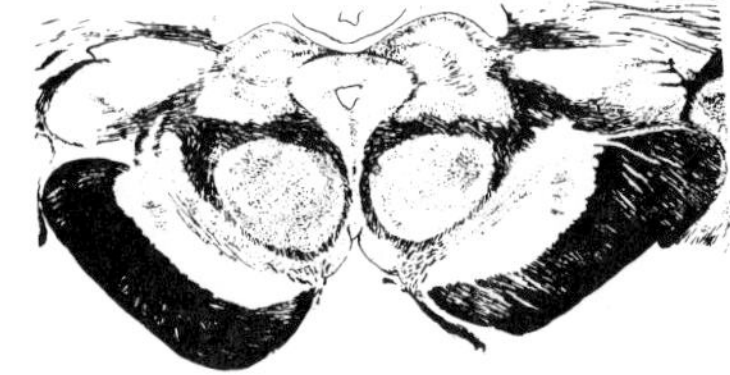

22.18. In addition to conducting impulses, nerves influence the mass of certain structures that they contact. This trophic influence is demonstrated by the observation that skeletal muscle atrophies when its nerve supply is ______.

22.14A. higher

22.15A. lower; upper

22.16A. laterally

22.17A. Left

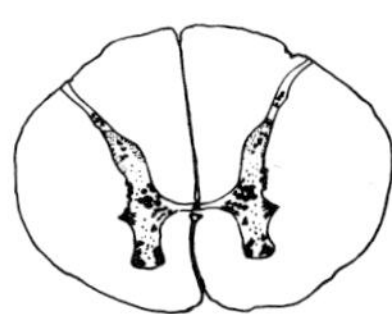

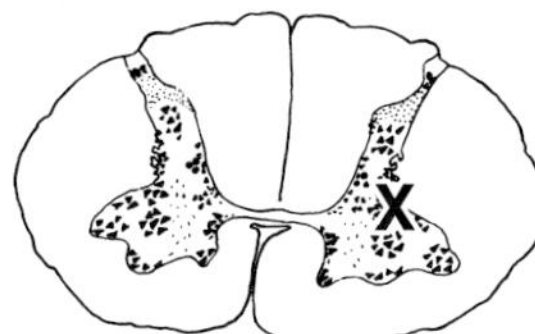

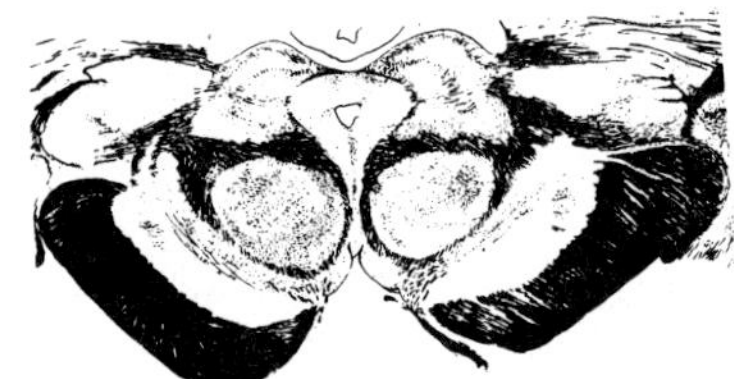

Right

22.18A. cut

22.19. If the indicated fibers are cut, some muscles become paralyzed and later atrophy. Place an "X" on the approximate location of cell bodies that directly innervate muscles of the left hand and fingers.

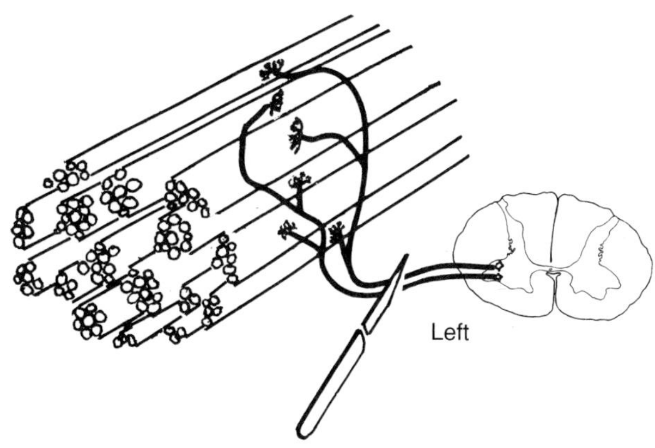

22.20. The nutritive, or trophic, influence requires direct contact between target organ, such as muscle, and its ______ supply.

22.21. Does lesion "X" in this sacral spinal cord section produce atrophy due to loss of trophic influence in leg muscles? ______ Explain your answer. ____.

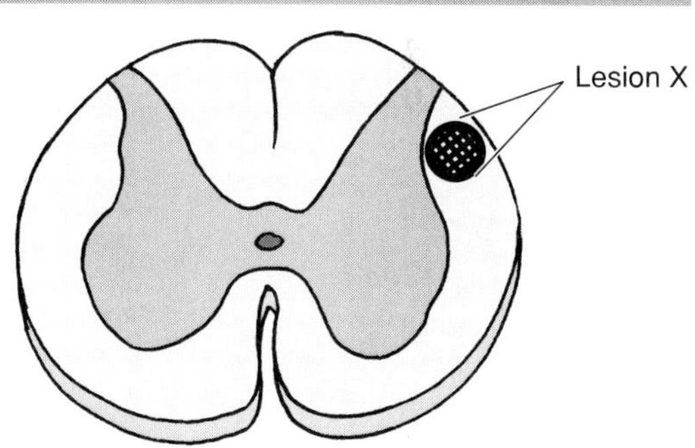

22.22. Atrophy of hand and finger muscles due to loss of trophic influence results from lesions of nerve number ______ on the diagram.

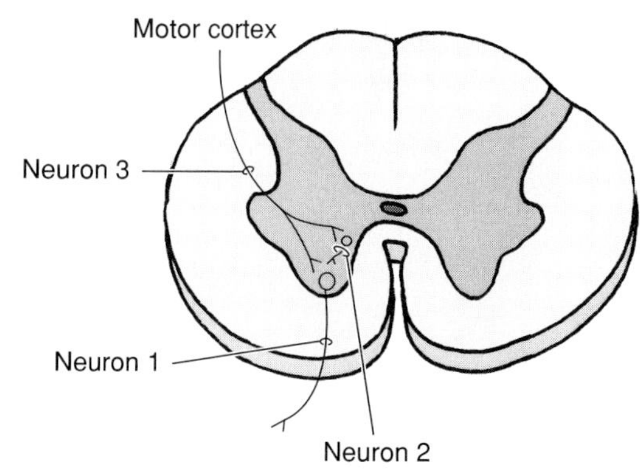

22.23. A lesion affecting the cell body or axon of the lower motor neuron leads to __________ and __________ of muscle. The major effect of an upper motor neuron lesion is __________.

22.19A.

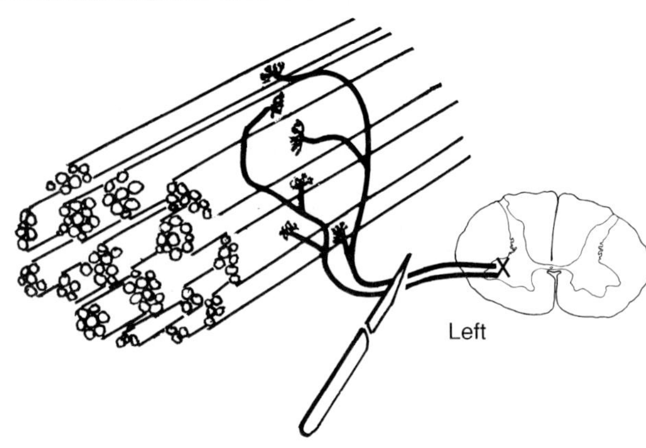

22.20A. nerve

22.21A. No; The injured corticospinal fiber is not in direct contact with the muscle.

22.22A. 1

22.23A. paralysis; atrophy; paralysis

22.24. A single axon usually branches and contacts ____________ skeletal muscle fibers. A "motor unit" is defined as: 1) the ______er motor neuron plus 2) all of the skeletal ____________ fibers that it innervates. A motor unit consists of how many types of components? ______

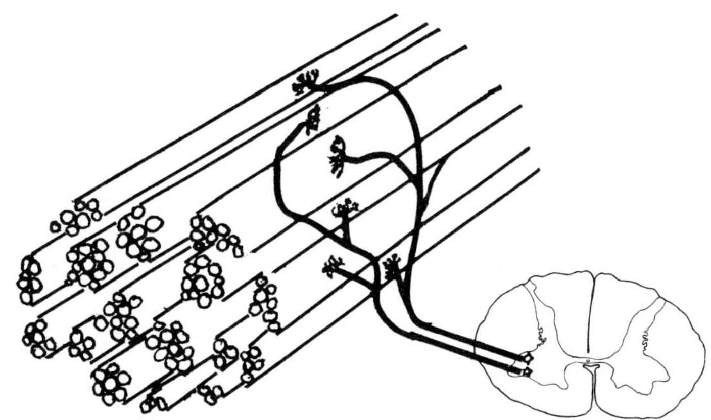

22.25. Some diseases, such as poliomyelitis, destroy lower motor neurons. On the left side of the diagram, blacken the tips of the paralyzed and atrophic muscle fibers connected with the destroyed (thin) neuron. These atrophic muscle fibers and destroyed neuron together form a m______ u______.

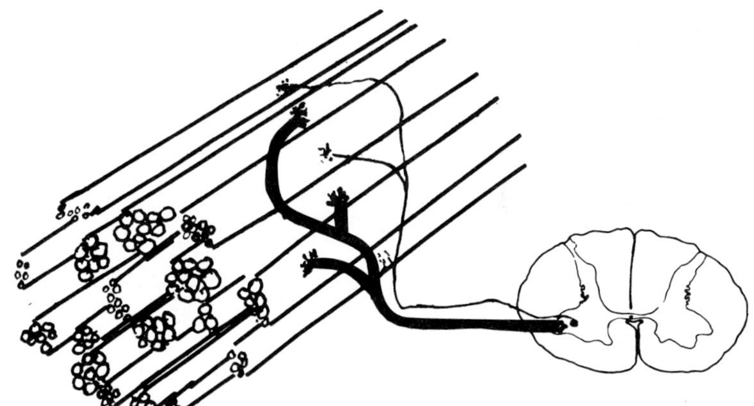

22.24A. multiple; lower; muscle; two

22.25A. motor unit

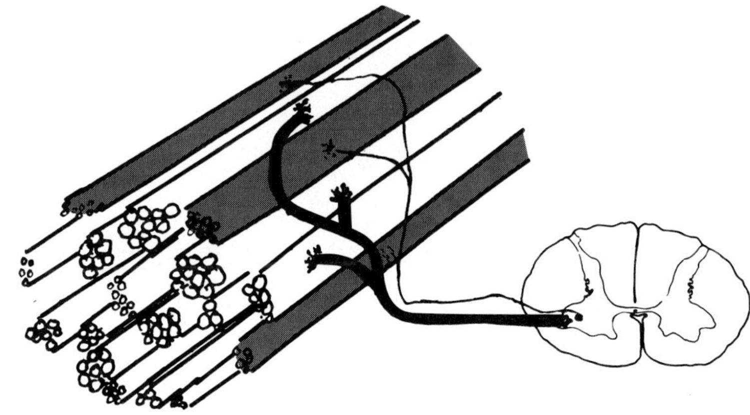

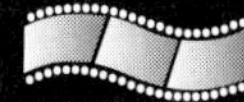

Animations

6. Axial Musculature (Chapters 8, 20)
10. Crude Movement (Chapters 7, 8, 13, 17, 18, 19)
11. Postural Movement (Chapters 7, 8, 13, 17, 18, 19)
18. Limbic (Chapter 15)
25. Basal Ganglia (Chapters 7, 10, 11, 13, 14, 15)
34. Higher Association Language (Chapter 3)
36. Higher Association Tracts and Areas (Chapter 3)

II BASAL NUCLEI

23 Identification of the Basal Nuclei

23.1. The interior of the lobes of the cerebral hemispheres consists partly of white matter and partly of well defined areas of gray matter known as the *basal nuclei*. The ______ate and lent __________ nuclei are the best known of the basal nuclei.

23.2. Label the caudate and lenticular nuclei on the diagram.

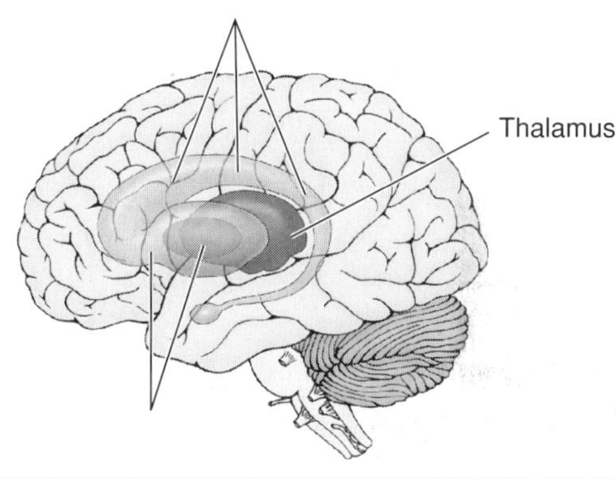

23.3. The *amygdala* may also be included as a component of the basal nuclei. Label the amygdala on the diagram.

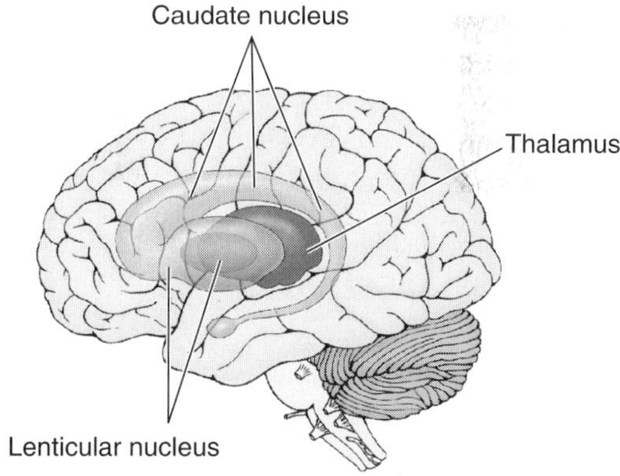

23.4. The pu______ and globus __________ together make up the *lenticular nucleus*.

23.5. The __________ forms the lateral part of the lenticular nucleus. The __________ pallidus forms the ______al part of the lenticular nucleus.

23.1A. caudate; lenticular

23.2A.

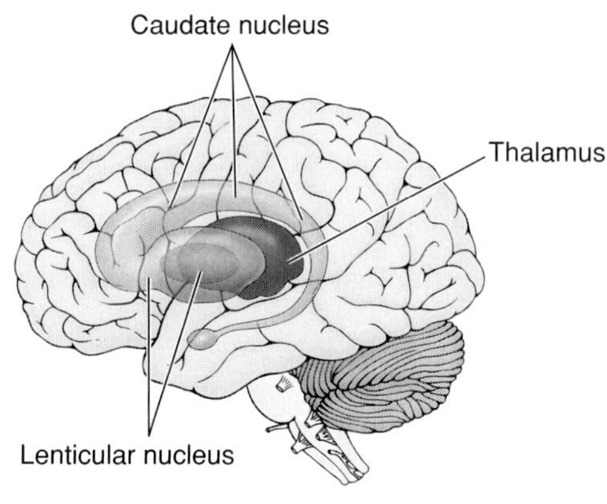

23.3A.

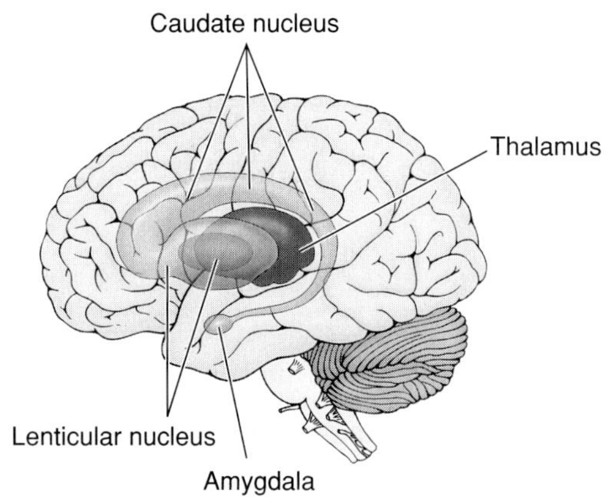

23.4A. putamen; pallidus

23.5A. putamen; globus; medial

23.6. Label the two parts of the lenticular nucleus.

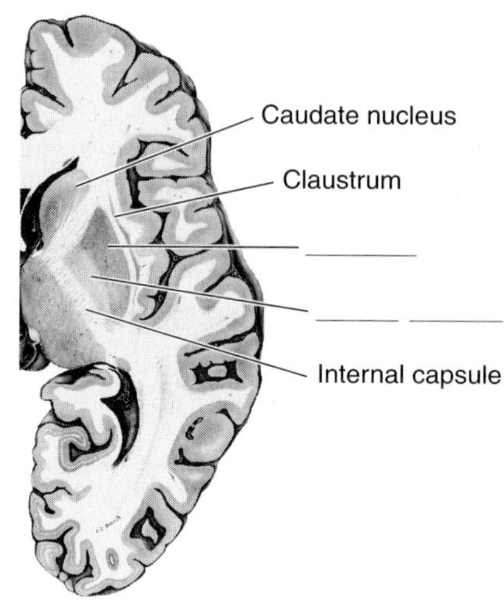

23.7. Cell bridges connect the putamen with all parts of the ____________ nucleus.

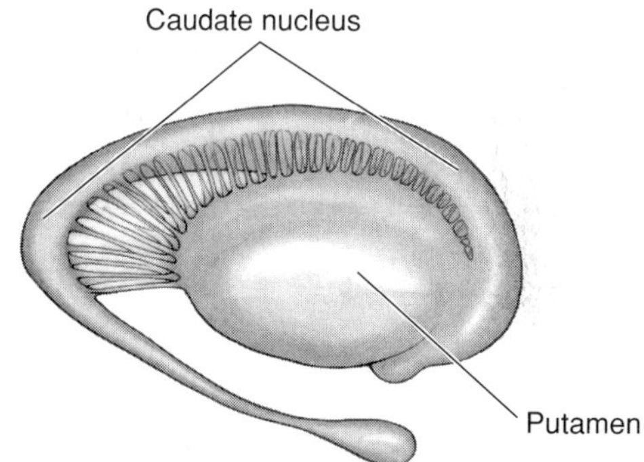

23.8. Numerous fibers from the cortical *surface* pass among the cell bridges that connect the caudate and putamen. Among them is a tract of fibers arising in the ________________ gyrus of the frontal lobe. Encircle and name this tract on the diagram.

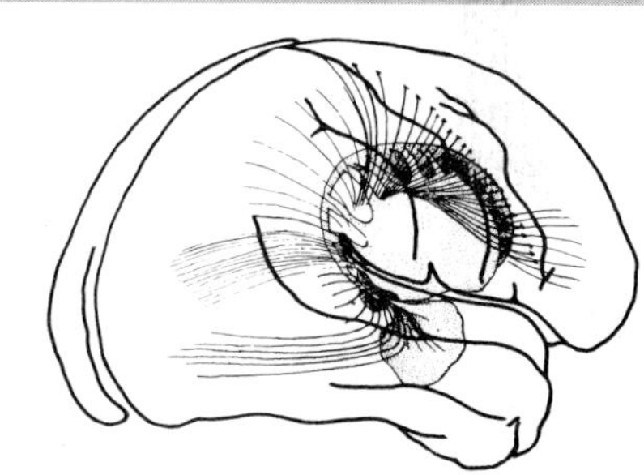

23.9. The fiber tracts that encapsulate the internal surfaces of the lenticular nucleus form the ______ternal ______sule.

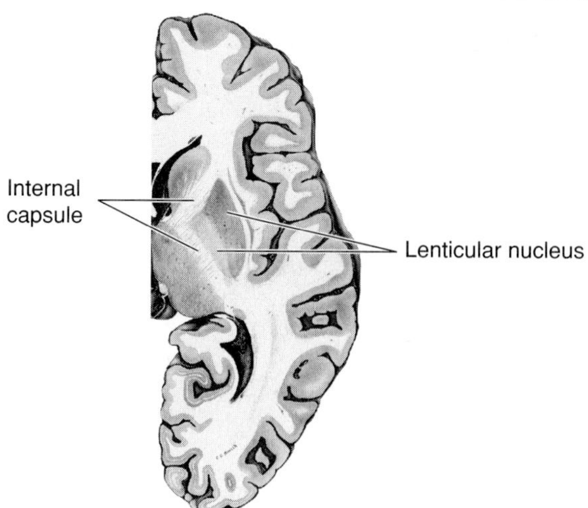

23.6A.

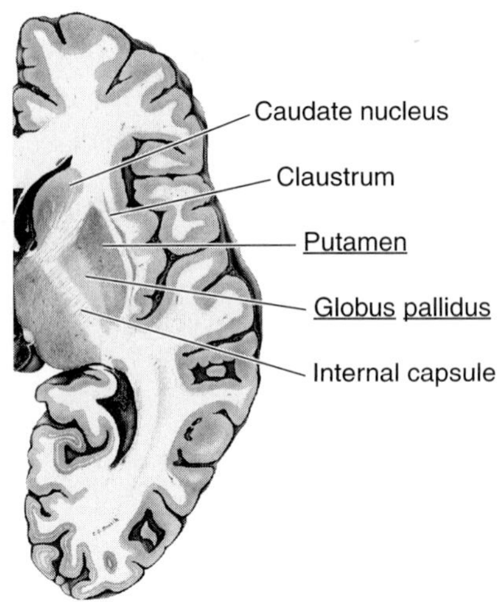

23.7A. caudate

23.8A. precentral

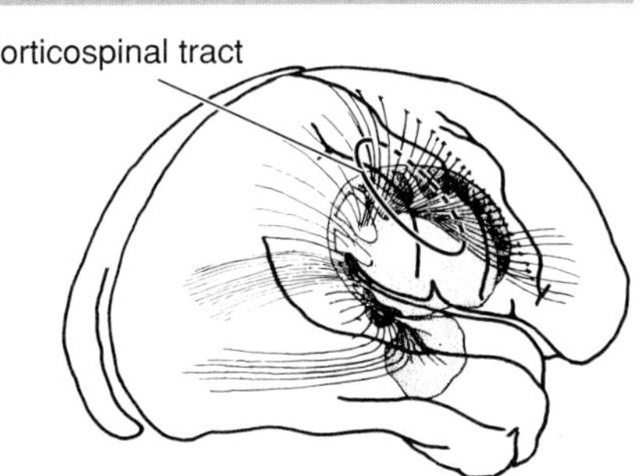

23.9A. internal; capsule

23.10. The internal capsule lies ______al to the globus pallidus and just ______al to the __________.

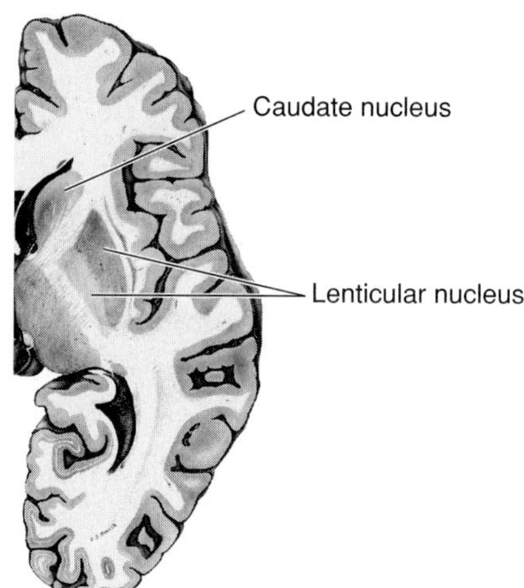

23.10A. medial; lateral; caudate

24 Connections of the Basal Nuclei

24.1. The basal nuclei play an important role in regulating motor functions by helping to initiate and terminate voluntary movements. They receive input from the ___________ ___________ and supply output signals to the ___________.

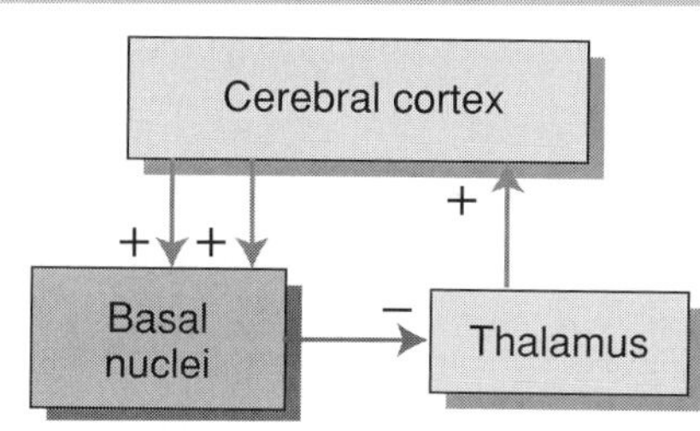

24.2. Cortical input to the basal nuclei is received by the caud ______ and ______ men. Because these two nuclei collectively form an area known as the striatum, the fibers traveling from cortex to the basal ganglia are termed cortico ___________ projections.

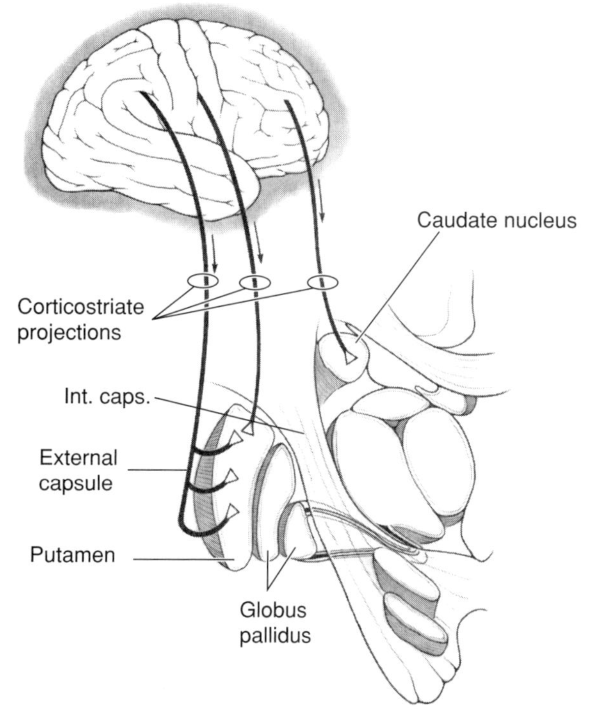

24.3. Output of the basal nuclei is generated by the ___________ pallidus, which regulates activity of the ___________.

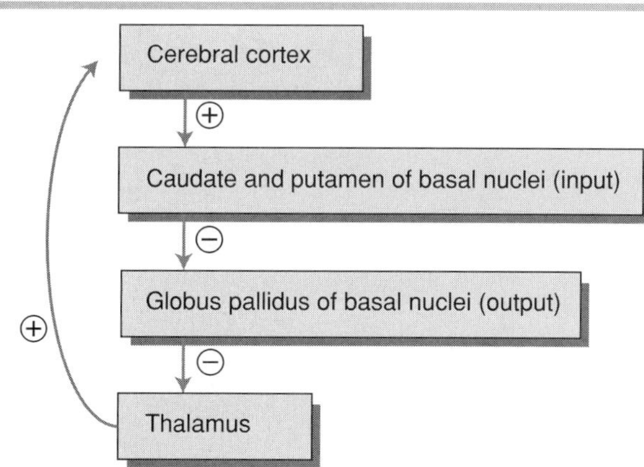

24.1A. cerebral cortex; thalamus

24.2A. caudate; putamen; corticostriate

24.3A. globus; thalamus

24.4. From the globus pallidus, there are two main pathways that reach the thalamus: the ________________ fasciculus and the ______ lenticularis.

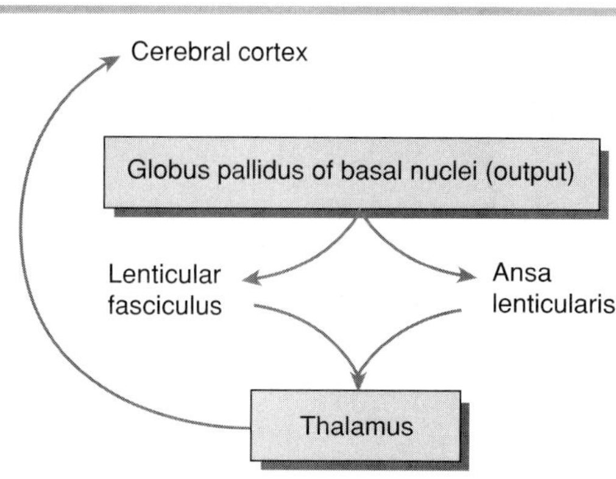

24.5. The *lenticular fasciculus* arises from the __________ __________, which passes through the posterior limb of the internal capsule and through the *subthalamus*, an area located ventral to the __________.

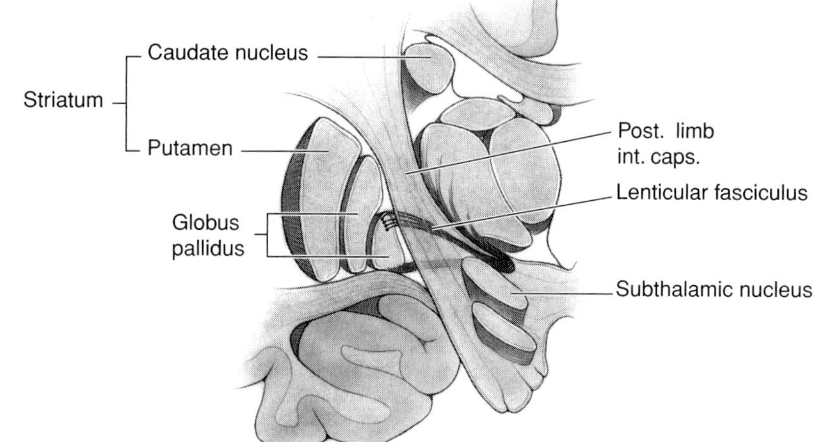

24.6. The ansa ________________ arises from the globus pallidus and travels anteriorly around the __________ capsule and into the subthalamus.

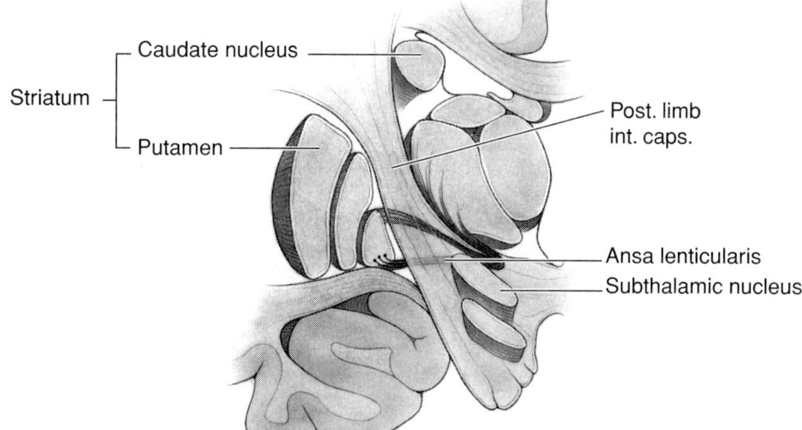

24.4A. lenticular; ansa

24.5A. globus pallidus; thalamus

24.6A. lenticularis; internal

24.7. Label the lenticular fasciculus and the ansa lenticularis on the diagram. The lenticular fasciculus and ansa lenticularis join to form the ____________ fasciculus, which projects to the *ventral anterior nucleus* (VAN) of the thalamus.

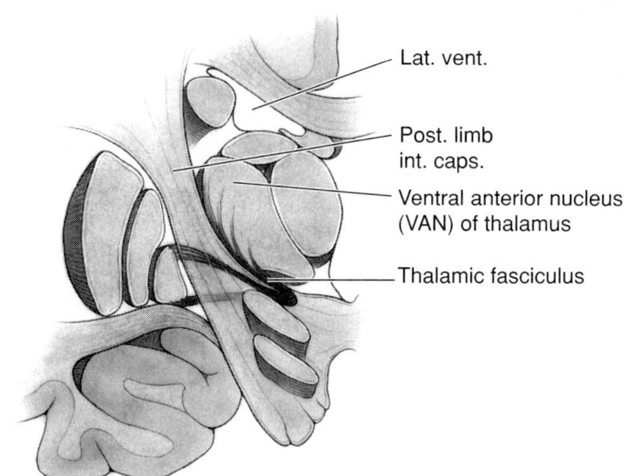

24.8. From the VAN (or ____________ ____________ nucleus) of the thalamus, ____________________ projections go to the *premotor area* of the cerebral cortex, which influences the activity of the primary motor cortex.

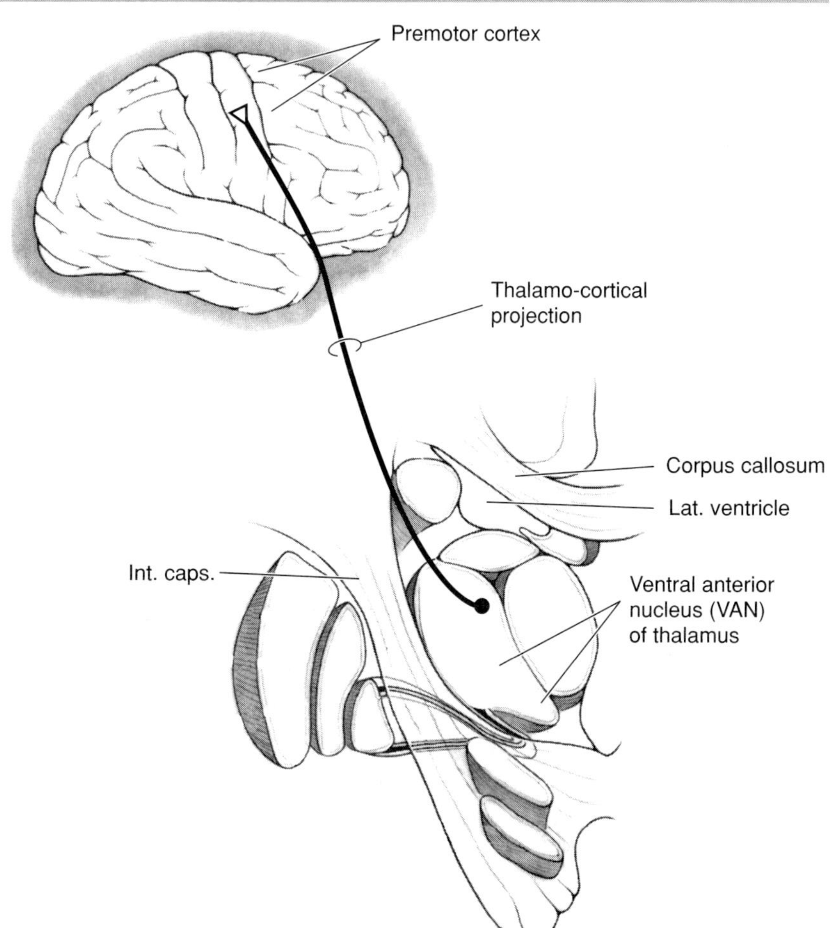

24.7A. thalamic

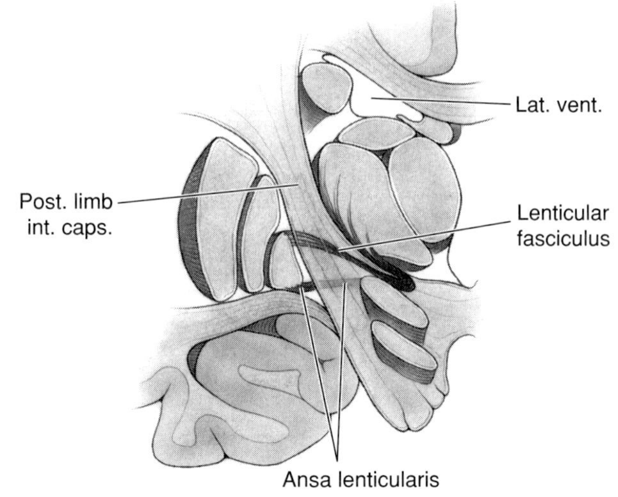

24.8A. ventral anterior; thalamo-cortical

24.9. Number the structures listed below in the proper sequence describing communications between the basal nuclei and cerebral cortex. Label the *input nuclei* of basal nuclei as "1."

_____ Caudate and putamen of basal nuclei
_____ Thalamic fasciculus
_____ Primary motor cortex
_____ Globus pallidus of basal nuclei
_____ Premotor cortex
_____ Lenticular fasciculus and ansa lenticularis
_____ Ventral anterior nucleus of the thalamus

24.10. Within the basal nuclei, there are many interconnections that function to regulate the output of this system. These intrinsic projections include: 1) *striato-pallidal projections* (located between the caudate/putamen and _________ _________); 2) *nigrostriatal tract* (located between the _____________ nigra and putamen); and 3) *subthalamic fasciculus* (located between the _____________ and globus pallidus).

24.11. Label the following pathways on the diagram: striato-pallidal, nigrostriatal, subthalamic fasciculus.

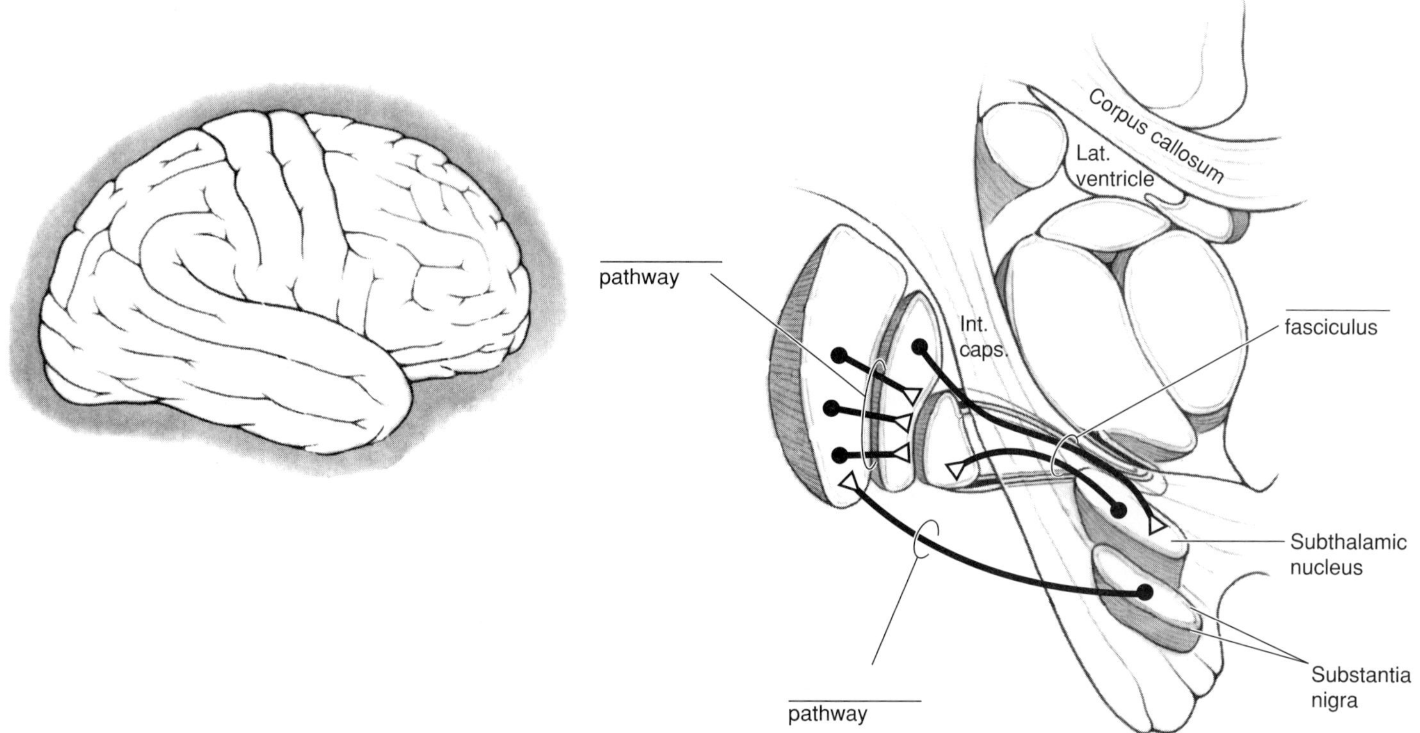

24.9A.

__1__ Caudate and putamen of basal nuclei

__4__ Thalamic fasciculus

__7__ Primary motor cortex

__2__ Globus pallidus of basal nuclei

__6__ Premotor cortex

__3__ Lenticular fasciculus and ansa lenticularis

__5__ Ventral anterior nucleus of the thalamus

24.10A. globus pallidus; substantia; subthalamus

24.11A.

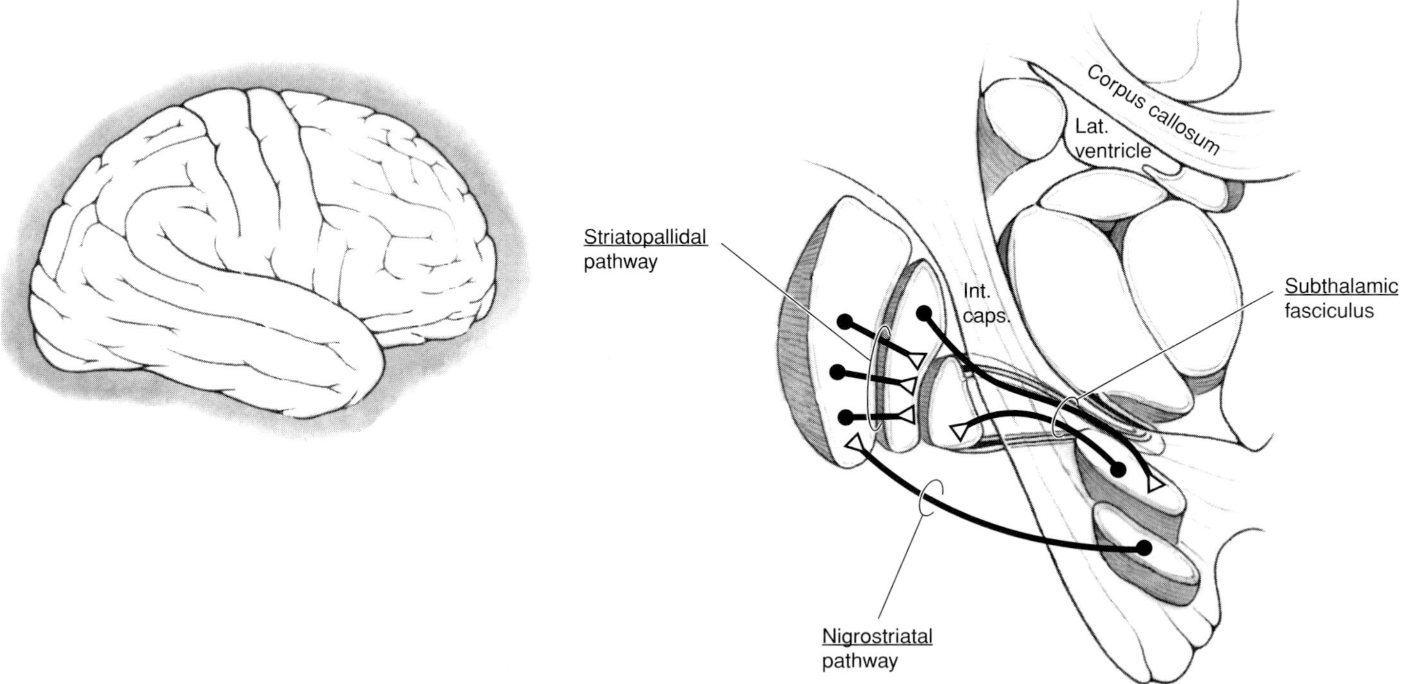

25 Circuits within and with the Cerebrum, Cerebellum, and Spinal Cord

25.1. The basal nuclei play an important role in helping to initiate and terminate ____________ movements. The primary function of the basal nuclei is to provide feedback to the ____________ to control motor responses.

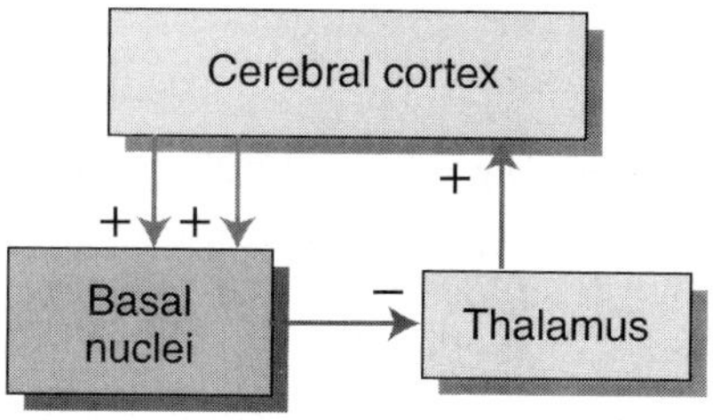

Cerebral cortex
+ +
Basal nuclei
−
+
Thalamus

25.2. Much of the output of the basal nuclei is funneled through the ____________. The basal nuclei ____________ the excitatory input to the cortex. Hyperactivity of the basal nuclei results in ______er movements, whereas lesions of basal nuclei produce ____________________ movements at rest.

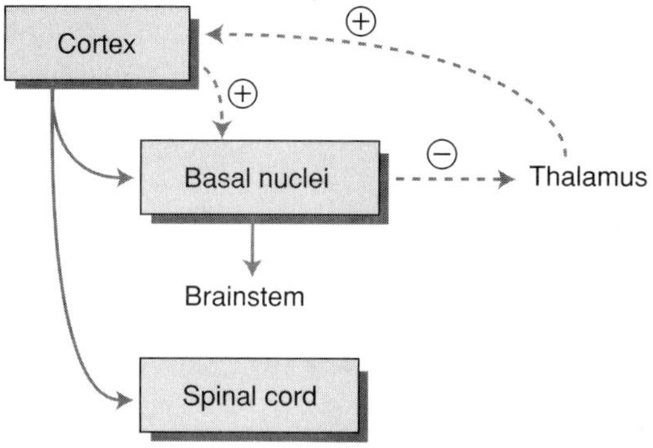

Cortex
⊕
⊕
Basal nuclei
⊖
Thalamus
Brainstem
Spinal cord

25.3. The cerebral ____________ and ______ nuclei provide crude motor commands that descend to the brainstem and the spinal cord. Control mechanisms in the ____________um, ______ stem and ____________ cord serve to fine-tune descending pathways to ensure smooth coordinated movement.

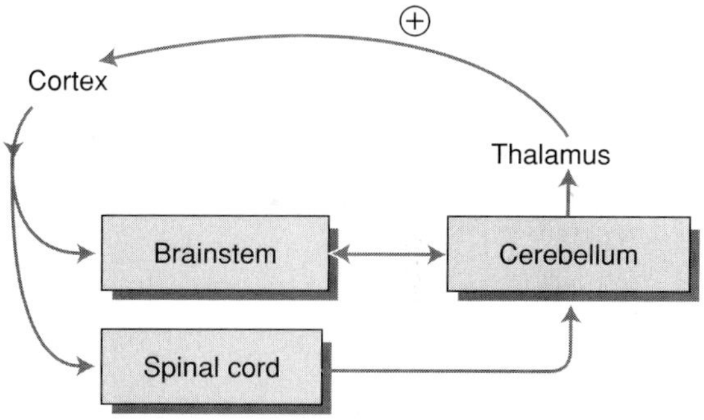

⊕
Cortex
Thalamus
Brainstem
Cerebellum
Spinal cord

25.4. The basal nuclei and cerebellum control different aspects of ____________ activity and are considered together as control circuits. They both receive input from the ____________ and send info back to it through the ____________.

25.5. Basal nuclei are concerned with activation and inhibition of ______ commands, whereas the ____________um plans and executes coordinated movements, adjusts motor performance, and is involved in learning motor tasks.

25.1A. voluntary; cortex

25.2A. thalamus; reduce; slower; involuntary (excessive)

25.3A. cortex; basal; cerebellum; brainstem; spinal cord

25.4A. motor; cortex; thalamus

25.5A. motor; cerebellum

25.6. The cerebellum compares motor commands with actual execution of movement, functioning to detect errors. Cerebellar inputs are sideloops of paths from the motor ____________, _______ nuclei, and spinal_______.

25.7. Cerebellum receives ____________ input from tendons, joints, and auditory, vestibular, and visual systems. The cerebellum receives ouput from the ______ cortex, ______ nuclei, and ____________. Cerebellar efferents descend to exert an inhibitory influence on the pyramidal and ______ pyramidal paths.

25.8. The cerebellum corrects motor performance through output to ____________ nuclei via *red nucleus, vestibular nuclei, superior colliculus*, and *reticular formation*. The cerebellum also projects to the cortex through the *ventral lateral* nucleus of the ____________.

Cerebral cortex
Ventral lateral nucleus of thalamus
Superior colliculus
Red nucleus
Reticular formation
Vestibular nuclei

25.9. The motor cortex sends projections to brainstem that run *outside the corticospinal (pyramidal) tract* to regulate lower motor neurons in the spinal cord. These *extrapyramidal paths* originate in the red ____________, ____________ colliculus, vest____________ nuclei, and reticular formation. All of these areas also receive input from the cerebellum and are involved in the maintenance of posture, muscle tone, and coordination.

Cortex
Red nucleus
Vestibular nuleus
Superior colliculus
Reticular formation
Pyramidal tract
Extrapyramidal tract
Spinal cord

25.6A. cortex; basal; cord

25.7A. sensory; motor; basal; brainstem; extrapyramidal

25.8A. brainstem; thalamus

25.9A. nucleus; superior; vestibular

26 Pathways of the Extrapyramidal System

26.1. Movement is controlled by spinal motor neurons that are influenced by the pyramidal system as well as by desc__________ extrapyramidal pathways in the brainstem and spinal cord.

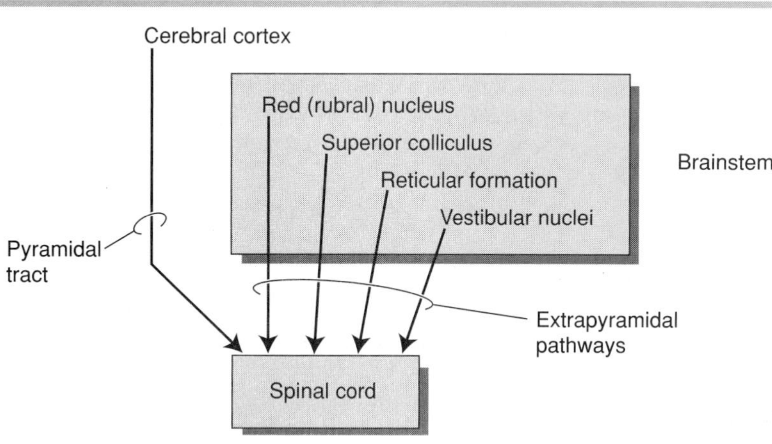

26.2. Four descending pathways contribute to the extrapyramidal motor system, including the __________spinal tracts, ret______spinal tracts, rubro__________ tract, and tectospinal tract. Label these tracts on the figure.

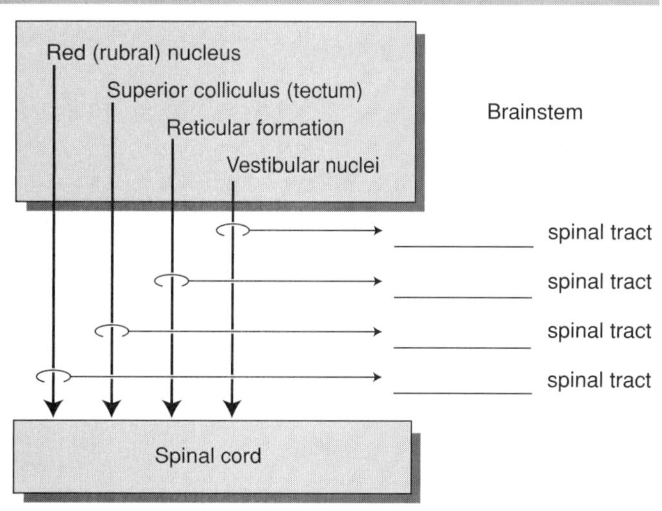

26.3. The vestibulospinal tract keeps body movements coordinated with the head when head position changes. Balance receptors in the ______ ear synapse in the vestibular nuclei, which are located at the junction of the ______ and __________ of the brainstem. These nuclei project to the __________ ______ via the vestibulospinal tract and are important for postural adjustments of trunk, neck, and limbs.

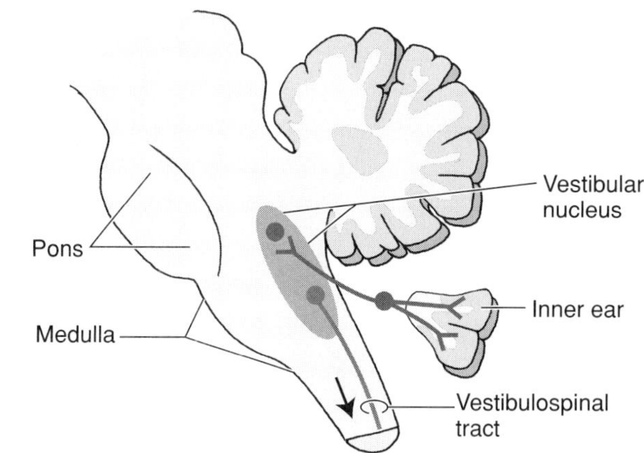

26.1A. descending

26.2A. vestibulospinal; reticulospinal; rubrospinal

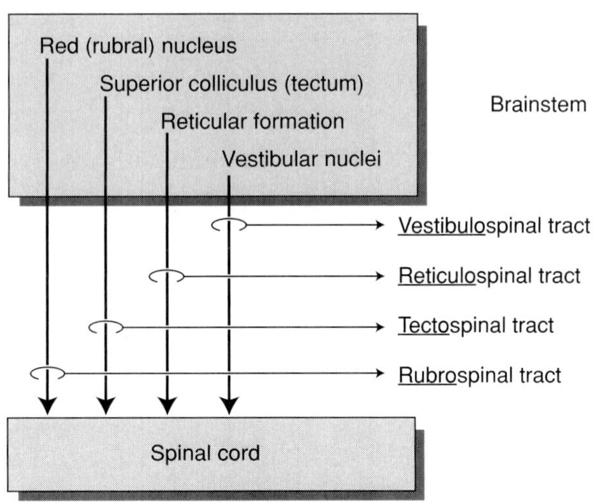

26.3A. inner; pons; medulla; spinal cord

26.4. The vestibulo__________ tract is split into medial and lateral pathways. The lateral vestibular nucleus gives rise to __________ ________________ tract, which descends __________ in ventral funiculi of the spinal cord to control __________ muscles of the trunk and proximal limb at all levels of the spinal cord.

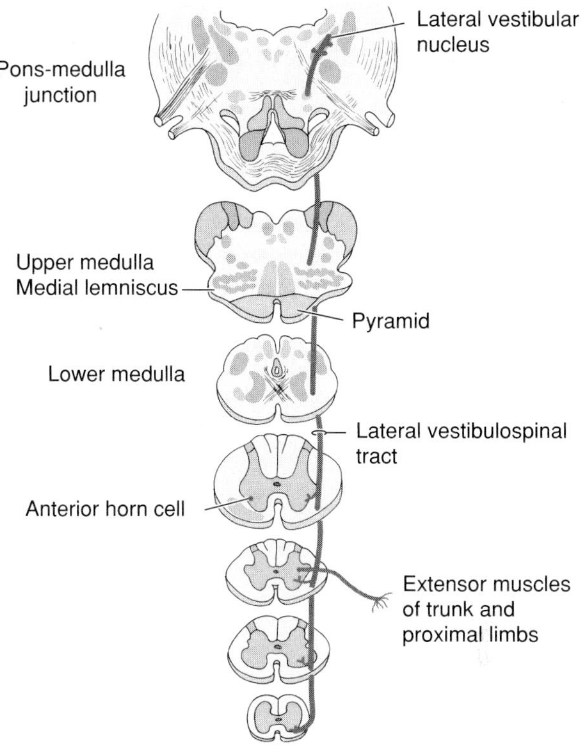

26.5. The __________ vestibulospinal tract arises from medial and inferior vestibular nuclei and descends bilaterally through the __________ ________________ fasciculus, adjusting head position in response to changes in posture.

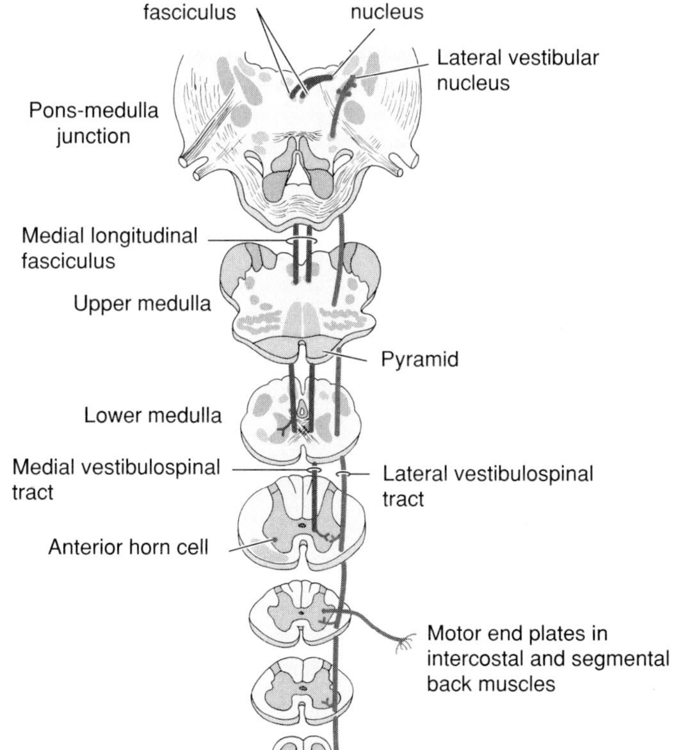

26.4A. vestibulospinal; lateral vestibulospinal; uncrossed (ipsilaterally); extensor

26.5A. medial; medial longitudinal

26.6. The reticulospinal tracts take origin from the __________ __________ in the brainstem, which is important for integrating sensory and motor cues. The reticular formation projects bilaterally to the spinal cord at all levels via the lateral ______________ tract, which innervates axial and proximal limb muscles. The lateral reticulospinal tract inhibits __________ spinal reflexes. By contrast, the __________ reticulospinal tract projects ipsilaterally to the cervical spinal cord and facilitates extensor spinal reflexes.

Pons
Medulla
Reticular formation
Facilitates extensors
Medial (pontine) reticulospinal tract
Lateral (medullary) reticulospinal tract
Inhibits extensors

26.7. Label the lateral and medial reticulospinal tracts on the diagram. These pathways innervate __________ muscles to maintain posture.

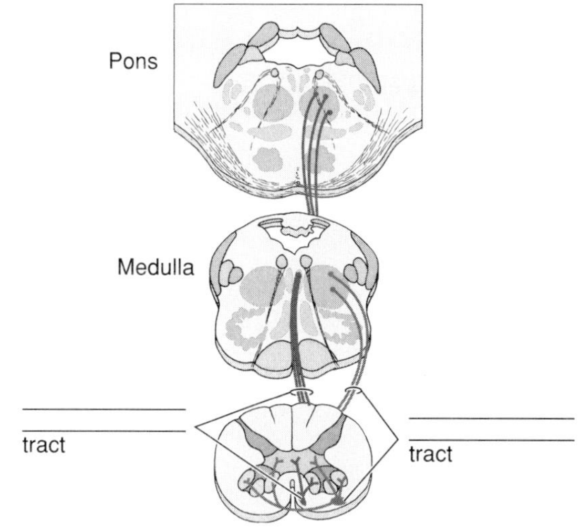

26.8. The *red (rubral) nucleus* is large structure in midbrain that receives projections from the motor and premotor cortex (areas 4 and 6). The ______________ tract arises from the red nucleus, crosses midline, and descends in the brainstem. It augments the function of the corticospinal tract by activating spinal motor neurons innervating distal __________ muscles, such as those of the upper limb.

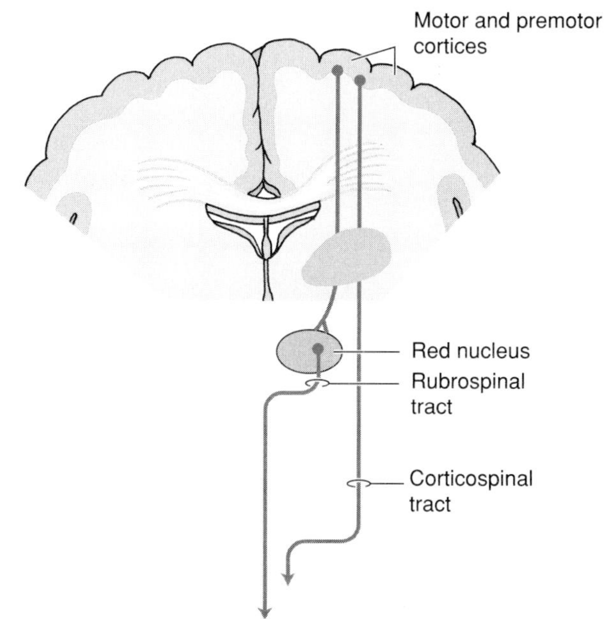

26.6A. reticular formation; reticulospinal; extensor; medial

26.7A. extensor

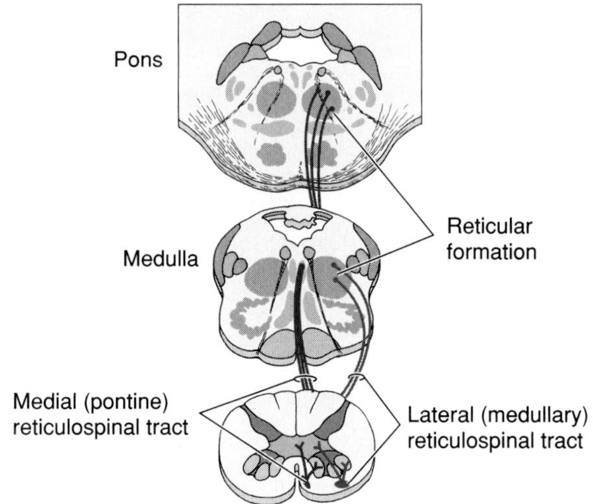

26.8A. rubrospinal; flexor

26.9. __________spinal and __________spinal tracts innervate neurons supplying axial muscles, whereas ______spinal fibers supply more distal flexor muscles.

26.10. Match the appropriate descriptor with the tracts on the left. More than one lettered option may be used for each tract.

______ Lateral vestibulospinal tract	A. Travels through medial longitudinal fasciculus
______ Rubrospinal tract	B. Innervates extensor muscles of trunk
______ Reticulospinal tract	C. Innervates distal flexor muscles
______ Medial vestibulospinal tract	D. Originates in the red nucleus of midbrain

26.11. The tectospinal tract originates in the __________ colliculus, located in the tectum of the midbrain. This pathway synapses in the cervical spinal cord, similar to the __________ vestibulospinal tract. The tectospinal tract functions to move the head in response to visual stimuli.

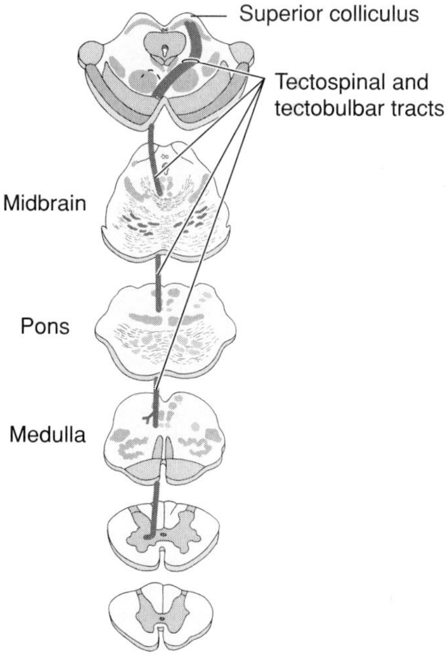

26.12. The vestibulospinal, reticulospinal, rubrospinal, and tectospinal tracts are all ______ pathways associated with the extra__________ system.

26.13. The ______________ tract and __________ ______________ tract are descending motor paths that reach only cervical spinal cord and control coordinate head and eye movements in response to stimuli. Together, these two tracts make up the descending part of the __________ ______________ fasciculus.

26.9A. Vestibulospinal; reticulospinal; rubrospinal

26.10A.

B	Lateral vestibulospinal tract	A. Travels through medial longitudinal fasciculus
C	Rubrospinal tract	B. Innervates extensor muscles of trunk
B	Reticulospinal tract	C. Innervates distal flexor muscles
A, B	Medial vestibulospinal tract	D. Originates in the red nucleus of midbrain

26.11A. superior; medial

26.12A. motor; extrapyramidal

26.13A. tectospinal; medial vestibulospinal; medial longitudinal

27 Blood Supply to the Basal Nuclei

27.1. Recall that two pairs of arteries supply blood to the brain, the ____________ carotid and vertebral arteries. Label these arteries on the diagram.

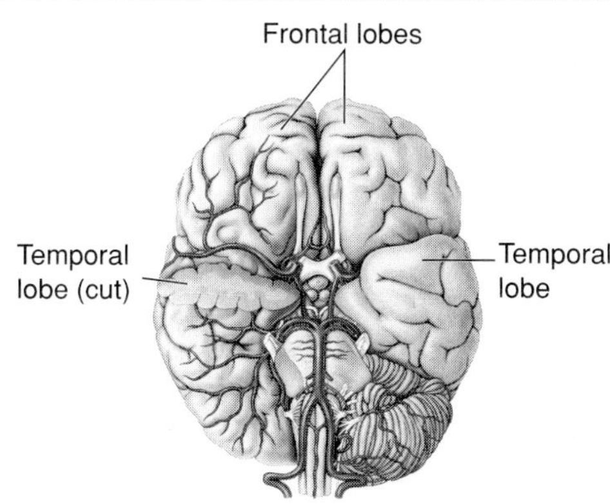

27.2. Each internal carotid artery splits into two terminal branches: the ____________ cerebral artery and the ____________ cerebral artery. Label them on the diagram.

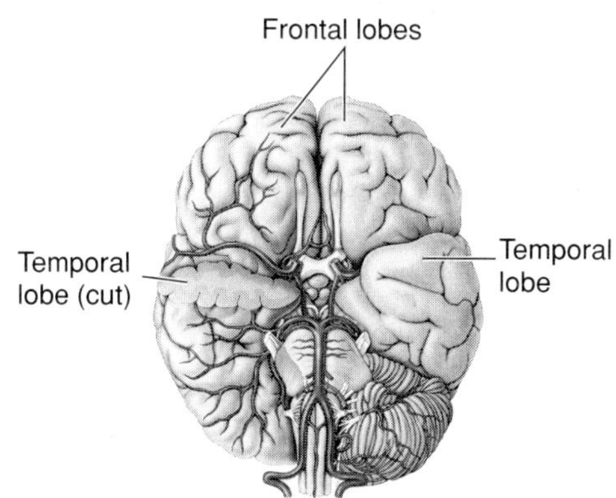

27.3. The blood supply to the basal nuclei arises from three sources: the internal carotid artery and the anterior and middle cerebral arteries. Label them on the diagram.

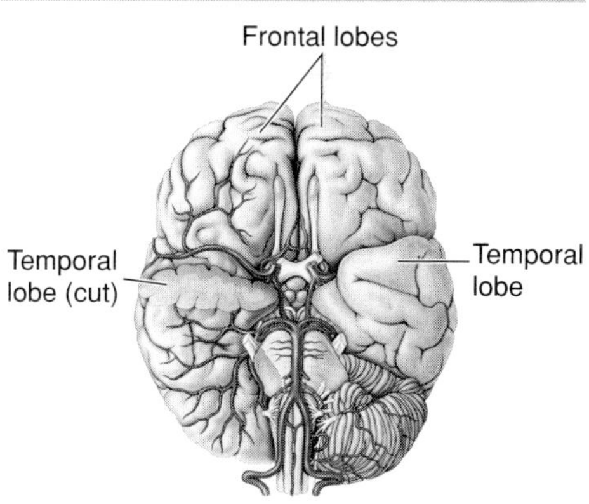

27.1A. internal

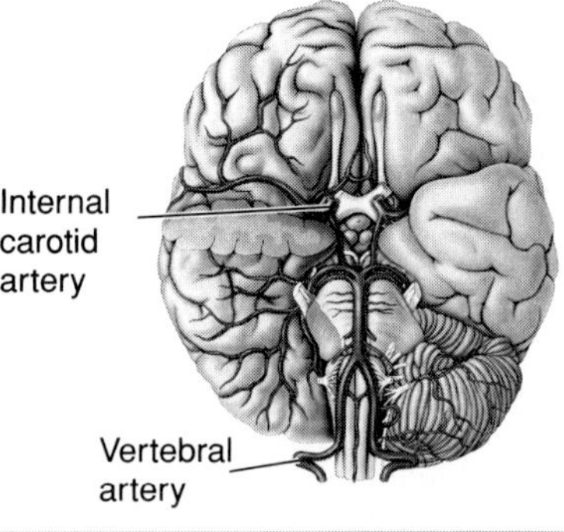

27.2A. anterior; middle

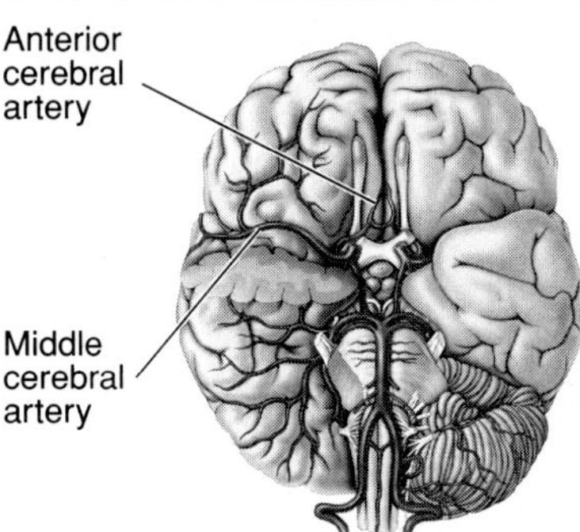

27.3A.

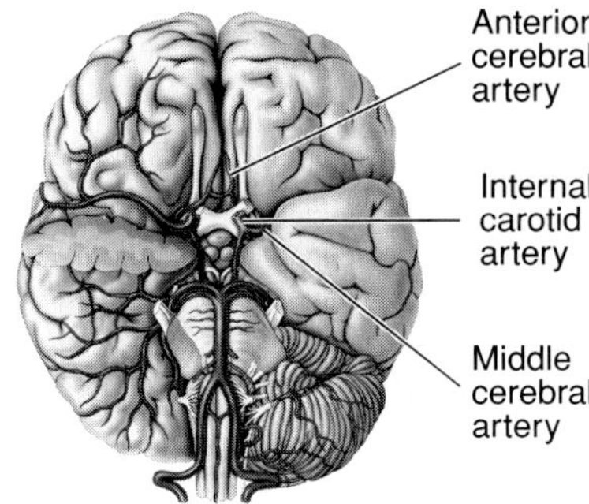

27.4. On this coronal section, label the internal carotid artery and its two terminal branches: the ____________ and ____________ cerebral arteries.

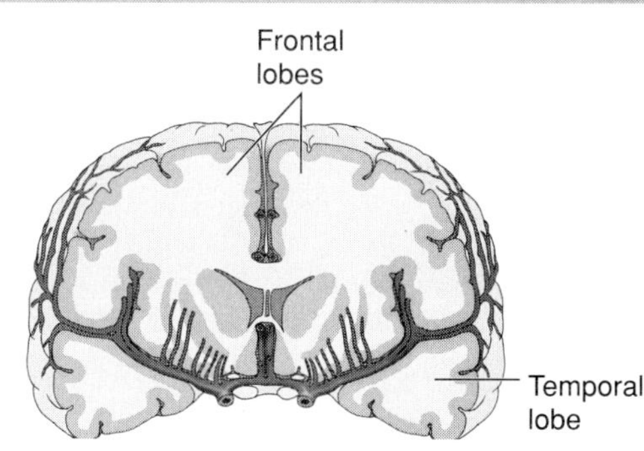

27.5. The basal nuclei primarily receive their blood supply from the middle cerebral artery via lenticulostriate *arteries*. Recall that the lenticular nucleus includes the ____________ and ____________ ____________, while the striatum consists of the ____________ and caudate nuclei.

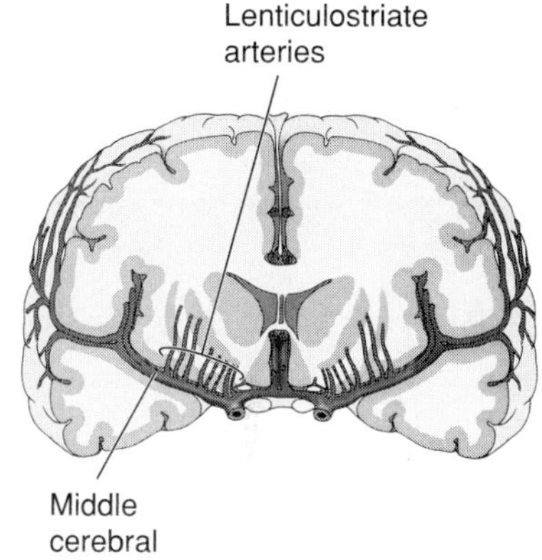

27.6. Label the middle cerebral and lenticulostriate arteries on the diagram.

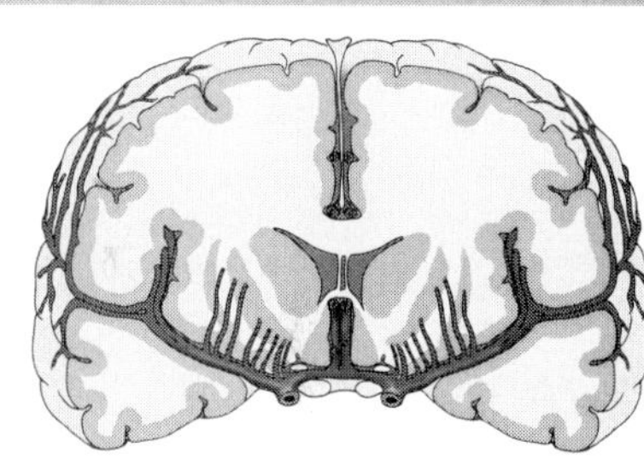

27.7. The internal carotid artery contributes blood to the globus pallidus via the ____________ choroidal artery, which arises near the optic chiasm. Label the lenticulostriate arteries and middle cerebral artery on the diagram.

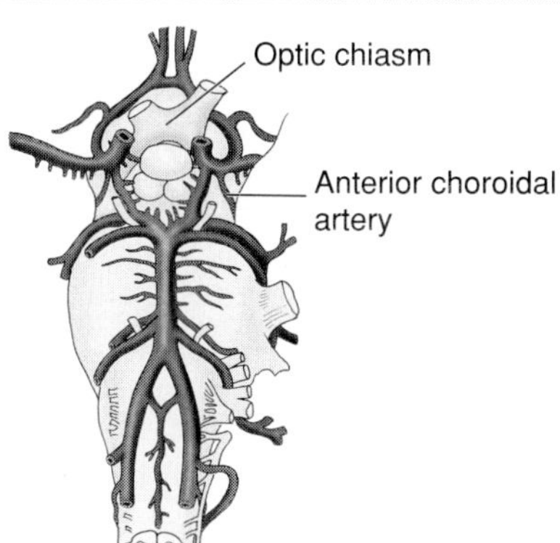

27.4A. anterior; middle

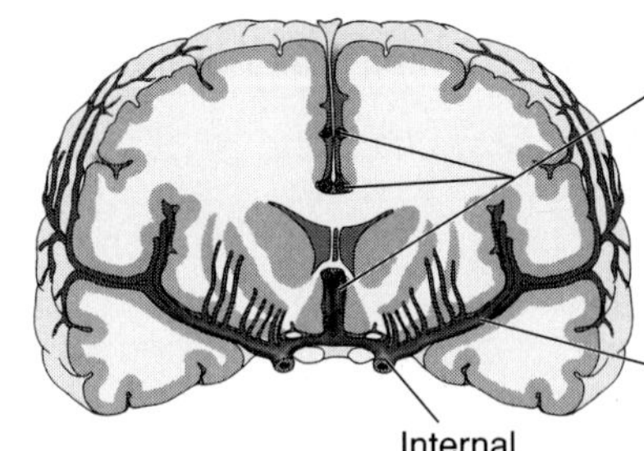

27.5A. putamen; globus pallidus; lenticular

27.6A.

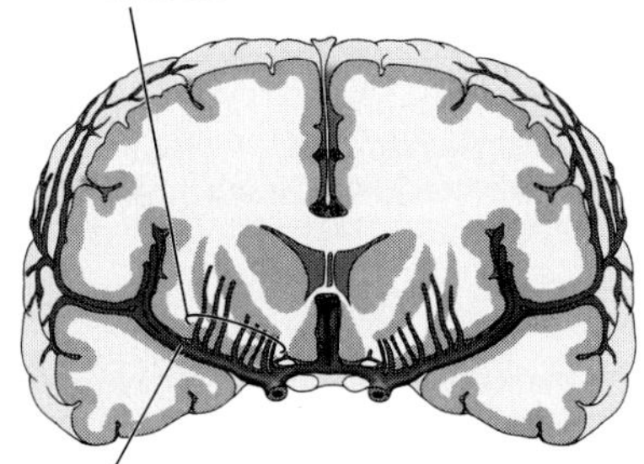

27.7A. anterior

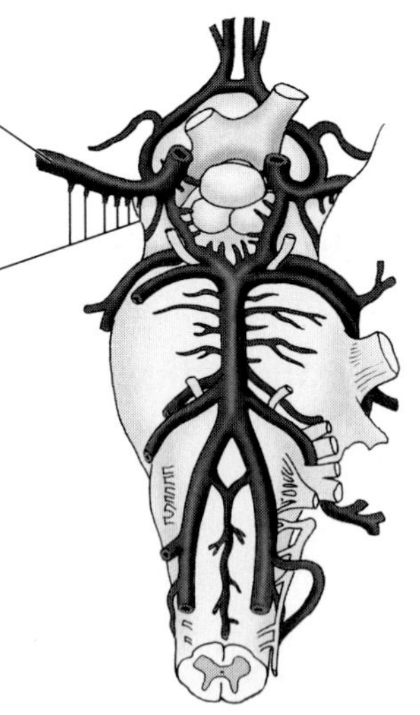

27.8. The anterior cerebral artery also contributes blood to the basal nuclei via the ____________ striate artery (also known as the ____________ artery of Huebner). This artery supplies blood to the head of the caudate and putamen.

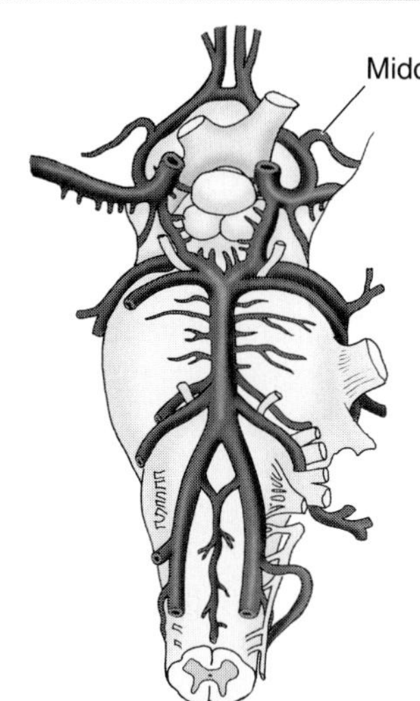

27.9. On this lateral view of the basal nuclei, label the anterior and middle cerebral arteries.

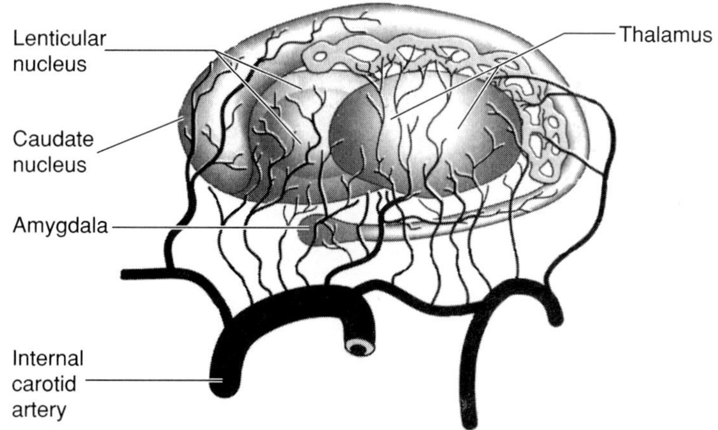

27.10. On the diagram, label the following arteries: 1) lenticulostriate arteries branching from the middle cerebral artery; and 2) medial striate artery arising from the anterior cerebral artery.

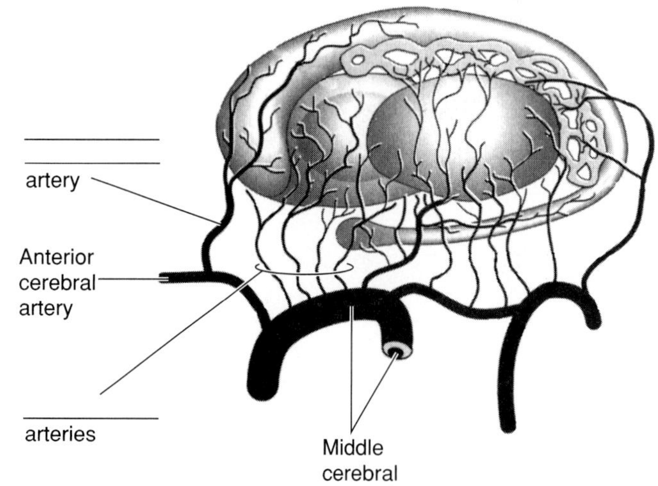

27.8A. medial; recurrent

27.9A.

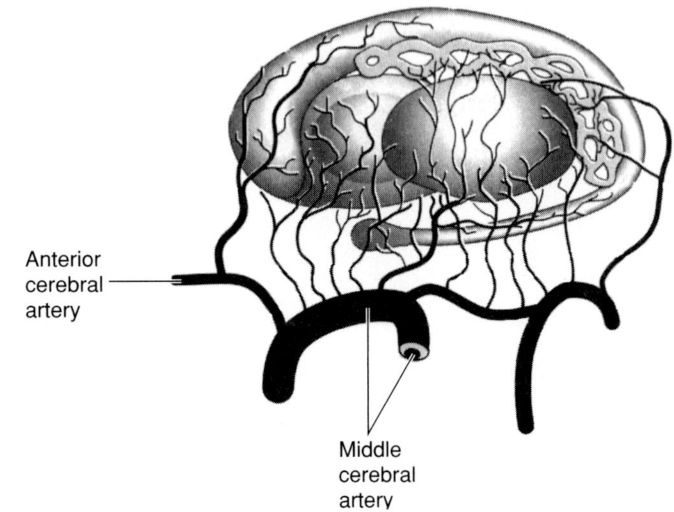

27.10A.

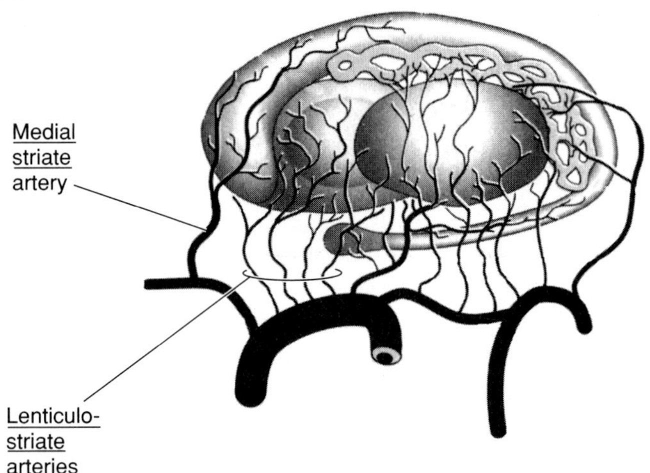

28 Clinical Signs of Basal Nuclei Damage

28.1. Output from the basal nuclei through the thalamus functions to ____________ the excitatory input to the motor cortex. Basal nuclei disturbances result in motor disturbances.

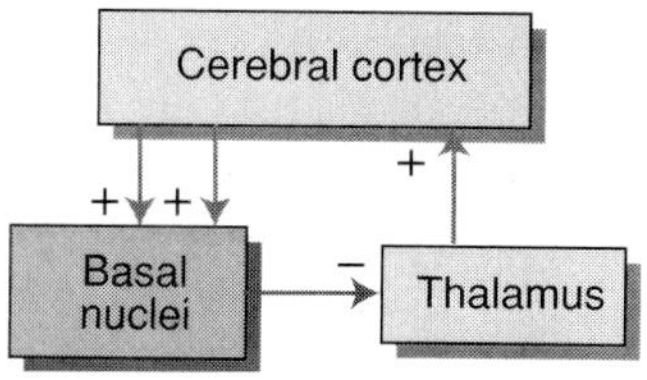

Cerebral cortex; + + (to Basal nuclei); Basal nuclei — (to Thalamus); Thalamus + (to Cerebral cortex)

28.2. There are both direct and indirect connections from the ______ nuclei to the thalamus. The *direct pathway* modulates the output of the basal nuclei to the ____________ ____________ to release thalamic inhibition of the cortex. This sequence of events facilitates movement.

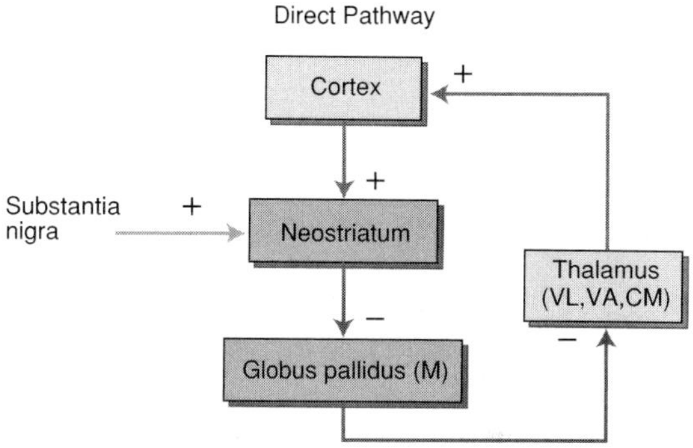

Direct Pathway

Cortex; + Neostriatum; Substantia nigra +; − Globus pallidus (M); − Thalamus (VL,VA,CM); + Cortex

28.3. The ____________ pathway uses the globus pallidus to ____________________ voluntary movements.

28.4. The *indirect pathway* involves cortical activation of the basal nuclei, which inhibits the subthalamus. The subthalamus activates the globus pallidus. The globus pallidus ____________ the thalamus, reducing motor cortical activation.

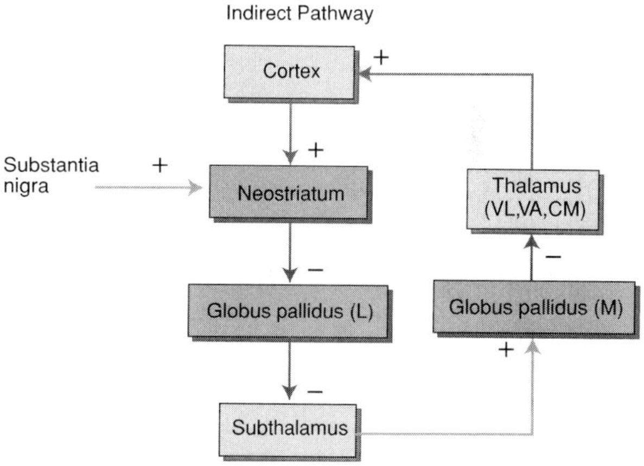

Indirect Pathway

Cortex; + Neostriatum; Substantia nigra +; − Globus pallidus (L); − Subthalamus; + Globus pallidus (M); − Thalamus (VL,VA,CM); + Cortex

28.5. The indirect pathway ____________ motor cortex, whereas the direct pathway ____________ motor cortex.

28.6. Malfunctioning of the basal nuclei results in movement disorders, known as *dyskinesias*. *Dys* refers to abnormal, and *kinesia* refers to ____________.

28.1A. reduce

28.2A. basal; globus pallidus

28.3A. direct; facilitate

28.4A. inhibits

28.5A. inhibits; activates

28.6A. movement

28.7. Dyskinesias, or abnormal movements, manifest in one of two ways: as either negative or positive symptoms. Negative signs (______kinetic symptoms) involve the inability of a patient to perform a movement (lack of movement), whereas positive signs (______kinetic symptoms) evoke unwanted motor activities (excessive movements).

28.8. Negative signs are characterized by the __________ ability to initiate movement. These signs include akinesia (lack of movement) and bradykinesia (slowness of movement) with increased muscle tone.

28.9. Negative signs, or ________________ dyskinesia, results from reduced excitation of the direct pathway. Increased inhibition of the __________ reduces motor activity.

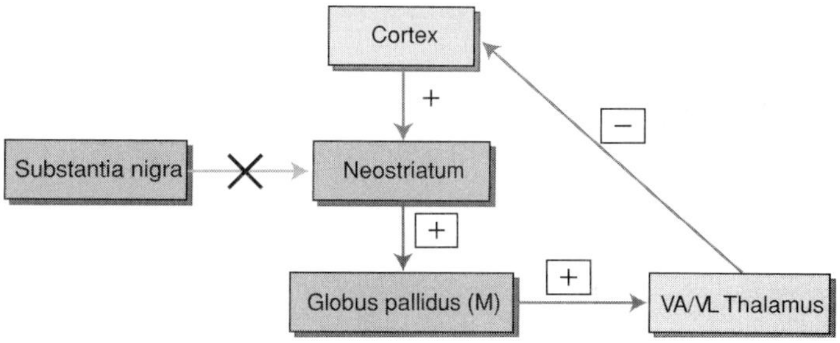

28.10. Positive signs are characterized by excessive involuntary movements and reduced muscle tone, resulting from diminished activation of the __________ pathway.

28.11. Reduced inhibition of the thalamus leads to __________ motor activity, characteristic of ______kinetic dyskinesias.

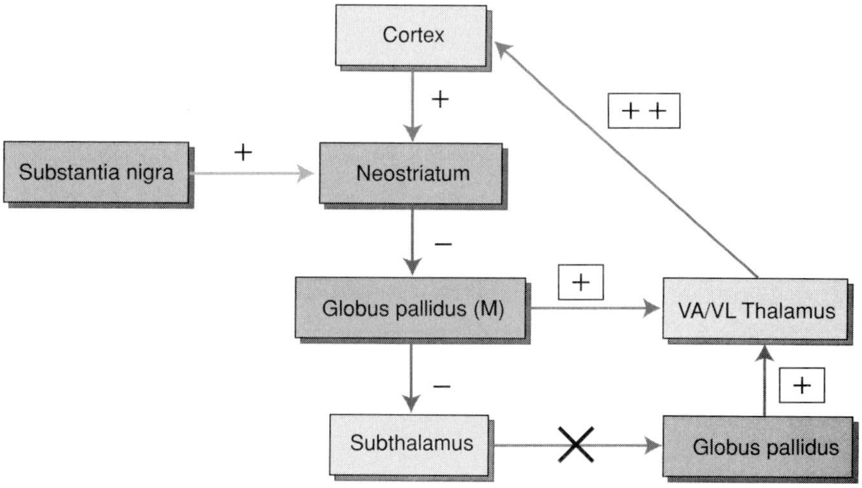

28.12. Note that dyskinesia is not equivalent to paralysis (muscle __________) or apraxia (inability to plan a __________), which are cortical problems.

28.7A. hypokinetic; hyperkinetic

28.8A. impaired

28.9A. hypokinetic; thalamus

28.10A. indirect

28.11A. excessive; hyperkinetic

28.12A. weakness; movement

29 Lesions of the Basal Nuclei

29.1. Hypokinetic dyskinesias involve ______ of movement, whereas hyperkinetic dyskinesias are characterized by ____________ movement.

29.2. Parkinson's disease is a ______kinetic movement disorder in which patients exhibit resting tremor, muscle rigidity, and bradykinesia.

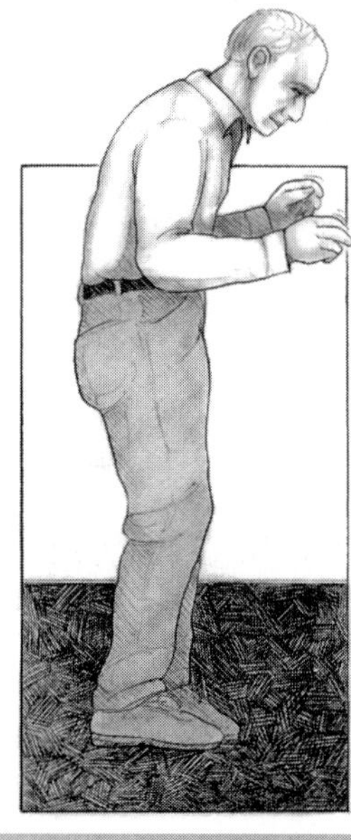

29.3. In Parkinson's disease, substantia nigral neurons degenerate, producing less dopamine. This affects both the direct and ___________ paths of the basal nuclei. Replacement therapy involves administering the dopamine precursor, L-DOPA, to patients. Dopamine is ineffective when administered exogenously because it cannot cross the blood- ______ barrier.

29.4. Huntington's chorea is an example of a ______kinetic dyskinesia. Chorea literally means "to dance," and these patients exhibit uncontrolled dance-like movements of the limbs.

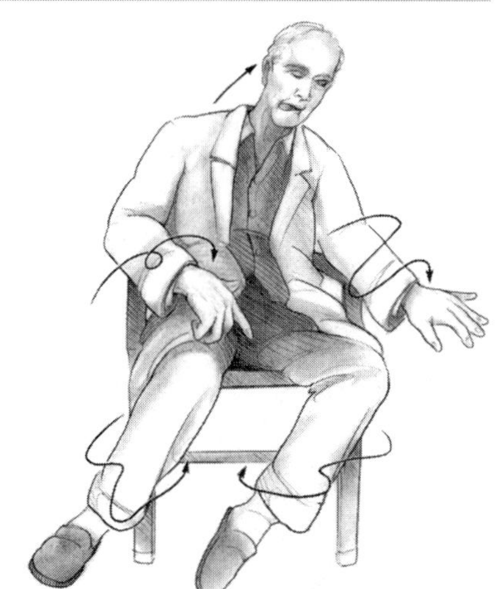

29.1A. lack; excessive

29.2A. hypokinetic

29.3A. indirect; brain

29.4A. hyperkinetic

29.5. Huntington's chorea affects the striatum, whereas Parkinson's disease targets the ________ ______.

29.6. Like Huntington's chorea, hemiballism is a ______kinetic disorder of the basal nuclei. Patients with hemiballismus often suffer from subthalamic nuclear stroke and exhibit b______istic movements of the limbs.

29.7. Damage to the subthalamic nucleus results in________________ of the contralateral extremities. The subthalamic nucleus reduces ________________ output of the globus pallidus, facilitating thalamic activation of the motor cortex.

29.8. Athetosis is similar to chorea, except the aberrant movements of the extremities are slow and writhing rather than __________. Like other dyskinesias, athetosis is caused by a lesion of the basal __________.

29.9. Dystonia is a variant of athe______ and involves sustained muscle contractions of the limbs, trunk, and neck, resulting in abnormal posture.

29.10. Tardive dyskinesia primarily affects muscles of the tongue and face. It differs from other dyskinesias in that it is not induced by lesions but, instead, by antipsychotic drugs that block dop______ transmission.

29.11. Match the appropriate classification on the right with the pathologies listed on the left.

A. Hyperkinetic disorder
B. Hypokinetic disorder

______ Hemiballism
______ Parkinson's disease
______ Athetosis
______ Tardive dyskinesia
______ Huntington's chorea

29.5A. substantia nigra

29.6A. hyperkinetic; ballistic

29.7A. hemiballismus; inhibitory

29.8A. ballistic; nuclei

29.9A. athetosis

29.10A. dopamine

29.11A.

A. Hyperkinetic disorder

B. Hypokinetic disorder

_A_ Hemiballism

_B_ Parkinson's disease

_A_ Athetosis

_A_ Tardive dyskinesia

_A_ Huntington's chorea

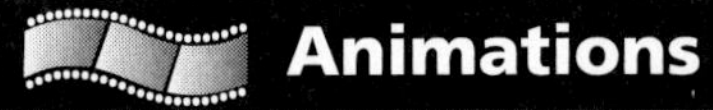

Animations

25. Basal Ganglia (Chapters 23, 24, 25, 26)
30. Vestibulocerebellum (Chapter 25)
31. Spinocerebellum (Chapter 25)
32. Neocerebellum (Chapter 25)

III CEREBELLUM

30 The Structure of the Cerebellum

30.1. Like the surface of the cerebral hemispheres, the surface of the cerebellum is composed of cerebellar neurons and is thrown into folds in order to increase surface area. Unlike the surface of the cerebrum, which exhibits raised ______i and grooves called s______i, the folia (folium = singular) of the cerebellum are separated by fissures.

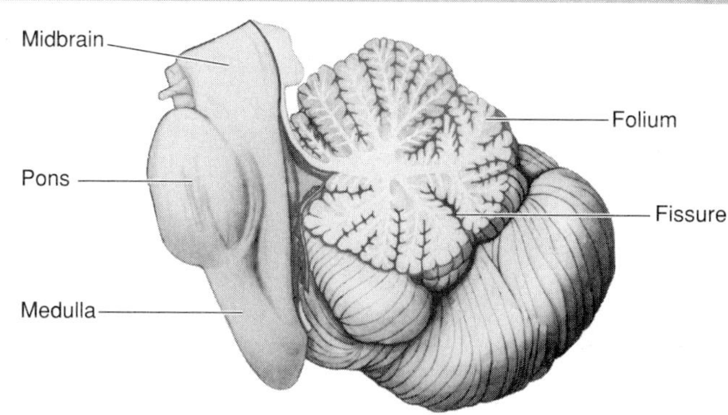

30.2. The deepest ____________ of the cerebellum divide it into lobes.

30.3. Like the cerebral cortex, the cerebellar cortex is ______ matter, which surrounds a core of ______ matter known as the medullary core of the cerebellum. Like the cerebral hemispheres, masses of cell bodies known as ____________ are contained within the white matter of the cerebellum—the deep cerebellar nuclei.

30.4. A deep posterolateral ____________ separates the flocculonodular lobe from the body of the cerebellum. A primary fissure subdivides the body of the cerebellum into an ____________ and a ____________ lobe.

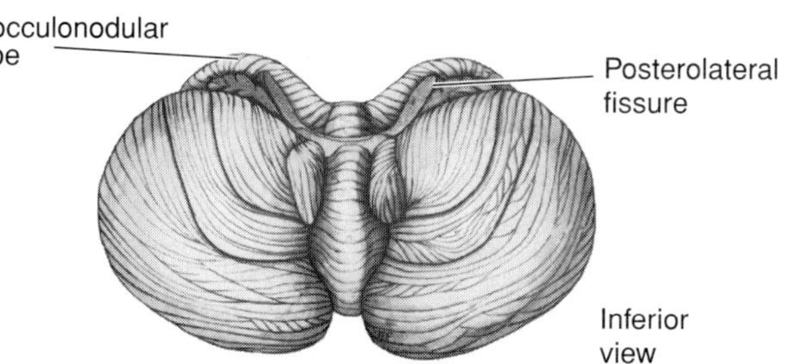

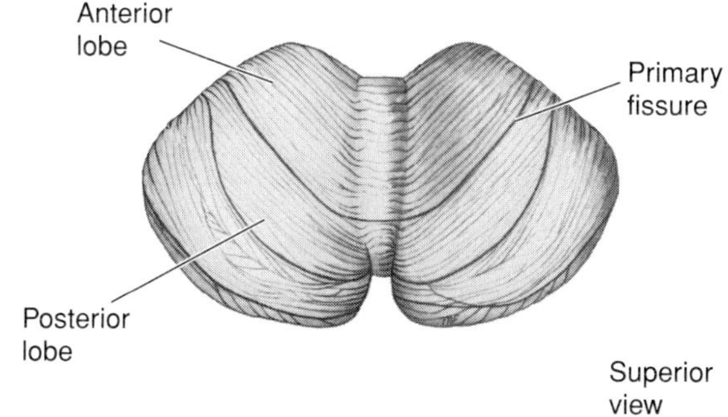

30.5. Label the lobes and fissure of the cerebellum indicated on the following image.

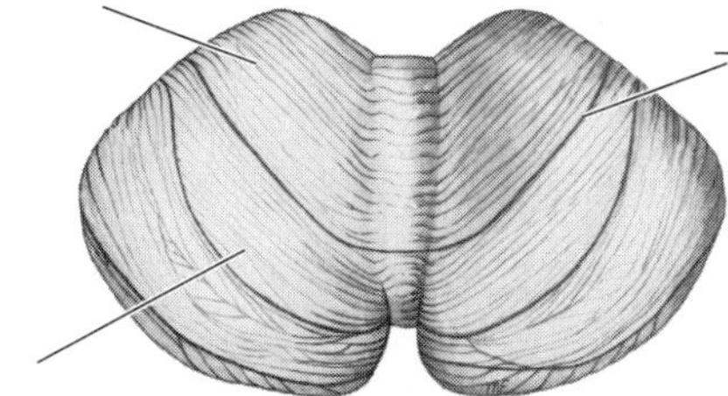

30.1A. gyri; sulci

30.2A. fissures

30.3A. gray; white; nuclei

30.4A. fissure; anterior; posterior

30.5A.

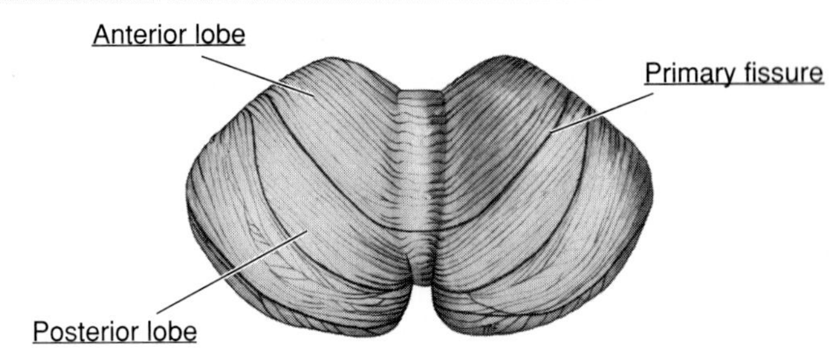

30.6. Label the lobe and fissure of the cerebellum indicated on the following image.

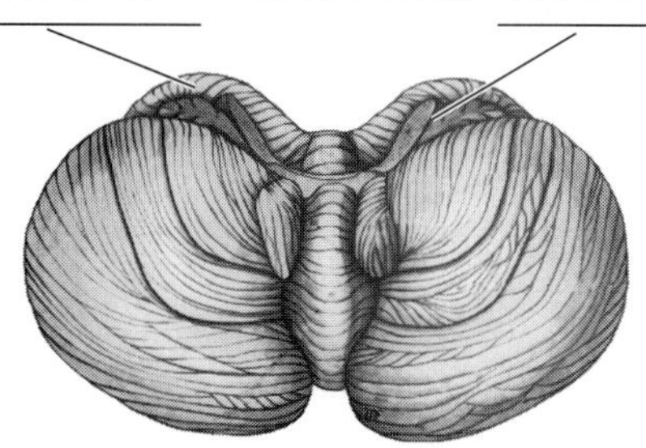

30.7. The __________ lobe is located anterior to the __________ fissure. The anterior lobe receives input from the ______cerebellar tracts that originated in the muscle spindles and Golgi tendon organs. It is important in maintaining synergy in trunk musculature and is involved in actions such as walking or standing.

30.8. Posterior to the __________ fissure is the __________ lobe. It receives input from motor areas of the cerebral cortex via pontine nuclei. The posterior lobe is primarily concerned with the coordination of voluntary ______ activity.

30.9. The __________ lobe is separated from the posterior lobe by the __________ fissure. The flocculonodular lobe is involved with maintaining equilibrium and as such receives input from the __________ibular system.

30.10. Match the lobe with the correct function by drawing lines between the columns.

posterior	equilibrium
anterior	coordination
flocculonodular	synergy of trunk musculature

30.11. The cerebellum may be divided morphologically, as described earlier, or into three longitudinally oriented functional zones. The zones are each associated with specific cerebellar __________ (accumulations of neurons inside the white matter __________ary core of the cerebellum).

30.6A.

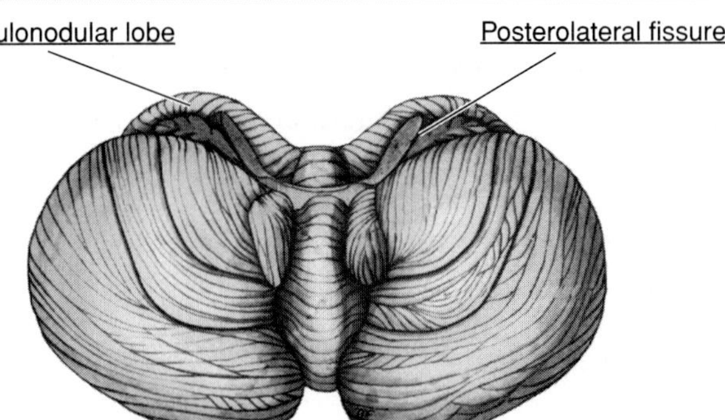

30.7A. anterior; primary; spinocerebellar

30.8A. primary; posterior; motor

30.9A. flocculonodular; posterolateral; vestibular

30.10A.

posterior	equilibrium
anterior	coordination
flocculonodular	synergy of trunk musculature

(Lines connect: posterior — coordination; anterior — synergy of trunk musculature; flocculonodular — equilibrium.)

30.11A. nuclei; medullary

30.12. The longitudinally oriented functional zones incorporate parts of the ____________, ____________, and __________________ lobes.

30.13. The medial-most zone is the median or vermal zone. *Vermis* refers to the worm-like appearance of the region. Circle and label the vermis on the image.

Superior view

30.14. The worm-like ____________ zone separates the __________________ hemispheres, which are subdivided into a more medial intermediate, or paravermal, zone and a more lateral zone.

30.15. Cerebellar zones are not clearly demarcated but, rather, are established based on connections with the deeply placed cerebellar ____________. The nuclei include the fastigial, interposed (emboliform and globose), and dentate.

30.16. Match the zone listed on the left with the cerebellar nuclei to which they are connected by drawing a line between the two columns.

vermal	emboliform
lateral	fastigial
paravermal	dentate
	globose

30.12A. anterior; posterior; flocculonodular

30.13A.

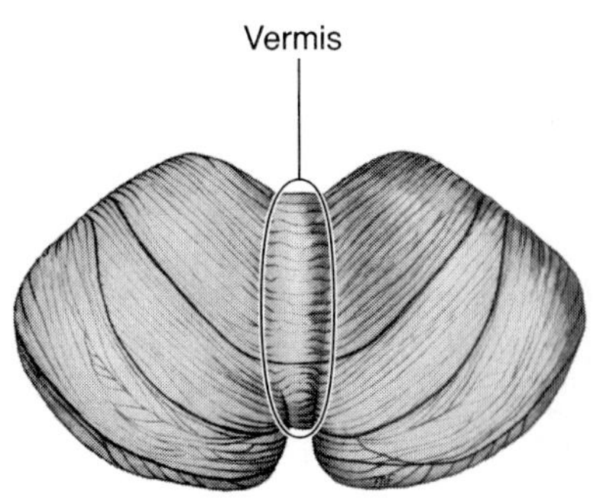

30.14A. vermal; cerebellar

30.15A. nuclei

30.16A.

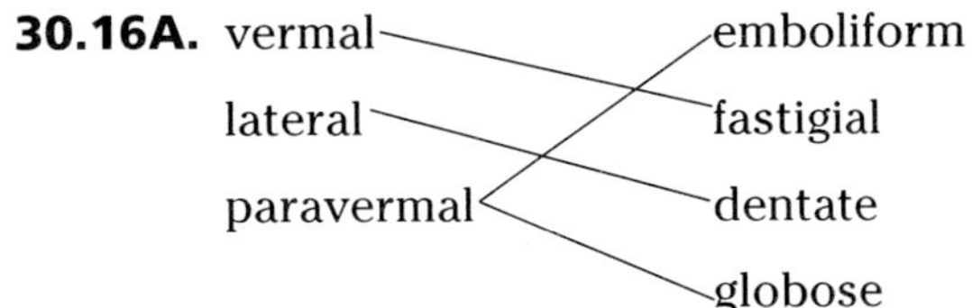

30.17. Beside each deep cerebellar nucleus identified on the following diagram, indicate with which zone it is associated.

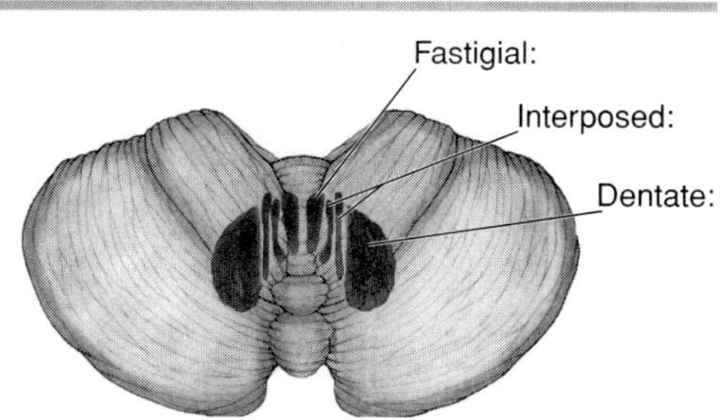

30.18. The cerebellar cortex has a three-layered arrangement. The outer molecular layer contains mostly fibers (mainly dendrites) of cerebellar neurons. The ___________ layer also contains stellate (star-shaped) and basket (basket-shaped) cells.

30.19. The Purkinje cell layer lies deep to the ___________ layer. Finally, the innermost layer is the granule cell layer, which is found between the ___________ cell layer and the ___________ core of the cerebellum.

30.20. The only output from the cerebellar cortex is via the Purkinje cells. The ___________ cells are inhibitory to the deep cerebellar nuclei.

30.21. Afferents to the cerebellar cortex are from two fiber types: 1) climbing fibers, which synapse directly on ___________ cells (found in the Purkinje cell layer); and 2) mossy fibers, which first synapse on granule cells (found in the granule cell layer) that then contact ___________ cells. The parallel fibers of the granule cells and the climbing fibers are both excitatory to the Purkinje cells, while input from the basket and stellate cells (both of which are found in the molecular cell layer) is ___________________.

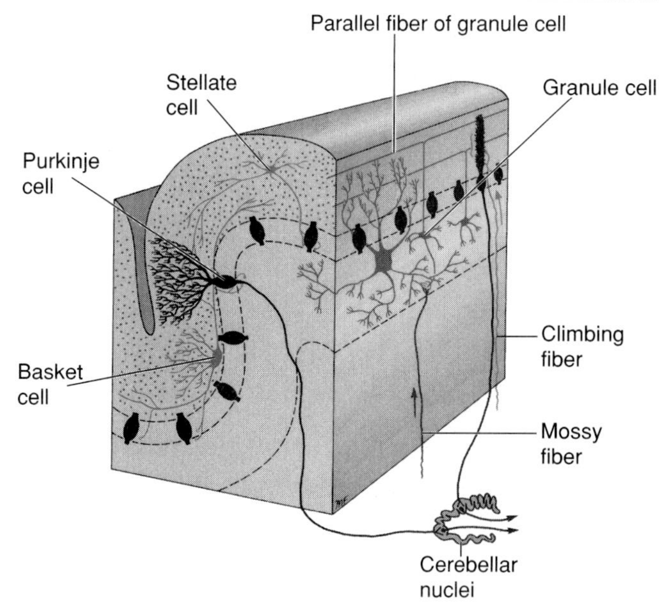

30.22. The ___________ cell axons are the only exit from the ___________ar cortex. However, very few of these axons actually leave the cerebellum; instead, they are inhibitory to the deep ___________ar nuclei, the axons of which form the majority of cerebellar output.

30.17A.

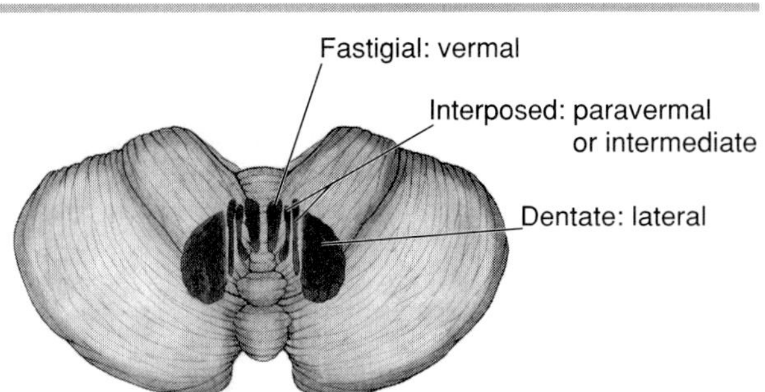

30.18A. molecular

30.19A. molecular; Purkinje; medullary

30.20A. Purkinje

30.21A. Purkinje; Purkinje; inhibitory

30.22A. Purkinje, cerebellar, cerebellar

30.23. Label the layers of the cerebellar cortex on the following diagram.

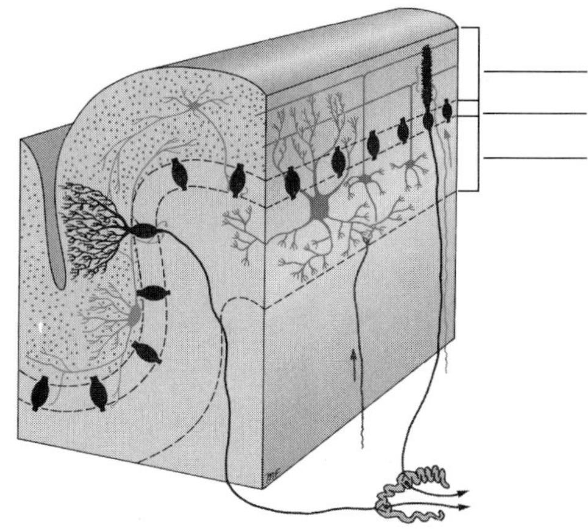

30.24. Label the basket, stellate, Purkinje, and granule cells on the following diagram.

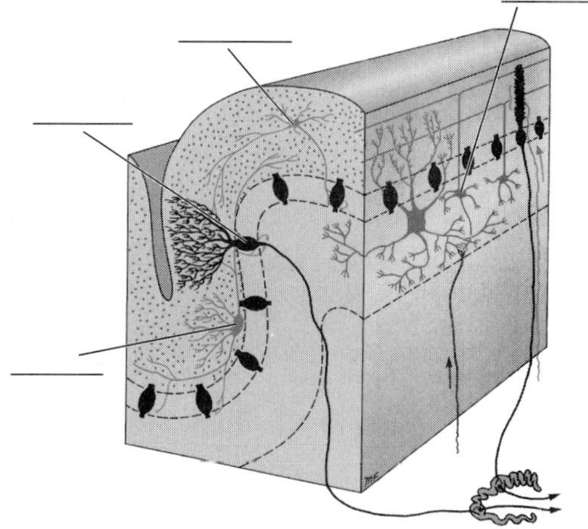

30.25. Place a "+" next to each cell that is excitatory and a "−" next to each cell that is inhibitory.

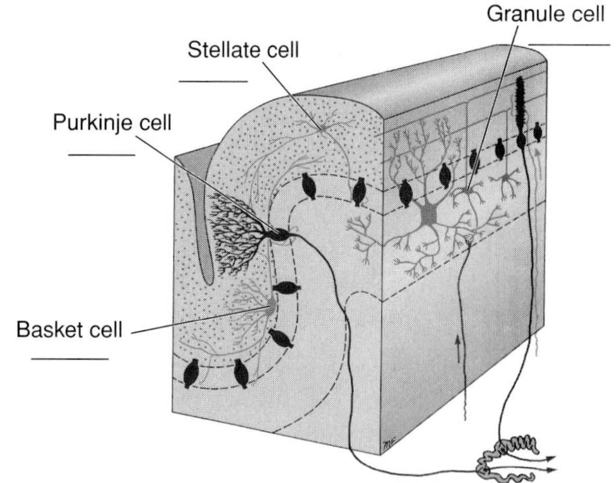

30.23A.

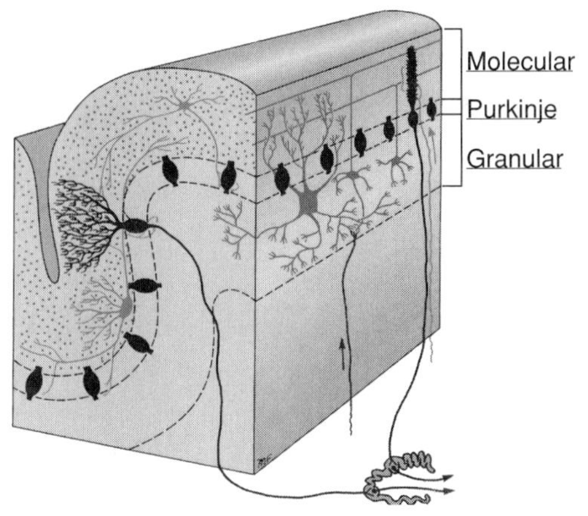

30.24A.

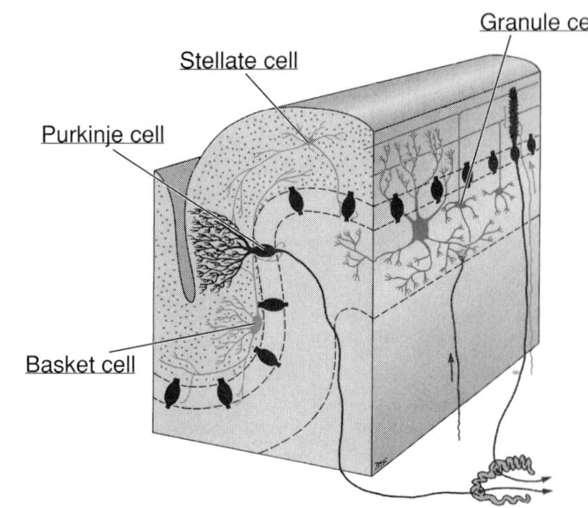

30.25A.

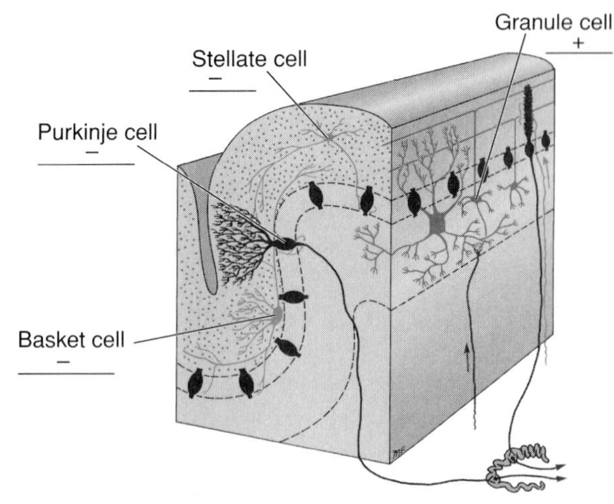

31 Cerebellar Peduncles

31.1. The cerebellum is attached to the brainstem by three large fiber tracts known as ___________ar peduncles. The peduncles are named for their position relative to one another: superior, middle, and ___________.

31.2. Identify the three cerebellar peduncles on the following diagram.

Posterior Anterior

____

____

____

31.3. The inferior cerebellar peduncle connects the cerebellum with the inferior division of the brainstem, the ___________.

31.4. The ___________ cerebellar ___________ is often divided into two parts: 1) a restiform body, which contains afferent fibers; and 2) a juxtarestiform body, which contains both ___________ and ___________ fibers.

31.5. Afferent and efferent connections of the juxtarestiform body are part of the bidirectional communication between the cerebellum and the vestibular system. The remaining fibers passing through the ___________ ___________ ___________ are ___________. They include the ___________ spinocerebellars and fibers from the contralateral inferior olive (a bilateral prominence of the medulla).

31.6. The middle cerebellar ___________ connects the ___________ to the pons. Also known as the brachium pontis, the middle cerebellar peduncle is the largest of the _____ peduncles. The middle cerebellar peduncle contains almost exclusively fibers originating in the contralateral pons entering the cerebellum; therefore, it contains almost all _____fferent fibers.

31.1A. cerebellar; inferior

31.2A.

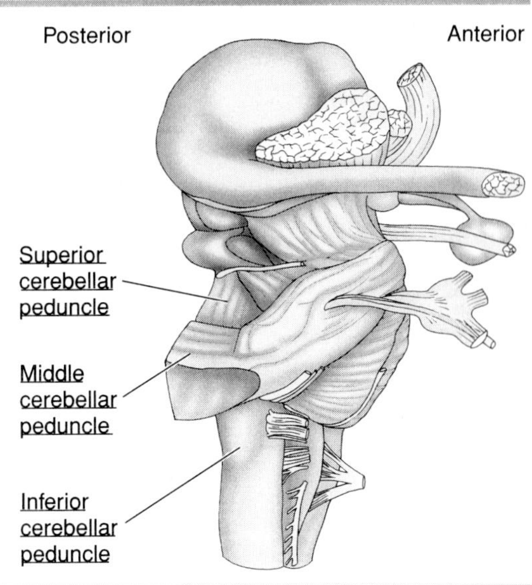

31.3A. medulla

31.4A. inferior; peduncle; afferent; efferent

31.5A. inferior cerebellar peduncle; afferent; dorsal (or posterior)

31.6A. peduncle; cerebellum; three (or cerebellar); afferent

31.7. The __________ cerebellar __________, also known as the brachium conjunctivum, connects the cerebellum to the rostral pons and __________ midbrain. The superior cerebellar peduncle contains the major ______fferent or outflow pathways from the cerebellum.

31.8. Label the cerebellar peduncles on the following diagram. Draw an arrow to indicate the direction of the majority of fibers carried within each.

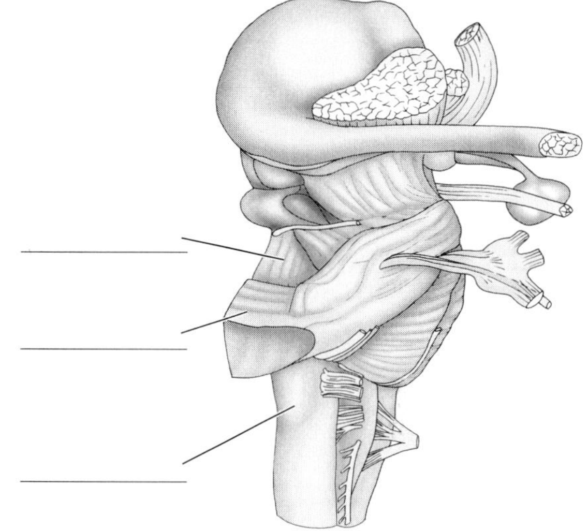

31.9. On the following diagram, label each peduncle and write a short description of the fibers found within.

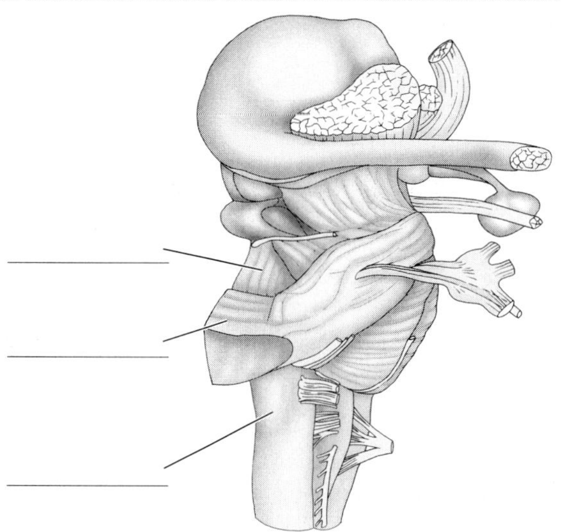

31.7A. superior; peduncle; caudal; efferent

31.8A.

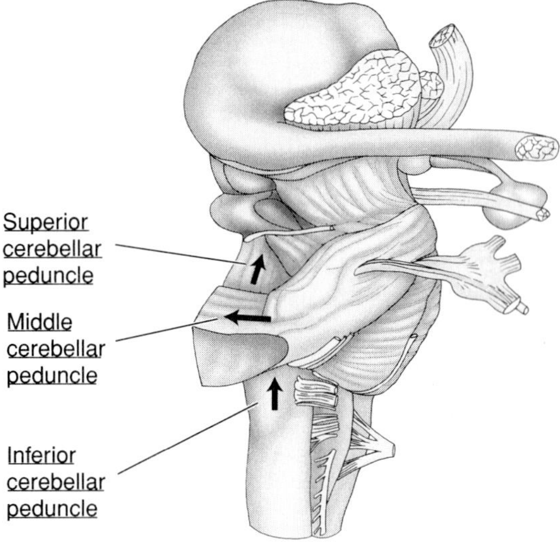

31.9A.

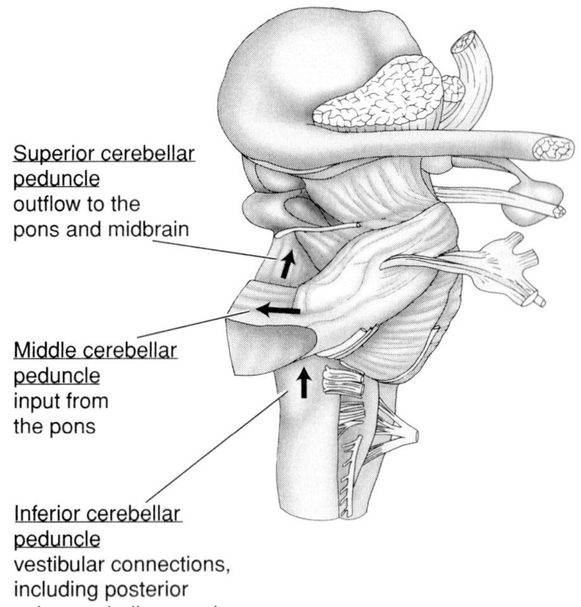

32 Cerebellar Pathways

32.1. Generally speaking, the cerebellum exerts its influence on motor systems ipsilaterally. For example, ascending pathways such as the posterior spinocerebellars do not cross as they ascend to the cerebellum. Anterior spinocerebellars cross in the cord and then cross back as they enter the cerebellum to the ________________ side.

32.2. It is useful to consider cerebellar pathways in relation to their function. The cerebellum is involved in: 1) equilibrium, 2) the coordination of voluntary movement, and 3) postural control and muscle tone. Thus, we can consider the connections involved with the __________cerebellum, neocerebellum, and _____cerebellum.

32.3. The __________cerebellum assists with equilibrium and balance as well as the coordination of eye movements. Fibers from the vestibular nuclei and ganglia enter the cerebellum via the juxtarestiform body of the __________cerebellar __________. The fibers pass to the flocculonodular lobe of the cerebellar cortex as _____ fibers.

32.4. The flocculo__________ lobe also receives input from the superior colliculus and the visual cortex; therefore, it receives a large amount of information dealing with __________.

32.5. The __________nodular lobe projects to the vestibular nuclei and thereby indirectly affects eye movements via the vestibular nuclei's projections to the MLF (__________ ________________ ________________) and the spinal cord via the vestibulo__________ tracts.

32.6. _____cerebellar connections are known as either: 1) cerebrocerebellar connections, indicating their origin in the cerebral cortex; or 2) the _____cerebellar pathway, indicating the location of the cells entering the cerebellum from the pons.

32.1A. ipsilateral (or same)

32.2A. vestibulocerebellum; spinocerebellum

32.3A. vestibulocerebellum; inferior; peduncle; mossy

32.4A. flocculonodular; vision

32.5A. flocculonodular; medial longitudinal fasciculus; vestibulospinal

32.6A. Neocerebellar; pontocerebellar

32.7. The neocerebellum is involved with the initiation, planning, and timing of voluntary ______ activity. Impulses originating in the cerebral cortex terminate on the ______ine nuclei. Pontine nuclei send their axons into almost all parts of the cerebellar cortex via the __________ cerebellar peduncle. The pontocerebellar fibers cross the midline to the __________lateral cerebellar hemisphere. On the diagram, draw the pontocerebellar fibers crossing the midline to enter the middle cerebellar peduncle.

Middle cerebellar peduncle

Pontine nuclei

32.8. The output cells of the cerebellar cortex, the __________ cells associated with the neocerebellum, project to the dentate __________. ______fferent fibers from the dentate nucleus travel in the superior cerebellar __________ to the thalamus, red nucleus, and inferior olivary nucleus.

32.9. Efferent fibers from the dentate nucleus are functionally reciprocated in the form of ______fferents returning from target structures back to the dentate nucleus, directly and indirectly. This completes a functional loop that allows the cerebellum to modify and influence ______ activity.

32.10. ______ cerebellar pathways are involved with postural control and muscle tone, particularly related to the limb girdles. The spinocerebellum involves the vermis and paravermal regions of cerebellar cortex, as these areas receive input from the __________ ______.

32.11. The vermis projects to the fastigial nucleus, one of the ______ __________ar nuclei. The fastigial nucleus affects the spinal ______ indirectly via the vestibular nuclei (vestibulospinal fibers) and through projections to the ventral lateral nucleus of the __________, which projects to the cerebral __________ that gives rise to cortico__________ fibers affecting the trunk musculature.

32.12. The interposed nuclei, including the __________ and ______________, receive input from the paravermal region of the cerebellar cortex. The interposed nuclei project to the ventral lateral nucleus of the thalamus (as does the __________ nucleus) and to the red nucleus, which gives rise to rubro__________ tracts in order to influence limb musculature.

32.13. In the blank after each deep cerebellar nucleus, indicate the relevant functional division of the cerebellum.

fastigial __________ dentate __________

globose __________ emboliform __________

32.7A. motor; pontine; middle; contralateral

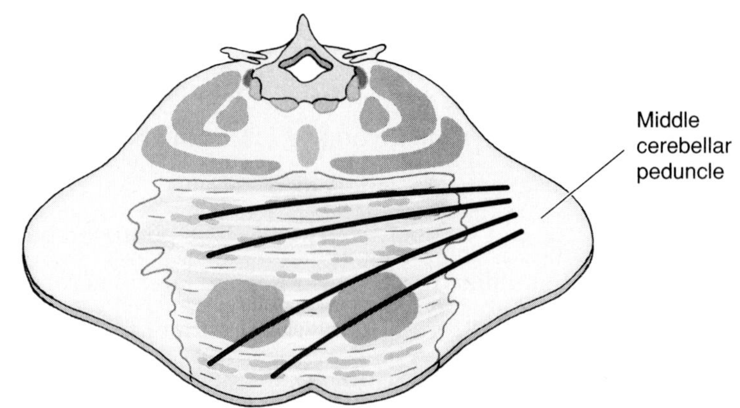

32.8A. Purkinje; nucleus; Efferent; peduncle

32.9A. afferents; motor

32.10A. Spinocerebellar; spinal cord

32.11A. deep cerebellar; cord; thalamus; cortex; corticospinal

32.12A. globose; emboliform; fastigial; rubrospinal

32.13A.

fastigial – spinocerebellum

globose – spinocerebellum

dentate – neocerebellum or cerebrocerebellum

emboliform – spinocerebellum

33 Blood Supply to the Cerebellum

33.1. The cerebellum has a rich blood supply from several branches of the vertebrobasilar arterial system. The ___________ artery runs on the anterior surface or "base" of the pons and is formed inferiorly by the junction of the paired ___________ arteries that ascend via foramina in the transverse processes of cervical vertebrae.

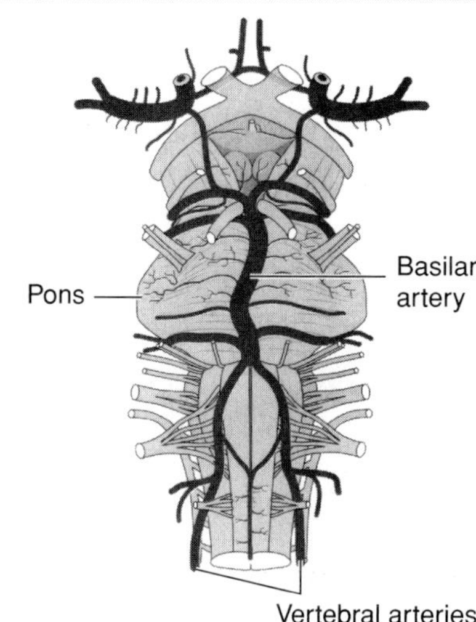

33.2. The superior cerebellar artery, a branch of the basilar artery, supplies the ___________ aspect of the cerebellum, particularly the anterior lobe. The superior cerebellar artery also supplies the ___________ cerebellar peduncle.

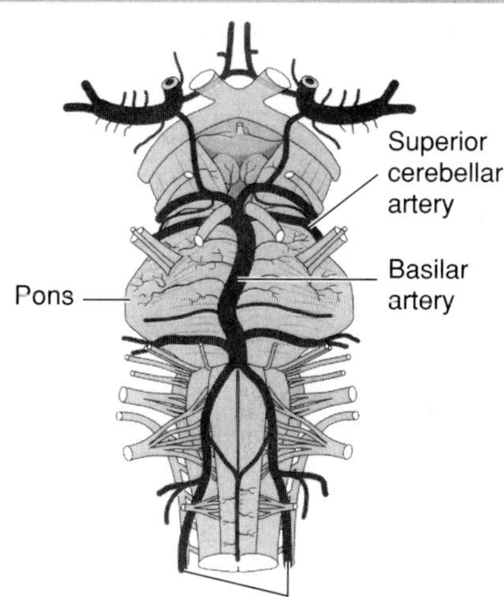

33.3. More caudal branches of the ___________ artery, the anterior inferior cerebellar arteries, supply the majority of blood to the cerebellum, including the posterior lobe. The ___________ ___________ cerebellar artery also supplies the ___________ and ___________ cerebellar peduncles and typically gives rise to the labyrinthine artery.

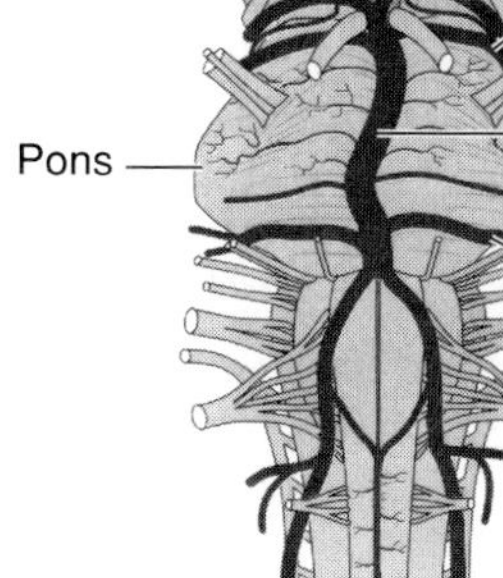

33.1A. basilar; vertebral

33.2A. superior; superior

33.3A. basilar; anterior inferior; middle; inferior

33.4. The remainder of the cerebellum, which includes the inferior aspect, is supplied by the ____________ ____________ cerebellar artery, which is a branch of the vertebral arteries.

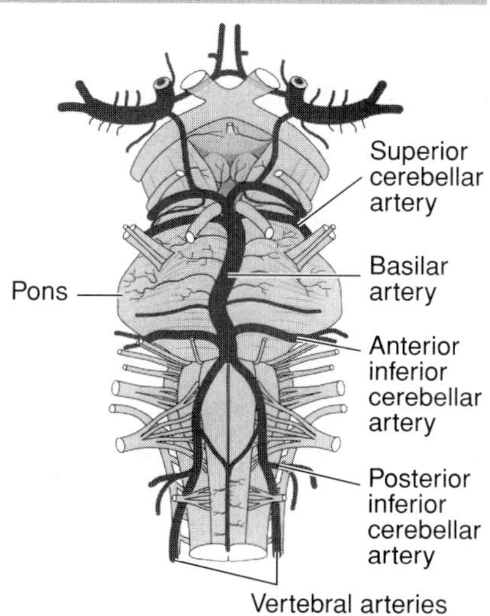

33.5. The posterior inferior cerebellar artery supplies the flocculo____________ lobe, some blood to the inferior cerebellar peduncle, and branches to the brainstem and spinal cord.

33.6. Label the arteries indicated on the following image.

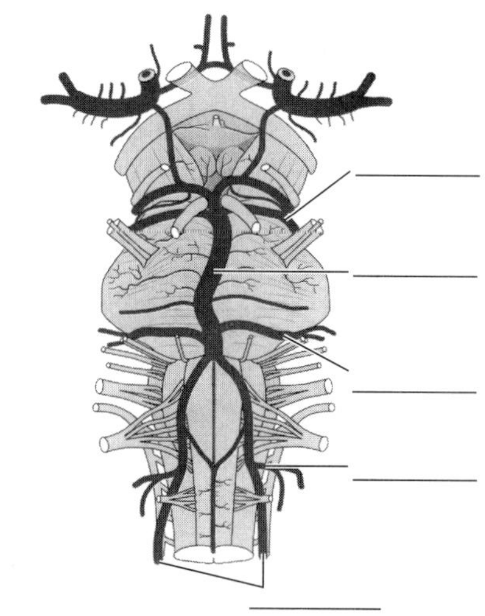

33.7. Next to each labeled artery, indicate the area of the cerebellum it supplies.

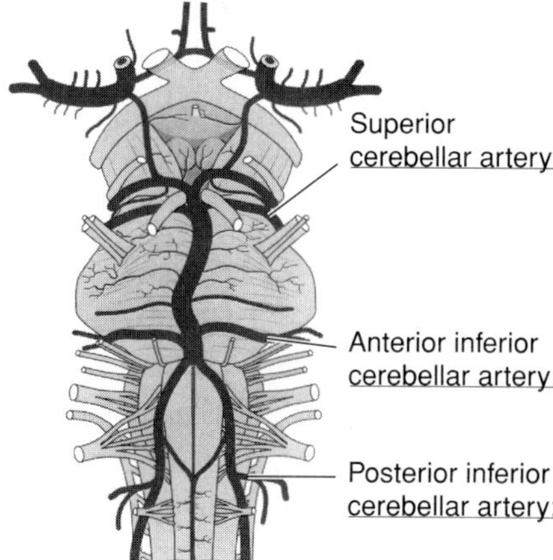

33.4A. posterior inferior

33.5A. flocculonodular

33.6A.

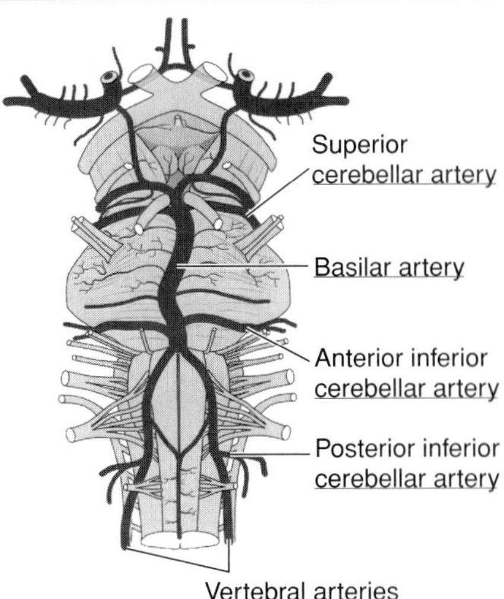

33.7A.

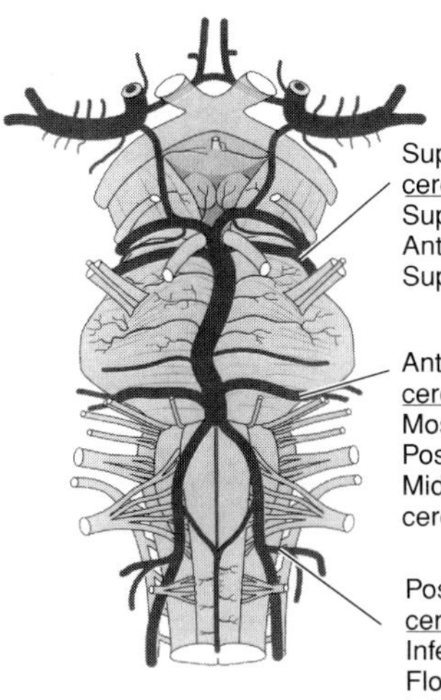

34 Cerebellar Lesions

34.1. As we have already learned, the cerebellum is an integral part of the motor system; therefore, cerebellar lesions (i.e., from blockage of the superior cerebellar, posterior ___________ cerebellar or ___________ inferior cerebellar arteries) will not cause appreciable ___________ deficits. Cerebellar lesions produce disturbances in muscles that are otherwise normally innervated. Lesions result in abnormal control and or regulation of ___________ activity.

34.2. Posterior inferior cerebellar artery lesions have a great affect on the flocculonodular lobe or ___________ulocerebellum. A tumor or other space-occupying lesion near the cerebellopontine angle or near the emergence of CN VIII will also affect the vestibulocerebellum and ___________nodular lobe.

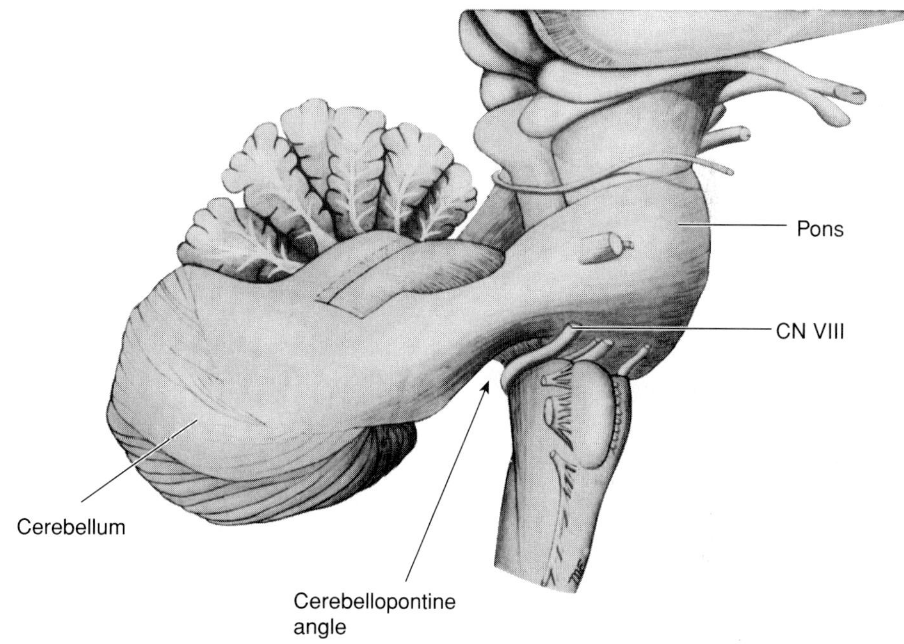

34.3. As may be expected, vestibulocerebellar damage produces problems with ___________ium and balance, mainly in the trunk.

34.4. Anterior lobe lesions, functionally related to ______ cerebellar deficits may occur as a result of blockage of the ___________ cerebellar artery. ___________ lobe lesions are often related to alcoholism and malnutrition. The resulting deficits are typically manifested as gross ______ disturbances of the trunk and lower limbs.

34.5. Neocerebellar or cerebrocerebellar lesions typically affect the lateral hemispheres of the cerebellum. The inferior cerebellar artery is the main source of blood to the lateral hemispheres. Blockage of the ___________ inferior cerebellar artery often produces unilateral problems and may involve the ___________ cerebellar peduncle—the primary outflow pathway of the cerebellum.

34.1A. inferior; anterior; sensory; muscle (or motor)

34.2A. vestibulocerebellum; flocculonodular

34.3A. equilibrium

34.4A. spinocerebellar; superior; Anterior; motor

34.5A. anterior; superior

34.6. Other areas that may be affected from a lesion of the __________ inferior __________ar artery include the __________ nucleus—the main deep cerebellar nucleus associated with the lateral hemispheres. The loss of learned, fine movements may result from damage to either the lateral hemisphere or the associated deep nucleus—the dentate.

34.7. Circle the areas supplied by the anterior inferior cerebellar artery.

Lateral hemisphere

Interposed nucleus

Flocculonodular lobe

Vermis

Posterior lobe

Anterior lobe

Dentate nucleus

Fastigial nucleus

Superior cerebellar peduncle

Middle cerebellar peduncle

Inferior cerebellar peduncle

34.6A. anterior; cerebellar; dentate

34.7A.

Lateral hemisphere

Interposed nucleus

Flocculonodular lobe

Vermis

Posterior lobe

Anterior lobe

Dentate nucleus

Fastigial nucleus

Superior cerebellar peduncle

Middle cerebellar peduncle

Inferior cerebellar peduncle

35 Clinical Signs of Cerebellar Damage

35.1. Cerebellar damage produces disturbances in the control and regulation of ______ activity. Each functional division of the cerebellum incorporates multiple structural regions; therefore, discreet functional deficits are not commonly seen. Deficiencies associated with the anterior lobe, flocculonodular lobe, or neocerebellar lesions are more characteristic of cerebellar malfunction.

35.2. Flocculonodular lobe lesions, as you may expect, manifest themselves as ____________ar system problems. Flocculonodular lobe pathologies arise from cerebellopontine tumors (typically form where cranial nerves VII and VIII emerge from the brainstem), inferior cerebellar artery lesions, and medulloblastomas.

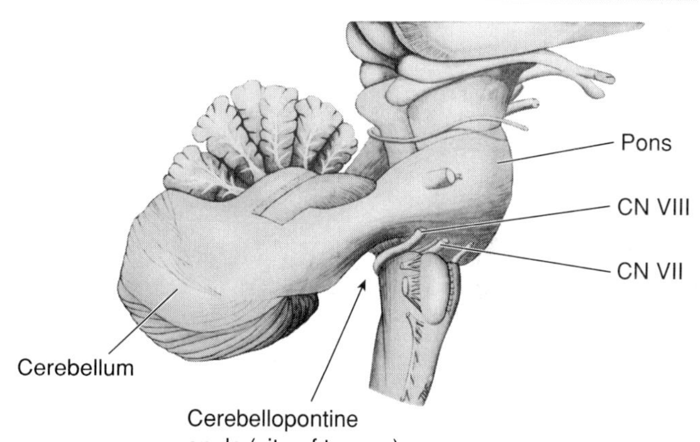

35.3. ____________cerebellum or ____________nodular lobe damage leads to trunkal dysequilibrium, affecting the trunk and gait. The trunk sways when walking and is unsteady when standing. Individuals with flocculo____________ lobe damage walk on a wide base and stagger, yet they have normal muscle tone and reflexes.

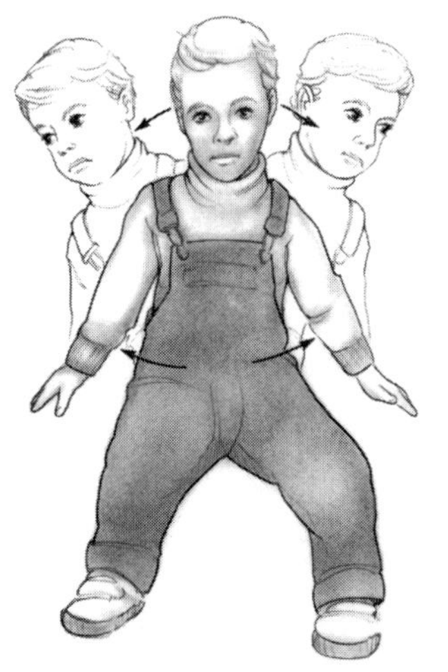
Trunk sways
from side to side
Stands on wide base

35.4. On the following diagram of the inferior aspect of the cerebellum, shade the area involved in flocculonodular lobe lesions.

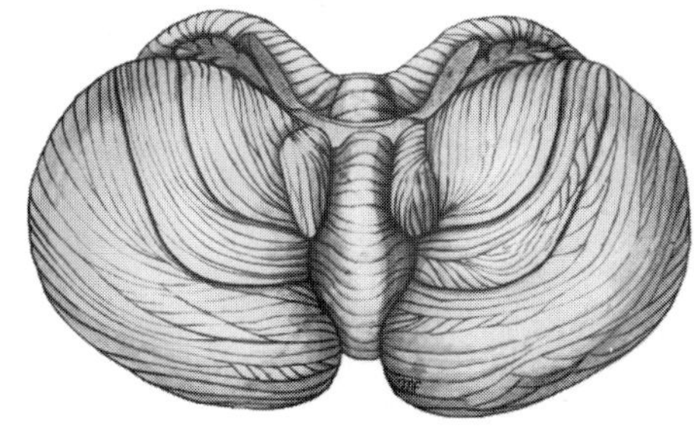

35.1A. <u>motor</u> (or muscle)

35.2A. <u>vestibul</u>ar

35.3A. <u>Vestibulo</u>cerebellum; <u>flocculo</u>nodular; flocculo<u>nodular</u>

35.4A.

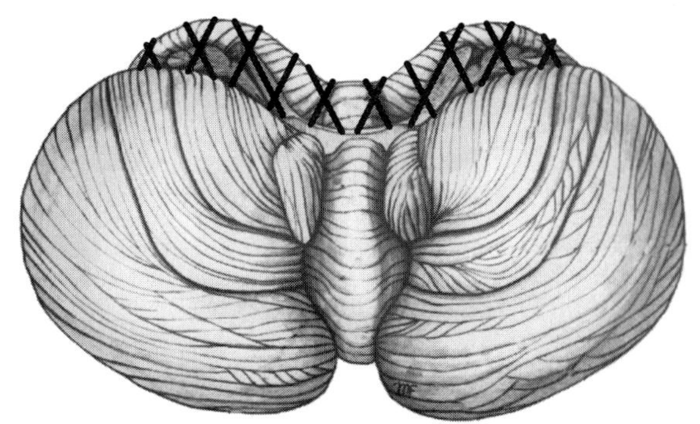

35.5. Ataxia is a disruption of the coordination of ______ movements, which is particularly evident in the limb girdles, resulting in a broad-based, unsteady gait. Anterior lobe lesions result in ______ia and may be related to malnutrition subsequent to alcoholism. Characteristics of the lesion include ataxia of the lower limbs and trunk and problems with muscle coordination during walking and standing.

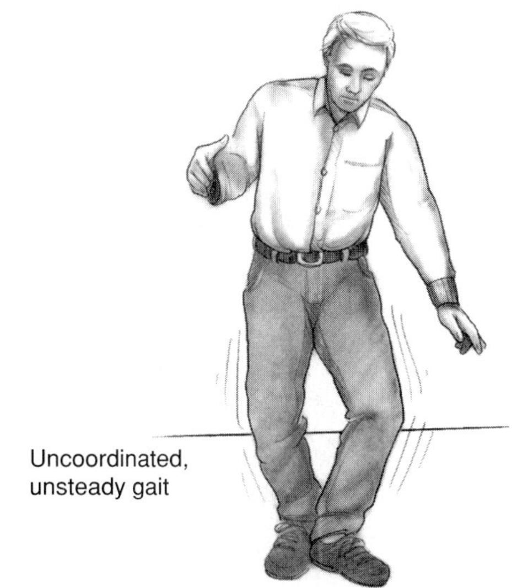

35.6. Shade the anterior lobe on the following superior view of the cerebellum.

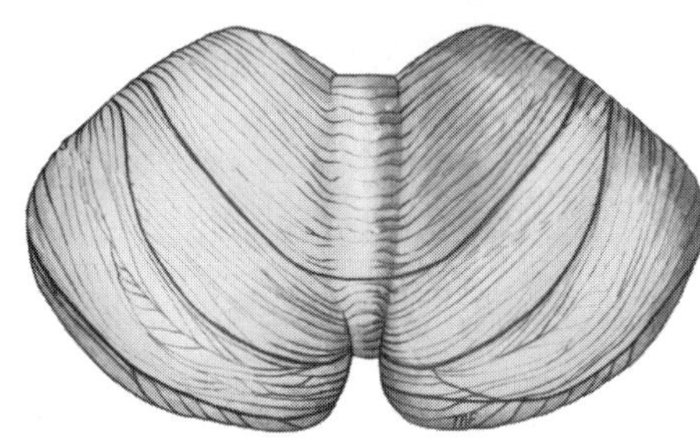

35.7. The loss of learned, fine skills may be a sign of ______cerebellar damage. The neocerebellum is housed in the __________ hemispheres of the cerebellum. Pathologies here may also involve the anterior lobe and vermis depending upon the nature and extent of the damage.

35.8. Shade areas that may be involved in neocerebellar damage on the superior view of the cerebellum.

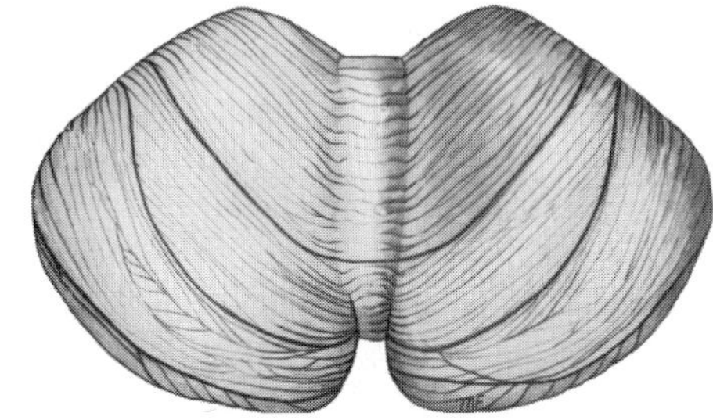

35.9. Each lateral hemisphere is supplied with blood by one __________ __________ cerebellar artery. Neocerebellar pathologies are often unilateral and occur as a result of the disruption of blood flow.

35.5A. motor; ataxia

35.6A.

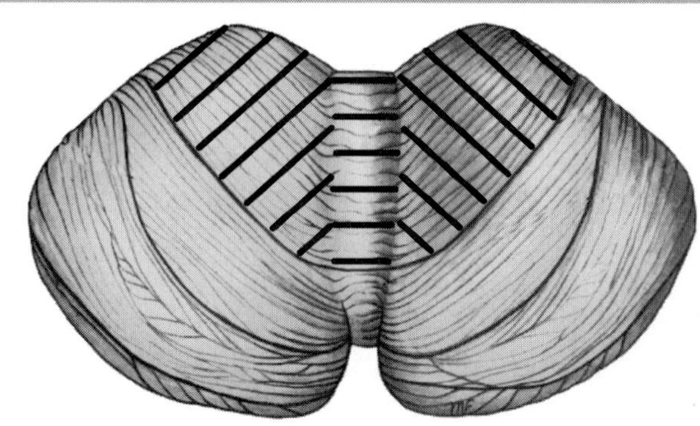

35.7A. neocerebellar; lateral

35.8A.

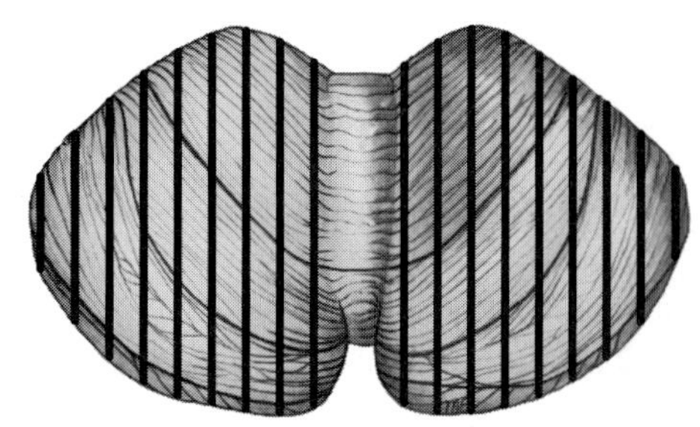

35.9A. anterior inferior

35.10. ______cerebellar damage may also involve the deep cerebellar nucleus associated with the neocerebellum, the ____________ nucleus, or the ____________ cerebellar peduncle, the primary outflow pathway for the cerebellum.

35.11. Neocerebellar damage is most evident in the loss of fine, rapid movements of the upper ______, resulting in intention tremor, but typically also affects fine motor skills including speech and eye movement.

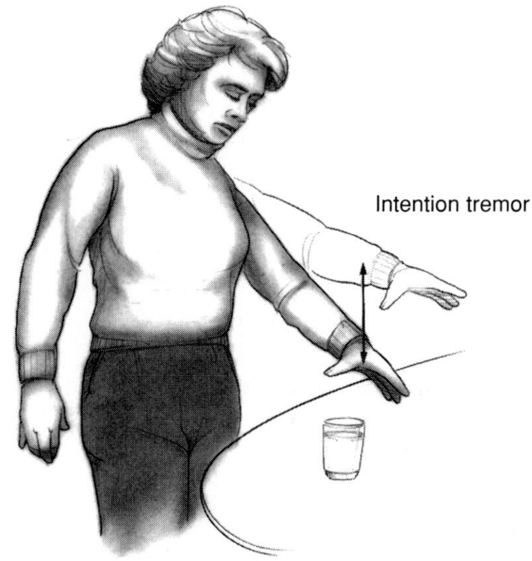

35.12. Widespread hypotonia (decrease in muscle tone) and hyporeflexia (reduced stretch reflexes) result in pendular reflexes (limb swings back and forth after initiating reflex), which are also symptoms of ______cerebellar syndrome.

35.10A. Neocerebellar; dentate; superior

35.11A. limb

35.12A. neocerebellar

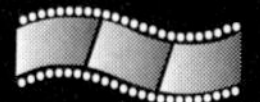

Animations

30. Vestibulocerebellum (Chapters 30, 31, 32)
31. Spinocerebellum (Chapters 30, 31, 32)
32. Neocerebellum (Chapters 30, 31, 32)

IV DIENCEPHALON

36 Divisions of the Diencephalon

36.1. On the diagram, label the midbrain, pons, and medulla; corpus callosum; interventricular foramen; cerebral aqueduct; and fourth ventricle.

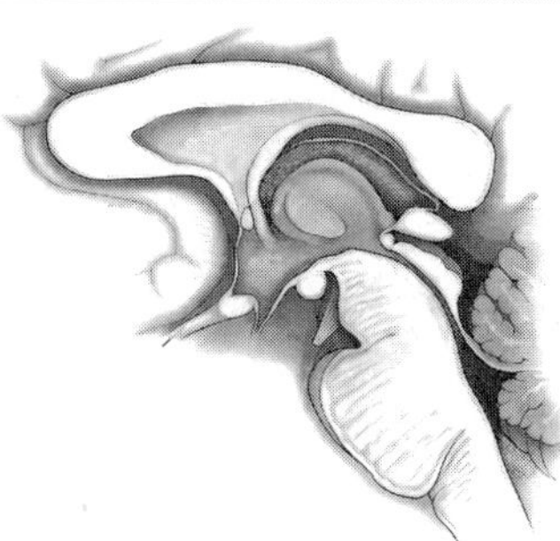

36.2. The diencephalon consists of four parts: the thalamus, ______thalamus, ______ thalamus, and ______ thalamus.

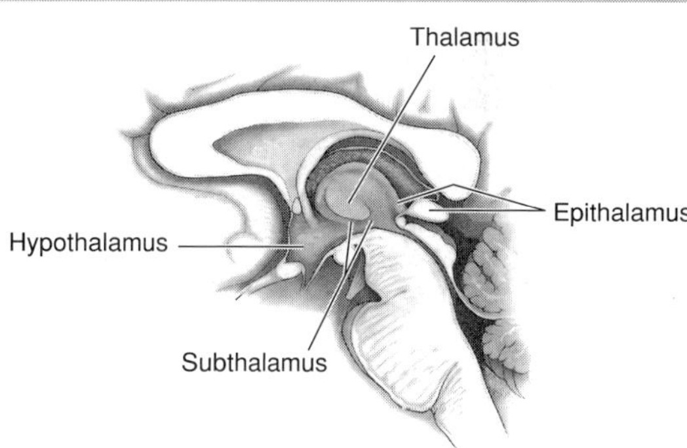

36.3. The anterior boundary of the diencephalon is the ____________ commissure and the lamina ____________________. Lamina terminalis forms the anterior wall of the ______ ventricle.

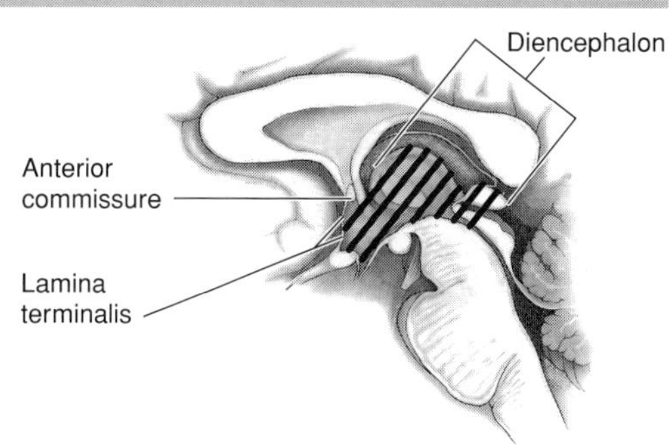

36.4. The anterior commissure joins the left and right ____________ lobes.

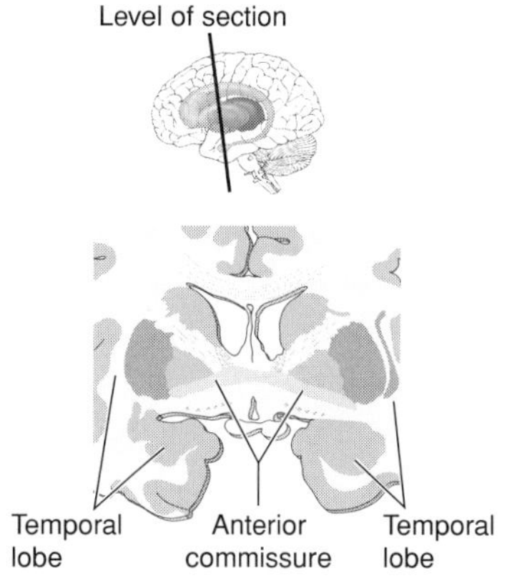

36.1A.

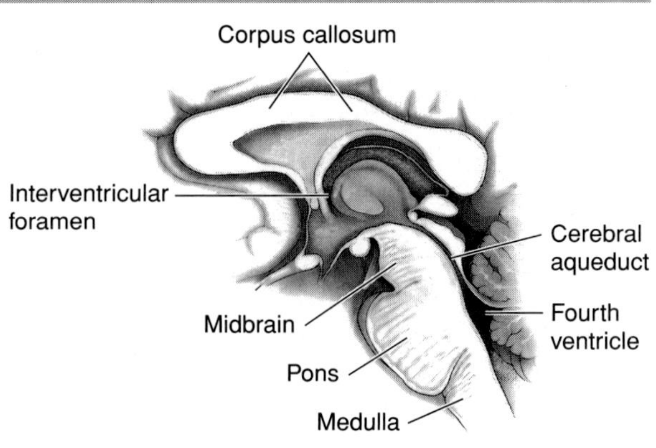

36.2A. subthalamus; epithalamus; hypothalamus

36.3A. anterior; terminalis; third

36.4A. temporal

36.5. Posteriorly, the diencephalon ends at the __________ commissure, which is located superior to where the third ventricle is continuous with the __________ __________ of the midbrain.

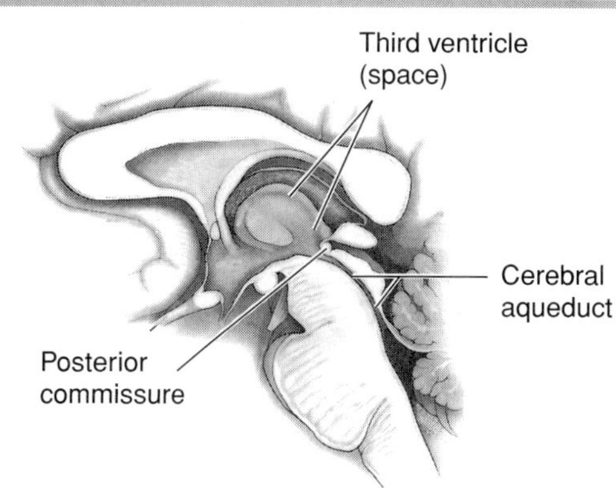

36.6. On this dorsal view of the brain, the third and lateral ventricles have been exposed by dissection from above. Label these two cavities on the diagram. The anterior and posterior commissures limit the third ventricle; label them on the diagram.

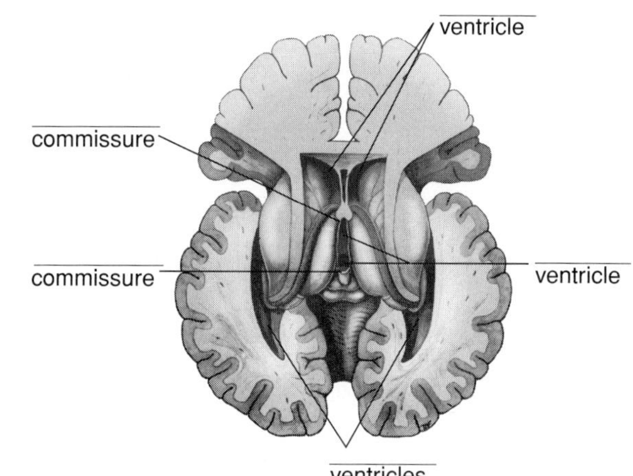

36.7. Identify the caudate nucleus, putamen, and thalamus on the diagram.

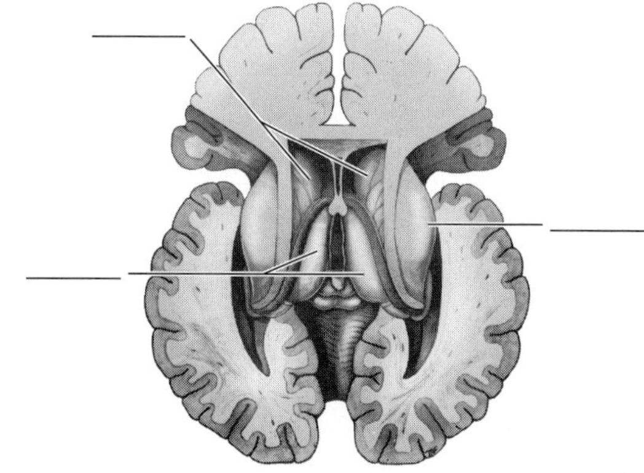

36.8. The lateral border of the diencephalon is the __________ capsule, while the medial border is the midline __________ ventricle.

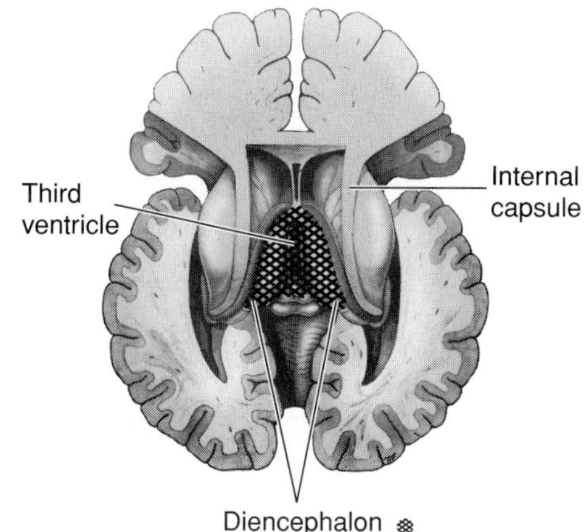

36.5A. posterior; cerebral aqueduct

36.6A.

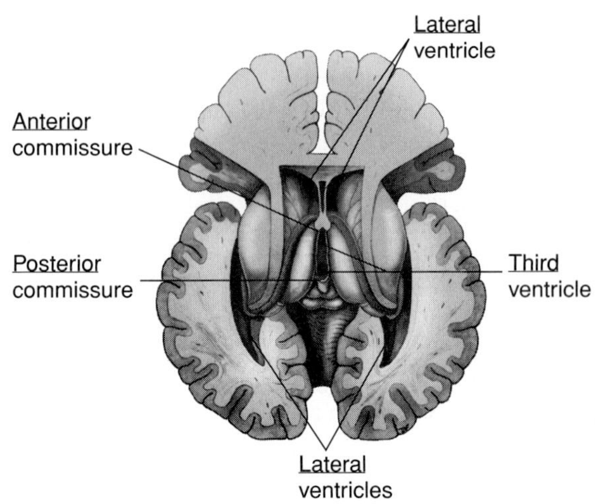

36.7A.

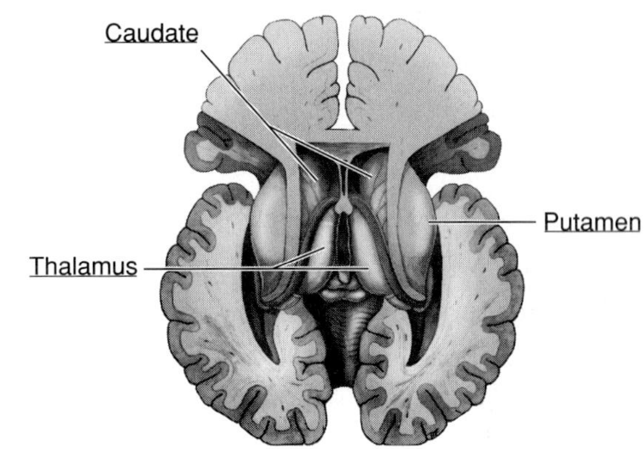

36.8A. internal; lateral

36.9. The ______ ventricle lies between the left and right sides of the diencephalon.

36.10. Superiorly, the diencephalon is bounded by the ____________, a thick bundle of white matter extending from hippocampus to mammillary body. The fornix is largely covered by the corpus ____________ and the cerebral ____________.

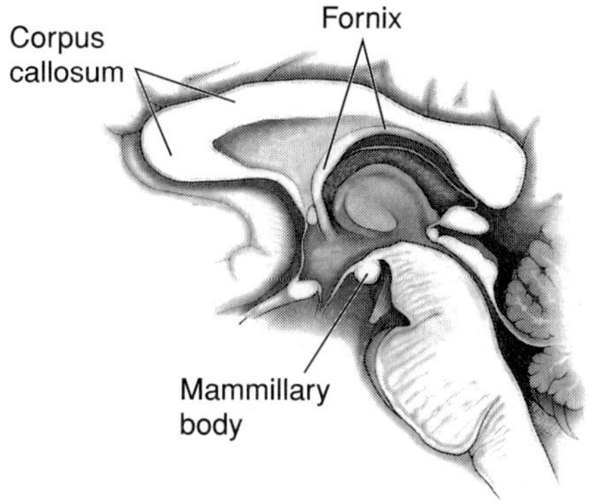

Corpus callosum
Fornix
Mammillary body

36.11. Inferiorly, the diencephalon is exposed at the base of the brain, where it communicates with the pituitary gland (hypophysis) via the ____________________.

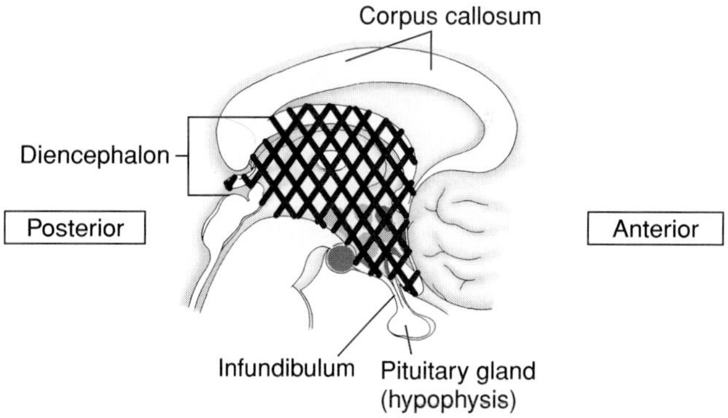

Corpus callosum
Diencephalon
Posterior
Anterior
Infundibulum
Pituitary gland (hypophysis)

36.12. On this ventral view of the brain, label the cerebral peduncles of the midbrain and the pons. From this perspective, identify several gross structures associated with the diencephalon, including the mammillary bodies (breast-shaped bodies), infundibulum (funnel-shaped), optic chiasm (cross), and optic tracts.

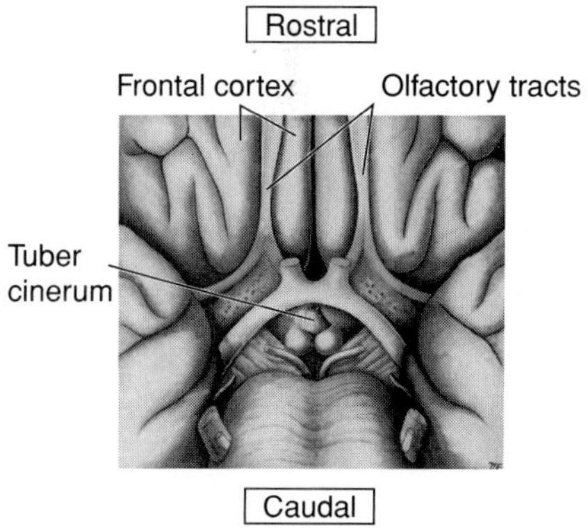

Rostral
Frontal cortex
Olfactory tracts
Tuber cinerum
Caudal

36.13. Match the structures listed on the right with the appropriate boundary of the diencephalon on the left.

A Third ventricle	______ Superior
B. Lamina terminalis	______ Inferior
C. Internal capsule	______ Anterior
D. Fornix	______ Posterior
E. Optic tract	______ Medial
F. Pineal gland	______ Lateral

36.9A. third

36.10A. fornix; callosum; cortex

36.11A. infundibulum

36.12A.

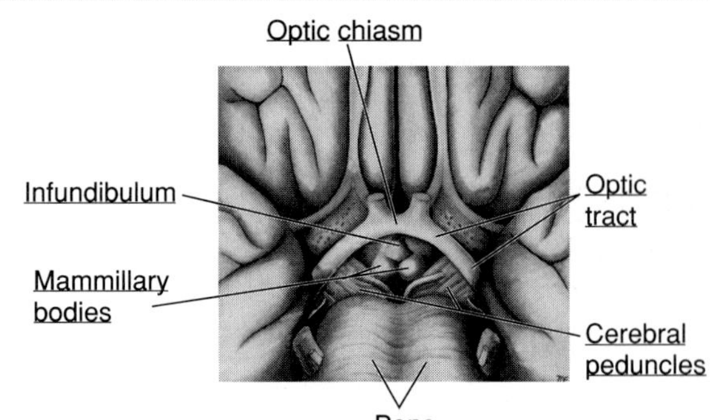

36.13A.

A. Third ventricle	D	Superior
B. Lamina terminalis	E	Inferior
C. Internal capsule	B	Anterior
D. Fornix	F	Posterior
E. Optic tract	A	Medial
F. Pineal gland	C	Lateral

36.14. The diencephalon is made up of two large regions, including the thalamus and ______ thalamus, which are separated by the __________________ sulcus, a groove in the lateral wall of the ______ ventricle.

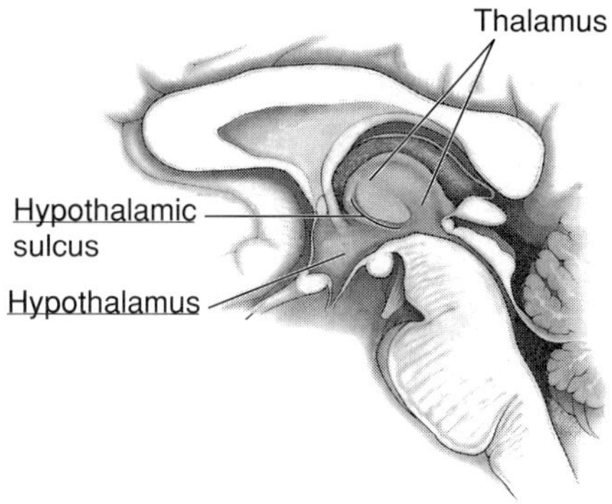

36.15. All sensory information except the sense of smell must pass through the thalamus en route to the ____________. The thalamus is formed by two egg-shaped masses connected in midline by the __________________ adhesion. Fill in the blanks on the diagram.

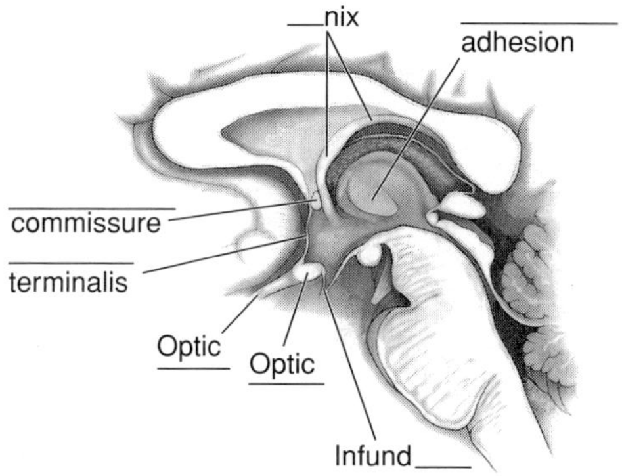

36.16. A terminal furrow, known as the stria __________________, separates the thalamus from the head of the ____________ nucleus. The ______ terminalis travels from the ____________ in the temporal lobe to the hypothalamus and neighboring areas. Label the blanks on the diagram.

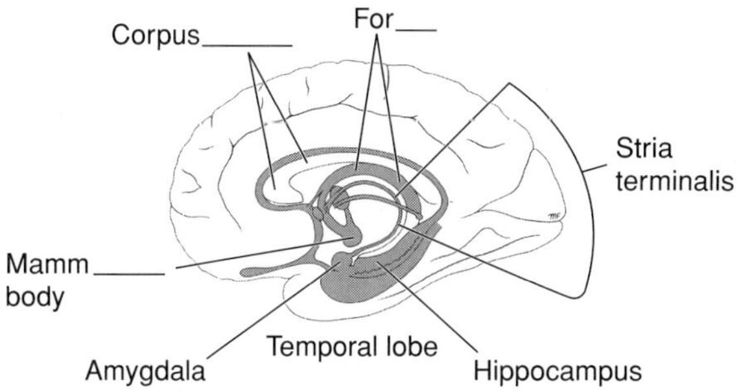

36.17. Each side of the thalamus is organized into groups of nuclei defined by a strip of white matter known as the ____________ ____________ lamina.

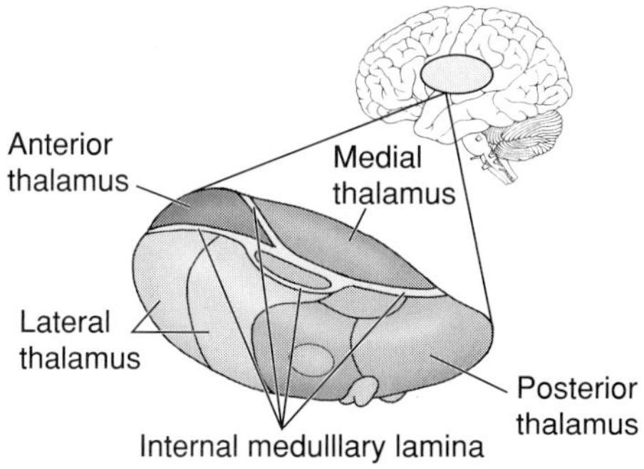

36.14A. hypothalamus; hypothalamic; third

36.15A. cortex; interthalamic

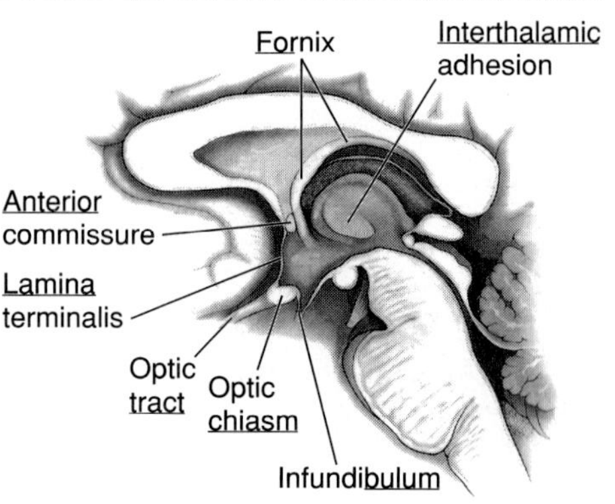

36.16A. terminalis; caudate; stria; amygdala

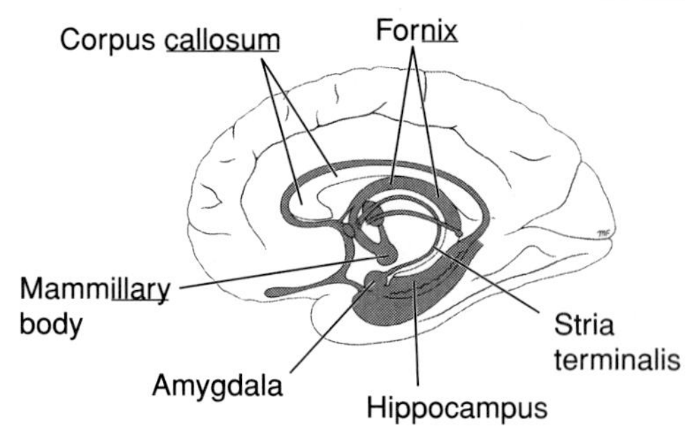

36.17A. internal medullary

36.18. Label the thalamus and hypothalamus on the diagram. The hypothalamus forms the ventral wall and floor of the ______ ____________ and is positioned inferiorly to the hypothalamic sulcus.

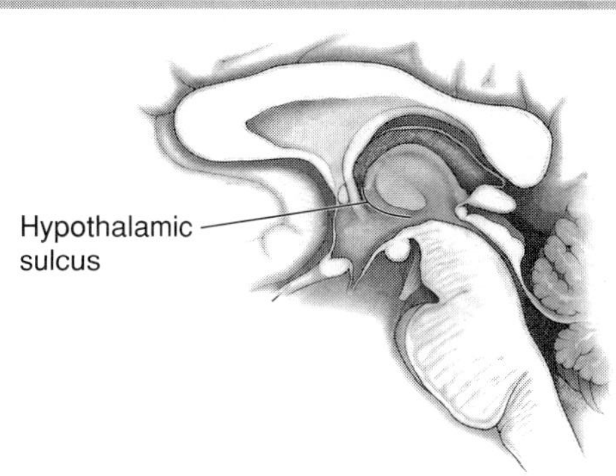

36.19. The hypothalamus is situated between the ______ chiasm anteriorly and the ____________ bodies posteriorly.

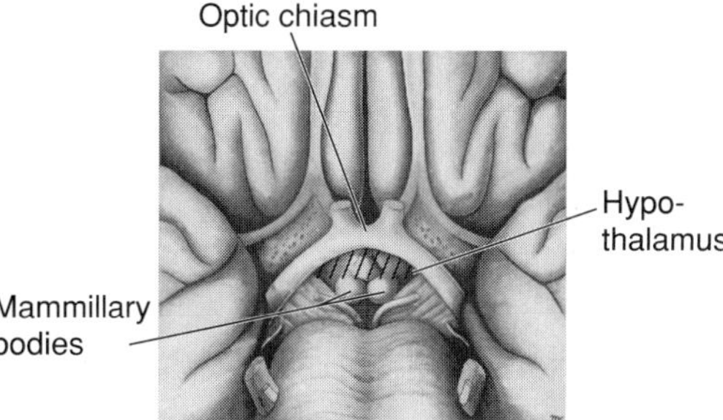

36.20. The hypothalamus is located medial to the ____________ capsule and subthalamus. Label all blanks on the diagram.

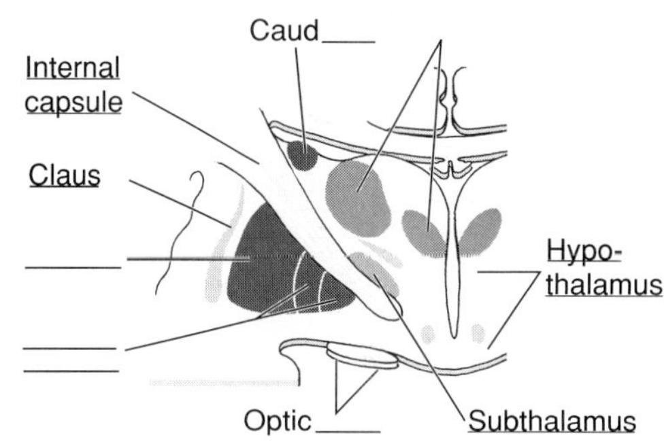

36.21. On the left diagram, label the thalamus, hypothalamus and subthalamus. The subthalamus controls ______ activity and includes the ______ thalamic nuclei, red nuclei, and substantia ______.

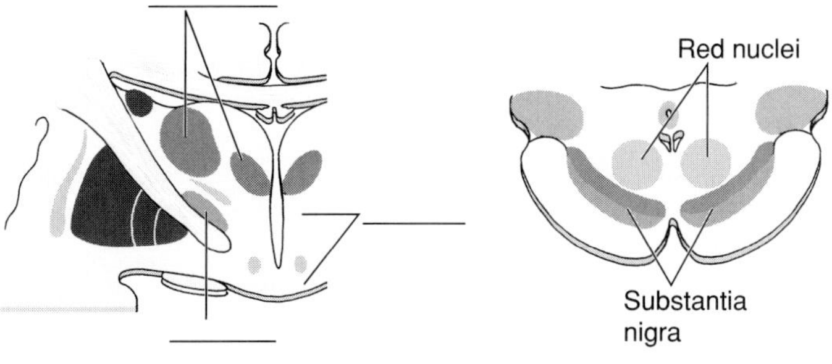

36.18A. third ventricle

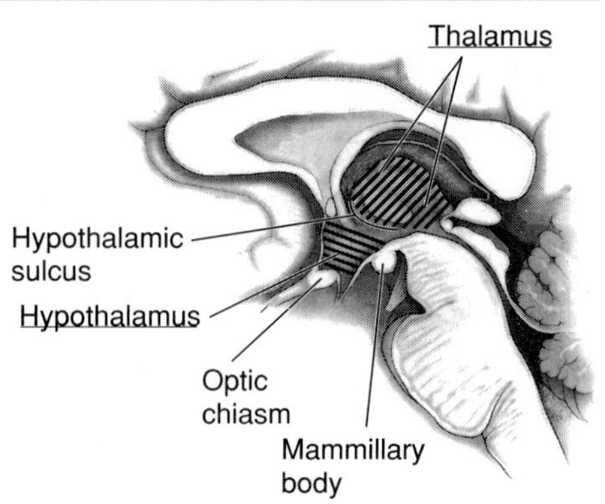

36.19A. optic; mammillary

36.20A. internal

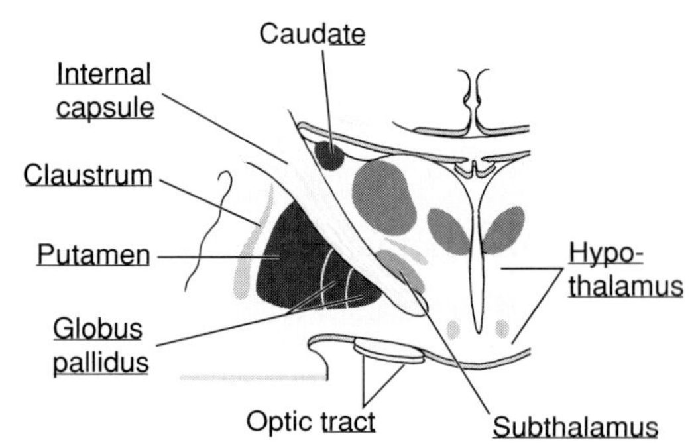

36.21A. motor; subthalamic; nigra

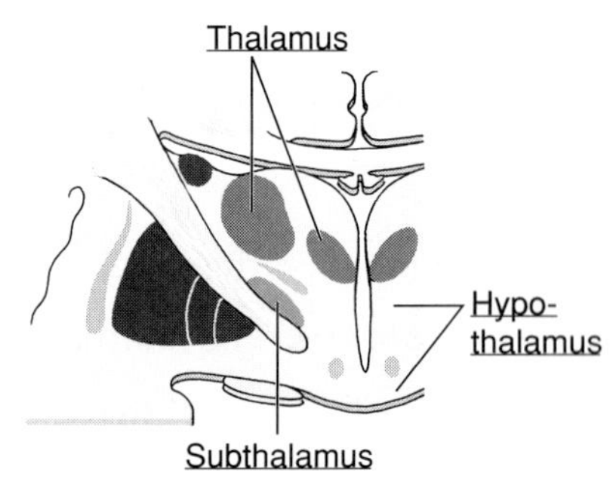

36.22. The tegmentum of the midbrain is continuous with the subthalamus of the diencephalon. The subthalamus is a lens-shaped structure. The subthalamus is __________ to the thalamus, lateral to the ________________, and __________ to the internal capsule and cerebral peduncles.

36.23. The zona incerta is positioned between the sub__________ and __________. It is a continuation of the midbrain's reticular formation and projects to many structures, including the cerebral __________.

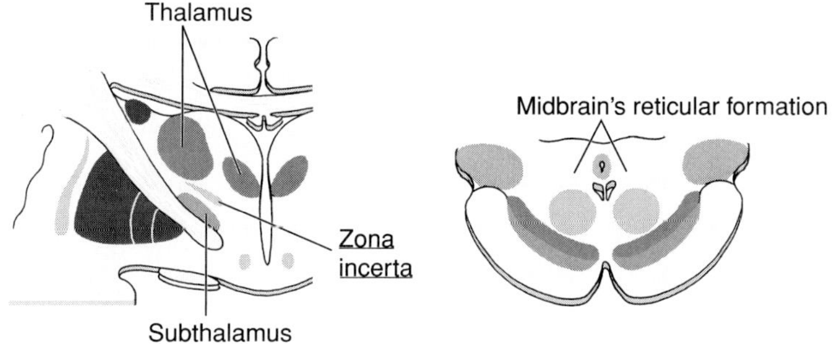

36.24. The four parts of the diencephalon are the: 1) __________; 2) ________________; 3) ________________; and 4) epithalamus. The epithalamus includes the hab______, stria ________________, and __________ gland.

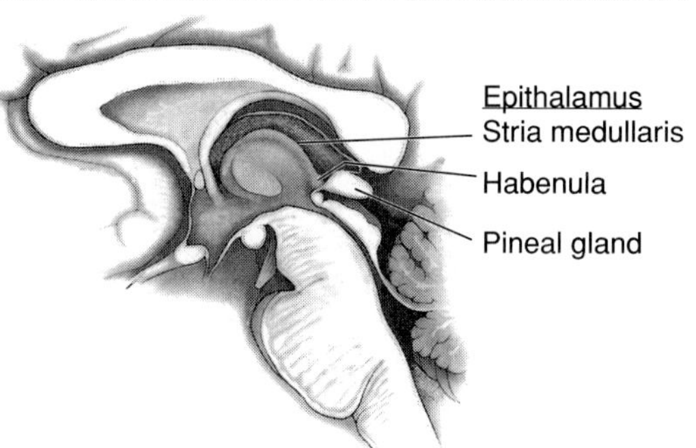

36.22A. inferior; hypothalamus; medial

36.23A. subthalamus; thalamus; cortex

36.24A. thalamus; hypothalamus; subthalamus; habenula; medullaris; pineal

36.25. The pineal gland is known as the “seat of the soul” and is located rostral to the superior colliculi of the ____________. Label the indicated structures on the diagram.

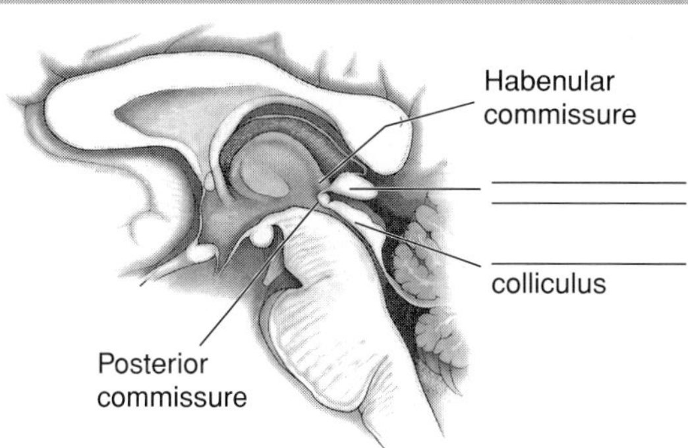

36.26. The pineal gland is named for its resemblance to a pinecone in shape. It functions as an endo______ organ involved in reproductive cycles. The pineal releases mel____________ at high rates during periods of darkness. It accumulates “brain sand” with age, which is opaque and thus a useful radiological landmark.

36.27. Superior to the pineal is the ____________ commissure; inferior to the pineal is the ____________ commissure. The pineal gland is responsible for circadian rhythms through the release of melatonin.

36.28. The habenula is a bilateral structure, located rostral to the ____________ gland. The habenulae are connected by the ____________ commissure.

36.25A. midbrain

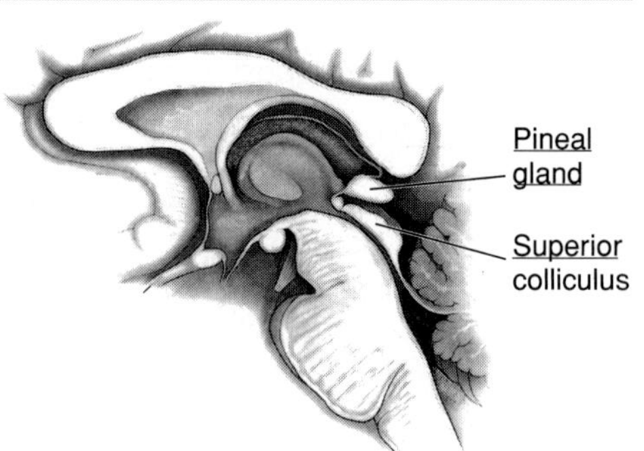

36.26A. endocrine; melatonin

36.27A. habenular; posterior

36.28A. pineal; habenular

37 Connections of the Diencephalon

37.1. Thalamus literally means "inner chamber" in Greek. Label the thalamus on the diagram.

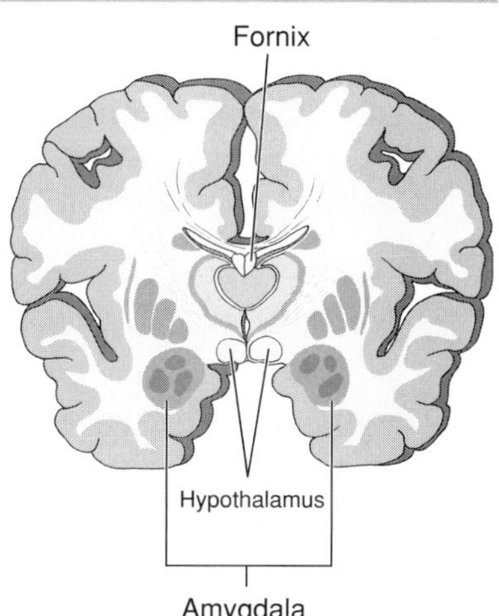

37.2. Most regions of the thalamus project reciprocally to the ______ lateral cerebral ____________, so that the thalamus and cortex can regulate one another. Some thalamic nuclei have focal connections with the cortex (specific thalamic nuclei); other thalamic nuclei exhibit widespread connections to the cortex (non ____________ thalamic nuclei).

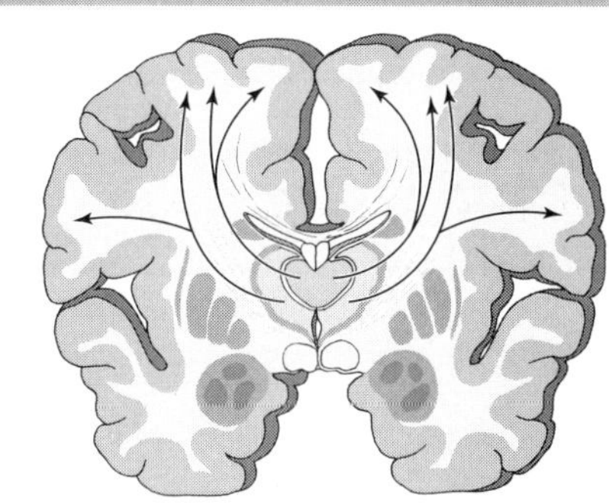

37.3. Specific sensory relay nuclei include the ventral posterior thalamic nuclei and medial and lateral geniculate nuclei. The ventrolateral nuclei relay somatic sensory information from the head as well as the trunk and limbs to the __________________ gyrus (areas 1 to 3) of the cerebral cortex.

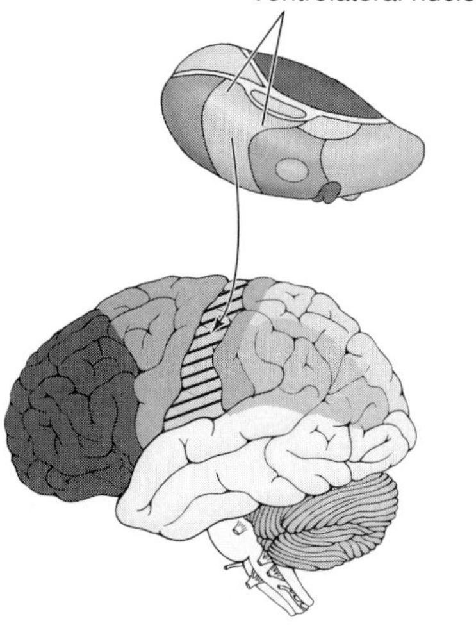

37.1A.

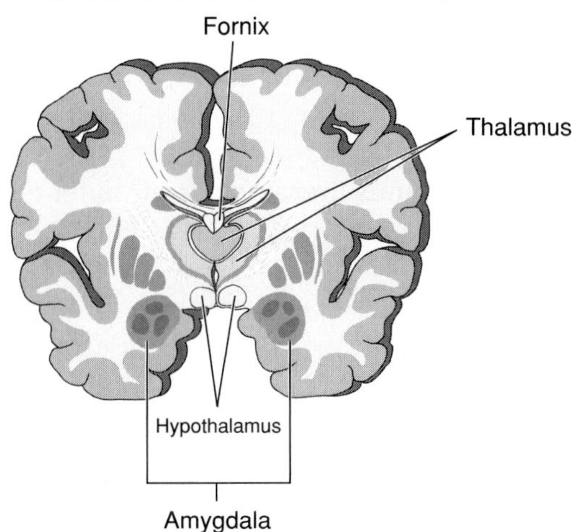

37.2A. ipsilateral; cortex; nonspecific

37.3A. postcentral

37.4. The medial geniculate nucleus receives auditory input from the inner ear and sends efferent fibers to the ____________ cortex (areas 41 to 42) of the temporal lobe. The lateral geniculate nucleus receives visual input from the retina and projects to the ____________ cortex (area 17) of the occipital lobe.

37.5. The anterior nucleus is the relay nucleus of the limbic system, receiving fibers from the ____________________ tract and projecting to the ____________ gyrus. This nucleus functions in emotion and recent memory.

37.6. Specific motor relay nuclei include the ventral anterior and ventral lateral nuclei, which receive input from the cerebellum and basal nuclei and project to the motor cortex (Brodmann's area ______) and premotor cortex (Brodmann's area ______). These motor relay nuclei influence both ____________ and ______ planning.

37.7. In addition to specific relay nuclei, the thalamus also contains association nuclei, such as dorsomedial and pulvinar. Association nuclei project to broad areas of ____________________ cortex including the prefrontal cortex and the parieto-occipito-temporal association cortex.

37.4A. auditory; calcarine

37.5A. mammillothalamic; cingulate

37.6A. 4; 6; movement; motor

37.7A. association

37.8. The DM (dorsomedial nucleus) has reciprocal connections with the ______frontal cortex and is involved in affect and foresight. Damage to the DM produces deficits seen in prefrontal lobo______.

37.9. Nonspecific thalamic nuclei project to widespread areas of the cerebral __________ and bas______ nuclei. They receive afferent input from the basal nuclei, ______ellum, ret__________ formation, and pain pathways (such as the spinothalamic pathway).

37.10. The reticular formation projects to the cerebral cortex via the __________ to function in arousal. Nonspecific nuclei regulate levels of cortical excitability and are one way that the reticular system influences the __________ __________.

37.11. Hypothalamic connections are concerned with endo______, auton______, emotional, and somatic functions. It has reciprocal connections with the limbic system, visceral and somatic nuclei, and efferent output to the pit__________ gland.

37.12. The hypothalamus receives sensory input from visceral and somatic structures, the retina, olfactory epithelium, __________ lobe and hippo__________, amyg______, thal______, and midbrain.

37.8A. prefrontal; lobotomy

37.9A. cortex; basal; cerebellum; reticular

37.10A. thalamus; cerebral cortex

37.11A. endocrine; autonomic; pituitary

37.12A. frontal; hippocampus; amygdala; thalamus

37.13. The hypothalamus projects ______ferent fibers to the brainstem and spinal cord to influence the autonomic nervous system, thalamus, ret____________ system, and lim______ formation.

37.14. In coronal section, the fornix divides the hypothalamus into two regions: medial and lateral. Draw a vertical line through the fornix and label the medial and lateral hypothalamus.

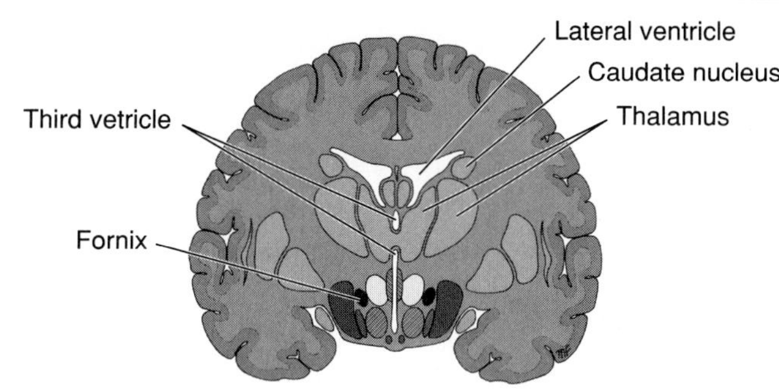

37.15. The medial hypothalamus regulates hormone release from the anterior ____________ and projects into the ____________ pituitary, releasing oxytocin and vasopressin. The lateral hypothalamus connects to the cortex and amy______, linking the autonomic system with behavior.

37.16. The major projections of the hypothalamus travel through the fornix, mammillo____________ tract, stria ____________, ventral amygdalo______ pathway, and medial ____________ bundle.

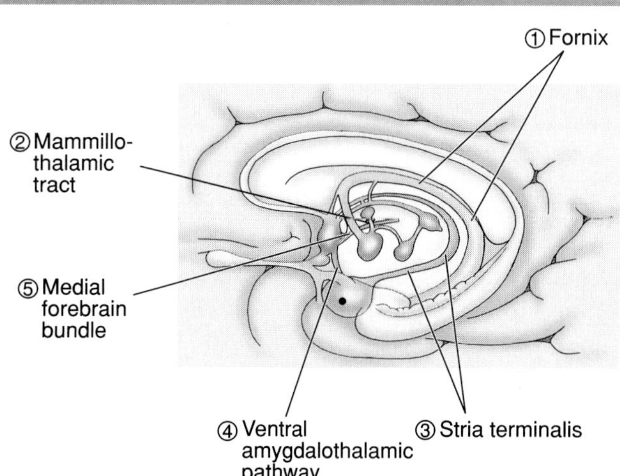

37.17. The fornix bounds the diencephalon superiorly and is formed by a thick bundle of white matter extending from the *hippocampus* to the *mammillary body*. Label the fornix on the diagram.

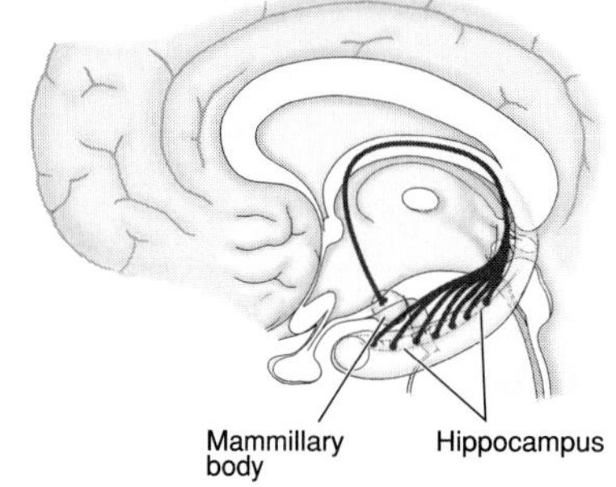

37.13A. efferent; reticular; limbic

37.14A.

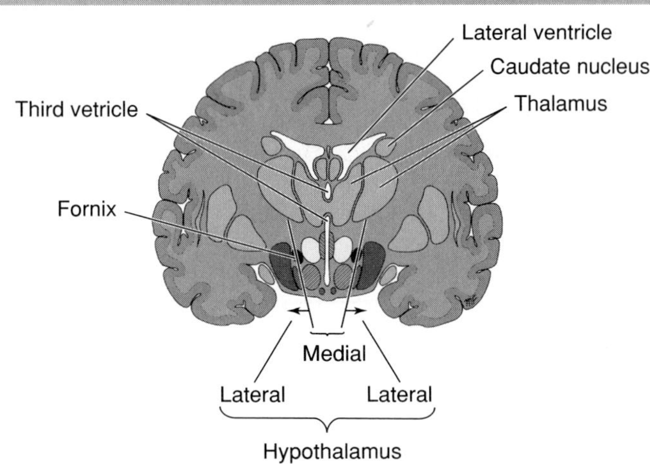

37.15A. pituitary; posterior; amygdala

37.16A. mammillothalamic; terminalis; amygdalofugal; forebrain

37.17A.

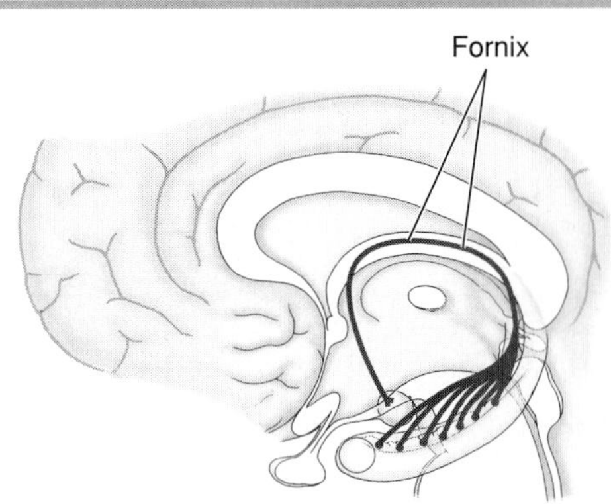

37.18. The fornix is largely covered by the corpus ____________ and the cerebral ____________. The fornix is easily recognizable in looking at the gross diencephalon as a C-shaped band.

37.19. The mammillothalamic tract carries efferent projections from the ____________________ bodies to the ____________ nucleus of the thalamus, ultimately signaling back to the ____________________.

37.20. The stria terminalis originates in the ____________ and projects in part to the hypo____________. The amygdala uses the ____________ ____________________ pathway to project to the hypothalamus.

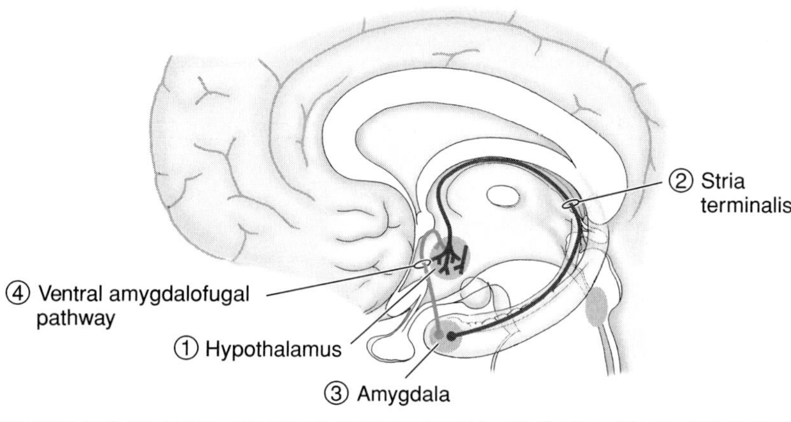

37.21. The medial forebrain bundle connects the hypothalamus with the forebrain (including the septal area) and brainstem. Label the medial forebrain bundle on the diagram.

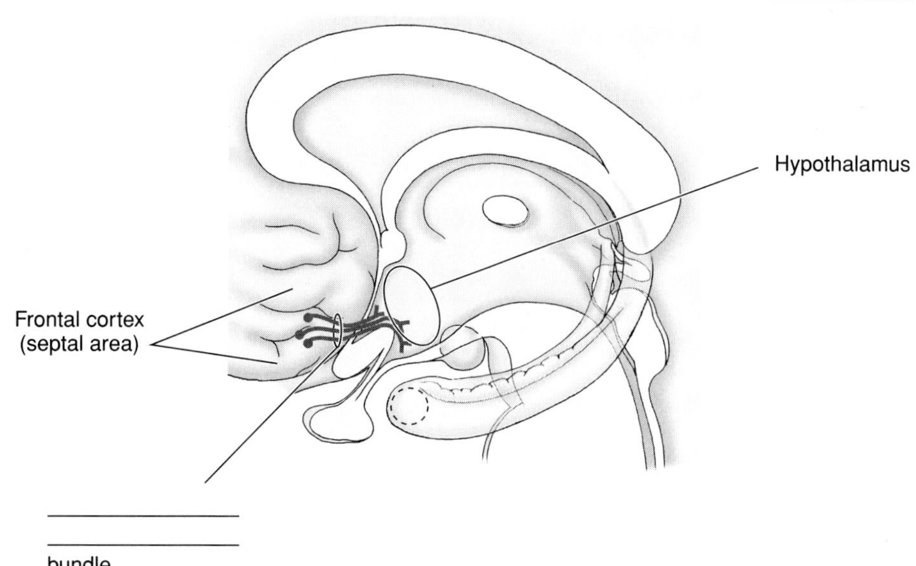

37.18A. callosum; cortex

37.19A. mammillary; anterior; hippocampus

37.20A. amygdala; hypothalamus; ventral amygdalofugal

37.21A.

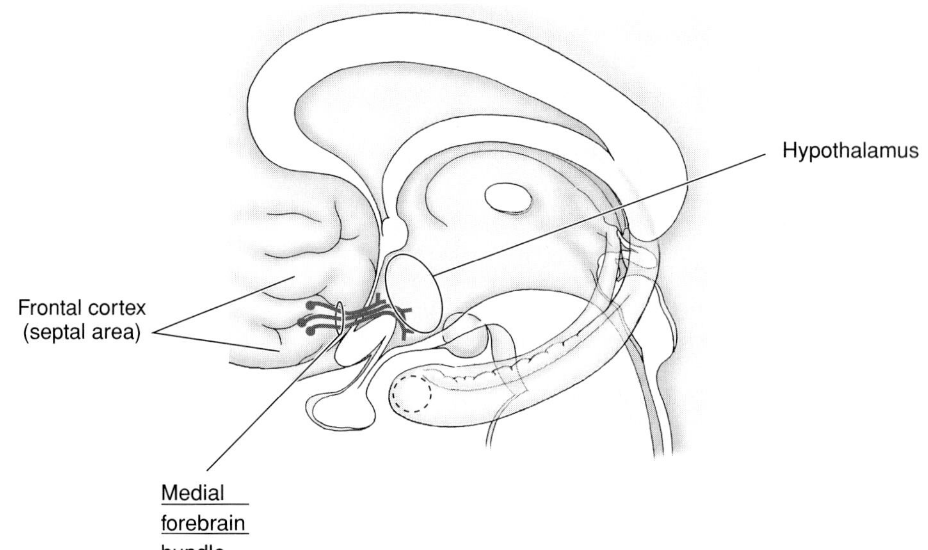

37.22. The septal area is a relay nucleus of the ________________ to the ________________. It receives fibers from the hippocampus via the __________ and projects to the medial and lateral hypothalamus.

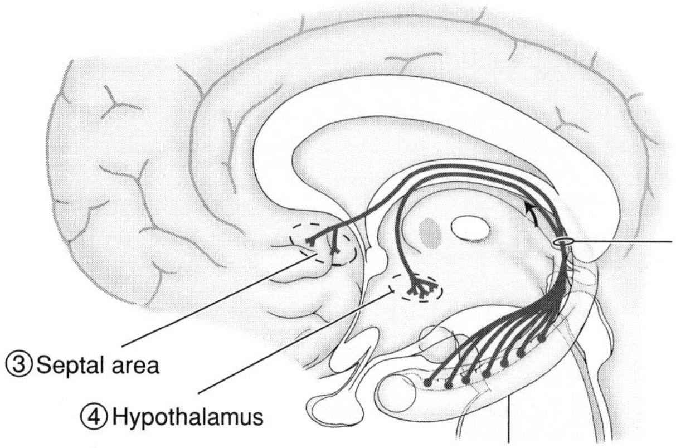

37.23. To review the connections of the thalamus and hypothalamus, match the structure on the left with the appropriate connections on the right.

A. Retina to calcarine cortex	_____	Medial forebrain bundle
B. Mammillary bodies to cingulate gyrus	_____	Fornix
C. Hypothalamus to septal area	_____	Lateral geniculate nucleus
D. Somatosensory input from head to cortical area 3	_____	Medial geniculate nucleus
E. Inner ear to temporal lobe	_____	Anterior nucleus of thalamus
F. Hippocampus to mammillary body	_____	Ventral nuclei of thalamus

37.24. The subthalamus contains the rostral portions of the _____ nucleus and substantia _____ in the midbrain.

37.25. Somatosensory pathways en route to the thalamus travel through the sub__________, along with pathways associated with the cerebellum and the basal nuclei. The subthalamus exhibits reciprocal connections with the __________ pallidus, regulating motor activity through the basal nuclei.

37.26. The subthalamic nucleus regulates the output of the _____ nuclei. Most afferent projections to the subthalamus arise from the __________ __________.

37.22A. hippocampus; hypothalamus; fornix

37.23A.

A. Retina to calcarine cortex	C	Medial forebrain bundle
B. Mammillary bodies to cingulate gyrus	F	Fornix
C. Hypothalamus to septal area	A	Lateral geniculate nucleus
D. Somatosensory input from head to cortical area 3	E	Medial geniculate nucleus
E. Inner ear to temporal lobe	B	Anterior nucleus of thalamus
F. Hippocampus to mammillary body	D	Ventral nuclei of thalamus

37.24A. red; nigra

37.25A. subthalamus; globus

37.26A. basal; globus pallidus

37.27. When subthalamic activity increases, it enhances the ____________________ influence of its efferent target, the globus pallidus, on the thalamus. Damage to the subthalamus increases ____________________ movements.

37.28. The epithalamus consists of the hab______, stria ____________________, and pineal gland. The epithalamus receives ______ ferent input from the amygdala and hippocampus. The epithalamus projects ______ ferent fibers to the midbrain, thalamus, and reticular formation to influence olfaction as well as visceral and somatic sensation.

37.29. The habenula has two pathways associated with it. The *stria medullaris* provides afferent fibers to the habenula from the hypothalamus, forebrain, and anterior thalamus. The stria medullaris originates in the ____________ system. The *habenulopeduncular tract* (fasciculus retroflexus) is the efferent output from the ____________ to the interpeduncular nucleus of the tegmentum. The interpeduncular nucleus is positioned between the cerebral ____________.

37.27A. inhibitory; spontaneous

37.28A. habenula; medullaris; afferent; efferent

37.29A. limbic; habenula; peduncles

38 Thalamic Nuclei and Relationships

38.1. The thalamus is divided into anterior, medial, and lateral regions by the ___________ medullary lamina.

38.2. Label the internal medullary lamina on the diagram. Identify the anterior, medial, and lateral regions of the thalamus.

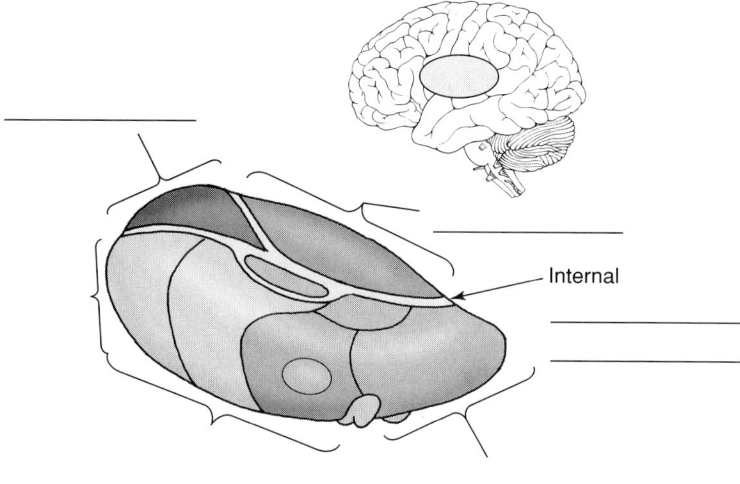

38.3. While the ___________ ___________ lamina partitions the thalamus intoanterior, medial, and lateral sections, the ___________ medullary lamina surrounds the thalamus.

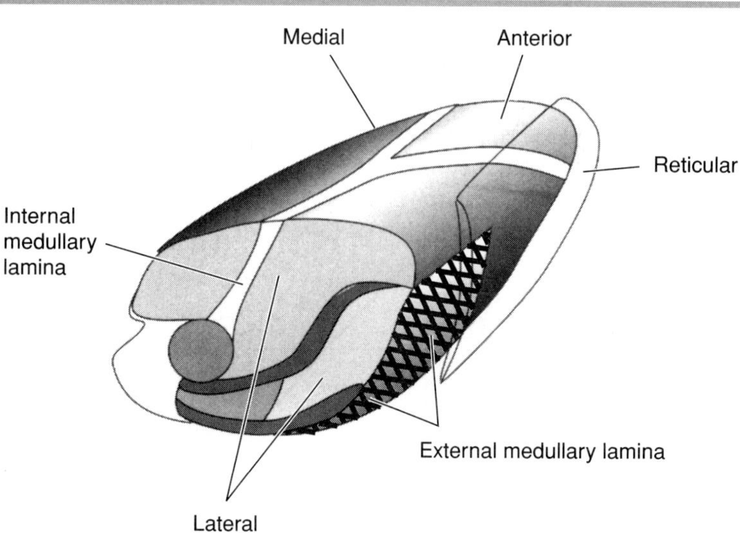

38.4. The external ___________ lamina surrounds the thalamus, separating its ___________ nuclei from the other thalamic regions.

38.5. The anterior thalamic nuclei are partially enclosed by a split in the internal ___________ ___________. The anterior thalamus relays limbic information to the cortex.

38.1A. internal

38.2A.

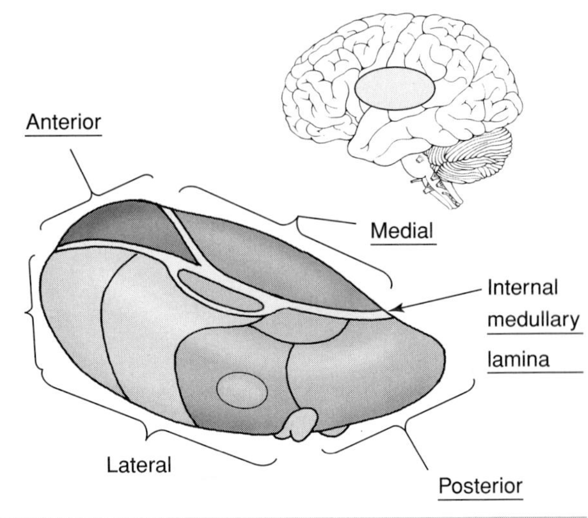

38.3A. internal medullary; external

38.4A. medullary; reticular

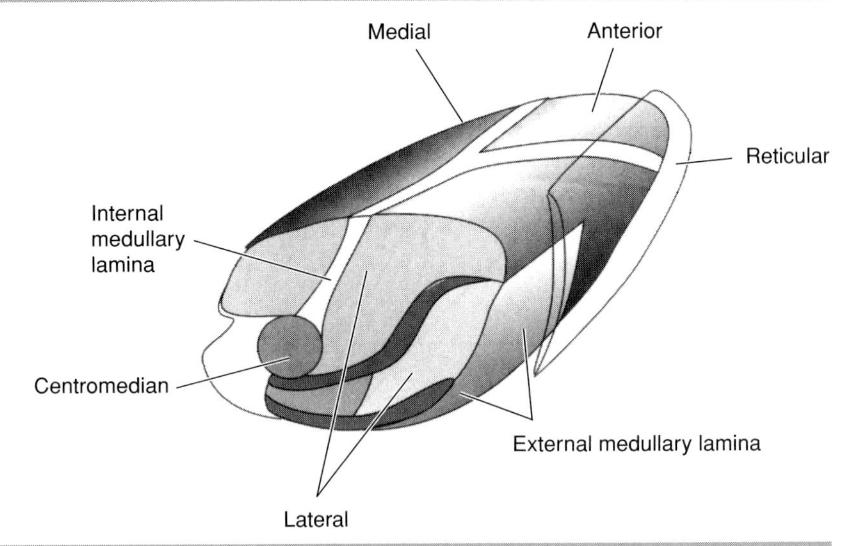

38.5A. medullary lamina

38.6. The anterior nuclei project into the ____________ ventricle as the anterior tubercle, adjacent to the ____________________ foramen.

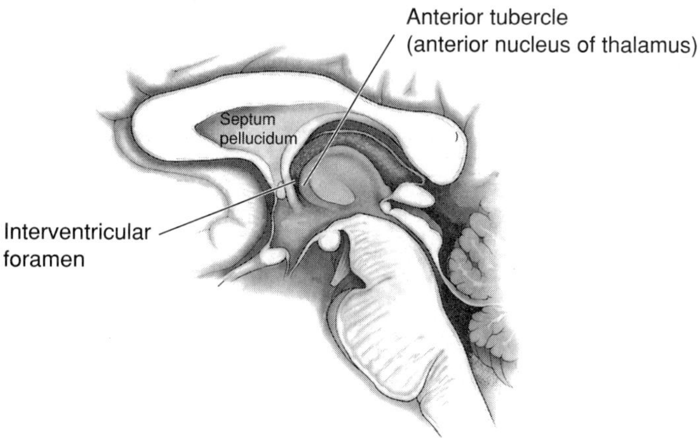

Anterior tubercle (anterior nucleus of thalamus)
Septum pellucidum
Interventricular foramen

38.7. The anterior thalamus receives input from both the mam____________ bodies via the ____________________ tract and from the temporal cortex and hippocampus via the ____________.

38.8. The anterior and medial thalamic nuclei are divided by the ____________ ____________ ____________.

The most prominent medial thalamic nucleus is the dorsomedial nucleus, which projects to the frontal lobe.

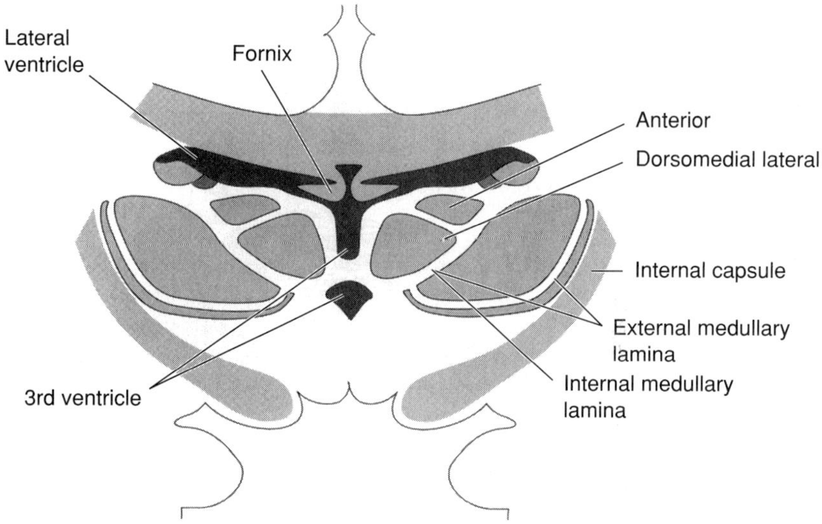

Lateral ventricle
Fornix
Anterior
Dorsomedial lateral
Internal capsule
External medullary lamina
Internal medullary lamina
3rd ventricle

38.9. The dorsomedial nucleus is located ____________ to the anterior nucleus of the thalamus.

38.10. Patients with damage to the dorsomedial nucleus have a flat emotional tone and anterograde amnesia, consistent with its projections to the ____________ lobe. These symptoms are similar to those observed in patients who have had prefrontal lobotomies.

38.6A. lateral; interventricular

38.7A. mammillary; mammillothalamic; fornix

38.8A. internal medullary lamina

38.9A. posterior

38.10A. frontal

38.11. Lateral thalamic nuclei make up the bulk of the thalamus and are divided into ____________ and dorsal tiers. The dorsal thalamic nuclei include the lateral dorsal, lateral posterior, and pulv______.

38.12. The pulvinar is the largest thalamic nucleus. It is located at the ____________ pole of the thalamus. The pulvinar receives input from the superior colliculus of the ____________ and projects to visual association areas.

38.13. The internal ____________ ____________ divides the thalamus into anterior, ____________, and lateral regions. The primary medial thalamic nucleus is the __________________. The lateral thalamic nuclei are organized into two groups: ____________ and ____________.

38.14. In the lateral group of thalamic nuclei, there are three ventral nuclei aligned along the anterior-posterior axis. List them:

____________ ____________

____________ ____________

____________ ____________

Ventral anterior nucleus (VAN)

Ventral lateral (ventrolateral nucleus)

Ventral posterior (ventroposterior nucleus)

38.15. Ventral anterior nuclei receive afferent input from the ______ nuclei and substantia ______.

Basal nuclei
Substantia nigra } → VA nucleus → Area 6 (Premotor cortex)

38.16. The ventral anterior nucleus of the thalamus initiates ____________ by way of connections with the ____________ cortex, or Brodmann's area 6.

38.11A. ventral; pulvinar

38.12A. caudal (or posterior); midbrain

38.13A. medullary lamina; medial; dorsomedial; dorsal; ventral

38.14A. In any order: ventral anterior; ventral lateral; ventral posterior

38.15A. basal; nigra

38.16A. movements; premotor

38.17. Ventral lateral nuclei connect ______ nuclei and cerebellum with the primary motor cortex in the ______________ gyrus and premotor cortex in the __________ lobe.

Cerebellum → VL nucleus → Primary motor cortex (area 4)
Basal nuclei → VL nucleus → Premotor cortex (area 6)

38.18. Ventral posterior nuclei can be divided into lateral and medial regions, which relay ______________ information to the postcentral gyrus.

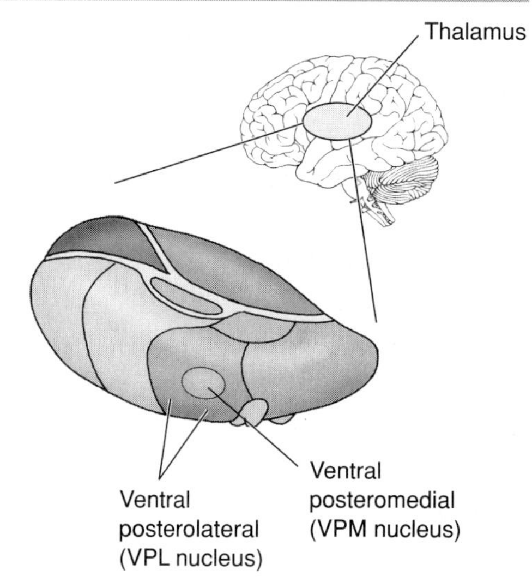

38.19. Somatosensory information from the head and the body is processed by different parts of the ventral posterior nuclei. The ventral postero __________ nucleus of the thalamus carries information from the body, while the ventral postero __________ nucleus of the thalamus carries information from the head.

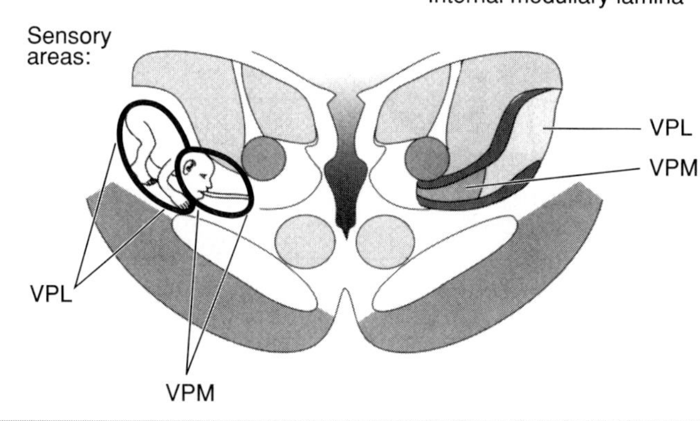

38.20. The geniculate nuclei are considered as an extension of the ventral thalamic nuclei. They are located at the __________ end of the thalamus. Indicate the level at which the thalamus was cut in the midbrain on the lower image. Label the medial and lateral geniculate nuclei on the lower image.

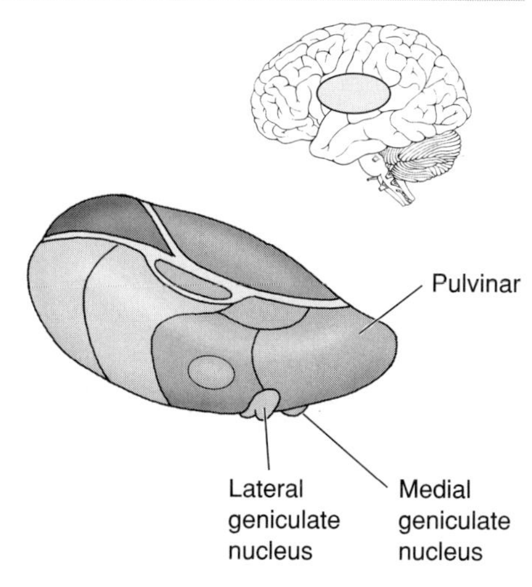

38.17A. basal; precentral; frontal

38.18A. somatosensory

38.19A. lateral; medial

38.20A. posterior

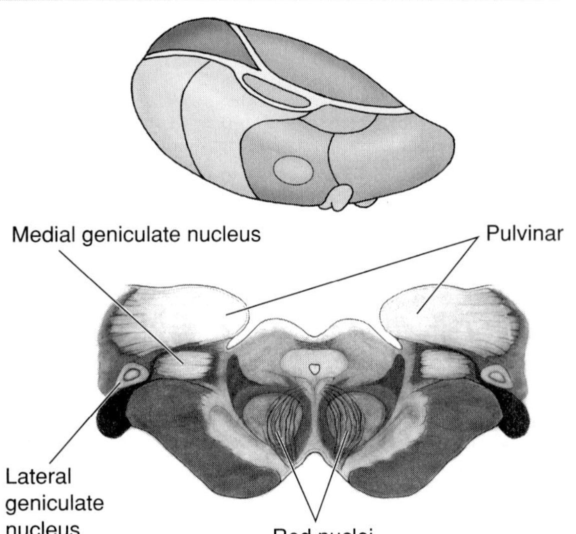

38.21. The medial geniculate nucleus is a relay system for the __________ system. The __________ geniculate nucleus is a relay system for the visual system.

38.22. The __________ __________ lamina splits to surround the intralaminar nuclei.

Intralaminar nuclei

38.23. The largest intralaminar nucleus is the centro __________ nucleus.

38.24. The centromedian nucleus is a round nucleus positioned medial to the __________ nuclei of the thalamus.

Third ventricle
Dorsomedial nucleus
VPL (ventroposterolateral nucleus)
Centromedian nucleus

38.25. The reticular nucleus is located between the __________ medullary lamina and the __________ __________. The reticular nucleus allows the cortex to regulate its afferent input for selective attention and arousal.

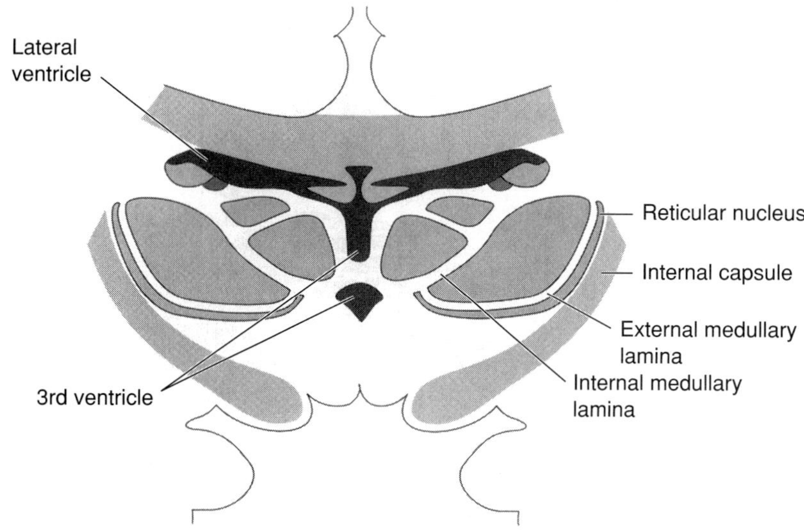

38.21A. auditory; lateral

38.22A. internal medullary

38.23A. centromedian

38.24A. ventral

38.25A. external; internal capsule

38.26 Match each descriptor with the appropriate thalamic nucleus.

_____ This structure divides the thalamus into anterior, medial, and lateral regions.

_____ This structure lies between the reticular nucleus of the thalamus and the internal capsule.

_____ This structure is a nonspecific thalamic nucleus.

_____ This thalamic nucleus projects primarily to the frontal lobe.

_____ This is the largest thalamic nucleus and projects nucleus to visual association areas.

_____ This nucleus conveys somatosensory information nucleus from the head to the postcentral gyrus.

_____ This nucleus links the cerebellum with the precentral gyrus.

_____ This thalamic nucleus relays limbic information to the cerebrum.

A. Anterior nucleus

B. Dorsomedial nucleus

C. Pulvinar

D. Ventral lateral nucleus

E. Ventral posterior medial nucleus

F. Ventral posterior lateral nucleus

G. Centromedian nucleus

H. Internal medullary

I. External medullary lamina

38.26A.

__H__ This structure divides the thalamus into anterior, medial, and lateral regions.

__I__ This structure lies between the reticular nucleus of the thalamus and the internal capsule.

__G__ This structure is a nonspecific thalamic nucleus.

__B__ This thalamic nucleus projects primarily to the frontal lobe.

__C__ This is the largest thalamic nucleus and projects to visual association areas.

__E__ This nucleus conveys somatosensory information from the head to the postcentral gyrus.

__D__ This nucleus links the cerebellum with the precentral gyrus.

__A__ This thalamic nucleus relays limbic information to the cerebrum.

39 Hypothalamic Nuclei and Relationships

39.1. A vertical line drawn through the ___________ divides the hypothalamus into lateral and medial regions in the coronal plane.

Lateral ventricle
Caudate nucleus
Third ventricle
Thalamus
Fornix
Hypothalamus

39.2. The ___________ hypothalamus initiates eating and increases water consumption.

39.3. The ___________ hypothalamus produces the releasing hormones that regulate pituitary activity.

39.4. On this sagittal section, circle and label the hypothalamus. Identify and label the optic chiasm, pituitary, tuber cinereum, infundibulum, and the mammillary body.

39.5. In the sagittal plane, the hypothalamic nuclei are grouped anterior to posterior by their relationship to the optic chiasm, tuber cinereum, and mammillary body. List these three areas from anterior to posterior:

1) ___________________

2) ___________________

3) ___________________

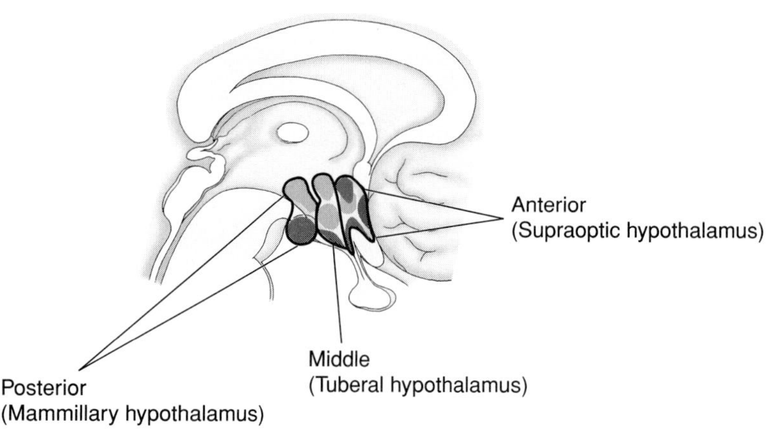

39.1A. fornix

39.2A. lateral

39.3A. medial

39.4A.

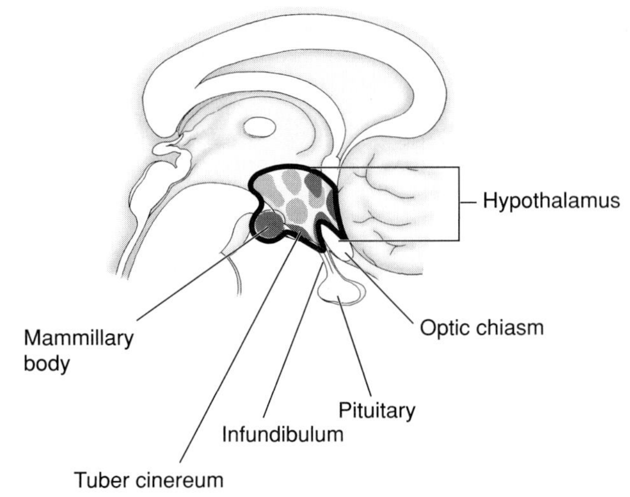

39.5A. 1) Anterior (supraoptic); 2) Middle (tuberal); 3) Posterior (mammillary)

39.6. The anterior, or ________________, hypothalamus is located superior to the ______ __________.

39.7. The tuberal (or __________) hypothalamus is superior to the ______ __________, which is defined as the superior aspect of the infundibular stalk joining the pituitary to the hypothalamus.

39.8. The posterior hypothalamus is superior to and includes the ________________ bodies.

39.9. The anterior hypothalamus lies between the __________ terminalis and the ______ __________. It contains the supra______ nucleus, which makes vasopressin (antidiuretic hormone), and the ______ ventricular nucleus, which makes oxytocin.

39.10. The pre______ nucleus lies anterior to the optic __________ and regulates temperature control. It merges with the anterior nucleus. They control the ________________ nervous system, producing effects including reduced blood pressure and heart rate and increased gastrointestinal activity.

39.11. The anterior hypothalamus also contains the ______chiasmatic nucleus located superior to the optic __________. This nucleus receives afferent input from the retina and regulates biological rhythms.

39.6A. supraoptic; optic chiasm

39.7A. middle; tuber cinereum

39.8A. mammillary

39.9A. lamina; optic chiasm; supraoptic; paraventricular

39.10A. preoptic; chiasm; parasympathetic

39.11A. suprachiasmatic; chiasm

39.12. Anterior to posterior, the middle hypothalamus is bounded by the ______ __________ and ______________ __________. Fill in the blank labels on the diagram.

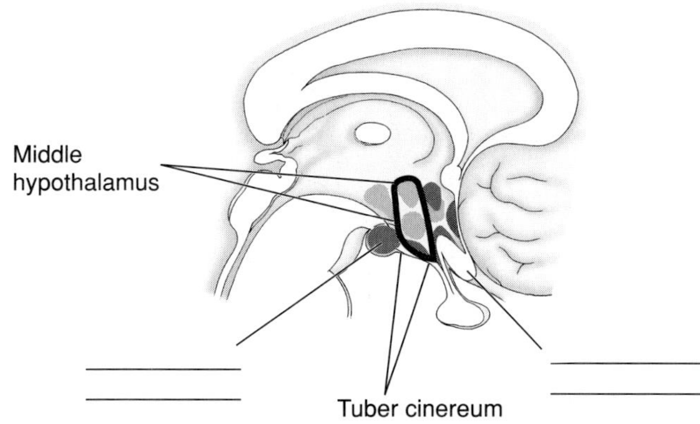

39.13. Draw a line from each structure on the left to the appropriate hypothalamic region on the right.

Mammillary bodies	Anterior hypothalamus
Infundibulum	Middle hypothalamus
Lamina terminalis	Posterior hypothalamus

39.14. The middle, or tuberal, hypothalamus, contains the arcuate nucleus. The arcuate (infund__________) nucleus regulates the activity of the anterior __________.

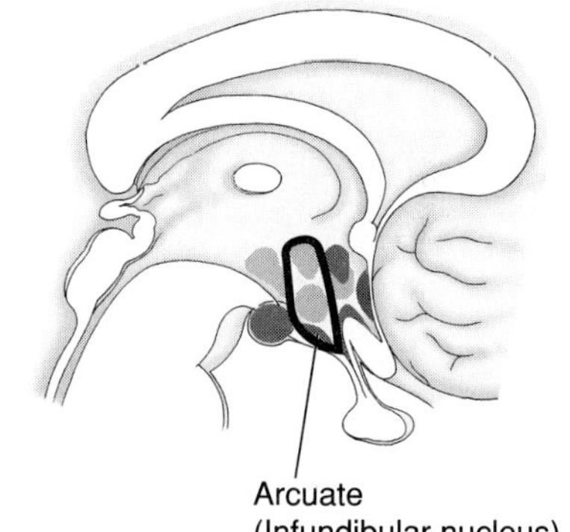

39.15. In addition to the arc______ nucleus, the middle hypothalamus also contains the __________medial and ______medial nuclei. These nuclei work with the lateral hypothalamus to regulate ______ and ______ consumption. The middle hypothalamus functions to inhibit eating and controls rage behaviors.

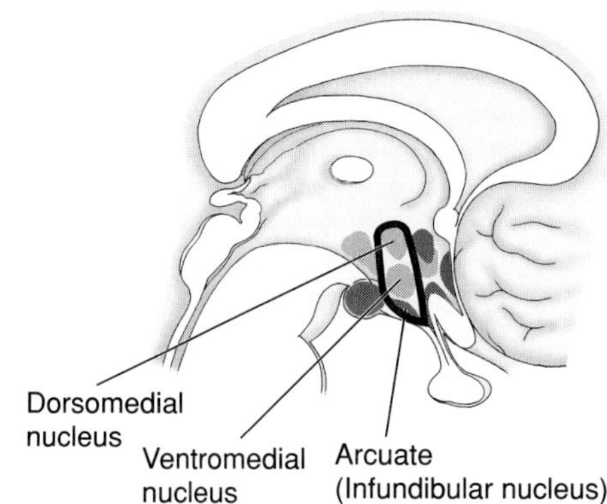

39.12A. optic chiasm; mammillary bodies

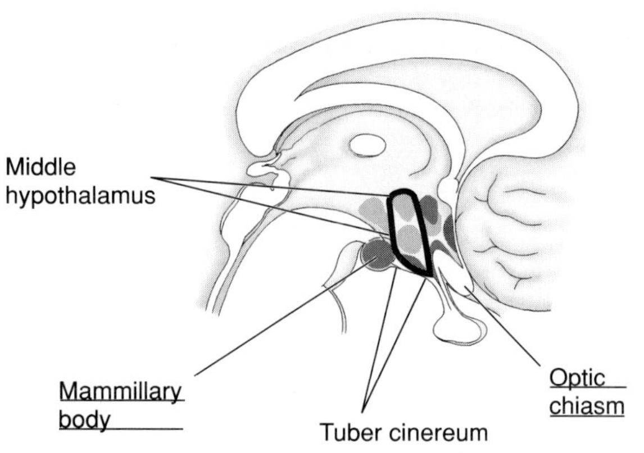

39.13A.

Mammillary bodies	Anterior hypothalamus
Infundibulum	Middle hypothalamus
Lamina terminalis	Posterior hypothalamus

39.14A. infundibular; pituitary

39.15A. arcuate; ventromedial; dorsomedial; food; water

39.16. Label the ventromedial and dorsomedial nuclei.

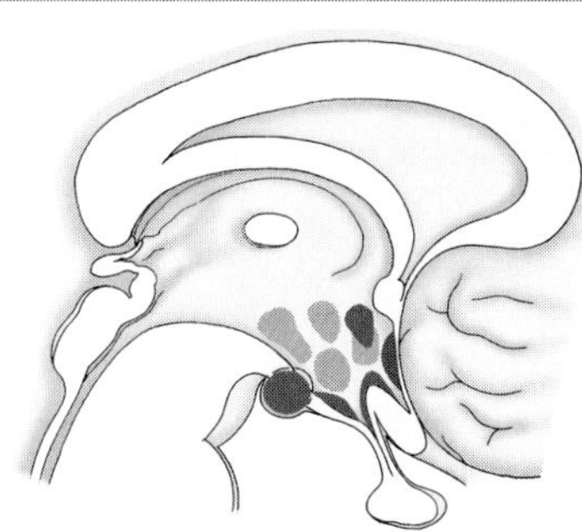

39.17. The posterior hypothalamus is formed by the mammillary bodies, which replace the __________________ nuclei posteriorly.

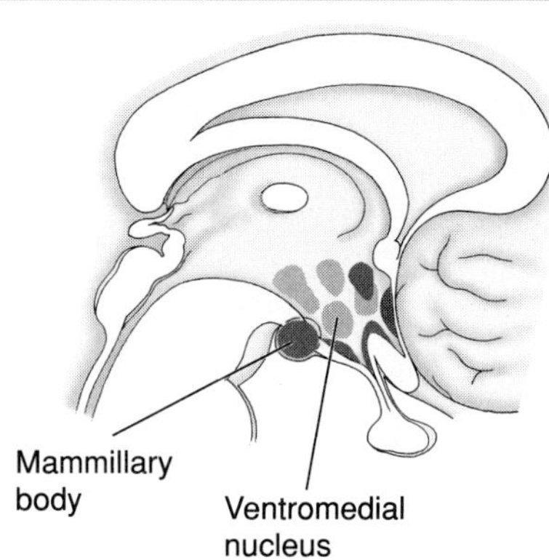

39.18. The mammillary bodies are part of the Papez circuit, which functions in emotion. The ______ circuit involves the following connections: hippocampus → ____________ → __________________ bodies → ____________thalamic tract → ____________ nucleus of thalamus → __________________ cortex → hippocampus.

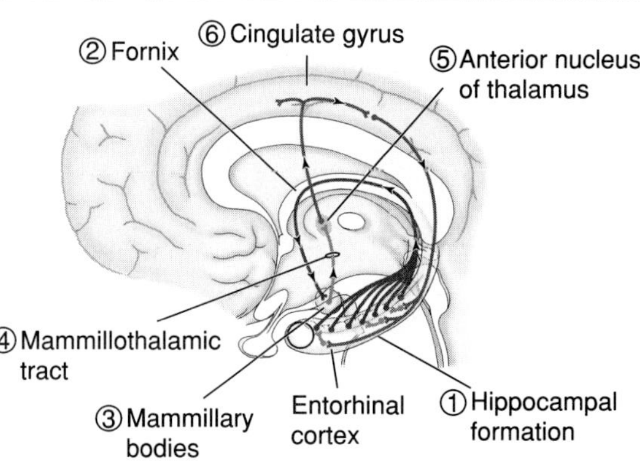

39.19. The ____________ nucleus of the hypothalamus functions in response to cold temperatures, whereas the ____________ nucleus of the hypothalamus functions in response to heat. The posterior nucleus also controls the sympathetic nervous system, ____________ heart rate and blood pressure.

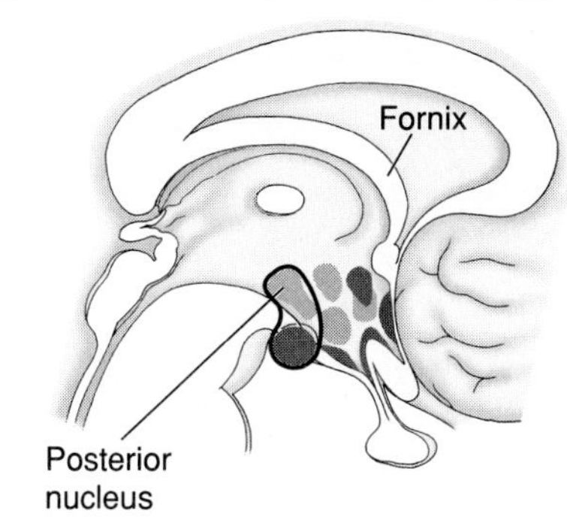

39.20. The ____________ splits the hypothalamus into medial and lateral regions.

39.16A.

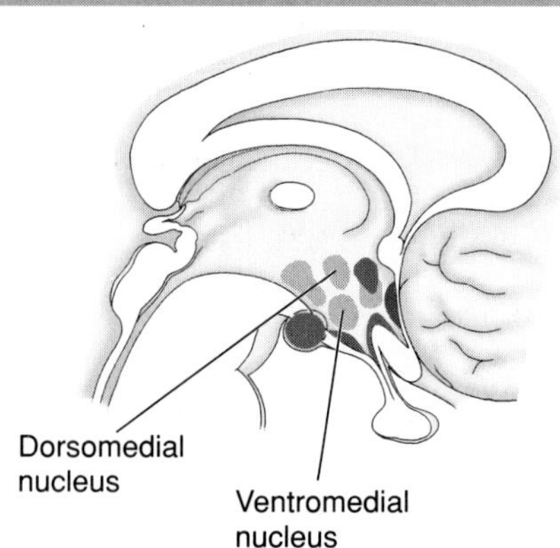

39.17A. ventromedial

39.18A. Papez; fornix; mammillary; mammillothalamic; anterior; entorhinal

39.19A. anterior; posterior; elevating

39.20A. fornix

40 Blood Supply to the Diencephalon

40.1. The diencephalon receives its blood supply by both the vertebrobasilar and internal carotid arterial systems. Label the basilar, posterior cerebral, posterior communicating, and internal carotid arteries on the diagram.

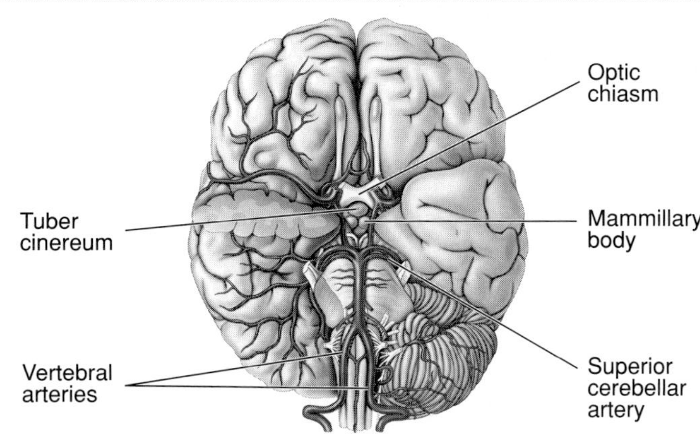

40.2. The thalamus is supplied largely by the posterior cerebral artery, which is a terminal branch of the ____________ artery. Label the thalamic branches of the posterior cerebral and posterior communicating arteries on the diagram.

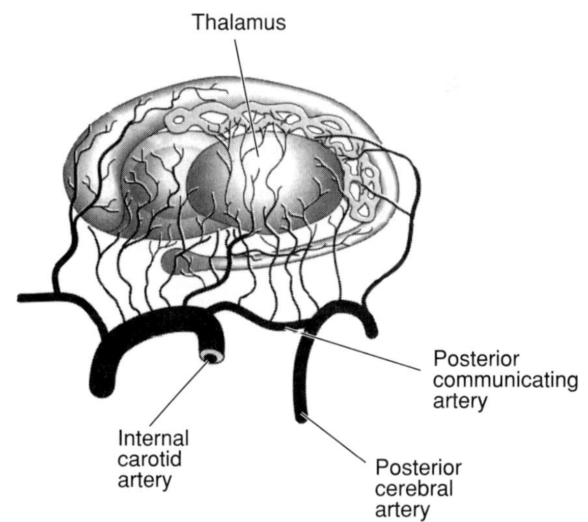

40.3. Thalamic branches also arise from the anterior ____________ artery from the ____________ carotid artery.

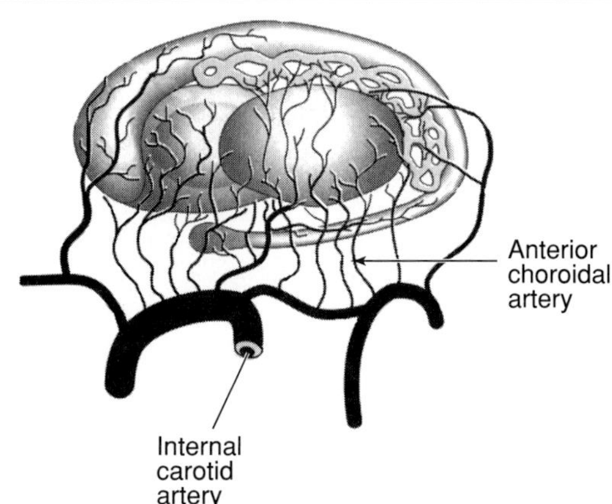

40.1A.

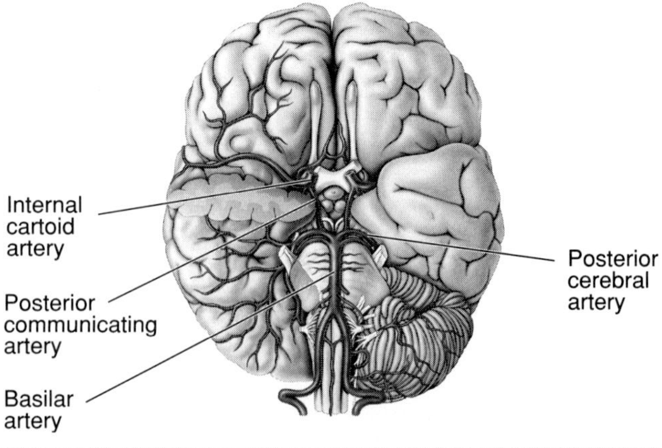

40.2A. basilar

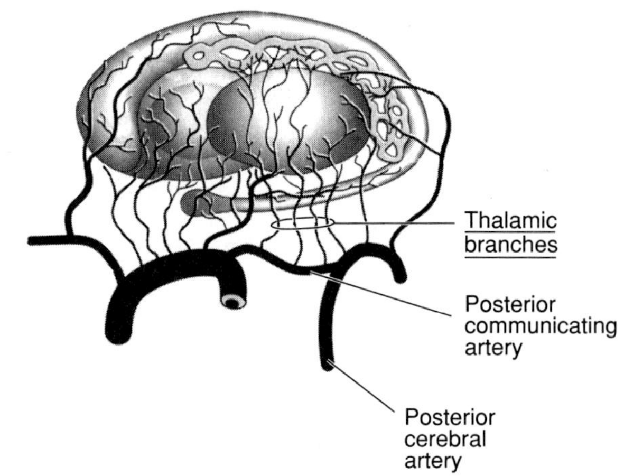

40.3A. choroidal; internal

40.4. The circle of ___________ gives rise to penetrating (central) arteries that supply the diencephalon. The anteromedial group of these penetrating arteries supplies the anterior hypothalamus.

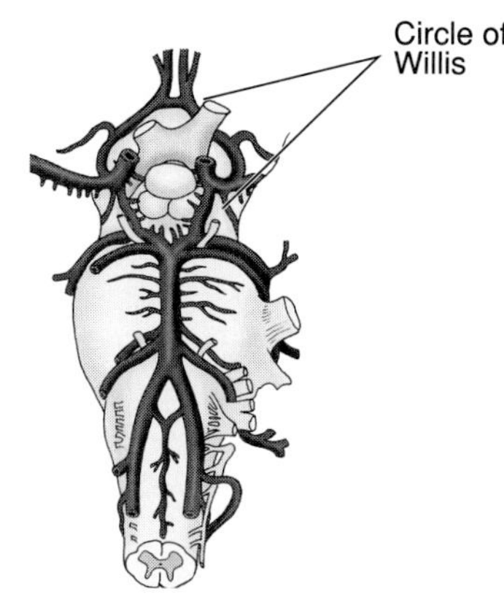

40.5. The posteromedial penetrating arteries from the circle of ___________ supply the anterior and medial thalamus, subthalamus, and middle and posterior hypothalamus. Identify the thalamus, subthalamus, and middle and posterior hypothalamus on the diagram.

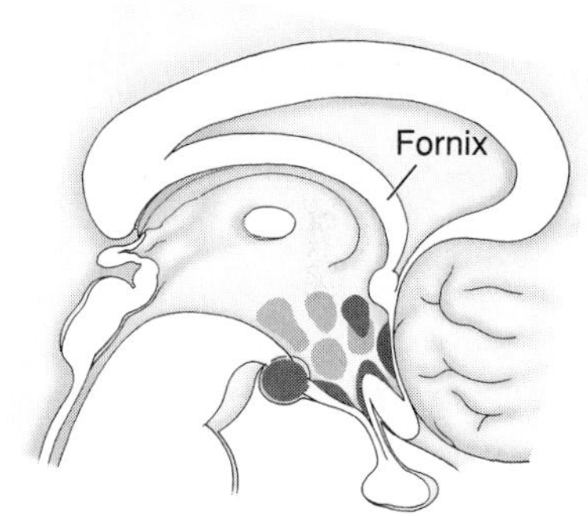

40.6. The posterolateral penetrating (central) arteries supply the geniculate nuclei, VPL (ventral posteromedial lateral nucleus of the thalamus), and pulvinar. Identify these areas on the diagrams.

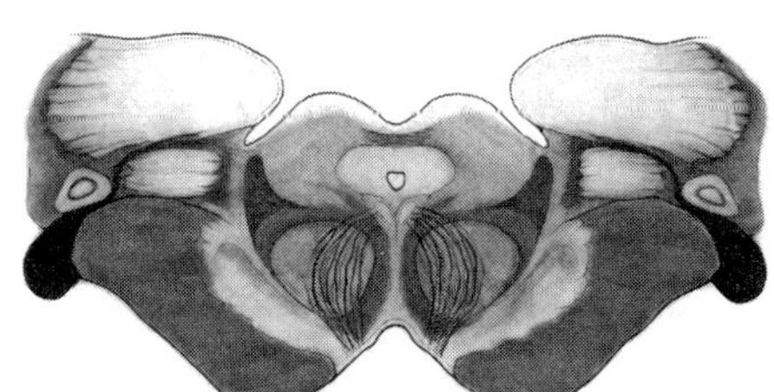

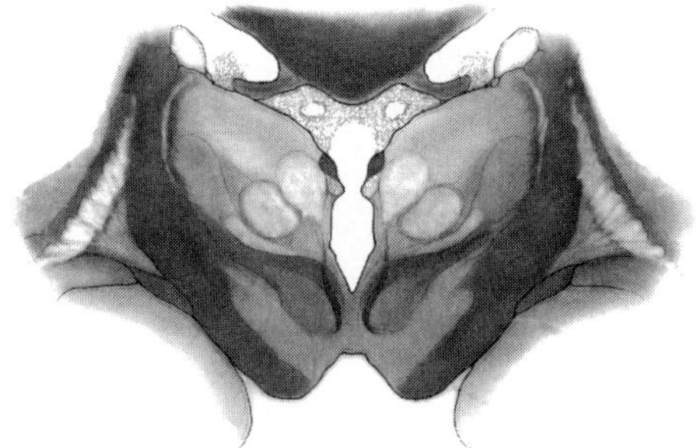

40.4A. Willis

40.5A. Willis

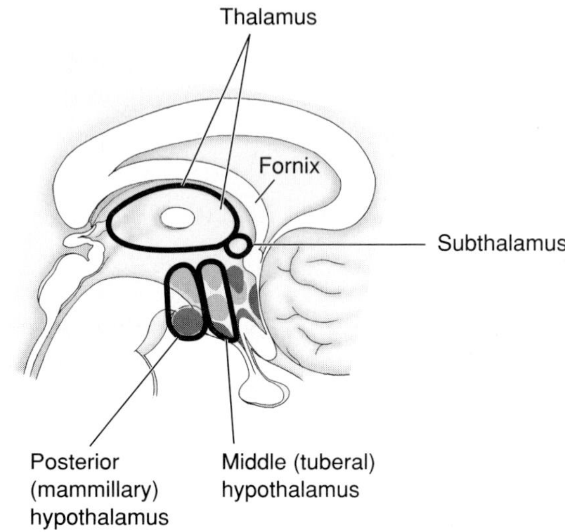

40.6A.

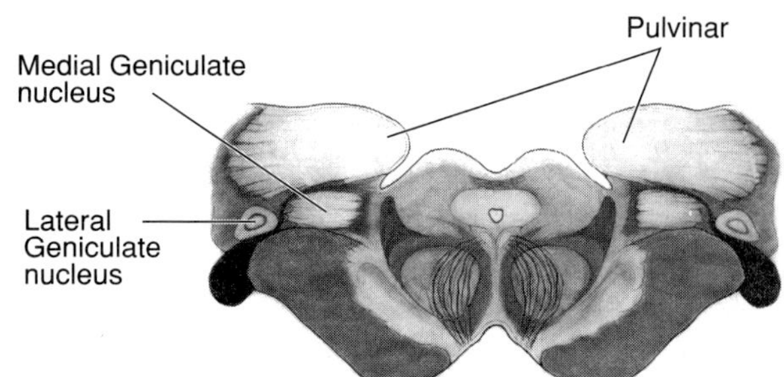

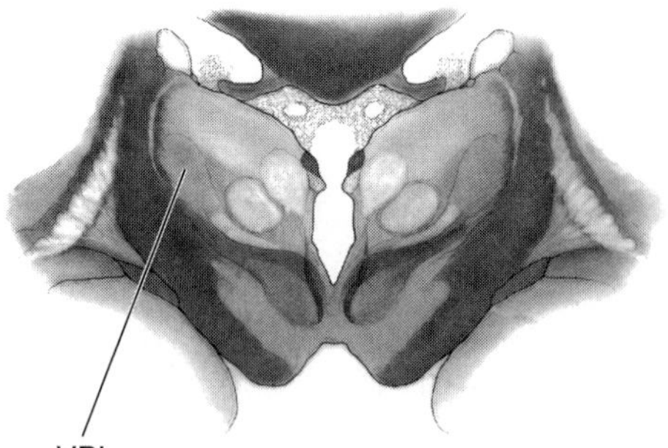

41 Lesions of the Diencephalon

41.1. Lesions of the thalamus produce ____________lateral hemianesthesia, with loss of all sensory modalities in the trunk, limbs, and face. This type of lesion may result from infarction due to hypertension or thrombosis of a branch of the ____________ cerebral artery.

41.2. Lesions of the thalamus will produce impaired sensation, including two types of touch—light or fine touch and ____________________touch—as well as ____________ception.

41.3. The initial ______anesthesia associated with thalamic lesions may be followed by a partial return of sensation with an unpleasant burning sensation known as thalamic pain syndrome.

41.4. Lesions of the hypothalamus may result from infection, trauma, or vascular pathologies. In addition, the hypothalamus is affected by tumors that grow up from the floor of the ______ ventricle or ____________ gland.

41.5. A common lesion is pituitary adenoma, which may grow to enormous sizes and compress the hypothalamus. An adenoma is a tumor derived from ____________________ cells.

41.6. Craniopharyngioma is another tumor of the pituitary, specifically of Rathke's pouch, that can affect the ______thalamus.

41.1A. contralateral; posterior

41.2A. discriminative; proprioception

41.3A. hemianesthesia

41.4A. third; pituitary

41.5A. epithelial

41.6A. hypothalamus

42 Clinical Signs of Damage to the Diencephalon

42.1. The thalamus receives sensory impulses from the ________________ side of the body. Lesions will be confined to this side and may impair all forms of sensation, including ______ touch, fine ________________ touch, and ___________ception.

42.2. Posterior thalamic lesions produce an unpleasant burning sensation known as __________ ______ syndrome. This pain is perceived by the patient without injury to the body.

42.3. Lesions of the subthalamus result in ______pyramidal signs, including ________________ movements of the ___________lateral extremities.

42.4. Pineal tumors alter reproductive function because __________ is antigonadotropic. Lesions of the posterior hypothalamus may also result in ______ disturbances.

42.5. Lesions affecting the hypothalamus may be seen in any type of medical practice since they result in problems with endocrine, visual, or homeostatic functions. Diabetes insipidus results from damage to neurons in the ________________ that make vasopressin. This disease is characterized by __________ urine production.

42.6. Hypothalamic lesions may result in a loss of sexual activity and genital ______plasia or atrophy.

42.7. Eating disorders commonly accompany hypothalamic tumors or lesions. Lesions of the ventro__________ hypothalamus result in increases in appetite and obesity, whereas lesions of the lateral hypothalamus result in ______ of appetite and emaciation.

42.8. Tumors located at the base of the brain that impinge on the ventromedial hypothalamus may also produce ______aggressive and __________ behaviors.

42.1A. contralateral; light; discriminative; proprioception

42.2A. thalamic pain

42.3A. extrapyramidal; involuntary; contralateral

42.4A. melatonin; sleep

42.5A. hypothalamus; copious (or increased)

42.6A. hypoplasia

42.7A. ventromedial; loss

42.8A. hyperaggressive; violent

42.9. Hypothalamic lesions that result in hypersecretion of corticotrophin-releasing hormone overstimulate the anterior pituitary. These patients have changes in sodium and water metabolism and ______tension.

42.10. Korsakoff's psychosis involves damage to mammillary bodies, the mammillothalamic tract, and the medial dorsal thalamus. This may result from chronic alcoholism and nutritional deficiency and can cause loss of __________.

42.9A. hypertension

42.10A. memory

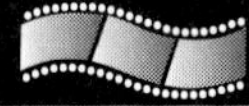

Animations

1. Pain and Temperature (Chapter 38)
2. Crude Touch (Chapter 38)
3. Fine Touch (Chapter 38)
4. Reflex Proprioception (Chapter 38)
16. Visceral Body (Chapter 38)
18. Limbic (Chapters 36, 37, 38)

V BRAINSTEM

43 Surface of the Brainstem

43.1. The brainstem is located within the ____________ crania fossa. It is continuous with the ____________ superiorly, where the midbrain merges with the thalamus, and the ____________ ______ inferiorly, at the level of the caudal medulla.

43.2. The brainstem is continuous with the spinal cord at the ____________ ____________ of the occipital bone, where the spinal cord enters the skull. The diencephalon is continuous with the brainstem at the ____________ ____________, a gap or deficiency in the falx cerebelli.

43.3. The brainstem is divided into three parts or divisions, the: ____________, ______, and ____________, from inferior to superior.

43.4. The brainstem contains the nuclei associated with many of the ______ cranial nerves.

43.5. The most ____________ division of the brainstem, the ____________, contains nuclei associated with cranial nerves VIII, IX, X, and XII.

43.6. The middle division of the brainstem, the ______, contains nuclei associated with cranial nerves V, VI, and VII.

43.7. The most ____________ division of the brainstem, the ____________, contains nuclei associated with cranial nerves III and IV.

43.1A. posterior; forebrain (or diencephalon); spinal cord

43.2A. foramen magnum; tentorial incisure

43.3A. medulla; pons; midbrain

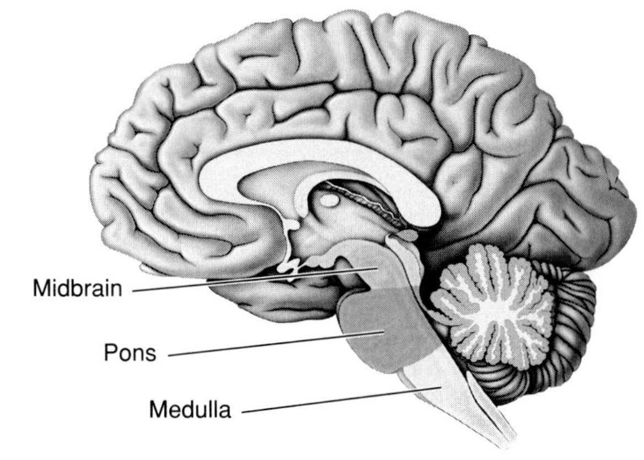

43.4A. 12

43.5A. inferior; medulla

43.6. pons

43.7A. superior; midbrain

43.8. Next to each cranial nerve, indicate the division of the brainstem it is most closely associated with:

III oculomotor: ____________

IV trochlear: ____________

V trigeminal: ______

VI abducens: ______

VII facial: ______

VIII vestibulocochlear: ____________

IX glossopharyngeal: ____________

X vagus: ____________

XII hypoglossal: ____________

43.9. The term "pons" is Latin for bridge. The pons serves as the bridge connecting the ____________ to the ____________________. The cerebellum is responsible for coordination of ______ activity.

43.10. The cerebellum covers the posterior aspect of the brainstem. The three large fiber bundles connecting the ____________ to the ____________________ are known as the cerebellar peduncles.

43.11. There are ______ sets of peduncles: superior, middle, and inferior. Place an S, M, and I on the appropriate peduncle in the diagram of the brainstem.

43.12. On the following diagram, label the thalamus, midbrain, pons, medulla, cerebellum, and spinal cord. Indicate the level of the tentorial incisure and foramen magnum by drawing a line at the appropriate level and labeling them accordingly.

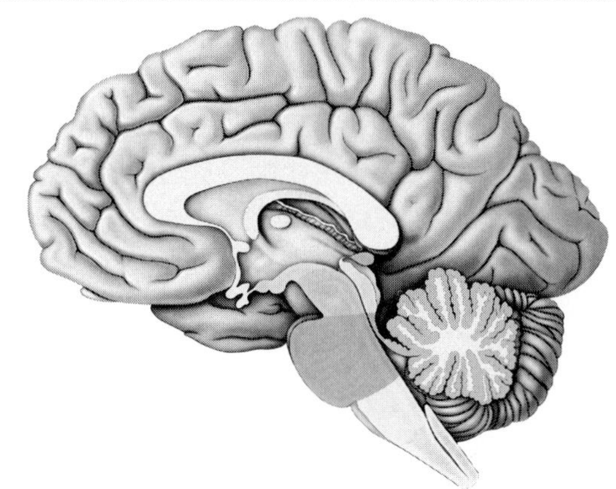

43.8A. midbrain; midbrain; pons; pons; pons; medulla; medulla; medulla; medulla

43.9A. forebrain; cerebellum; motor

43.10A. brainstem; cerebellum

43.11A. 3

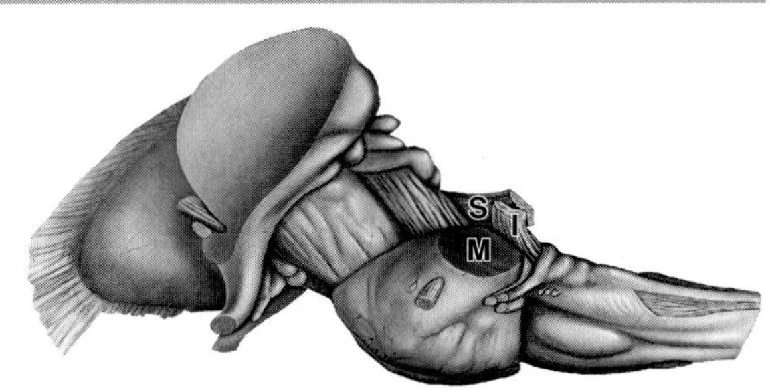

43.12A.

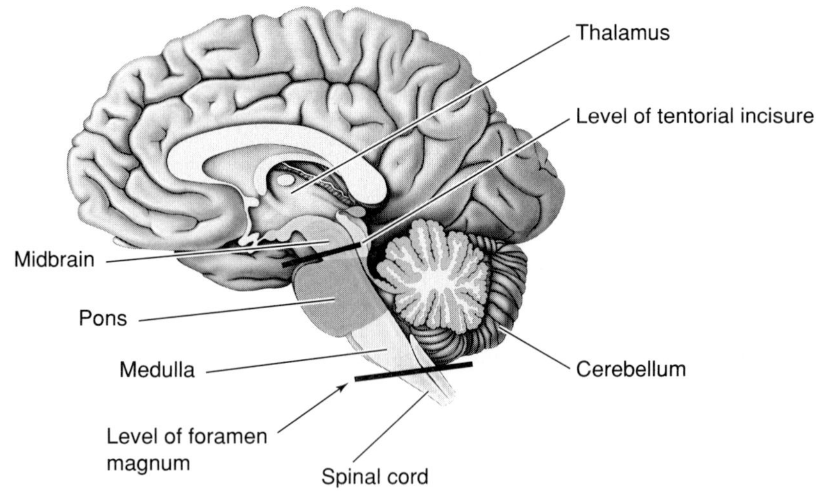

43.13. Place an X on the part of the diagram that acts as a bridge between the forebrain and the cerebellum. Place a Y on the part of the diagram that contains neurons associated with cranial nerve III. Place a Z on the part of the diagram that is continuous with the spinal cord at the __________ __________.

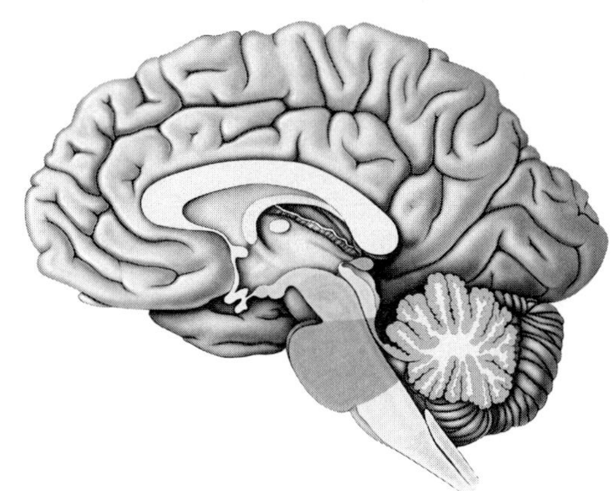

43.14. The __________ ______ of the spinal cord is indicated on the left image. The lower portion of the __________ contains a rostral prolongation of the central canal labeled on the second image. The central canal expands to form the __________ ventricle in the rostral __________.

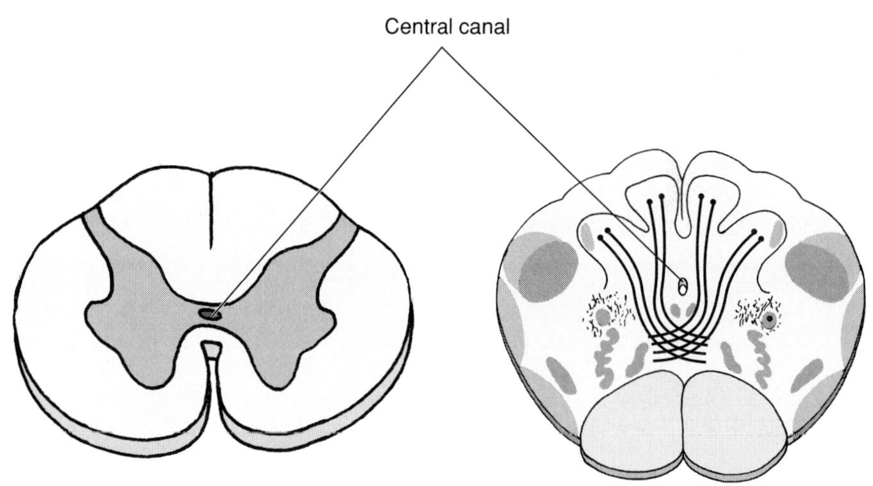

43.15. The rostral part of the medulla is known as the open part, as it opens to form the floor of the __________ __________. The fourth ventricle contains __________ ______ and extends __________ between the pons anteriorly and the __________ posteriorly.

43.16. Label the cerebrospinal fluid–filled space in all three images with the correct name, and then label each of the images.

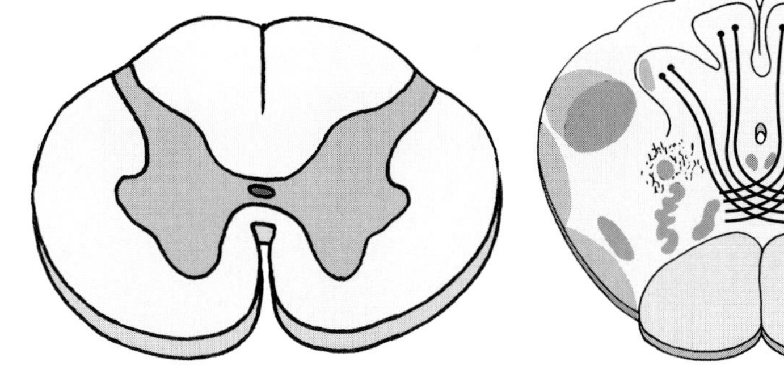

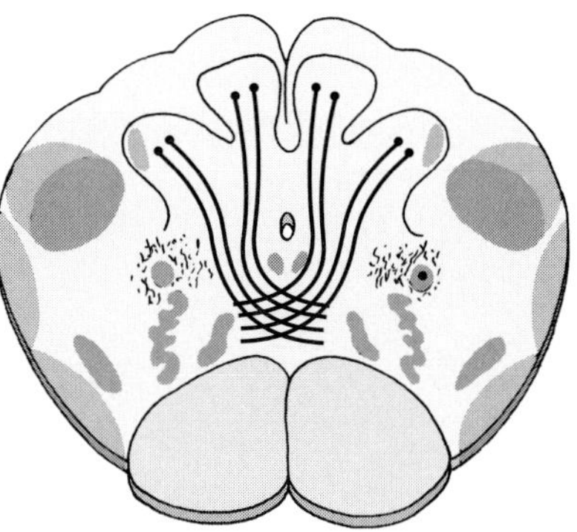

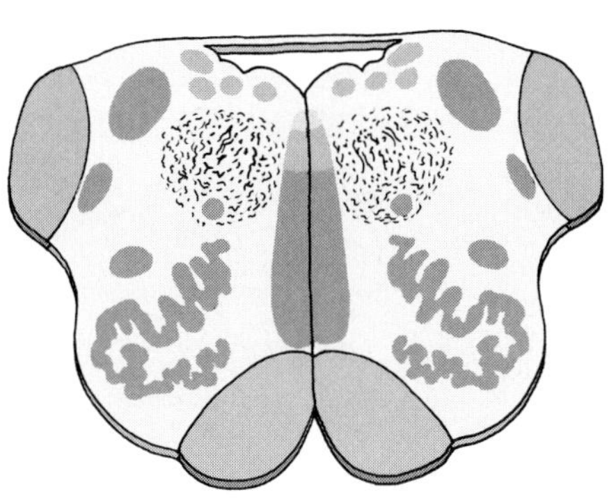

43.13A. foramen magnum

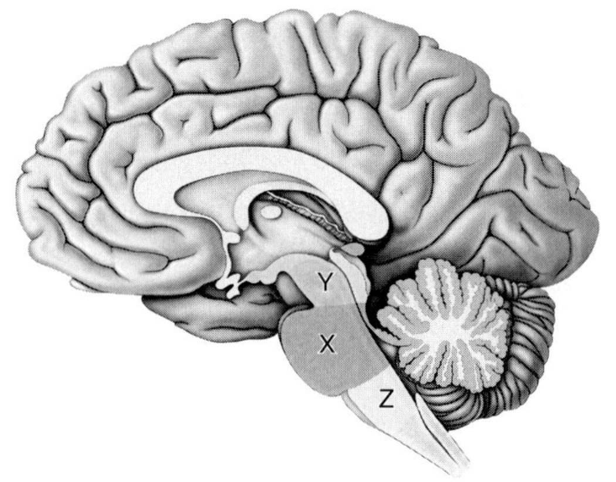

43.14A. central canal; medulla; fourth; medulla

43.15A. fourth ventricle; cerebrospinal fluid; superiorly (or rostrally); cerebellum

43.16A.

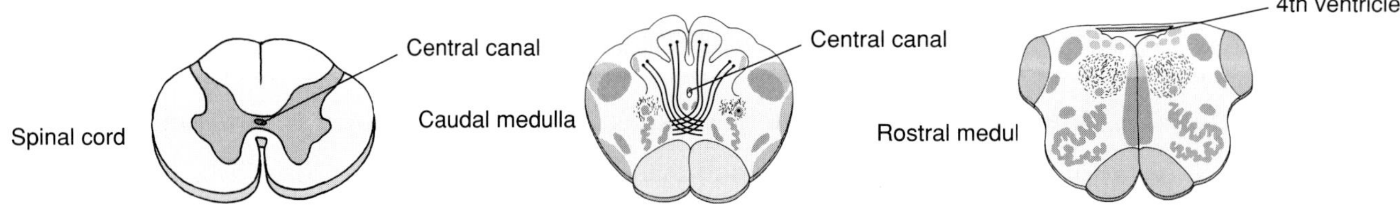

43.17. Moving ____________ or superiorly, the fourth ventricle narrows to form the cerebral aqueduct as it passes through the ____________.

43.18. A line drawn through the ____________________ ________ filled cerebral aqueduct divides the midbrain into a more ____________ roof (tectum) and a more anterior ______ (cerebral peduncle).

43.19. The ____________ or roof of the midbrain bears four elevations (two pairs; a superior and inferior pair)—the corpora quadrigemina—formed by the ____________ and ____________ colliculi.

43.20. Continuity between the spinal cord and caudal ____________ does not end with the presence of a CSF-filled ____________ ______. In fact, many of the surface landmarks also remain. For example, the ____________ ____________ ____________ found as a deep groove along the anterior aspect of the spinal cord continues along the anterior aspect of the ____________. Label the groove on the diagram.

Rostral medulla

43.21. Draw an arrow to indicate the location of the anterior median fissure. The P on the right diagram indicates the location of the pyramids (descending tracts), and the O indicates the location of the olives (also part of the motor system). Cranial nerve ______ emerges between the ____________ and the ______ in the preolivary sulcus.

L4 spinal cord level

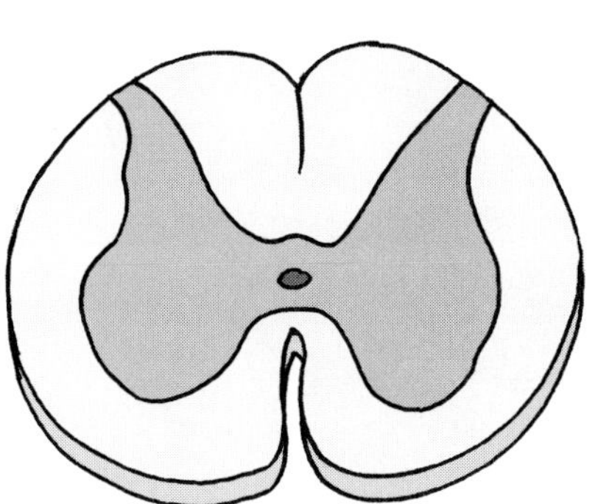

Rostral medulla

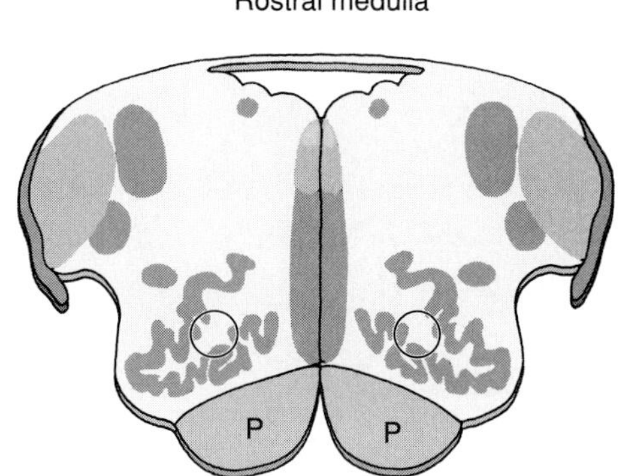

43.17A. rostrally; midbrain

43.18A. cerebrospinal fluid; posterior; floor

43.19A. tectum; superior; inferior

43.20A. medulla; central canal; anterior median fissure; brainstem (or medulla)

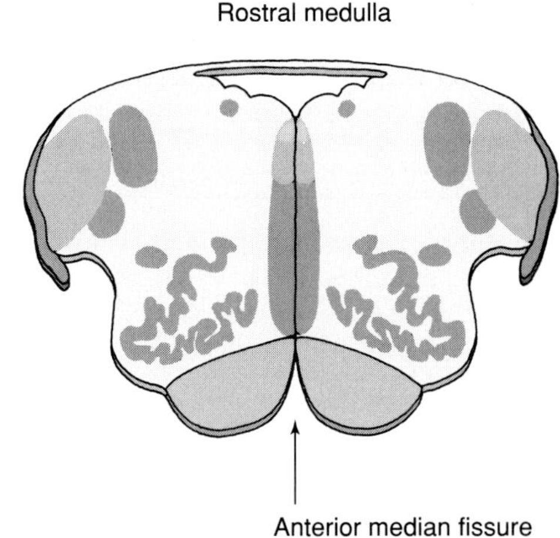

43.21A. XII; pyramid; olive

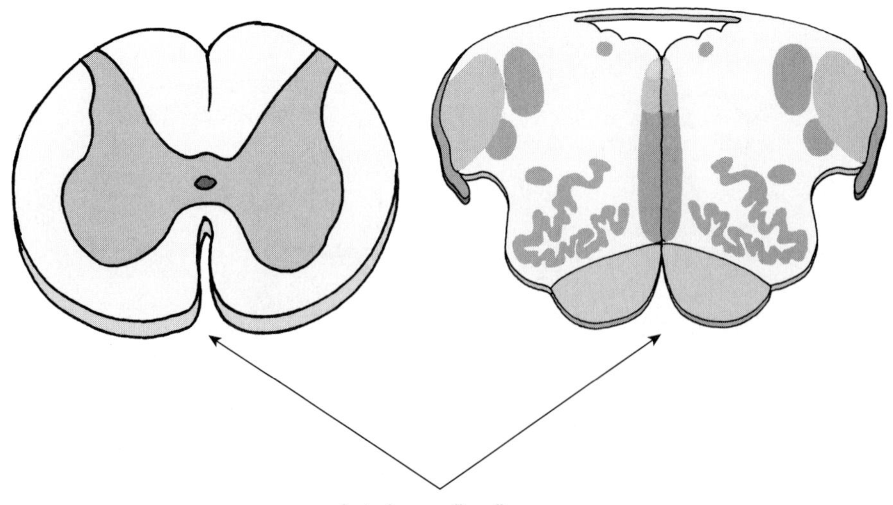

43.22. The ____________ ____________ ____________ becomes very shallow over the pons and contains the ____________ artery. The artery takes its name as it passes over the anterior-most portion of the pons, the basilar portion. The base of the pons is formed by transversally oriented fibers that form the ____________ cerebellar peduncles laterally.

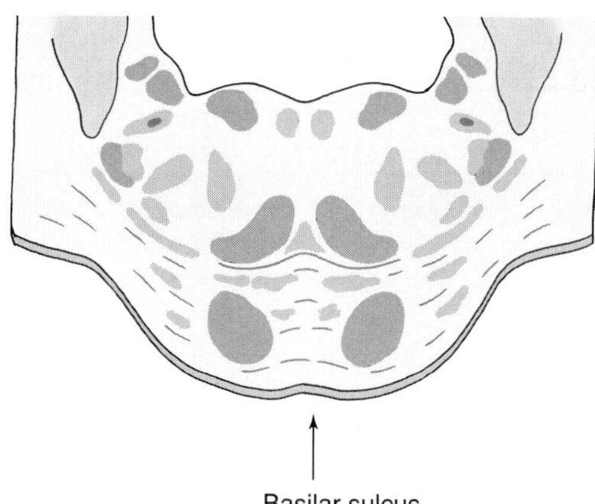

43.23. More superiorly, the shallow basilar sulcus is deepened over the anterior aspect of the ____________ to form the interpeduncular fossa; as the name indicates, this fossa separates the cerebral ____________.

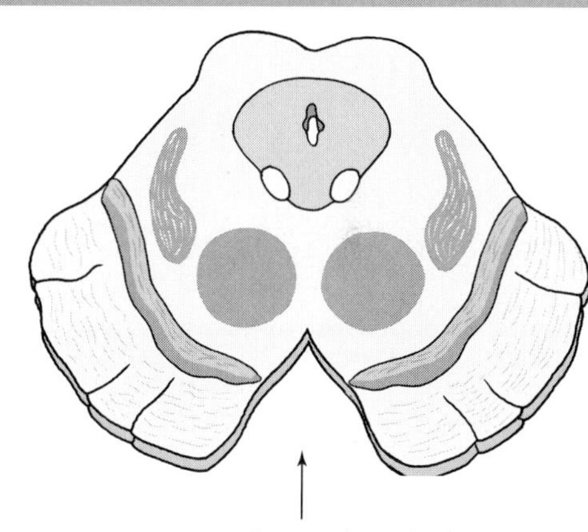

43.24. On the appropriate diagram(s), label the central canal, 4th ventricle, cerebral aqueduct, basilar sulcus, cerebral peduncles, basilar pons, olive, pyramids, anterior median fissure, and interpeduncular fossa.

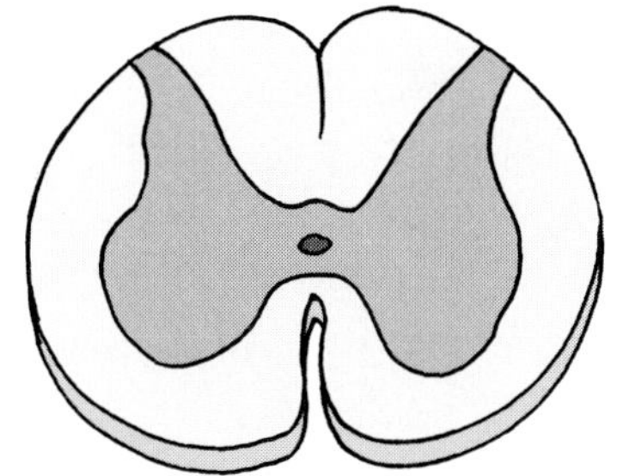

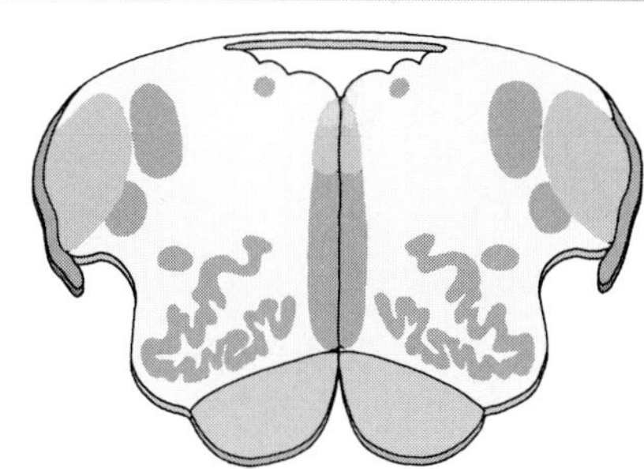

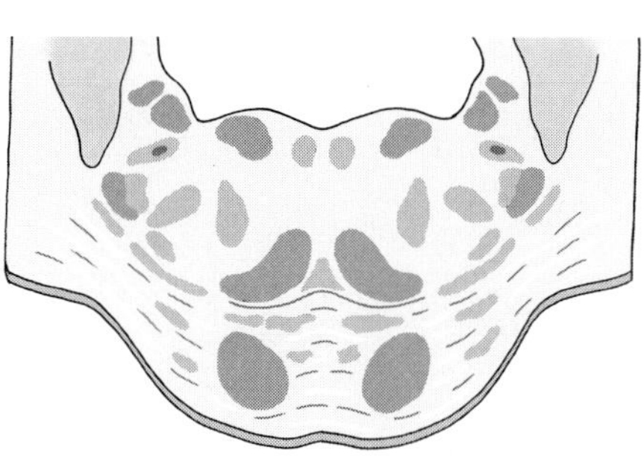

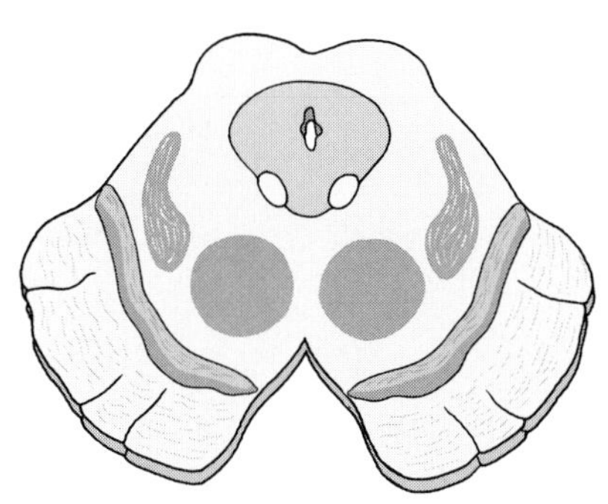

43.22A. anterior median fissure; basilar; middle

43.23A. midbrain; peduncles

43.24A.

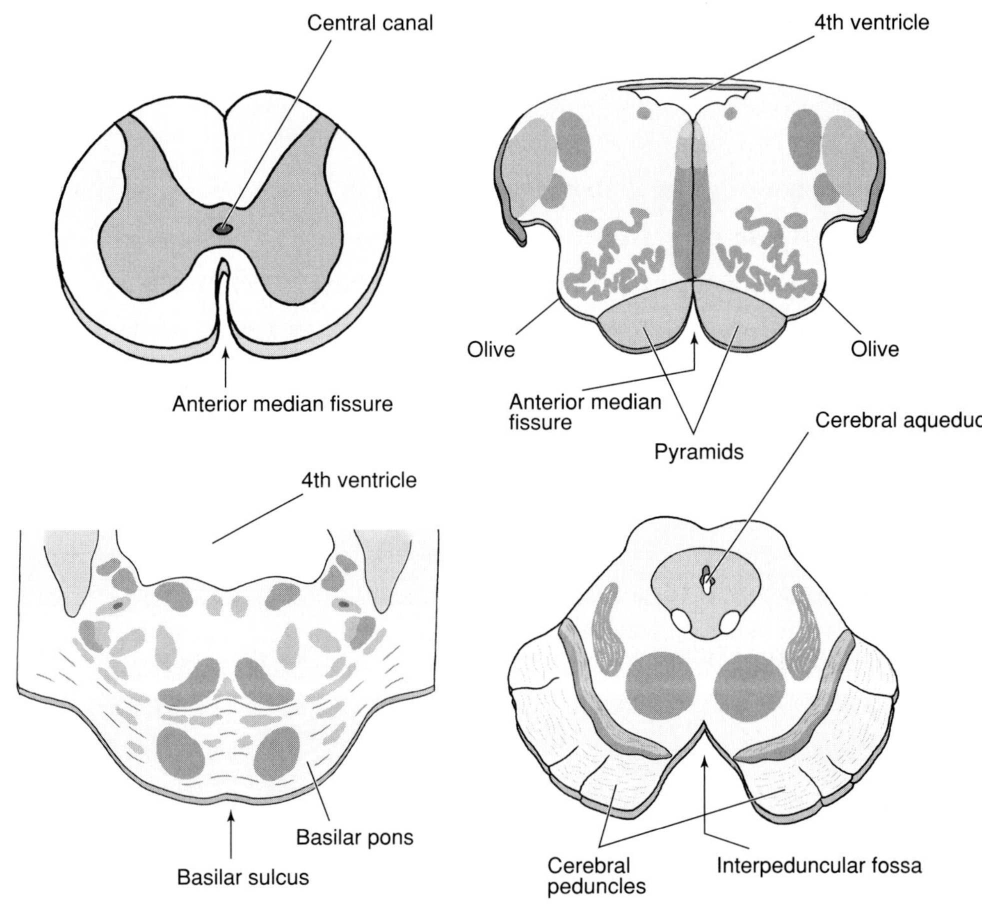

43.25. Match the structure on the left with the appropriate level/region on the right.

Cerebral peduncle: ________________ midbrain

Middle cerebellar peduncle: ________________ pons

Olive: ________________ medulla

CN XII: ________________ spinal cord

Pyramid: ________________

Basilar artery: ________________

Anterior median fissure: ________________

Fourth ventricle: ________________

Central canal: ________________

Interpeduncular fossa: ________________

43.26. The posterior median sulcus of the spinal cord can also be seen associated with the __________ aspect of the brainstem. It appears on the floor of the __________ ventricle, dividing it into two halves.

43.27. During development, neural folds come together to form a CSF-filled __________ ______. The regions more posterior to the newly formed canal are __________, while the _____ areas are located anteriorly in the spinal cord. In the brainstem, this process is incomplete. The folds do not fuse to form a central canal; rather, they remain open and form the __________ ventricle on the __________ aspect of the _____ and __________.

43.28. As a result of the lack of movement of the sensory areas to a __________ location as in the spinal cord, the sensory areas are located more __________ along the floor of the __________ ventricle, while the _____ areas remain more medially located on either side of the posterior __________ sulcus.

43.29. Along the floor of the fourth ventricle, evidence of the line dividing the _____ and __________ areas—the sulcus limitans—is seen in the form of small depressions called fovea. On the following diagram, place an M on the motor areas and an S on the sensory areas. Label the posterior median sulcus and the location of the sulcus limitans on the image.

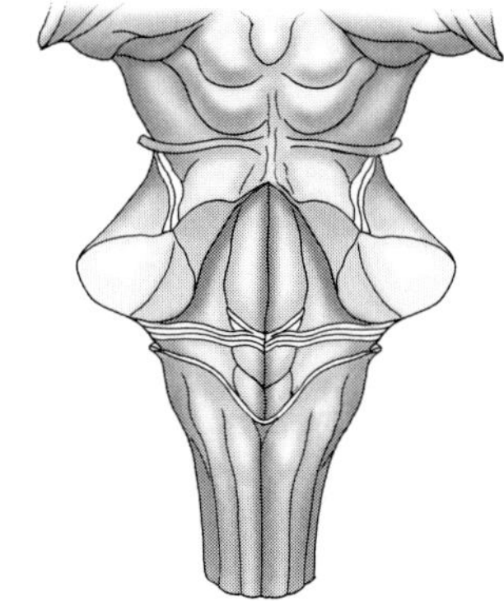

Posterior surface of the brainstem

43.25A. midbrain; pons; medulla; medulla; medulla; pons; spinal cord; pons (or medulla); spinal cord; midbrain

43.26A. posterior; fourth

43.27A. central canal; sensory; motor; fourth; posterior; pons; medulla

43.28A. posterior; laterally; fourth; motor; median

43.29A. motor; sensory

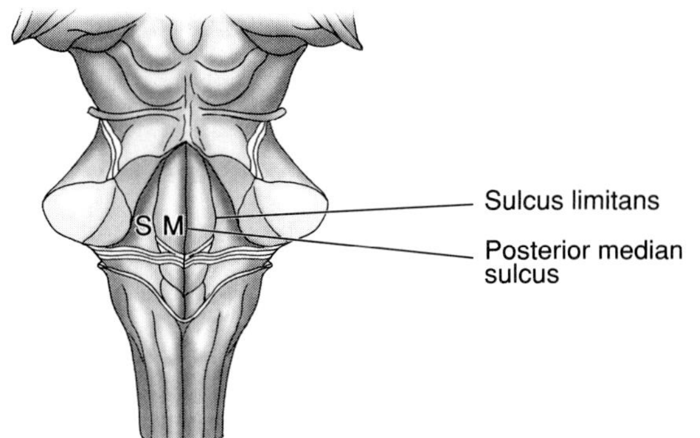

Posterior surface of the brainstem

44 Intrinsic Anatomy of the Brainstem

44.1. A useful way to study the brainstem is via cross sections. You saw many cross sections of the brainstem in the preceding chapter. Each level of the brainstem, the medulla, pons, and midbrain, has one or more "representative" cross sections. In each representative cross section, intrinsic structures can be identified. One representative cross section for each level appears below. Based on your knowledge of the external anatomy of the brainstem, label each of the three levels.

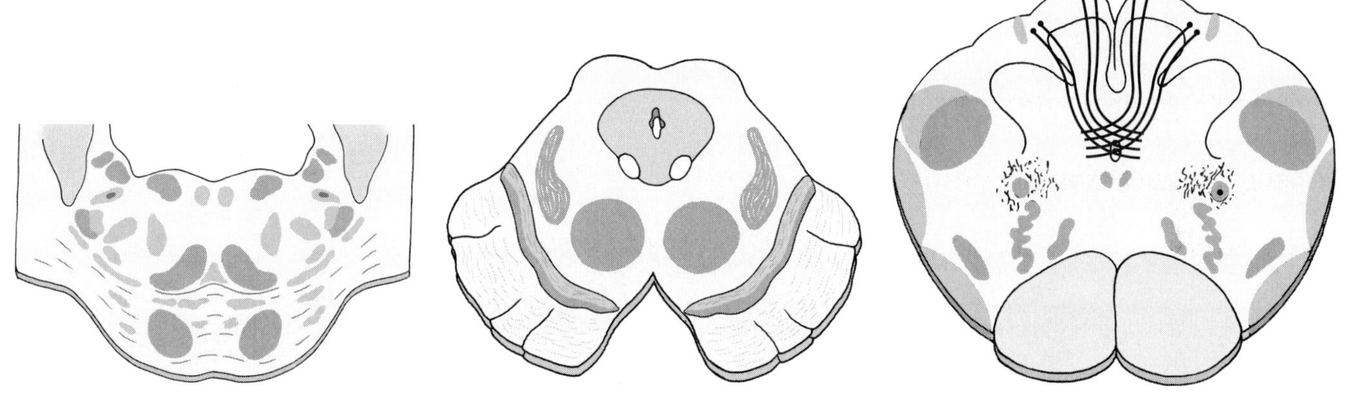

44.2. The medulla is often represented with several cross sections from top to bottom, a ______al medulla section, a middle section, and a ______al section. Based on your understanding that the ____________ medulla has the most in common with the spinal cord and the rostral medulla has the least in common, label each of the three sections below.

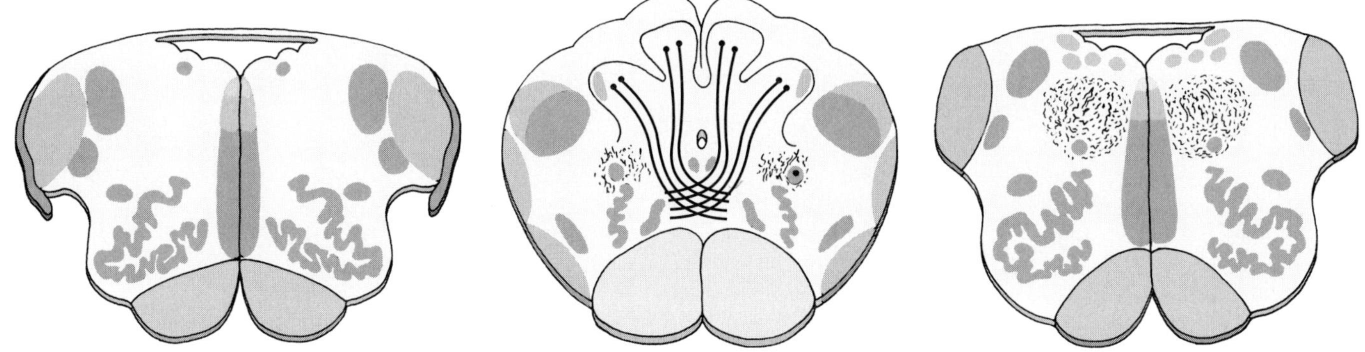

44.1A.

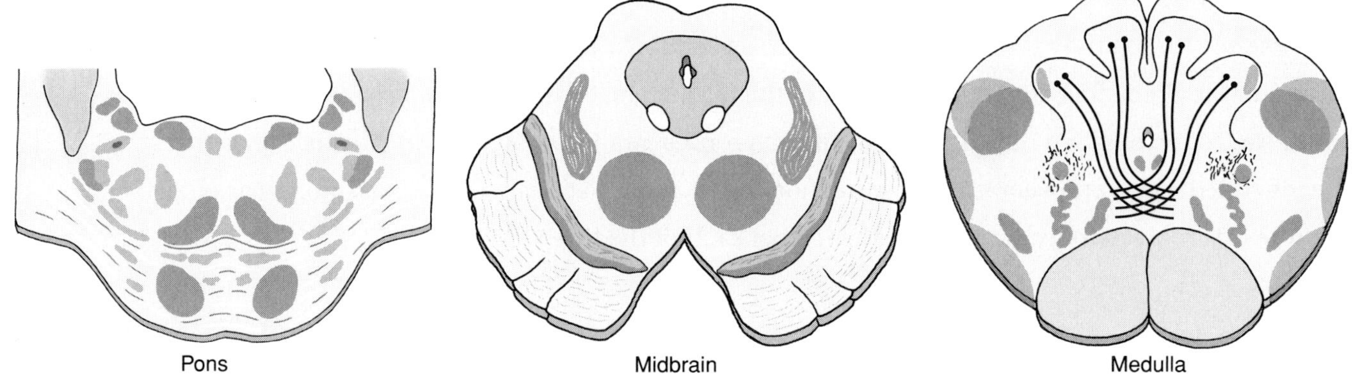

44.2A. rostral; caudal; caudal

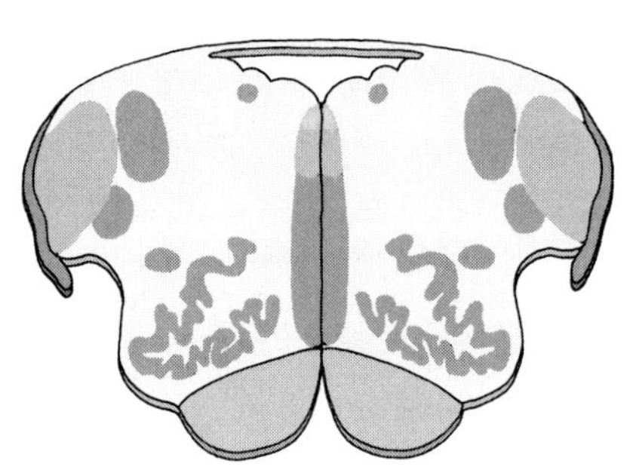

Rostral medulla

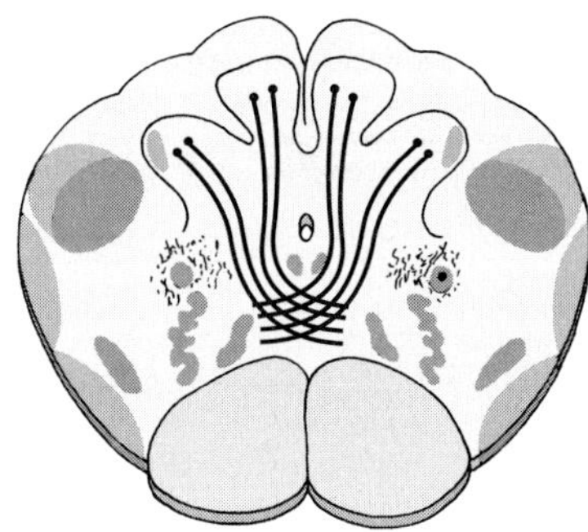

Caudal medulla

Mid - medulla

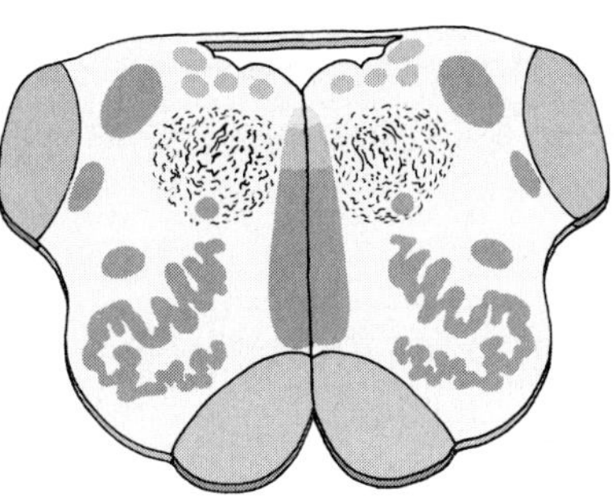

44.3. Cross sections through the medulla are easy to identify. The caudal medulla exhibits large pyramids (descending or ______ fibers) on its anterior aspect, while still possessing a CSF-filled ____________ canal, as seen in the spinal cord. Label these two structures on the diagram.

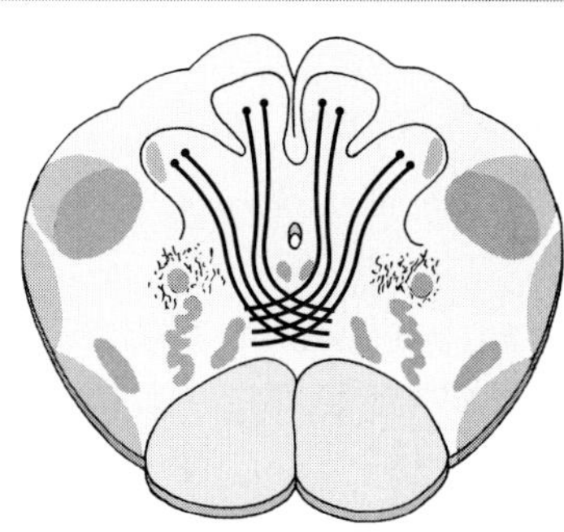

44.4. In the middle of the medulla, the central canal expands and moves ____________________ to form the 4th ventricle, and a large midline fiber bundle, the medial lemniscus, becomes evident. The medial lemniscus is made of crossed secondary fibers carrying fine touch, conscious proprioception, and vibratory sense from the ____________lateral side of the body. These modalities were carried in the ____________ columns in the spinal cord. Label the 4th ventricle and medial lemnisci on the diagram.

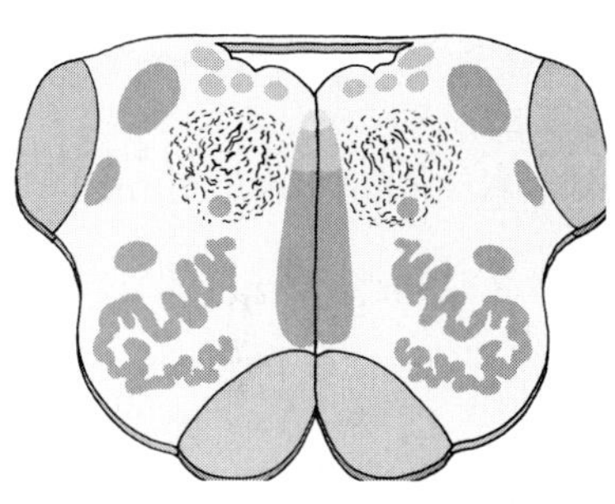

44.5. The ____________ medulla also exhibits the 4th ventricle and medial lemniscus; in addition, a prominent fiber bundle connecting it to the cerebellum appears on the lateral aspects—the inferior cerebellar peduncle. Label the 4th ventricle, medial lemniscus, and inferior cerebellar peduncle on the diagram.

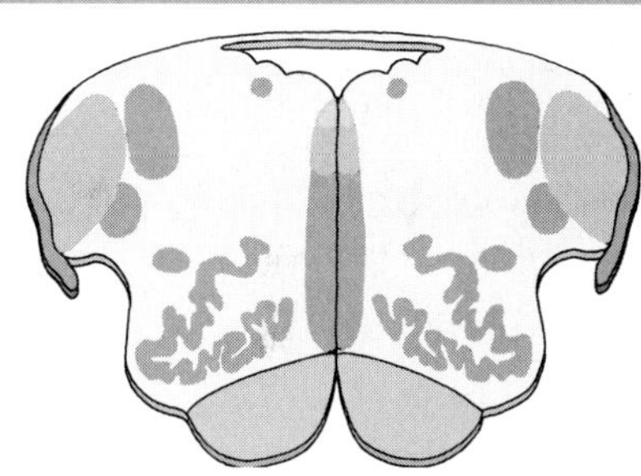

44.6. The ______, the middle division of the brainstem, has a unique expansion of its tegmentum (anterior aspect)—the base. The base of the pons is made primarily of many transversally oriented fibers. Label the base and tegmentum of the pons on the following diagram.

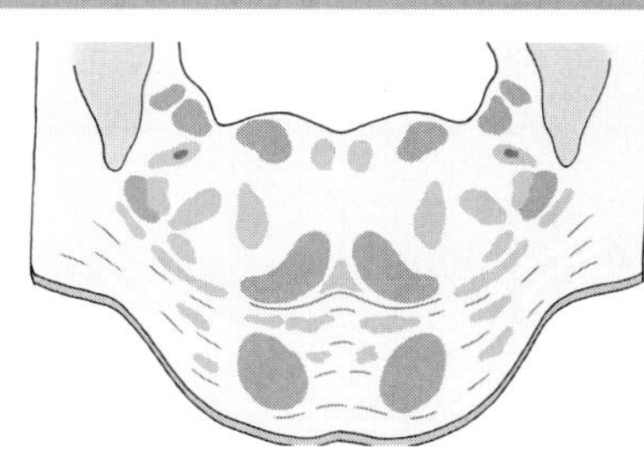

44.7. The most striking feature of the midbrain is the presence of two very large fiber masses on the ______ior aspect—the peduncles, which carry a host of ascending and descending fibers. The 4th ventricle has shrunk in size to form a CSF-filled tube, the cerebral aqueduct. Label the peduncles and the cerebral aqueduct on the diagram.

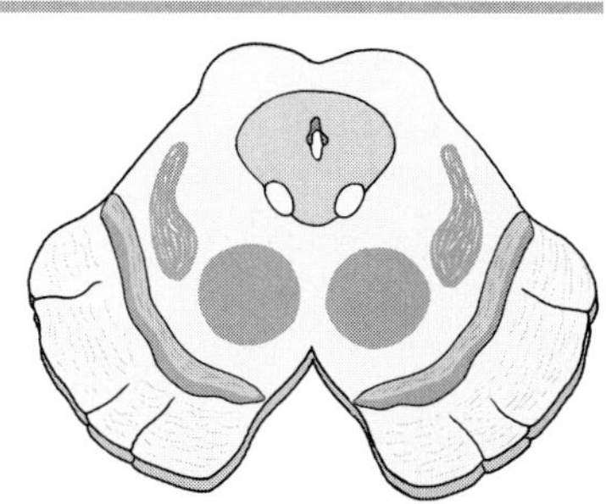

44.3A. motor; central

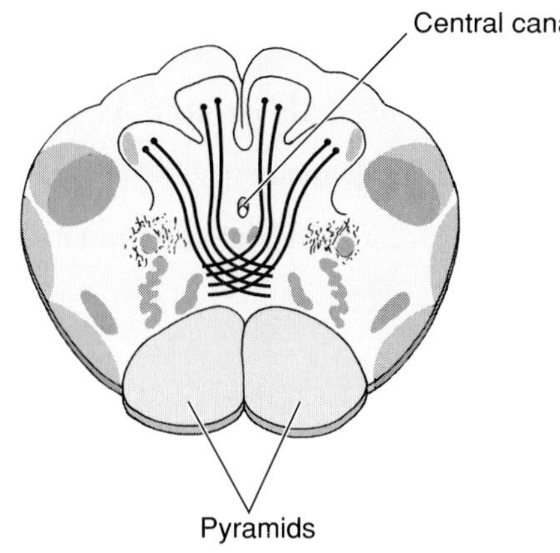

44.4A. posteriorly; contralateral; posterior

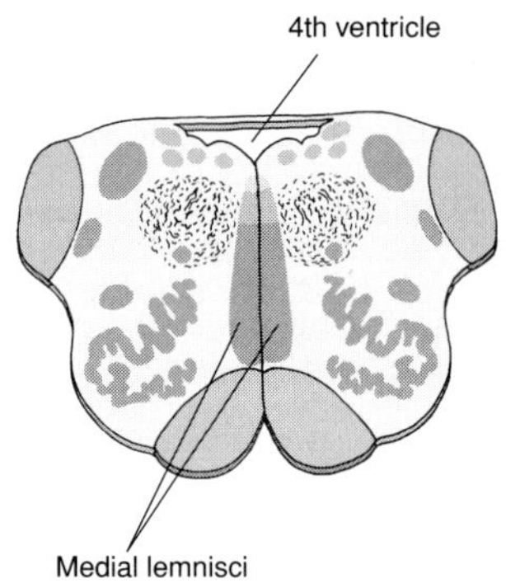

44.5A. rostral

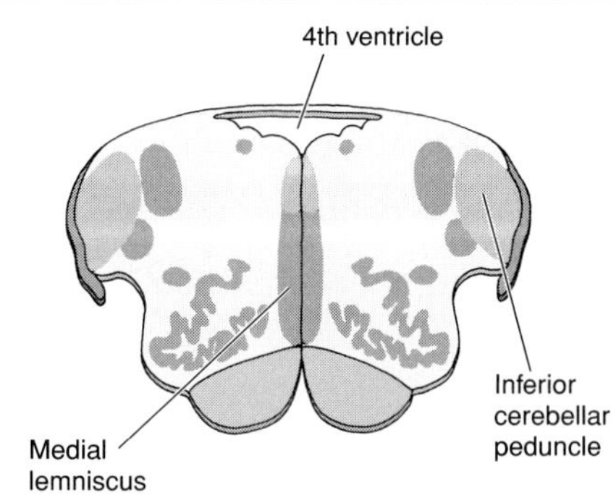

44.6A. pons

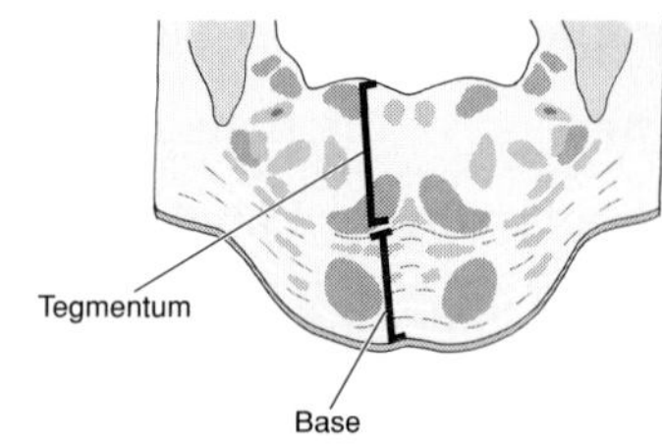

44.7A. anterior

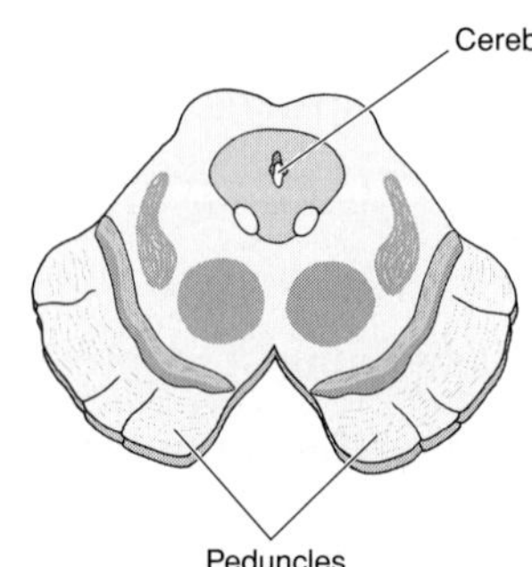

44.8. Although not necessarily exclusive to a section, the relatively unique characteristics of each section make identification of regions of the brainstem simple; in other words, certain structures are most prominent or first appear in a particular region and therefore serve as useful landmarks. For each structure listed below, identify whether it is a characteristic of the midbrain, pons, or medulla.

Peduncles: ________________

Medial longitudinal fasciculus: ________________

Inferior cerebellar peduncles: ________________

Base: ________________

Pyramids: ________________

Cerebral aqueduct: ________________

44.9. Extending the length of the brainstem, which includes the __________, ______, and __________ from superior to inferior, is the reticular formation. The __________ __________ may be conceptualized as the longitudinal core of the brainstem surrounded by tracts and nuclei in much the same way that a hot dog is surrounded by a bun.

44.10. The __________ __________ is composed of an extensive and poorly organized network of cells and fibers, which given its position in the center of the ______stem, makes it able to receive and project to a huge number of ascending (__________) and descending (______) tracts and nearby nuclei. Its position allows it to influence such things as consciousness, sleep, musculoskeletal reflexes, and the endocrine and the autonomic nervous systems.

44.11. Surrounding the reticular formation are the __________ nerve nuclei and the central pathways of their fibers as well as an extensive network of fibers "passing through" the brainstem towards more superior and inferior targets. Encircle the location of the reticular formation on the following diagrams.

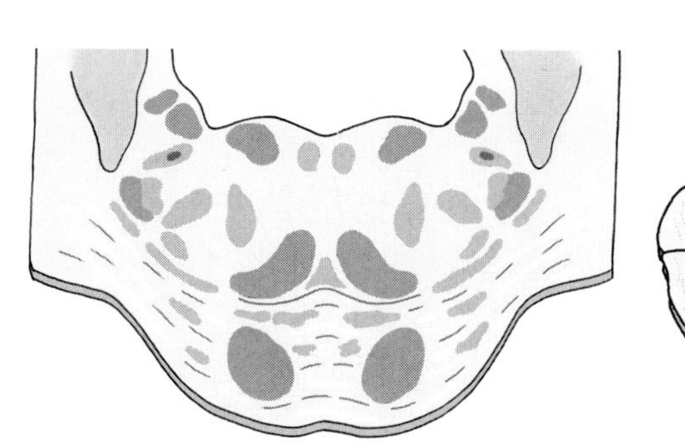
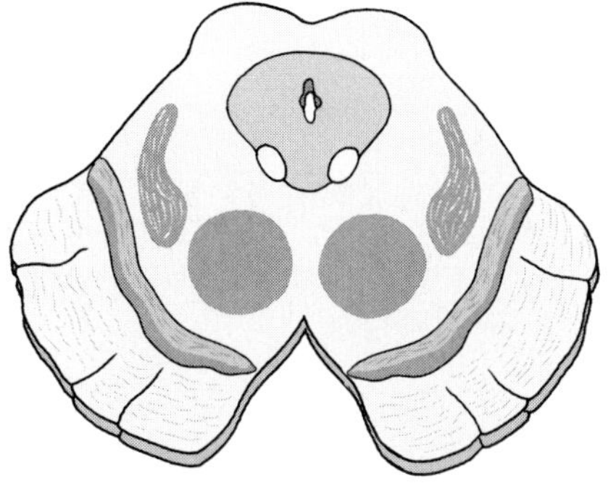
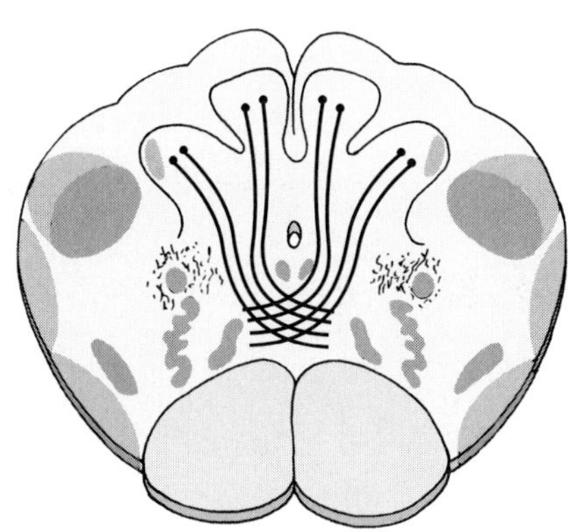

44.8A. midbrain; medulla; medulla; pons; medulla; midbrain

44.9A. midbrain; pons; medulla; reticular formation

44.10A. reticular formation; brainstem; sensory; motor

44.11A. cranial

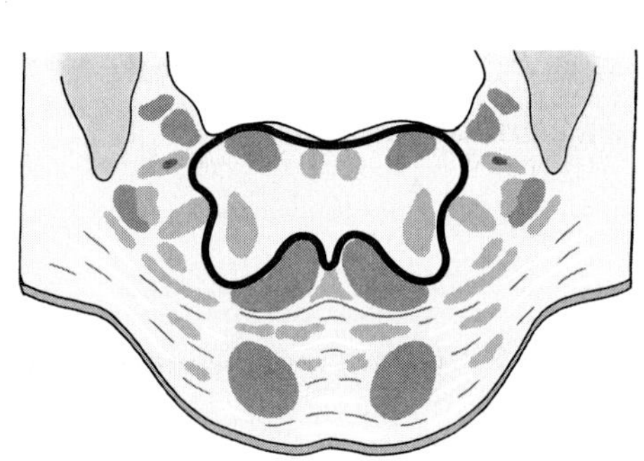

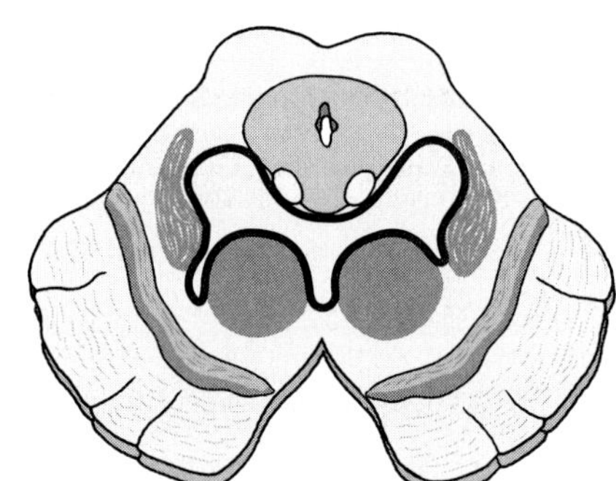

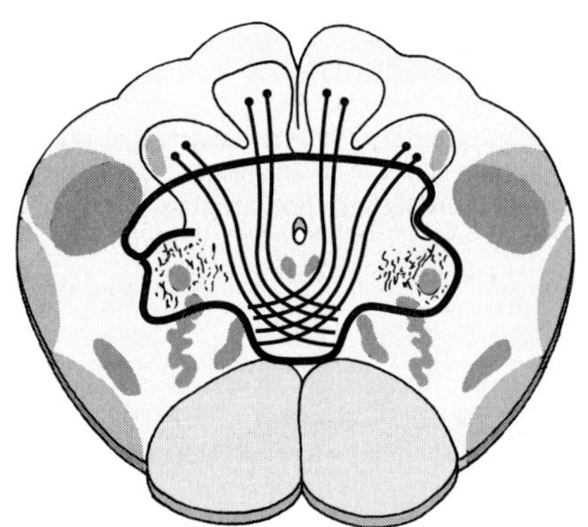

44.12. Within the ____________, the caudal-most part of the brainstem, many characteristics of the ____________ cord are still evident. Most of the ____________ horns of the spinal cord (the motor aspect) move posteriorly towards the central portion of the medulla, while the ____________ horns (sensation for the body) move laterally to become associated with the trigeminal system, which mediates ____________ for the head. Label the encircled regions on the section to indicate if they are more likely motor areas or sensory areas.

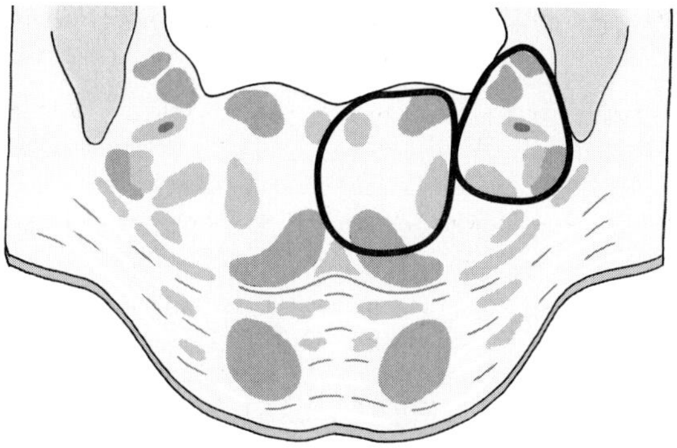

44.13. The ____________ columns, composed of the fasciculus gracilis and cuneatus, feed into their respective nuclei, the nucleus ____________ and nucleus ____________ in the medulla.

44.14. Closer to the midline in the upper sections of the medulla, there appears a pair of medial ____________. The ____________ lemniscus of each side contains ____________ary fibers mediating the dorsal column modalities from the nucleus gracilis (lower limb) and cuneatus (______ limb).

44.15. Label the encircled arcuate fibers leaving the nucleus gracilis and ____________ as they cross to form the ____________lateral ____________ ____________. Label the nucleus gracilis and cuneatus.

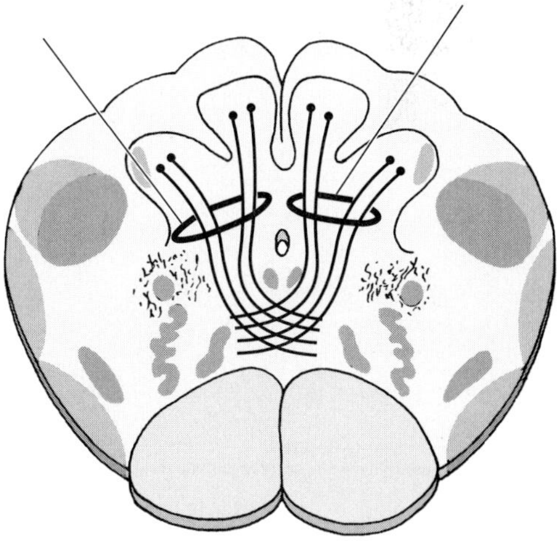

44.16. Further ____________, the middle division of the brainstem, the ______, is seen to possess a base region. The base contains a mass of crossing fibers that gives rise to the ____________ cerebellar peduncle. In addition to the crossing fibers, the base contains cell bodies—the pontine nuclei—and many ____________ing fibers on their way down to the spinal cord.

44.12A. medulla; spinal; anterior; posterior; sensation

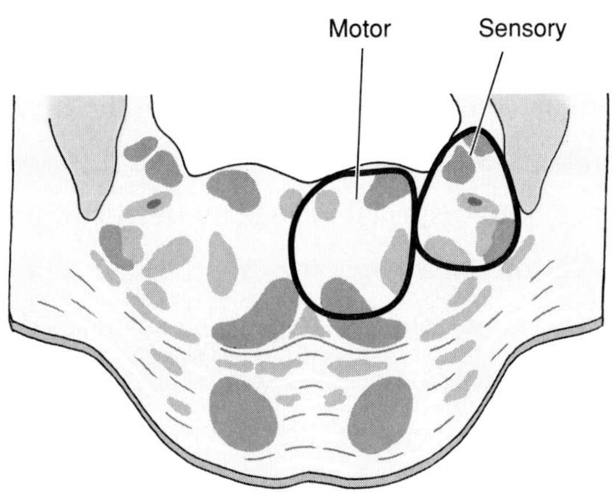

44.13A. dorsal (or posterior); gracilis; cuneatus

44.14A. lemnisci; medial; secondary; upper

44.15A. cuneatus; contralateral; medial lemniscus

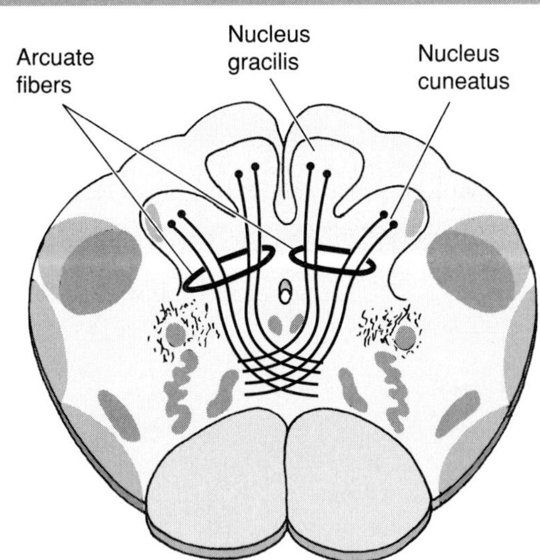

44.16A. rostrally; pons; inferior; descending

44.17. Other features of the pons are continuations of structures seen in the medulla, such as the __________ __________—the ascending fibers that began as the __________ columns of the spinal cord and other pathways passing rostrally to terminate in the __________.

44.18. From the following list of structures, circle all of the choices that are associated with the posterior or dorsal columns of the spinal cord.

Medial lemniscus

Pontine nuclei

Arcuate fibers

Inferior cerebellar peduncle

Nucleus gracilis

Pyramids

Central canal

44.19. In the midbrain, the ______ ventricle narrows to form the cerebral aqueduct. The cerebral aqueduct is surrounded by a mass of gray matter called the periaqueductal gray. The cells of the ________________ gray have a prominent role in pain modulation. Shade in the periaqueductal gray and label the cerebral aqueduct on the diagram.

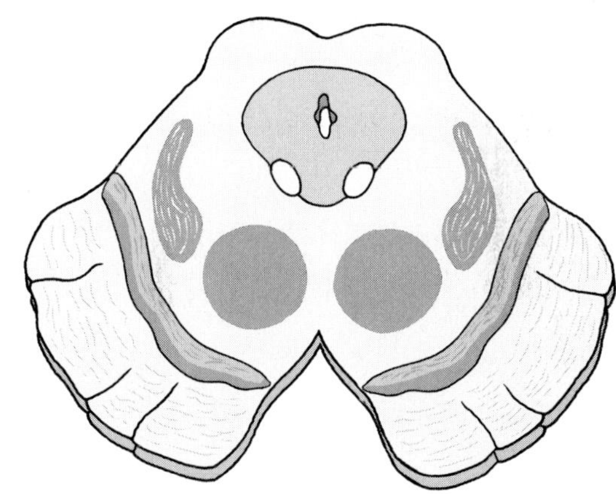

44.17A. medial lemniscus; dorsal (or posterior); thalamus

44.18A. Medial lemniscus; Arcuate fibers; Nucleus gracilis

44.19A. 4th; periaqueductal

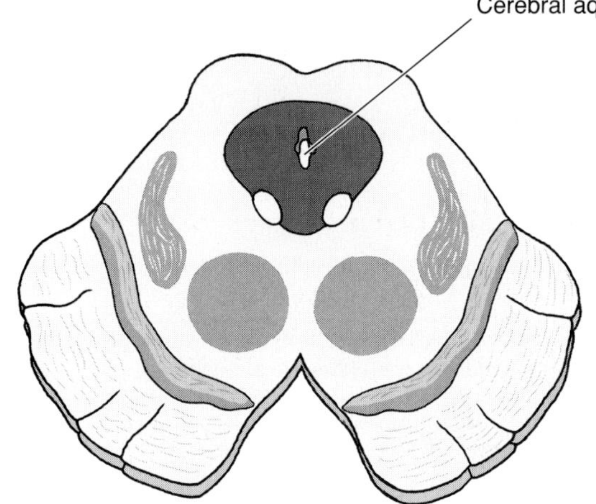

45 Blood Supply to the Brainstem

45.1. The brainstem blood supply originates in the pair of ___________ arteries that ascend through the transverse foramina of the cervical vertebrae (as the name implies). They enter the skull via the ___________ ___________, the large foramen that marks the transition from ___________ cord to brainstem.

45.2. The paired vertebral arteries merge at the pontomedullary junction to form a single basilar artery, named for its position along the ______ of the pons. The basilar artery terminates by dividing into two posterior cerebral arteries. Label the vertebral, basilar, and posterior cerebral arteries on the diagram.

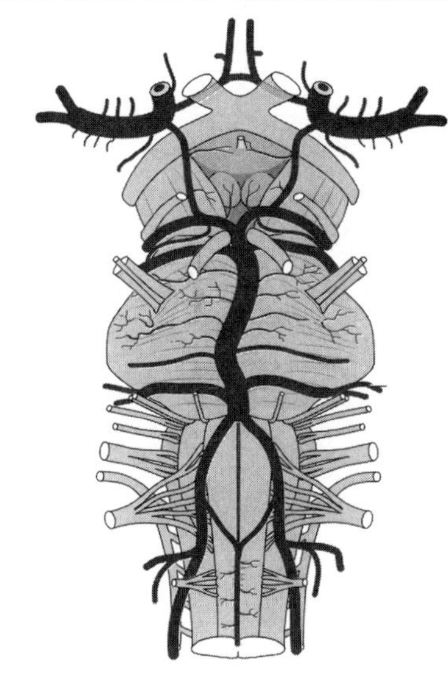

45.3. The most inferior division of the brainstem, the ___________, receives blood from multiple sources, all of which are branches of the vertebral or ___________ arteries.

45.4. The primary branches supplying blood to the medulla are the anterior and posterior spinal arteries. The ___________ spinal artery is found in the anterior median sulcus, while the pair of ___________ spinal arteries is found in the posterior lateral sulci on either side of the posterior median sulcus. Label the anterior and posterior spinal arteries, the anterior and posterior median sulci, and the posterior lateral sulci on the diagram.

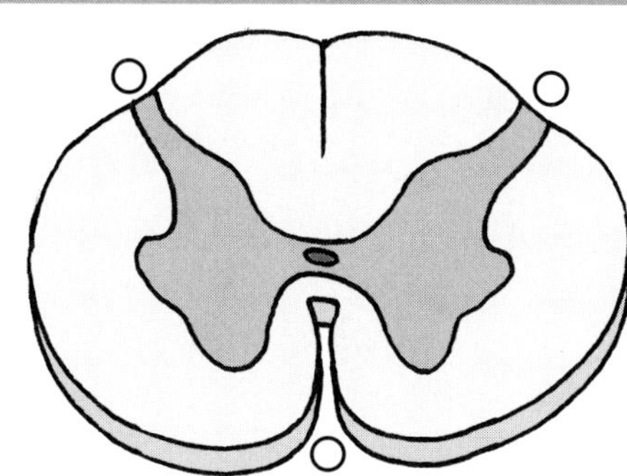

45.1A. vertebral; foramen magnum; spinal

45.2A. base

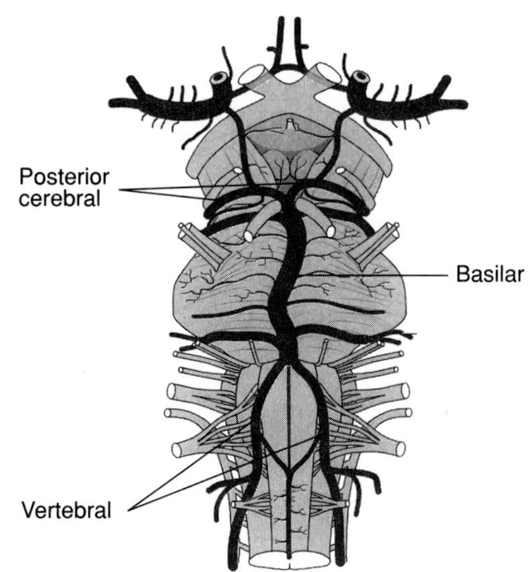

45.3A. medulla; basilar

45.4A. anterior; posterior

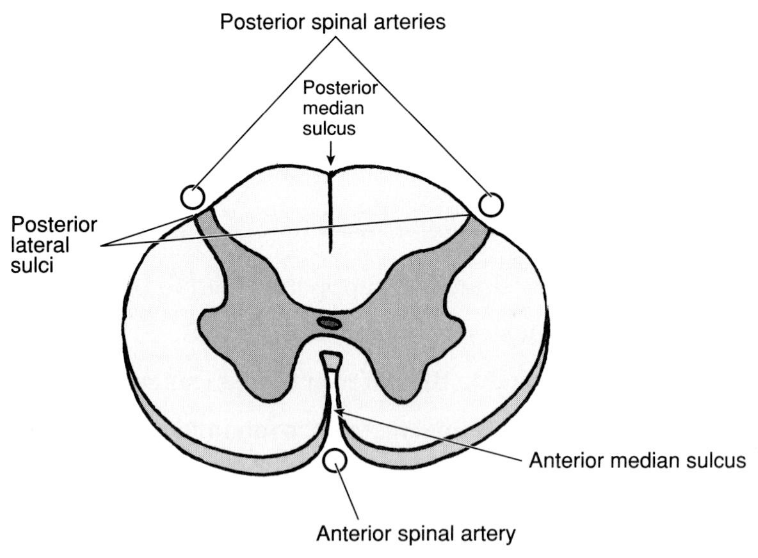

45.5. Branches of the spinal arteries penetrate the substance of the medulla, dividing it into vascular zones based on the regions they supply. These ____________ zones lead to predictable functional loss when their blood supply is compromised. The following sections illustrate the vascular zones of the medulla; circle and label the vascular zones in each section on the left side.

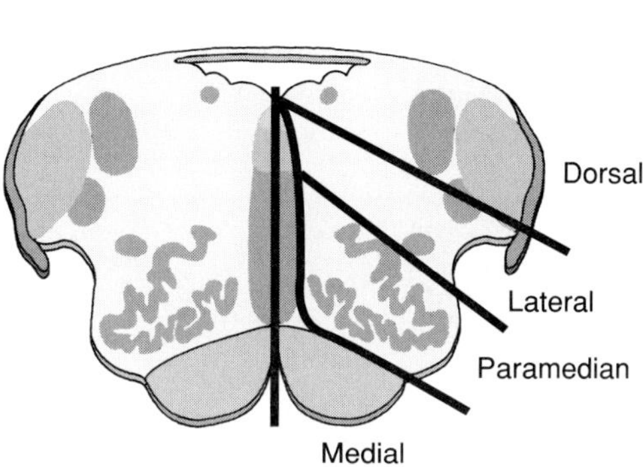

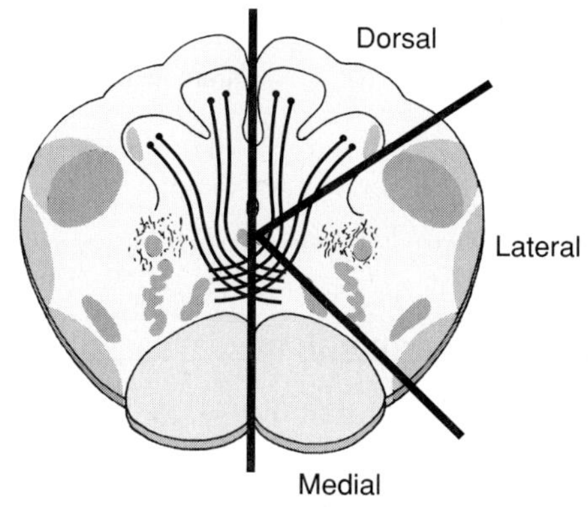

45.6. In the caudal medulla, there are three vascular zones that are all supplied by branches of the ____________ arteries. The branch to the medial vascular zone is particularly small and prone to problems. If the small artery feeding the ____________ ____________ zone becomes blocked, the ____________ and ____________ ____________ may be compromised, creating a predictable loss of motor function contralateral to the lesion (pyramid), a loss of dorsal column modalities ____________lateral to the lesion, and loss of CN XII, producing deviation of the tongue to the ______lateral side upon protrusion. Shade in the medial vascular zone on the diagram, and label the structures affected by a loss of blood and a loss of posterior column modalities on the left side of the diagram.

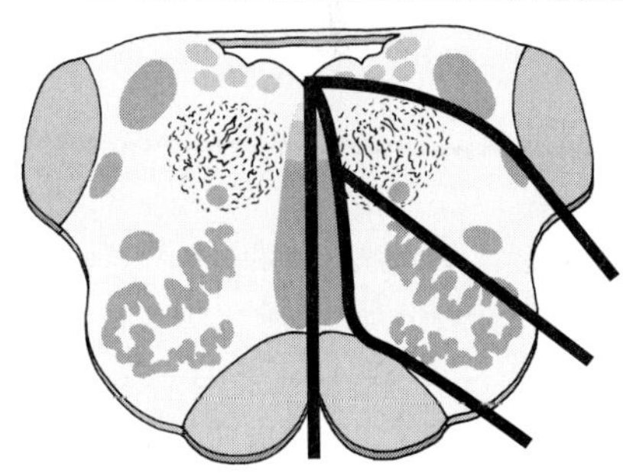

45.7. A blockage of the artery to the paramedian zone, which contains the ______, produces ______ problems.

45.8. Branches of the unpaired ____________ artery—pontine arteries—serve as the chief supply to the pons. The blood supply divides the ______ into four vascular zones. The superior cerebellar artery supplies the dorsal ____________ ______, which contains the superior cerebellar ____________, the main outflow of the cerebellum; thus, individuals with damage here suffer severe and obvious motor impairment.

45.5A. vascular

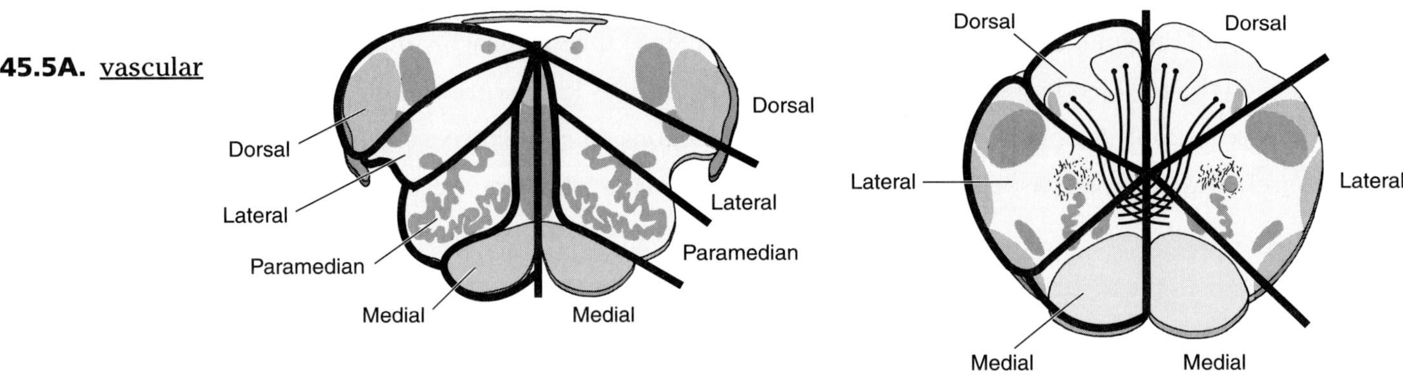

45.6A. vertebral; medial vascular; pyramid; medial lemniscus; contralateral; ipsilateral

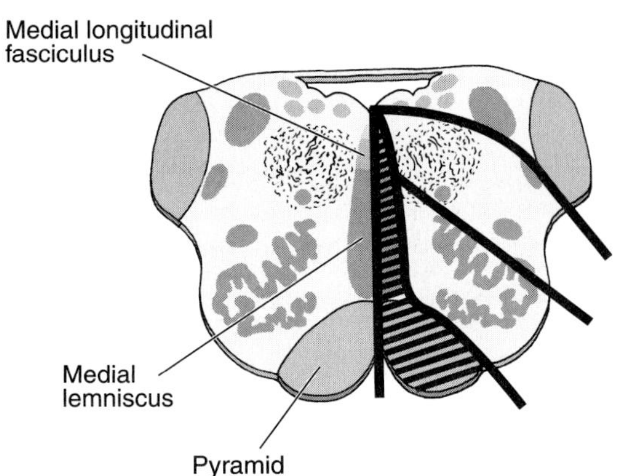

45.7A. olive; motor

45.8A. basilar; pons; vascular zone; peduncle

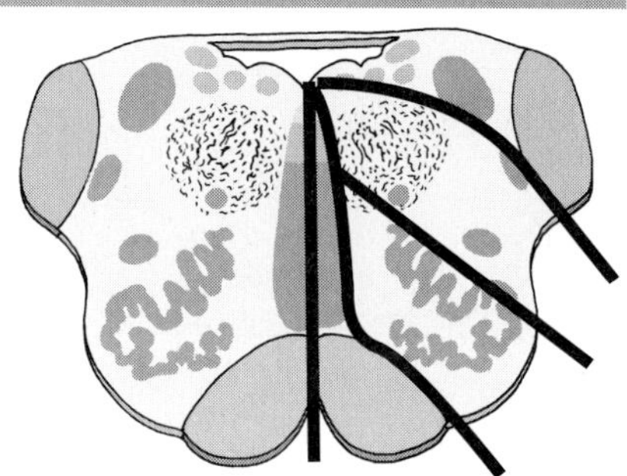

45.9. Shade in the medial vascular zone on the right side of the image, and label the structure affected by such a lesion on the left side of the image. Will the individual have sensory loss ipsilateral to the lesion? ______ Will the individual have motor loss contralateral to the lesion? ______ The medial longitudinal fasciculus is affected by this lesion; this will have an adverse affect on conjugate eye movements (coordination of the eyes as they attempt to move in concert).

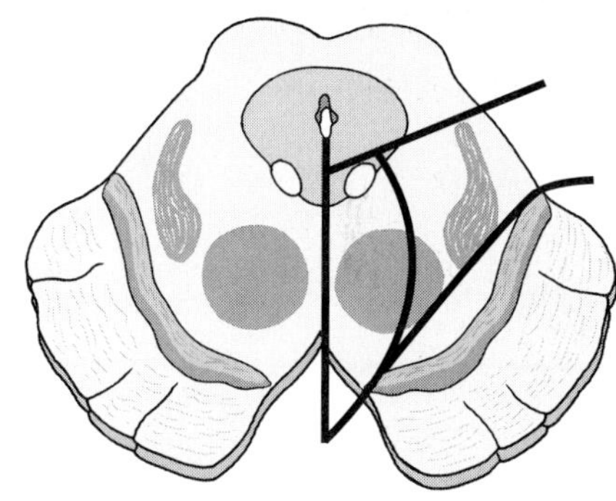

45.10. The midbrain is also divided into four vascular zones. Label them on the right side of the diagram.

45.11. The posterior inferior cerebellar artery is the primary supplier of blood to the paramedian vascular zone. Lesion of this artery has a devastating affect on the cerebral peduncles, which contain descending ______ fibers among other things. Also affected by this lesion are the substantia nigra (motor system) and the oculomotor nerve as it passes through the region. This collection of problems has been named Weber's syndrome. For each of the following structures, indicate whether the problem will be ipsilateral or contralateral for the lesion.

Extraocular muscle paralysis: ____________________

Arm paralysis: ____________________

Leg paralysis: ____________________

Chronically dilated pupil: ____________________

Drooping eyelid: ____________________

Tongue movement: ____________________

45.9A. No; Yes

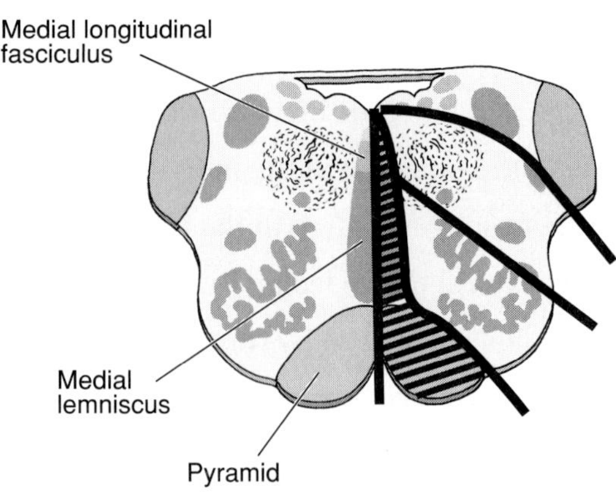

45.10A.

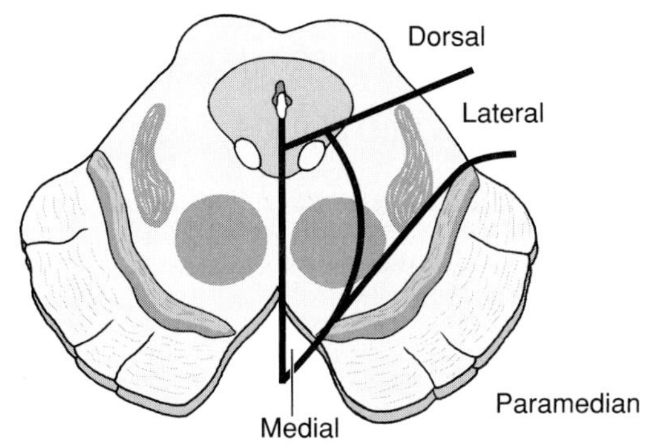

45.11A. motor; ipsilateral; contralateral; contralateral; ipsilateral; ipsilateral; ipsilateral

45.12. Label the following arteries on the diagram:

Anterior spinal
Vertebral
Basilar
Pontine
Superior cerebellar
Posterior cerebral

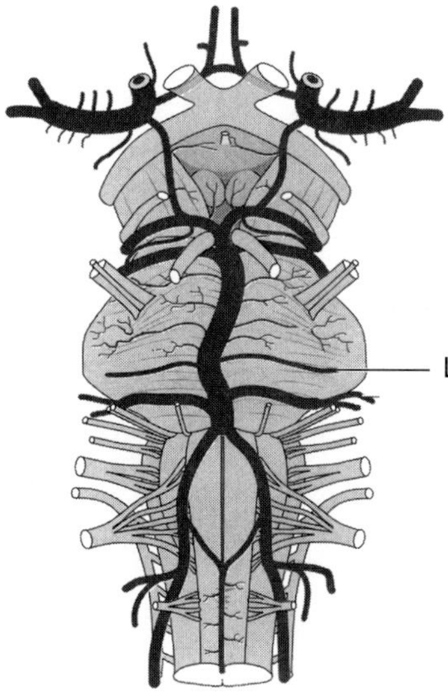

Labyrinthine

45.13. The tiny labyrinthine artery, a branch of the __________, constitutes the blood supply to the vestibular system; blockage here causes equilibrium problems and loss of balance.

45.14. For each artery listed, indicate its source—either the vertebral or basilar artery.

Pontine: __________________
Anterior spinal: __________________
Superior cerebellar: __________________
Labyrinthine: __________________
Posterior spinal: __________________

45.12A.

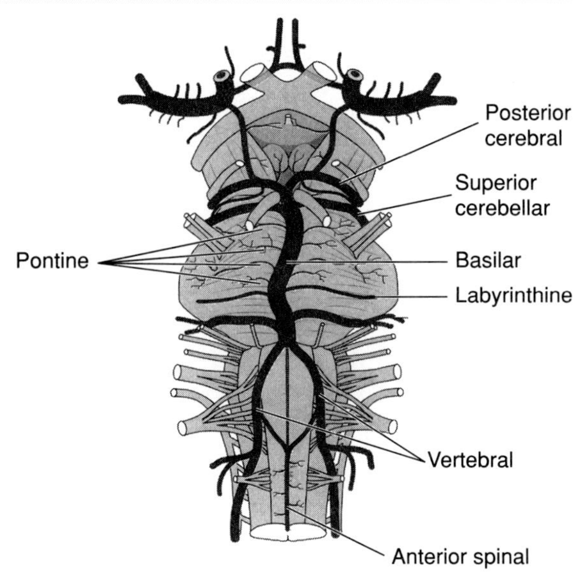

45.13A. basilar

45.14A. basilar; vertebral; basilar; basilar; vertebral

46 Brainstem: Spinocerebellar Components of the Lower Medulla

46.1. Some afferent nerves transmit impulses from skeletal *muscles* and *tendons* to the spinal cord. Skeletal muscle has both _____ferent and _____ferent innervation. Afferent impulses arising in skeletal muscles and __________ contribute to the regulation of muscle _____.

46.2. Afferent impulses influencing muscle tone in the left foot are carried along lumbar spinal nerves on the _____ side. The *primary* neuron cell bodies lie in lumbar __________ __________ on the _____ side.

46.3. The neurons drawn on the diagram convey information for the regulation of __________ _____. The afferent "message" reaches the secondary neuron from a ganglion cell neuron on the ______________ side.

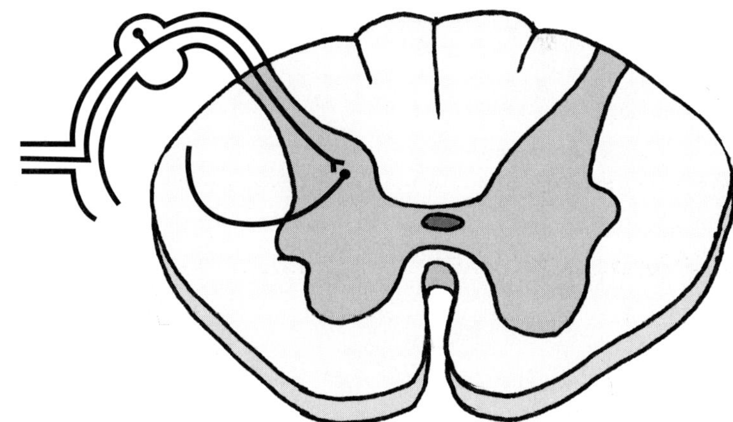

46.4. The primary neuron with endings in skeletal muscle may send branches that synapse directly with anterior horn cells to form the pathway for the *stretch reflex*. This reflex circuit is composed of only _____ neurons. Complete the afferent and efferent parts of the stretch reflex circuit on the diagram. Indicate the synapse in the anterior horn by the conventional sign (see figure).

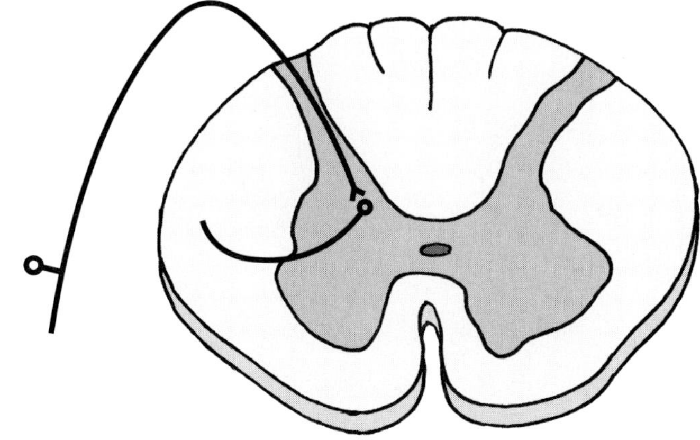

46.1A. afferent; efferent; tendons; tone

46.2A. left; spinal ganglia; left

46.3A. muscle tone; ipsilateral

46.4A. two

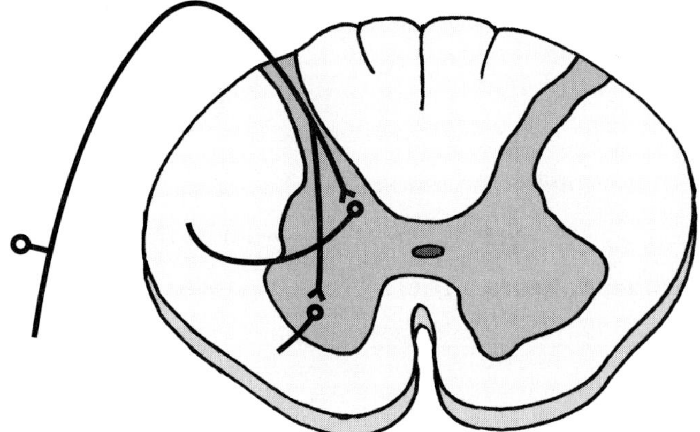

46.5. The term "dorsal," used with reference to the spinal cord of a four-legged animal, is the equivalent of the term ____________ for an upright vertebrate. In the afferent pathway influencing muscle tone, the secondary neuron cell bodies lie in the ____________ horn. Place an "X" on the right posterior horn. It receives the information from afferent neurons with endings in ____________ and ____________. Axons of the secondary neurons in this pathway enter the ________________ tracts of the cord mainly on the ________________ side as the sensory endings and terminate in the ________________.

RIGHT

46.6. Ipsilateral means *same* side; contralateral means *opposite* side. In somesthetic sensory pathways, the axon of the secondary neuron carries the message across to the ____________lateral side of the CNS. In the spinocerebellar pathway, from a given body part all the way to the cerebellum, the peripheral receptors and nerves and the secondary cell bodies and axons all lie mainly on the same or ______lateral side.

46.7. Two terms often used for the cells within the posterior horn that give rise to the spinocerebellar pathway are Clarke's nucleus/column and the nucleus dorsalis. The cell bodies with axons entering the spinocerebellar pathway are located in the ____________ horn (or ____________'s nucleus or nucleus ____________).

46.8. The term *Clarke's column* has the virtue of emphasizing that this prominent aggregate of cells in the anteromedial part of the Clarke's nucleus ____________ horn has the three-dimensional shape of an elongated *column*. In transverse section, the *column* appears as a *nucleus*.

46.5A. posterior; posterior; muscles; tendons; spinocerebellar; ipsilateral; cerebellum

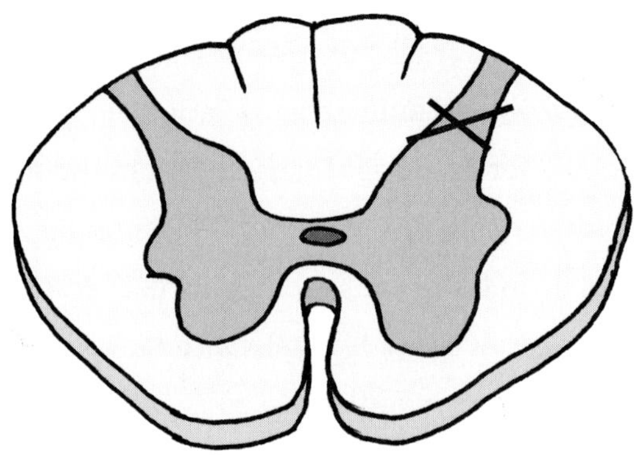

46.6A. contralateral; ipsilateral

46.7A. posterior; Clarke's; dorsalis

46.8A. posterior

46.9. The nucleus dorsalis is found at all levels of the *thoracic* spinal cord. It extends superiorly into the lowest segments of the cervical cord. Inferiorly, a few large cells typical of this nucleus are found in sections through upper lumbar levels of the spinal cord. Label the sections with "L," "C," and "T" to indicate Clarke's column at the lumbar, cervical, and thoracic levels, respectively.

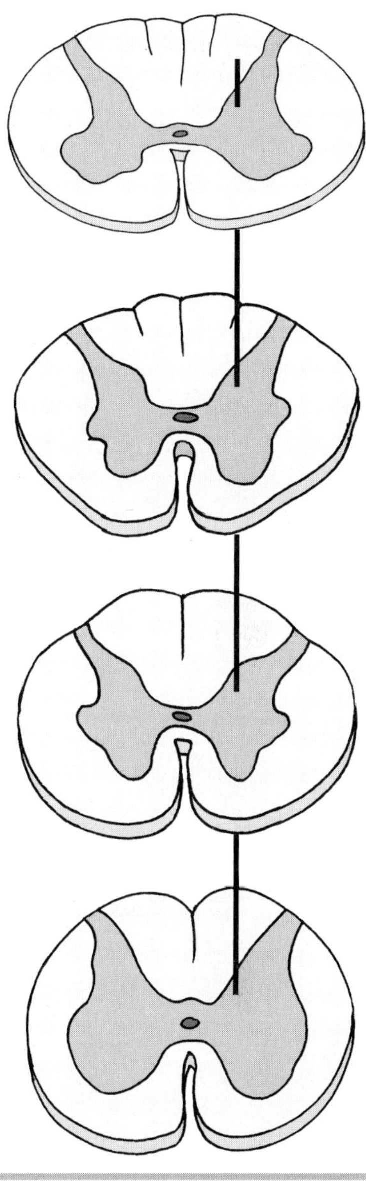

46.10. The cells of Clarke's column receive blood primarily from the __________ spinal artery, as they are located in the posterior horn.

46.11. Primary afferent neurons with endings in tendons or __________ transmit impulses across __________ to secondary neurons of the posterior horn. In order to reach these secondary neurons, which lie mainly in the __________ segments of the spinal cord, the incoming primary fibers from the *lower* limbs must ______scend before they terminate. Similar fibers from the arm must ______scend to C7, C8, and thoracic levels to synapse with neurons of the nucleus dorsalis.

46.9A.

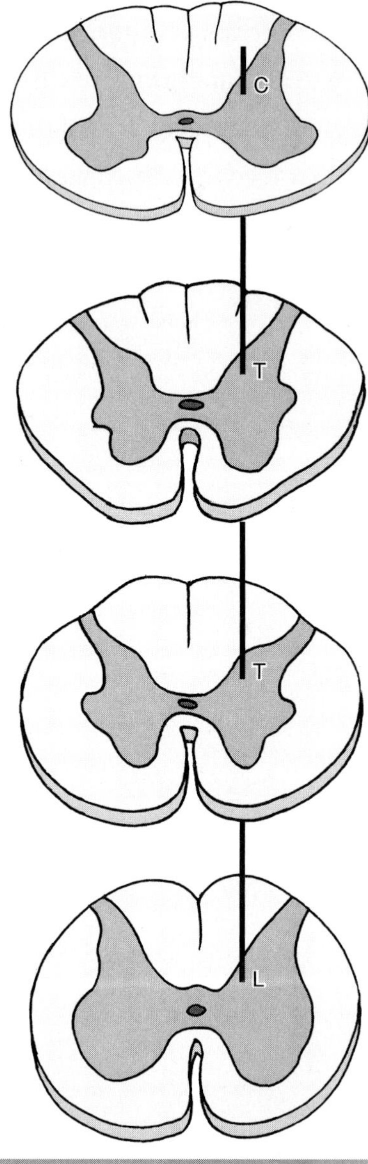

46.10A. posterior

46.11A. muscles; synapses; thoracic; ascend; descend

46.12. The nucleus dorsalis receives impulses transmitted by lumbar, thoracic, and lower cervical spinal nerves. Impulses influencing muscle tone in most of the *arm* and *neck*, which are destined for the cerebellum, do not pass to secondary neurons in the nucleus dorsalis. Instead, they enter the cord via *upper* cervical nerves and *ascend* to the accessory cuneate nucleus. Draw a primary afferent fiber passing from a ganglion cell at C2 and making synaptic contact with neurons in the ipsilateral accessory cuneate nucleus.

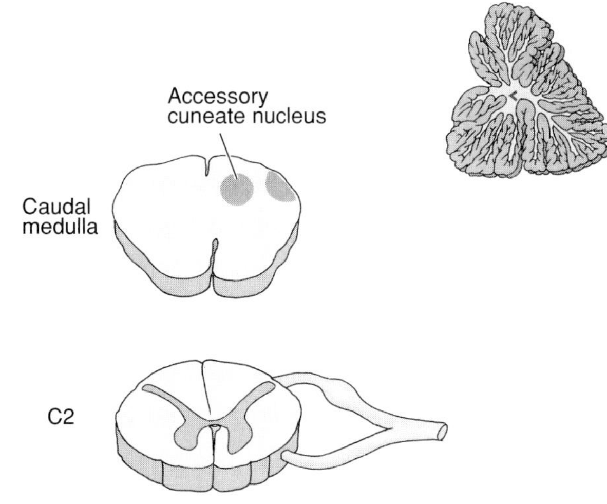

46.13. The accessory cuneate nucleus is located lateral to the nucleus cuneatus. It is seen on one side of this section. Place an "X" on the accessory cuneate nucleus.

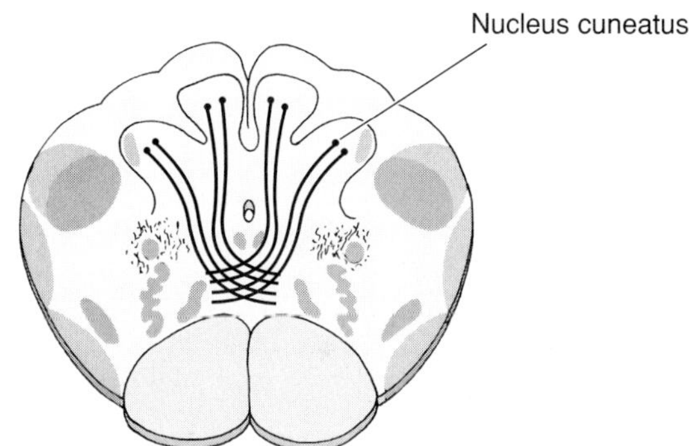

46.14. The accessory cuneate nucleus receives blood primarily from the posterior spinal artery. Label the posterior spinal artery on the diagram.

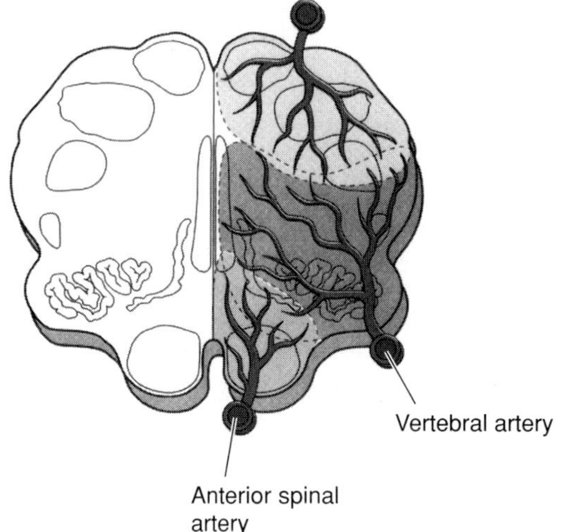

46.12A.

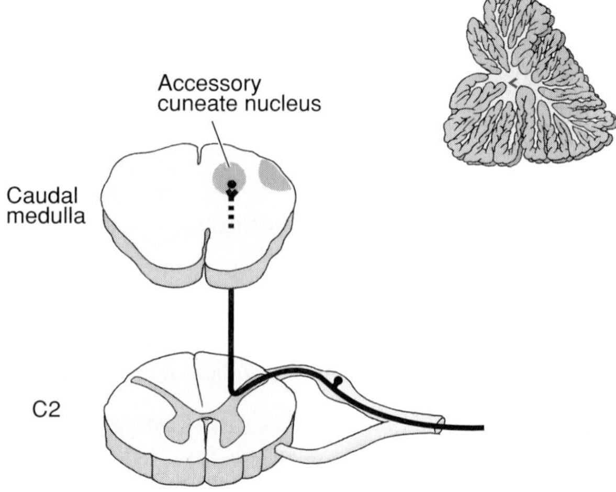

46.13A.

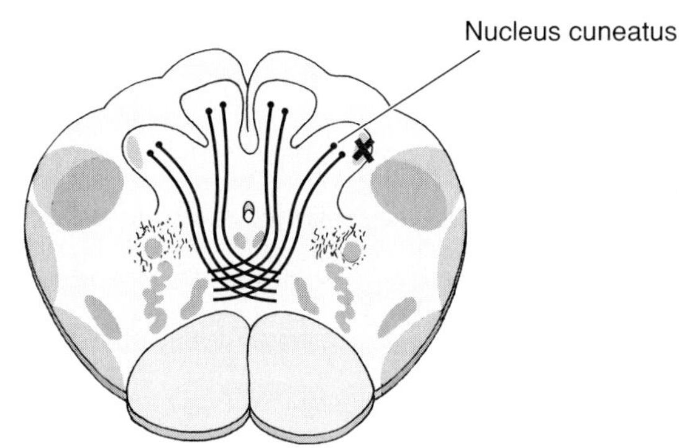

46.14A.

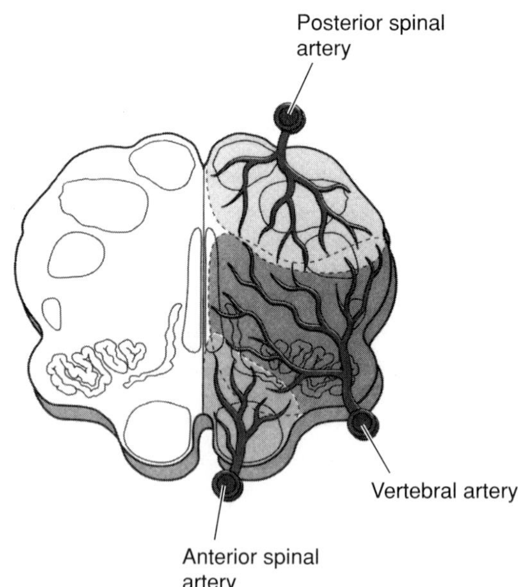

46.15. The encircled axons emerge from cell bodies in the __________ __________ nucleus and travel to the cerebellum with analogous axons of the __________________ tract.

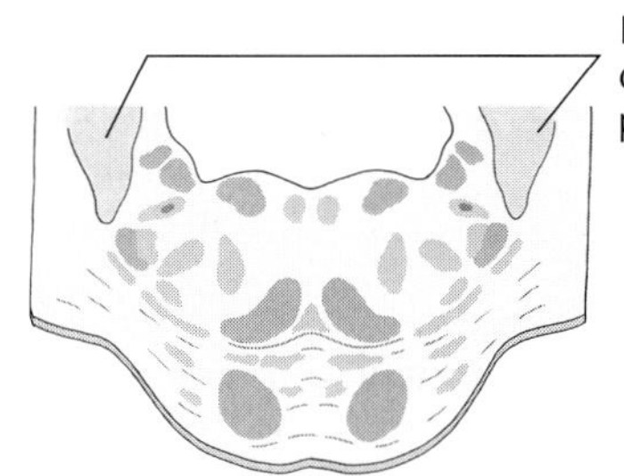

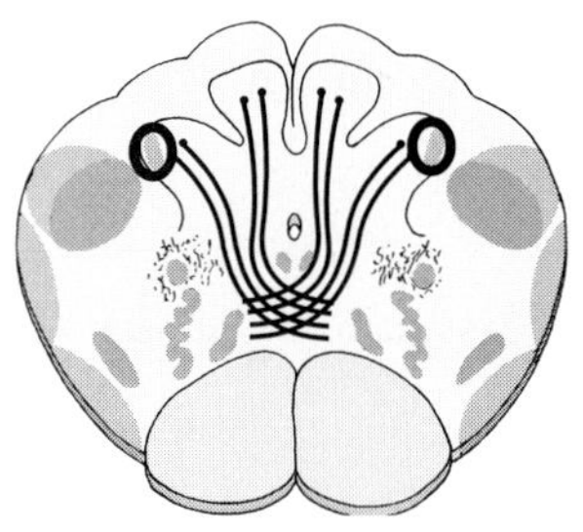

46.16. The __________ __________ nucleus relays information about tone in neck muscles just as the __________ __________ does for trunk and limb muscles. Both nuclei send impulses mainly to the ______lateral side of the cerebellum.

46.17. The two afferent fibers in the picture are ascending to the __________________. One fiber arises from a neuron in the posterior horn and transmits information arising in muscles and tendons of the trunk or the upper or lower ______. The other fiber comes from a neuron cell body in the __________ __________ nucleus and transmits information arising in muscles and tendons of the ______.

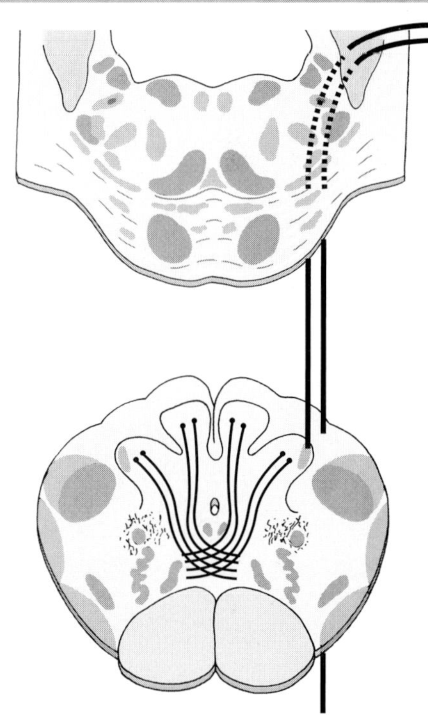

46.15A. accessory cuneate; spinocerebellar

46.16A. accessory cuneate; nucleus dorsalis; ipsilateral

46.17A. cerebellum; limbs; accessory cuneate; neck

46.18. A giraffe would be expected to have a large accessory cuneate nucleus because of the large number of primary neurons projecting from receptors located in the ___________ and ___________ of the long neck.

46.19. The more "rostral" part of the cerebellum, labeled "S," is the ______ior part. The cerebellum lies ___________ior to the brainstem.

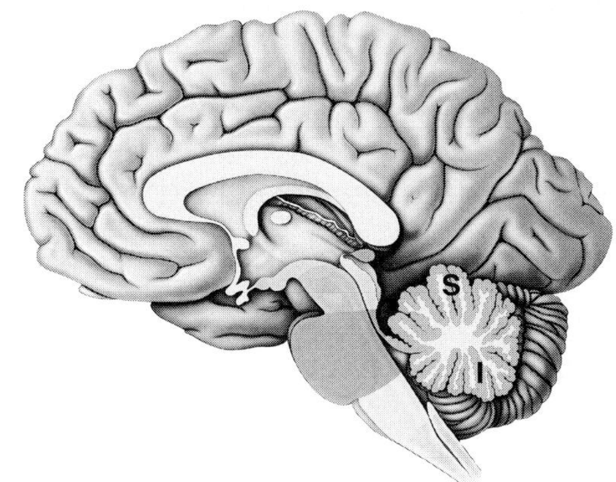

46.20. The ______ side of the head is shown in this midsagittal section. The colliculi (indicated with arrows) of the midbrain are named the left and right ___________ colliculi and the left and right ___________ colliculi.

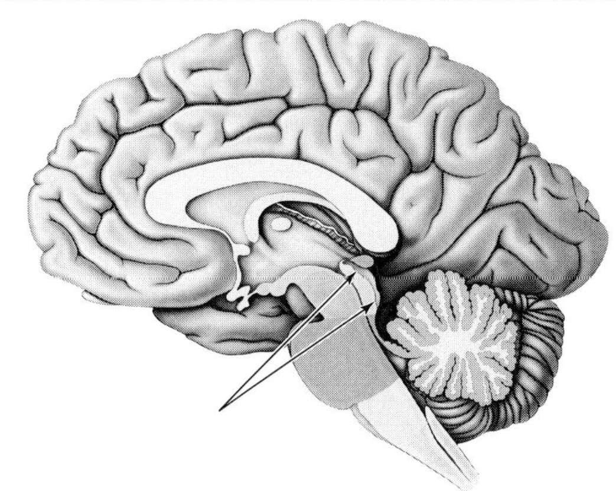

46.21. On the diagram, place an "S" on the superior part of the cerebellum, a "P" on the pons, an "SC" on the superior colliculi, and an "M" on the medulla.

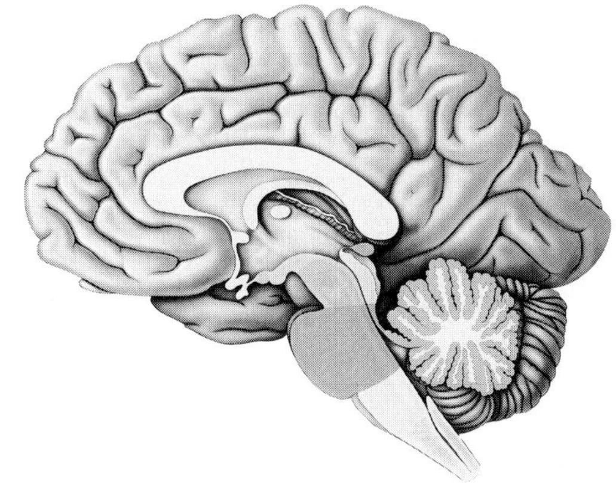

46.18A. muscles; tendons

46.19A. superior; posterior

46.20A. right; superior; inferior

46.21A.

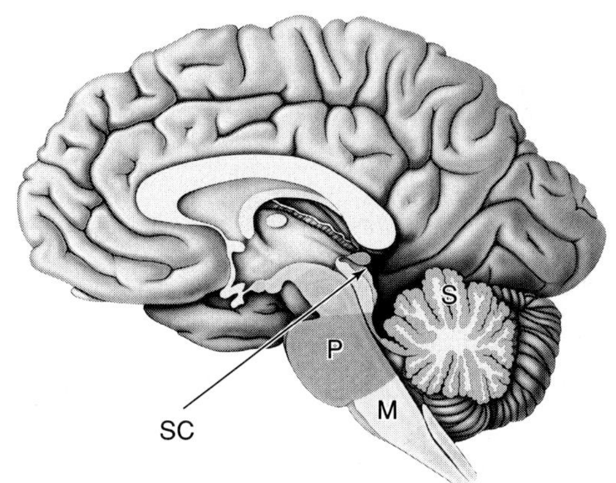

46.22. Both pictures represent the brainstem, but the cerebellum is missing from the bottom picture. On the *top* picture, encircle the four colliculi; place a "P" on the pons. On the *bottom* picture, place a "C" on the cut surface of the peduncle exposed by the removal of the cerebellum.

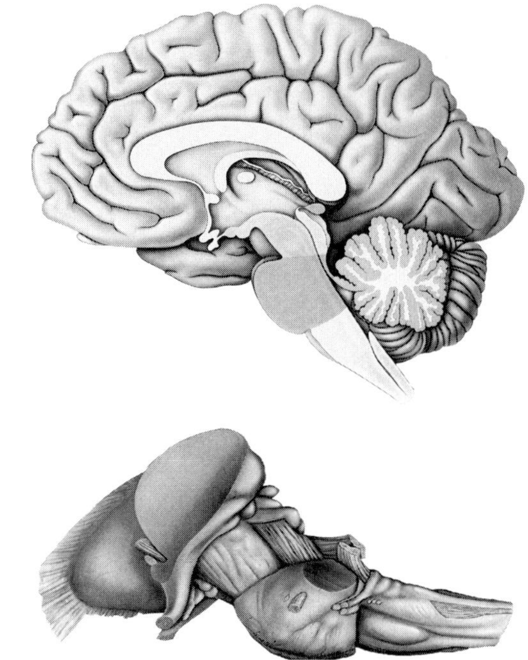

46.23. Three large bundles of fibers connect the brainstem and cerebellum; they are called the pillars or *peduncles*. On the diagram, label the peduncle connecting the spinal cord and the lower medulla to the cerebellum.

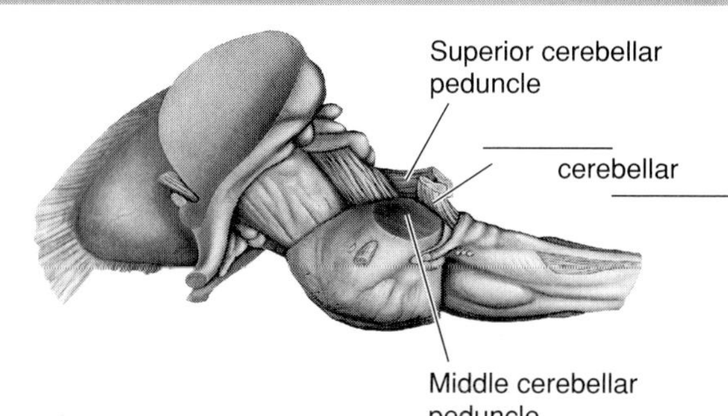

46.24. The pons and the cerebellar peduncles receive blood primarily from branches of the basilar artery. Label the pons on the diagram on the right.

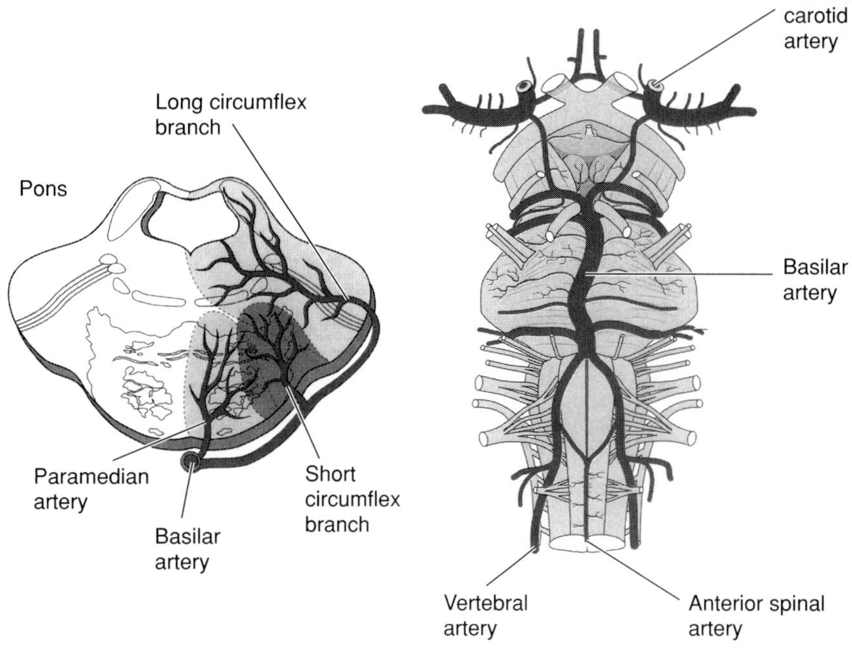

46.22A.

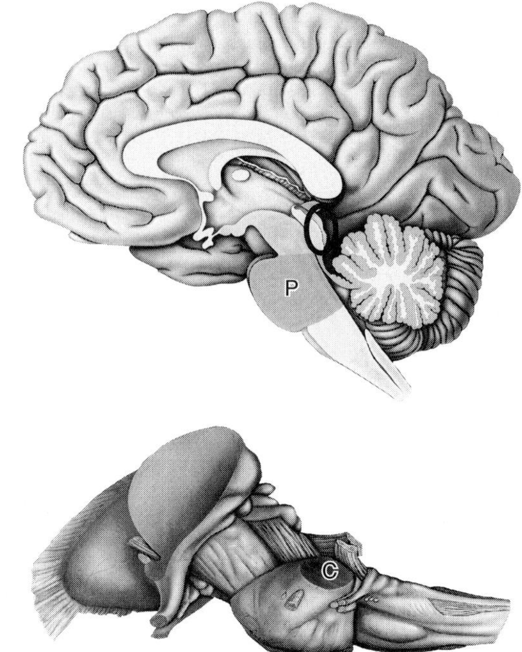

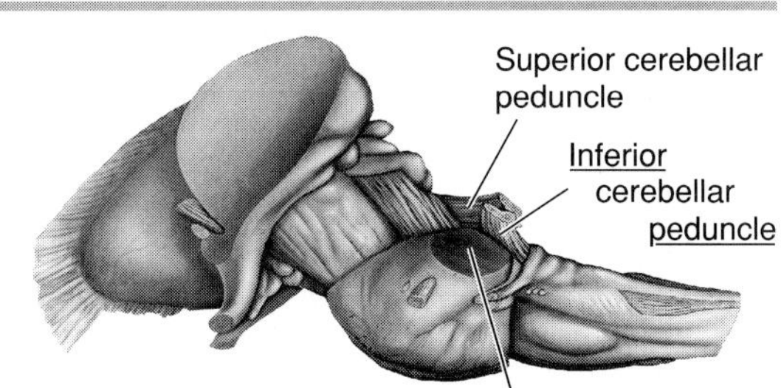

46.23A.

46.24A.

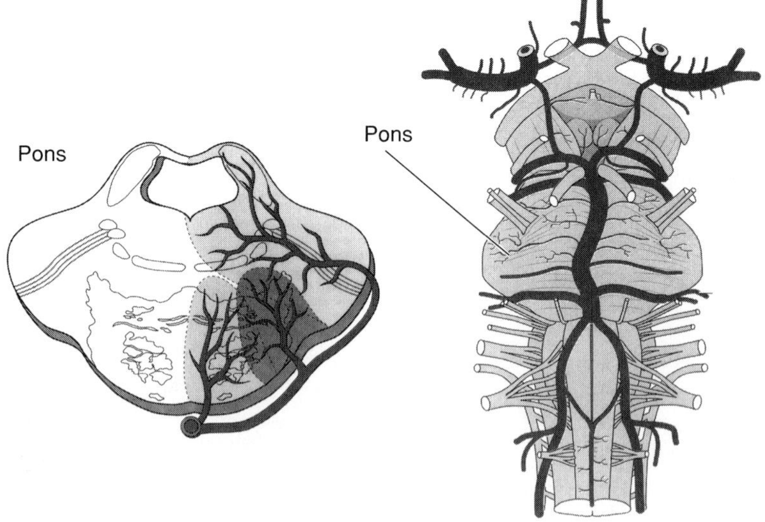

46.25. Complete the labels on the diagram.

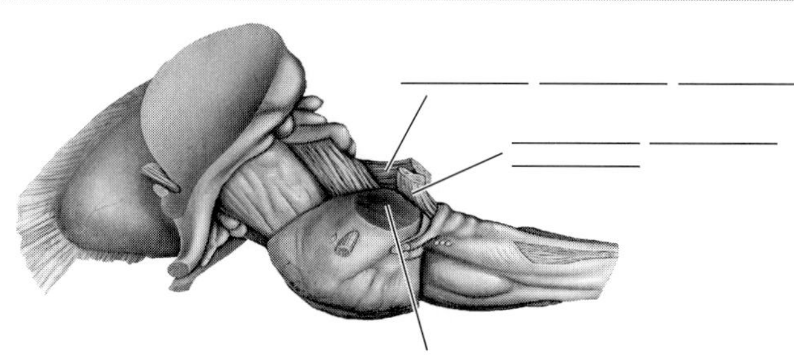

46.26. Place an "X" on the cut surface of the inferior cerebellar peduncle.

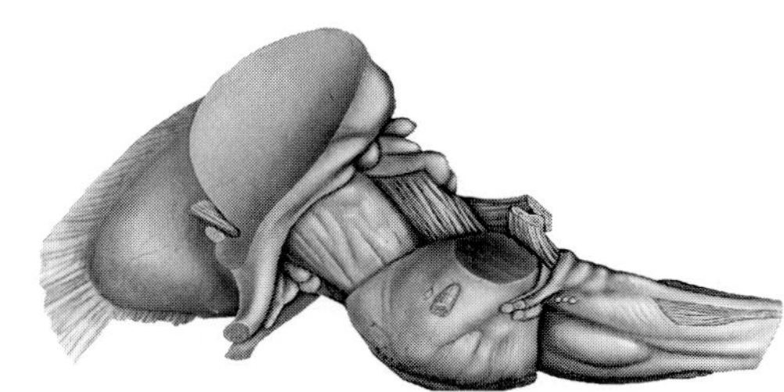

46.27. Most of the fibers in the spinocerebellar pathway come up from the spinal cord and reach the cerebellum via the ____________ cerebellar peduncle.

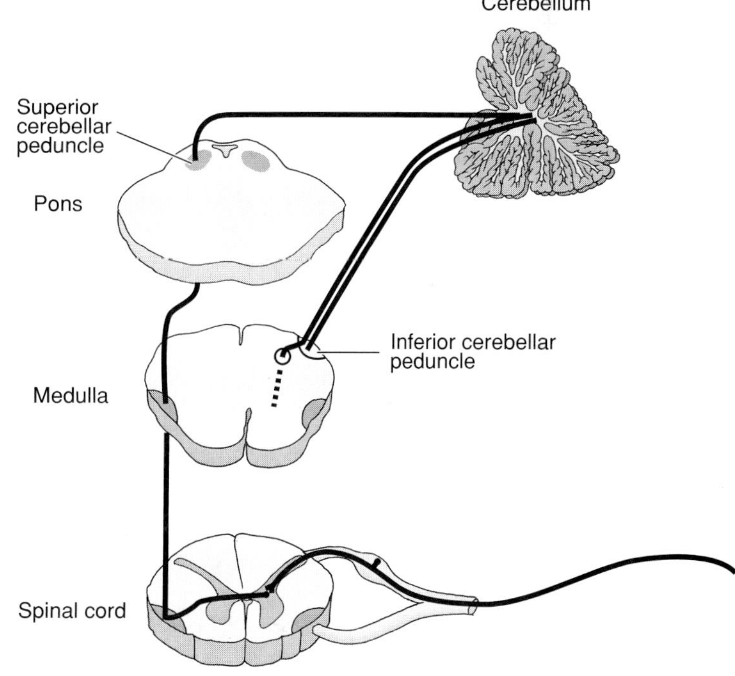

46.25A.

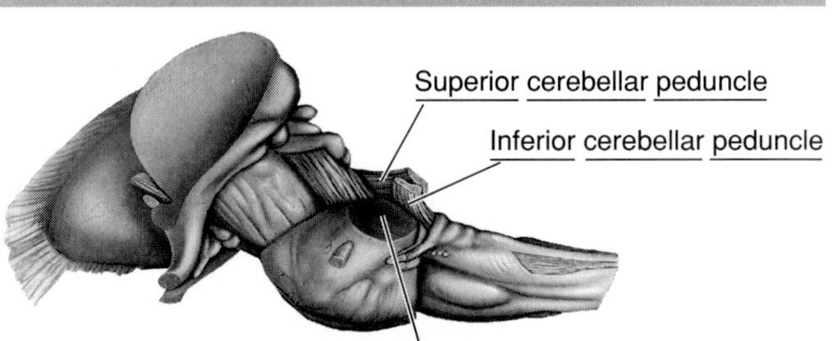

46.26A.

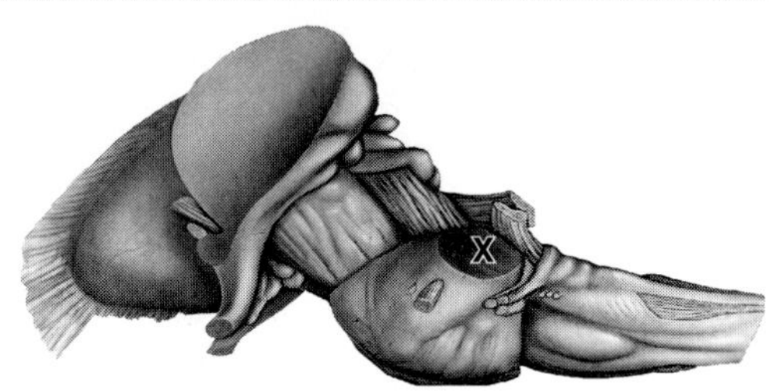

46.27A. inferior

46.28. Place an "S" in the encircled spinocerebellar tracts on both sections. Place an "A" on the encircled accessory cuneate nucleus.

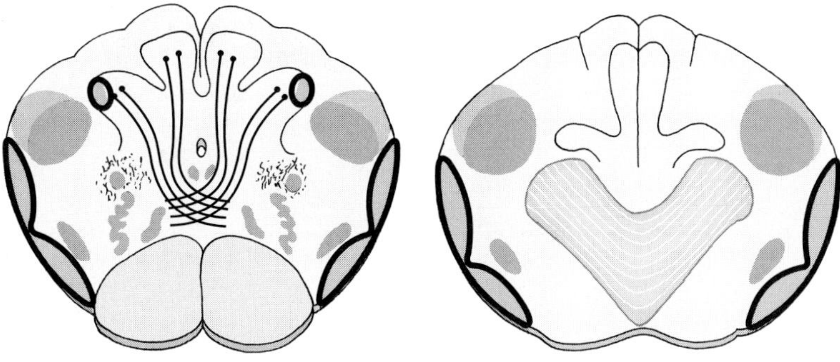

46.29. Draw a line through the sections in this picture to indicate the ascent of the right spinocerebellar tract into the cerebellum via the inferior cerebellar peduncle. Has this tract crossed the midline? ______

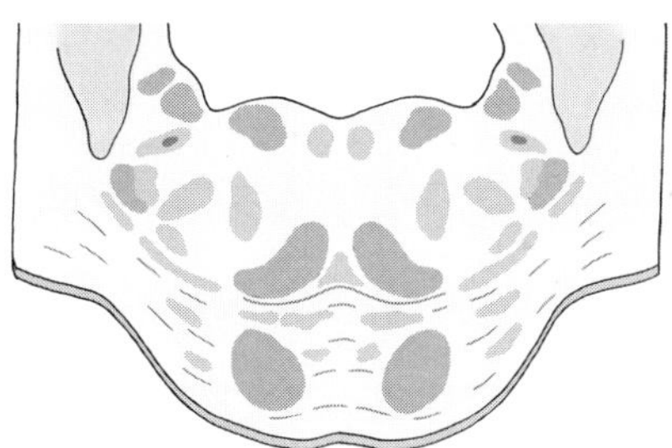

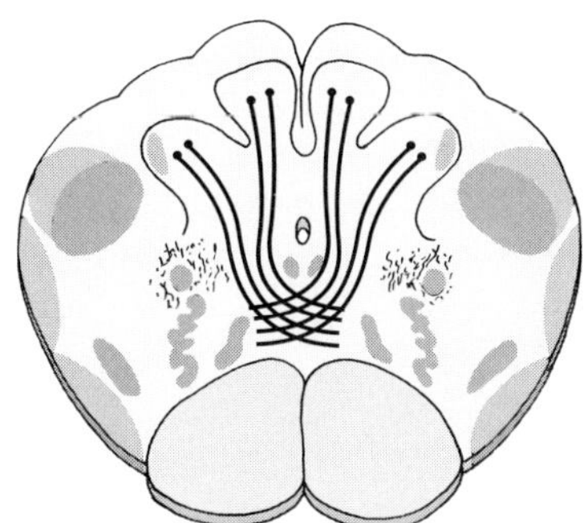

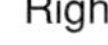

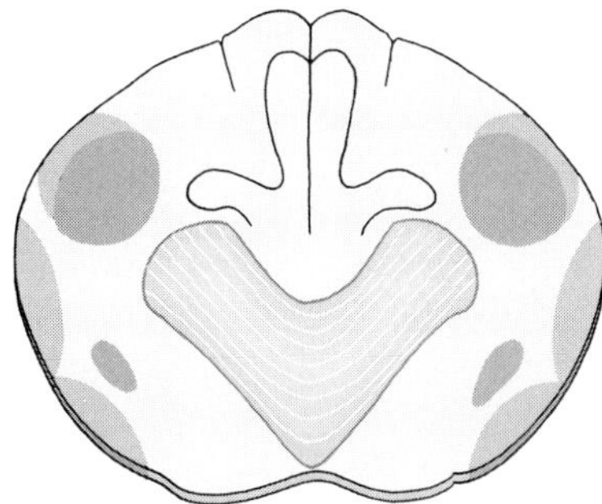

46.28A.

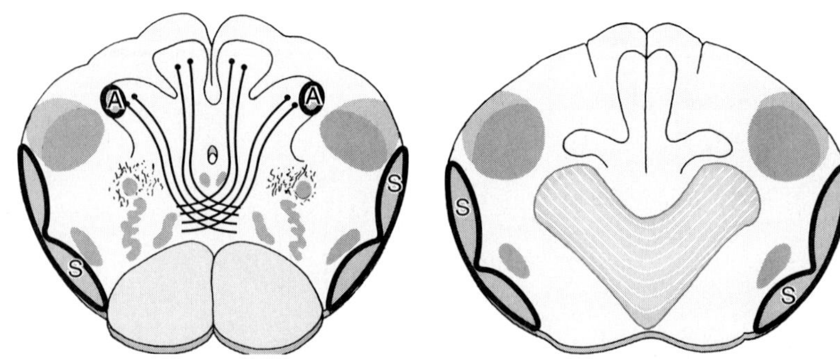

46.29A. No

Left

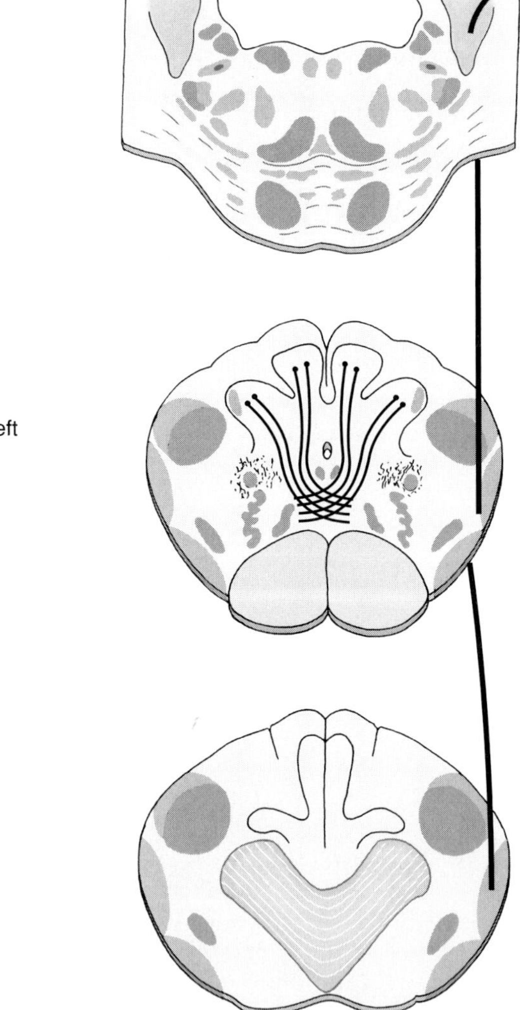

Right

46.30. Place an "X" on the right accessory cuneate nucleus. The accessory cuneate nucleus is in a very convenient position to project its axons to the cerebellum. Draw an axon projecting to the cerebellum from the accessory cuneate nucleus. Information about muscle ______ reaches the ______lateral side of the cerebellum via secondary afferent neurons with cell bodies in the ____________ ____________ nucleus and in the ____________ ______ of spinal cord gray matter.

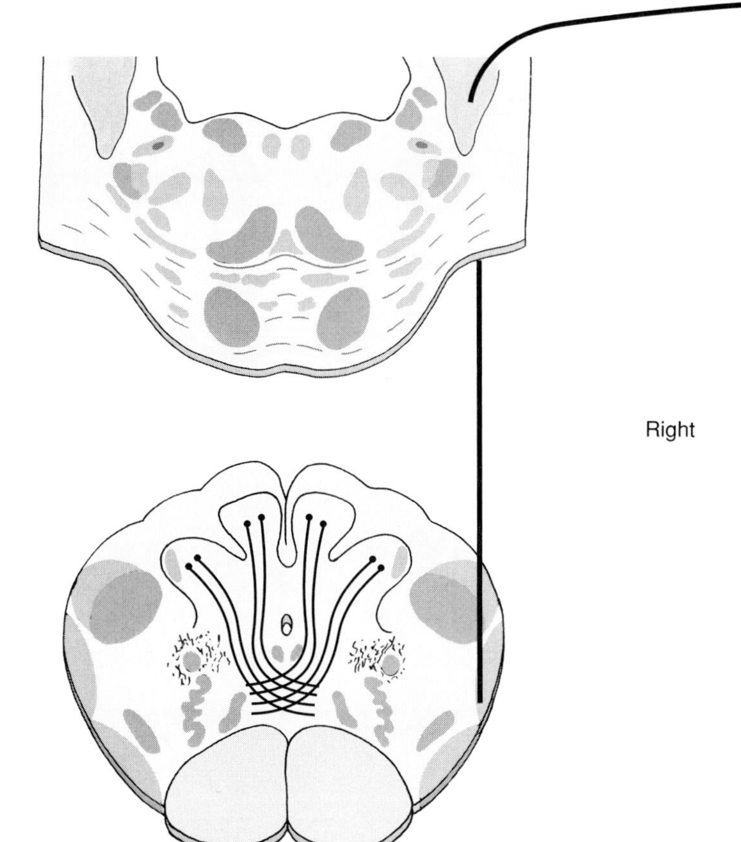

46.30A. tone; ipsilateral; accessory cuneate; posterior horn

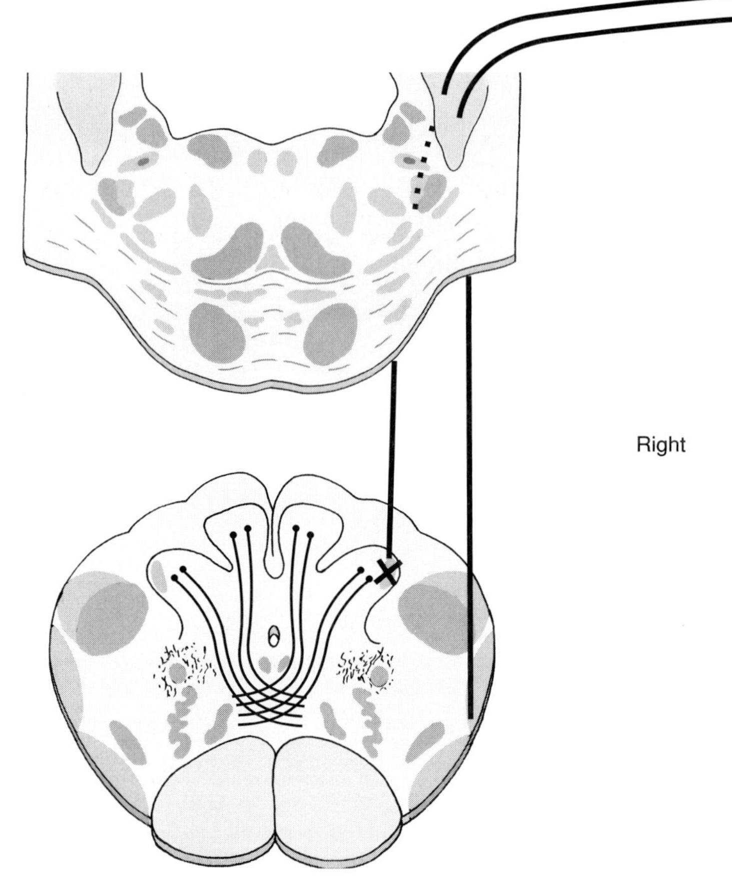

47 Brainstem: Transition from Spinal Cord to Medulla, with Emphasis on the Kinesthetic Pathway

47.1. The nucleus gracilis lies in the lower medulla. The primary axons that ascend the spinal cord and make synaptic contact with secondary neurons of the nucleus gracilis are axons of the fasciculus ____________. Axons of the fasciculus cuneatus terminate in the lower medulla in synaptic contact with neurons of the nucleus ____________.

47.2. Blockage of the posterior spinal artery would affect the blood supply to the nucleus gracilis and cause a lack of information regarding the ______thetic senses from the lower limb.

47.3. Information about muscle tone ordinarily does not reach consciousness; impulses may be relayed via the ____________ ____________________ peduncle to the ______lateral side of the cerebellum. Information about the kinesthetic senses ascends the spinal cord in the ____________ gracilis and cuneatus; these axons belong to neuron number ______ in the afferent pathway.

47.4. As the fibers of the posterior columns ascend into the medulla (passing in a predominantly ______ior direction), they run along the ____________ior surfaces of the nuclei gracilis and cuneatus. Label the two indicated nuclei in the section.

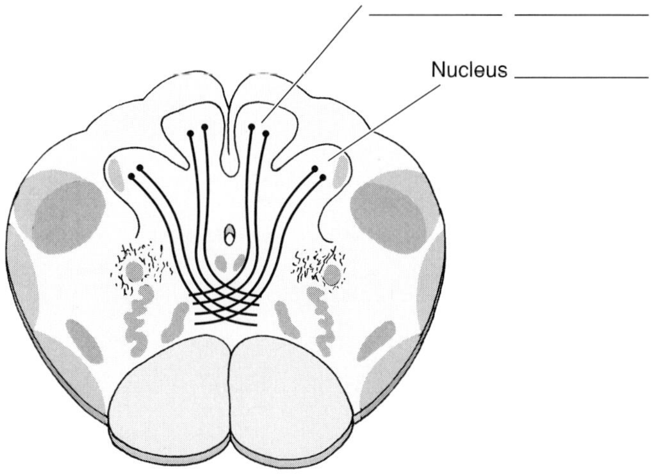

47.5. In the pathway for position sense, the neurons of the *nuclei* gracilis and cuneatus are the ____________ary neurons. Cell bodies of these neurons lie in the region of the brainstem called the ____________.

47.1A. gracilis; cuneatus

47.2A. kinesthetic

47.3A. inferior cerebellar; ipsilateral; fascicule; one

47.4A. superior; posterior

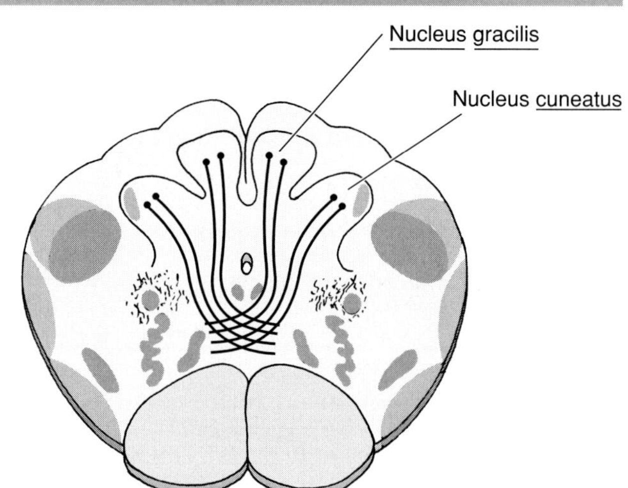

47.5A. secondary; medulla

47.6. At progressively higher levels of the lower medulla, the fasciculi gracilis and cuneatus gradually disappear and are replaced by ____________ with the same names. In the appropriate cross section(s) place an "X" on the cell bodies of *secondary* neurons mediating position sense in the left *hand.*

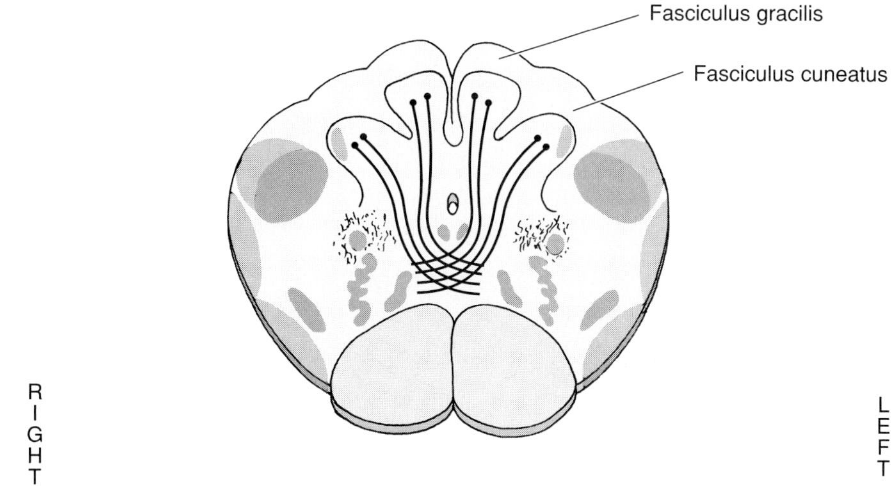

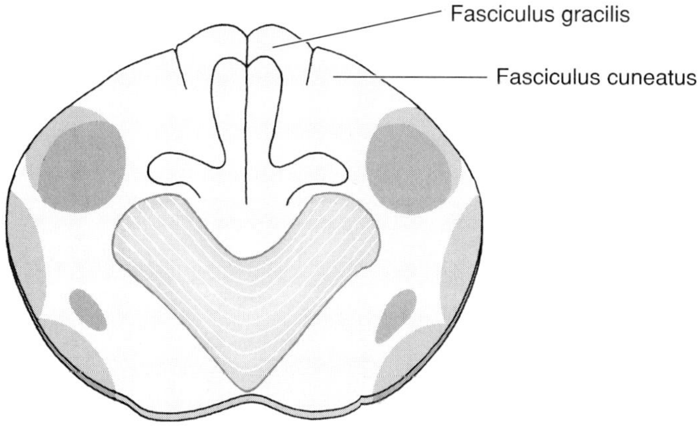

Fasciculus gracilis
Fasciculus cuneatus
RIGHT
LEFT
Fasciculus gracilis
Fasciculus cuneatus

47.7. In all sensory pathways, the *cell bodies* of primary and secondary neurons lie on the ______ side. In the pathway mediating pain in the left foot, the *cell body* of the secondary neuron lies in the ______ side of the lumbar spinal cord. In the pathway mediating position sense in the left foot, the *cell body* of the secondary neuron lies in the ______ side of the ____________.

47.8. In the pain and temperature pathways, the axon that crosses the midline belongs to the ____________ary neuron; it then ascends and synapses with a tertiary neuron whose cell body is in the ____________. In the kinesthetic pathway, the *axon* of the *secondary* neuron crosses the midline and terminates in synaptic contact with a ______iary neuron in the ________________ thalamus.

47.9. In the ascending pathway for cold in the right hand, the first synapse is in the posterior horn of the ____________ region of the ____________ ______. Kinesthetic fibers in the right hand make the analogous first synapse in the nucleus ____________ in the ____________. In both systems, the axons of the secondary neuron ascend slightly as they ______ the midline and then pass upward to their highest site of synapse in the ____________.

47.6A. nuclei

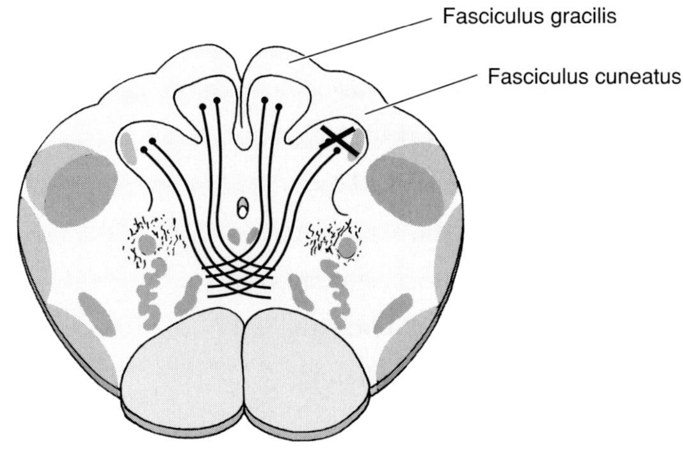

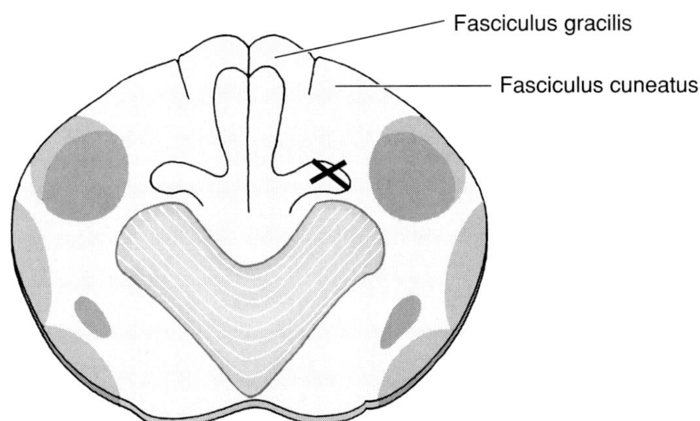

47.7A. same; left; left; medulla

47.8A. secondary; thalamus; tertiary; contralateral

47.9A. cervical; spinal cord; cuneatus; medulla; cross; thalamus

47.10. Label the central canal (CC) in each of the two lower cross sections. Most of the tissue posterior to the central canal in the cervical cord is ______ matter, and most of the tissue in the lower medulla is ______ (the nuclei ____________ and ____________). The most posterior structure higher in the medulla is the fluid-filled ______ ____________.

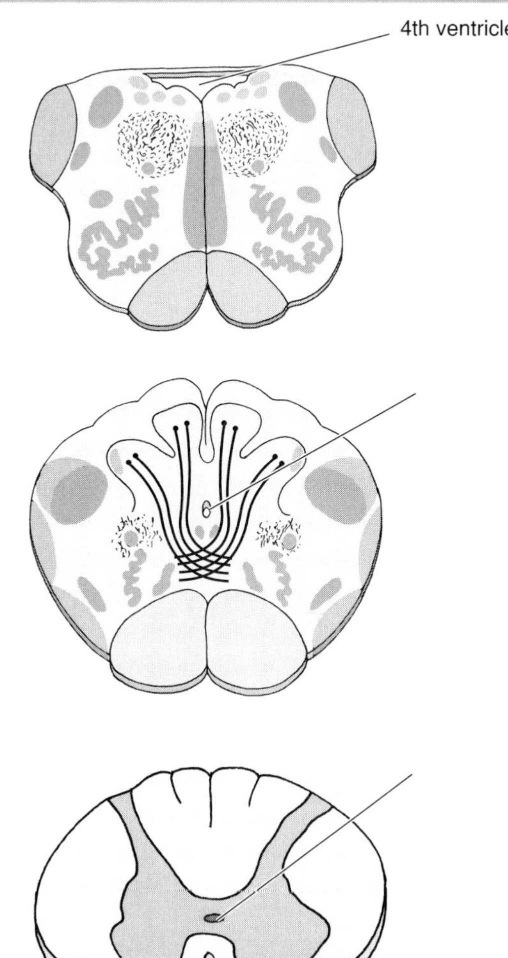

47.11. Draw a circle around the superior colliculi on both pictures. Anterior to the cerebellum are two regions of the brainstem, the ____________ and the ______. The fluid-filled cavity between these structures and the cerebellum is the ______ ____________.

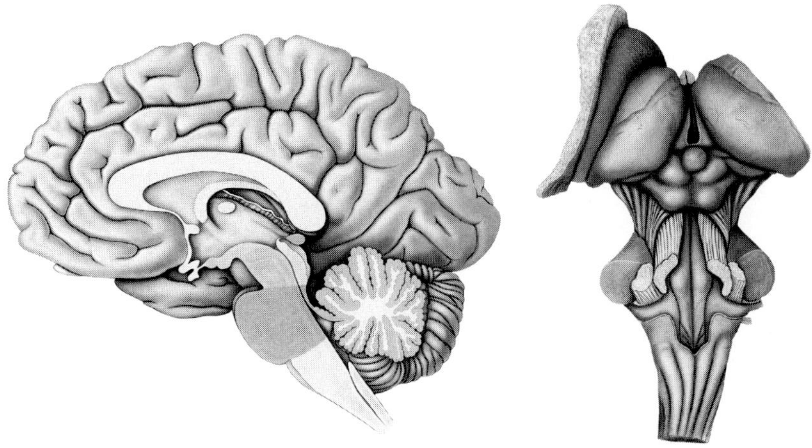

47.10A. white; gray; gracilis; cuneatus; 4th ventricle

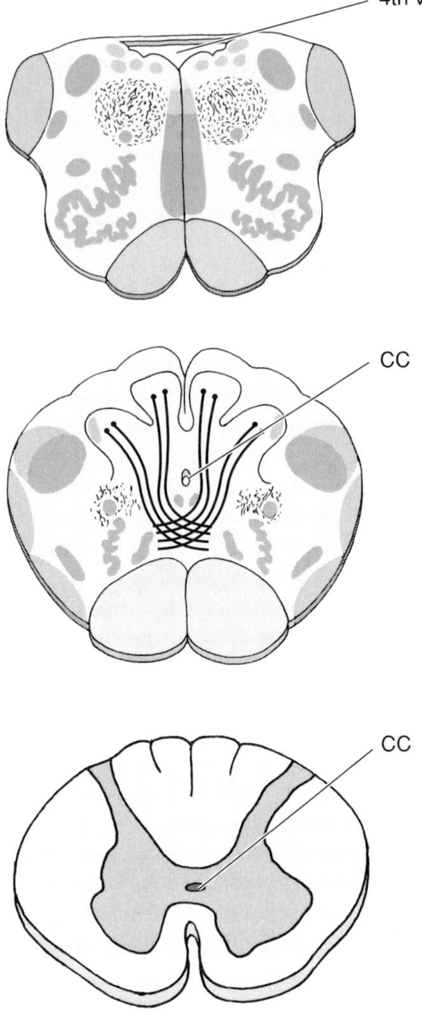

47.11A. medulla; pons; 4th ventricle

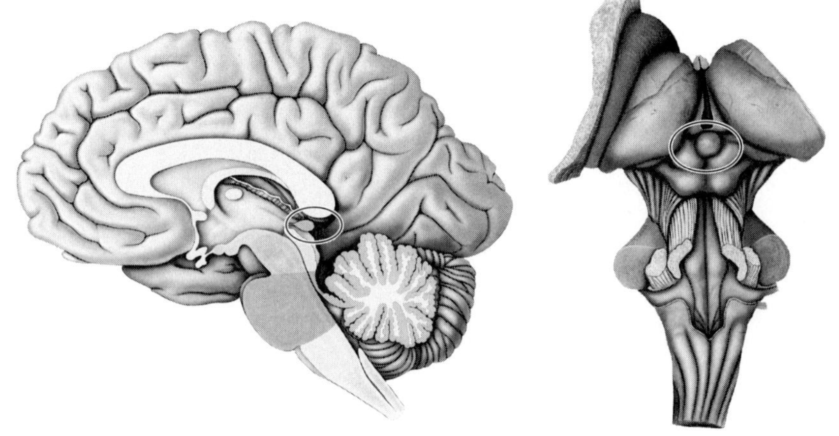

47.12. Kinesthetic impulses arising in the left arm and ascending toward the cortex first cross a synapse in the nucleus ____________ on the ______ side. As the axons *emerge* from the *nuclei* gracilis and cuneatus, do they travel in the same direction as the axons in the *fasciculi* gracilis and cuneatus? ______

47.13. Axons emerging along the length of the nuclei gracilis and cuneatus follow the course of an arc around the central canal. For this reason, they are called the ____________ ____________ fibers.

47.14. Encircle the right internal arcuate fibers and label the nuclei from which such fibers emerge.

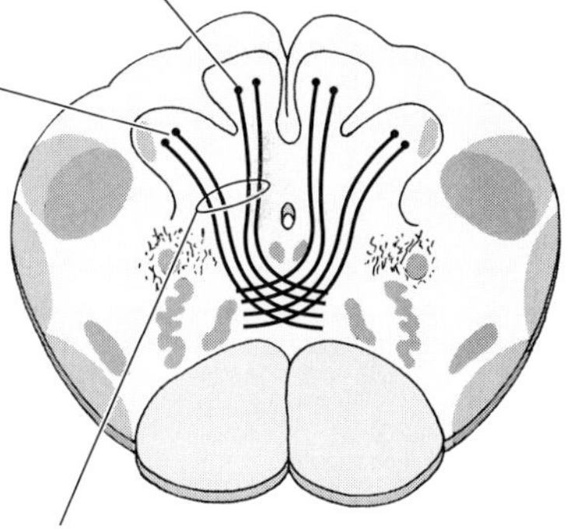

Left nucleus gracilis

Left nucleus cuneatus

Left internal arcuate fibers

47.15. When the internal arcuate fibers complete their arc, they turn sharply in a superior direction and continue uninterrupted all the way to the contralateral ____________. En route, the decussated fibers are given a new name, medial lemniscus. With an arrow, indicate the medial lemniscus.

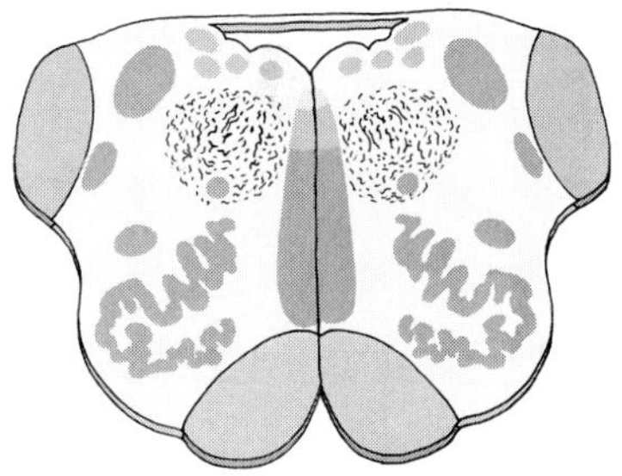

Medulla

47.16. Internal arcuate fibers from the left and right sides cross in the ________________ of the ____________ ____________.

47.17. In the kinesthetic pathway, the axon of the second neuron is initially called an ____________ ____________ fiber and then changes its name by becoming part of the ____________ ____________ on the ________________ side of the brainstem.

47.12A. cuneatus; left; No

47.13A. internal arcuate

47.14A.

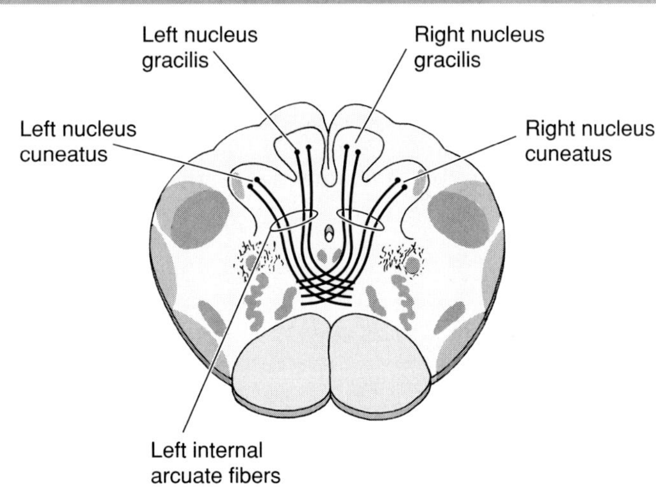

47.15A. thalamus

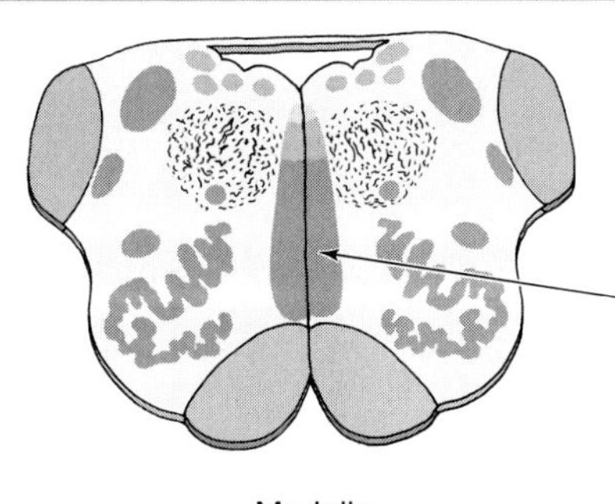

47.16A. decussation; medial lemniscus

47.17A. internal arcuate; medial lemniscus; contralateral

47.18. The medial lemniscus receives arterial supply primarily from branches of the vertebral arteries; __________ sense, ______ure, and ______ is lost in relation to the medial lemniscus from blockage of the vertebral artery.

47.19. Information in the right posterior columns of the spinal cord comes to the ______ side of the thalamus. In the kinesthetic pathway from the right foot, the first synapse is in the __________ __________ on the ______ side, and the next synapse is in the __________ on the ______ side.

47.20. As the internal arcuate fibers curve anteriorly and medially, they also curve in a somewhat ______ior direction. Most of the internal arcuate and medial lemniscus fibers cut in any given transverse section arose from cell bodies in a more ______ior section.

47.21. Circle the internal arcuate fibers on both sides of the left image and draw an arrow to the medial lemniscus on both sides of the right image.

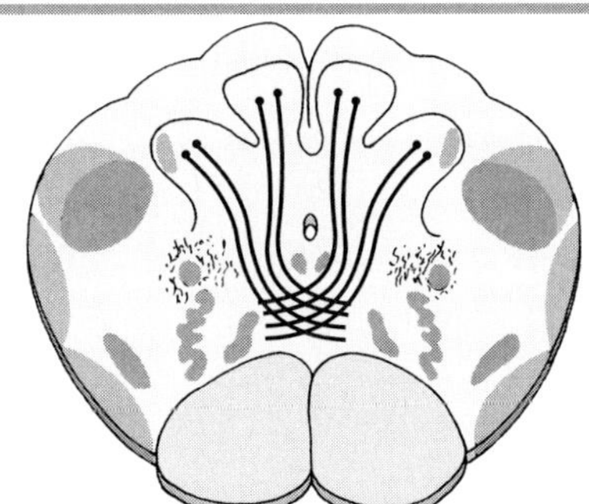

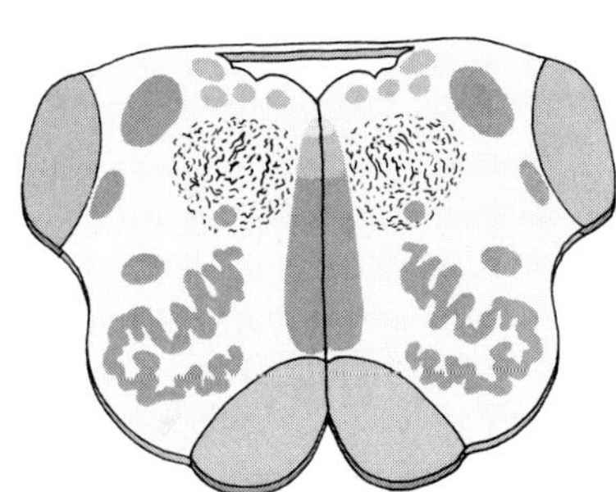

47.18A. position; pressure; touch

47.19A. left; nucleus gracilis; right; thalamus; left

47.20A. superior; inferior

47.21A.

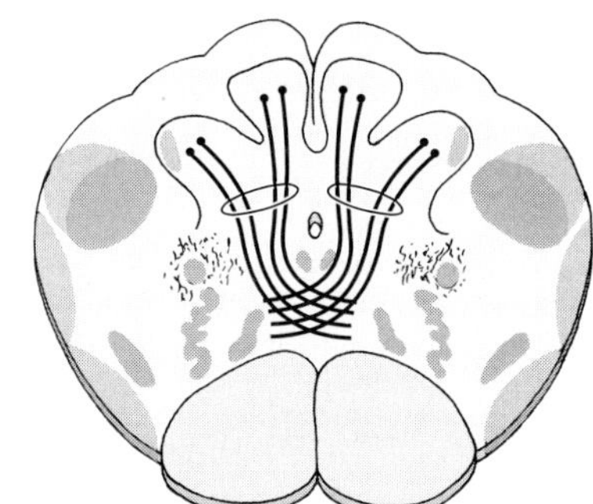

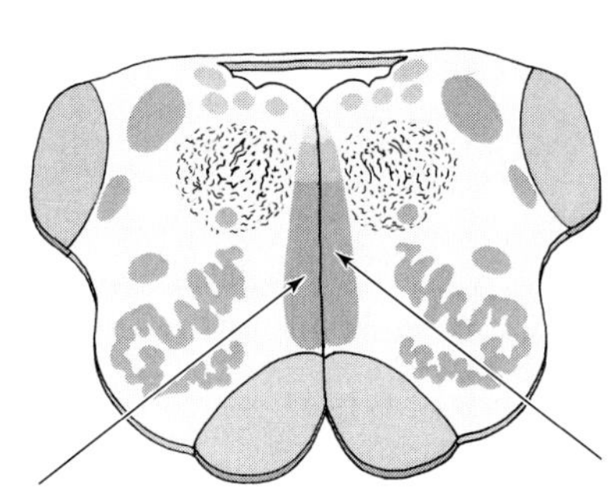

47.22. Label the nuclei gracilis (G) and cuneatus (C) on the right side of each picture. In the top section, label the fibers of the kinesthetic pathway with the name given to them in the first portion of their course after they leave cell bodies in the two nuclei.

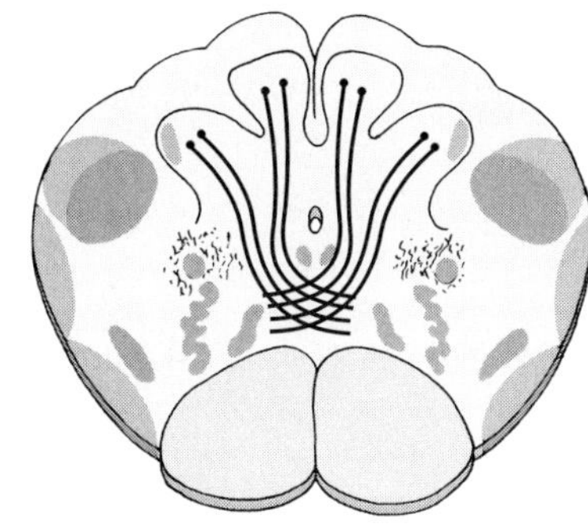

RIGHT

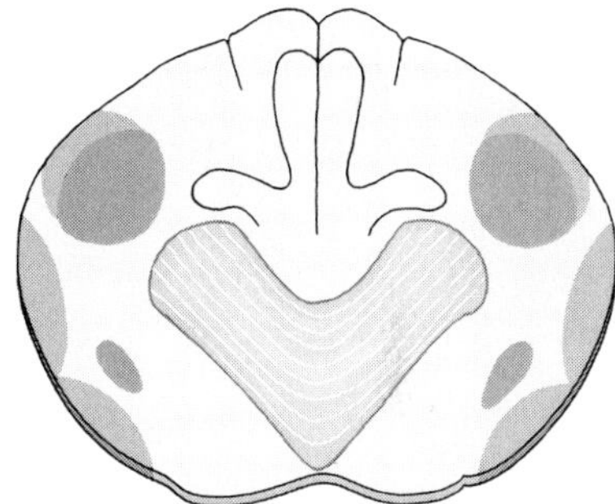

47.23. The fibers at "X" belong to the ____________ ____________. They arise from cell bodies in the nuclei gracilis and cuneatus on the ________________ side. The fibers marked "Y" arise mainly in the ____________ lobe of the cortex on the ________________ side.

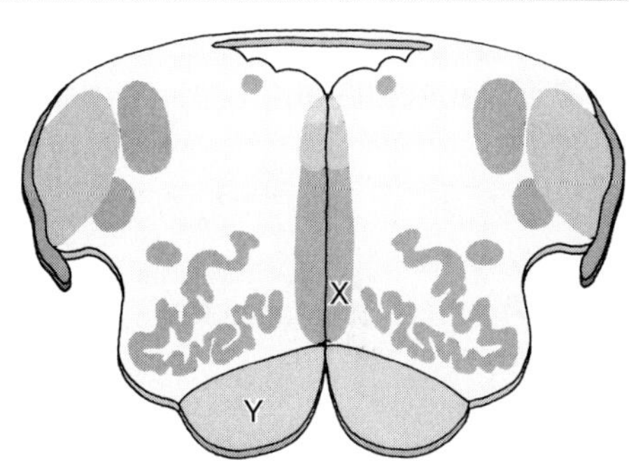

47.24. The internal arcuate fibers course obliquely to higher levels of the medulla at the same time that they form an arc from posterior to anterior positions. Label the internal arcuate fibers (IA) on the left picture and the medial lemnisci (ML) bilaterally on the right picture. At the level of the medulla, illustrated in the right picture, all internal arcuate fibers have entered the left or right ____________ ____________.

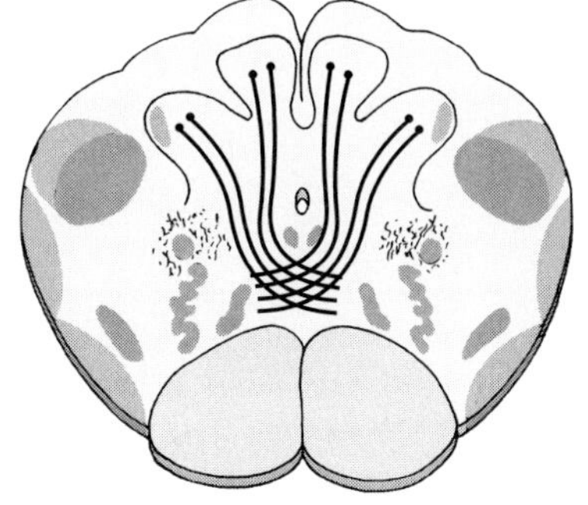

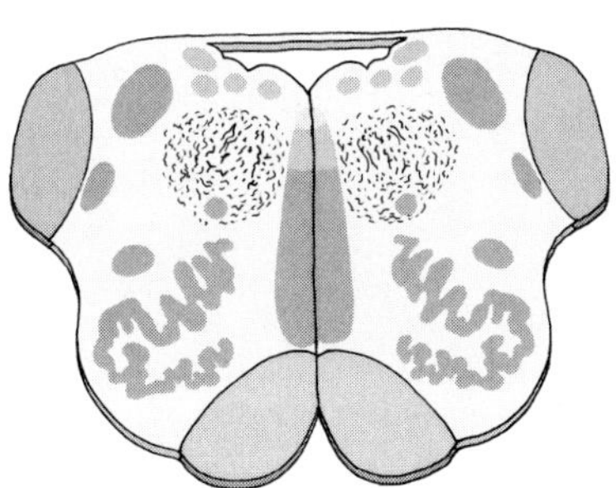

47.22A.

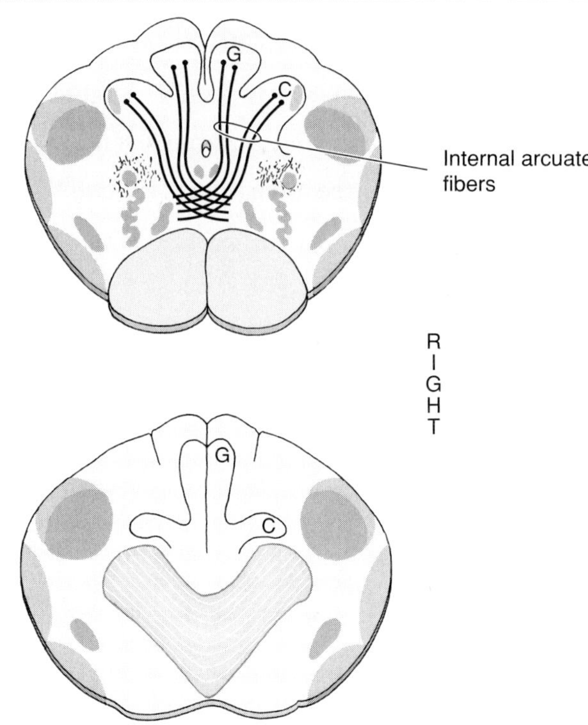

47.23A. medial lemniscus; contralateral; frontal; ipsilateral

47.24A. medial lemniscus

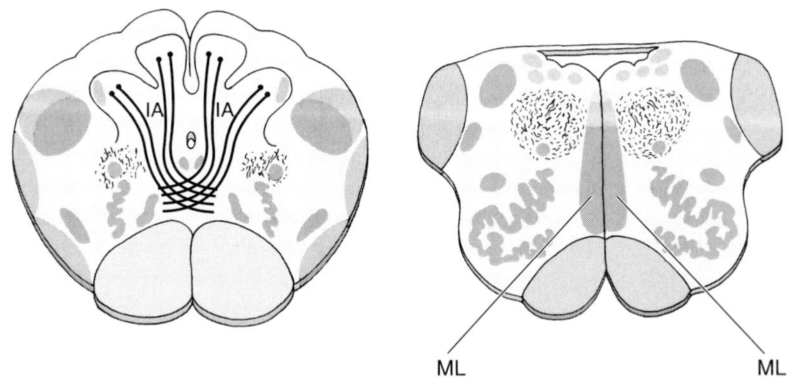

47.25. The arrow at this cervical cord level points to a headless "homunculus" representing the layout of one side of the body in the posterior columns. If a corresponding simple homunculus were drawn on the other side of the cervical section, the part of this body nearest the midline would be the ______.

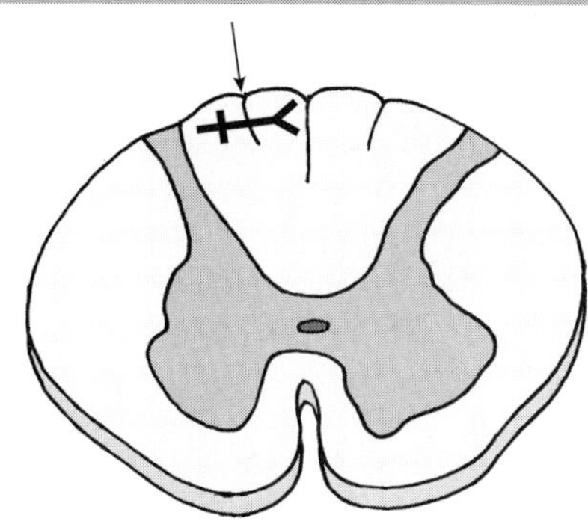

47.26. Kinesthetic impulses from the leg reach the nucleus gracilis and pass along its axons in a curving and mainly ______ior direction; forming the leg are __________ __________ fibers that ______ the midline and join the __________ __________. The *left* medial lemniscus carries somesthetic information from the ______ side of the body. The midline is crossed by axon number ______ in the afferent chain.

47.27. The most inferior *internal arcuate* fibers arise from the nucleus gracilis and carry kinesthetic information from the most __________ region of the body. Information from the arm passes along internal arcuate fibers at more ______ior levels.

47.28. The homunculus "stands upright" in the medial lemniscus of the medulla. Beyond the inferior olive, the "feet slide out from under him," so that information from the legs is transmitted along fibers __________ to those carrying information from the arms.

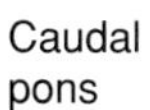

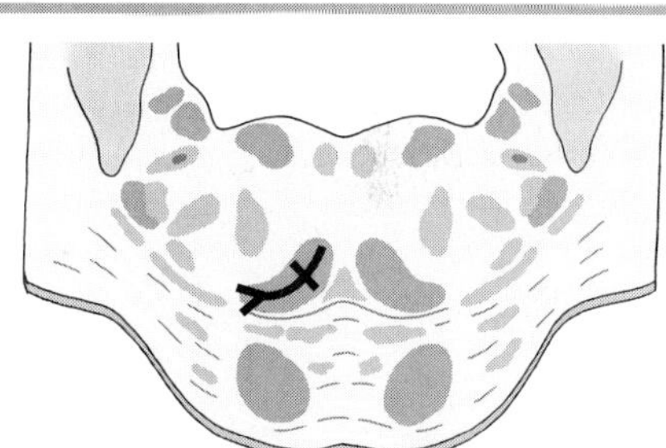

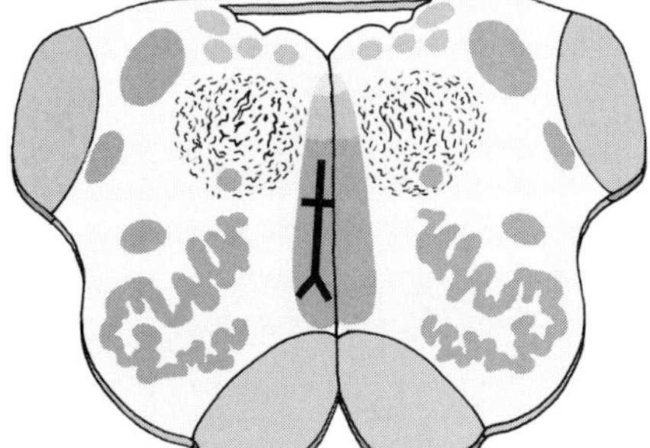

47.25A. foot

47.26A. anterior; internal arcuate; cross; medial lemniscus; right; two

47.27A. inferior; superior

47.28A. lateral

47.29. The somesthetic pathway exhibits somatotopic organization. Information from the left foot lies in the most ____________ part of the *posterior columns*, in the most ______ior part of the *medial lemniscus* in the mid and upper medulla, and in the most ____________ position in the medial lemniscus from the pons all the way to the ____________.

47.30. The primary neurons conveying information on *pain and temperature* senses from the left hand enter the cervical cord and synapse with secondary afferent cell bodies in the ____________ior horn. The secondary axons decussate in the ____________ ____________________ of the cord and ascend to the ____________ in the ____________ ____________________ tract on the ____________________ side.

47.31. In the left or right lateral spinothalamic tract, as in the left or right medial lemniscus, the fibers conveying information from the leg lie most ____________. This somatotopic organization is reversed in only one location: the ____________ ____________ of the spinal cord.

47.32. Comparing central pathways for *pain* and *position* sense in the fingers of the left *hand*: (1) nerve cell bodies in the posterior horn of the left side of the cervical cord correspond to nerve cell bodies in the nucleus ____________ of the ______ side of the lower ____________; (2) fibers in the anterior commissure correspond to the ____________ ____________ fibers; and (3) decussated secondary fibers in the right lateral spinothalamic tract correspond to secondary fibers in the ____________ ____________ on the ______ side of the brainstem.

47.33. On the section, draw outlines of the *right* lateral and *both* anterior spinothalamic tracts. All three transmit afferent information from the same side of the body, the ______ side.

LEFT

RIGHT

47.29A. medial; anterior; lateral; thalamus

47.30A. posterior; anterior commissure; thalamus; lateral spinothalamic; contralateral

47.31A. lateral; posterior columns

47.32A. cuneatus; left; medulla; internal arcuate; medial lemniscus; right

47.33A. left

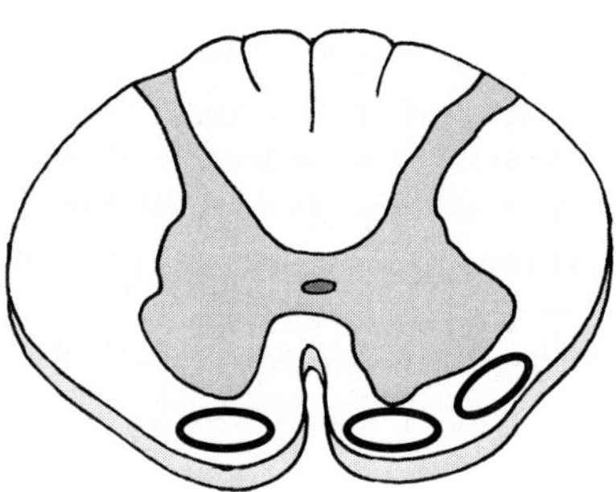

47.34. The diagram shows that pain and kinesthetic pathways are anatomically separated from each other in the spinal cord and most of the brainstem. In the upper medulla, the spinothalamic tract is well separated from the medial lemniscus and lies close to the posterior and lateral part of the ___________ _____. Both pathways become virtually confluent by the time they enter the ___________.

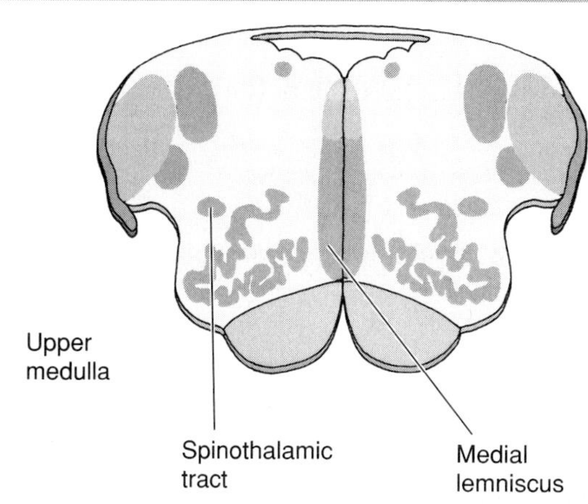

47.35. The name of the pathway serving for position sense, pressure, and touch is called the _______________ sensory pathway. The cell bodies of primary neurons in this pathway are in ___________ ___________. In this pathway, the midline is crossed by ___________ ___________ fibers arising in cell bodies of the nuclei ___________ and ___________. These are ___________ary afferent neurons. The secondary axons make synaptic contact with cell bodies of the tertiary neurons of the ___________.

47.36. At the junction of the spinal cord and the medulla, the fibers in the ___________ columns are passing superiorly toward the nuclei gracilis and cuneatus. On the anterior side, *descending* fibers of the left and right _______________ tracts are crossing to become the ___________ _______________ tracts of the cord.

47.37. The minimum number of neurons encompassed by the terms *spinal ganglion cell* and *fasciculus gracilis* is _____. The minimum number of neurons encompassed by the terms *nucleus gracilis*, *internal arcuate fiber*, and *medial lemniscus* is _____.

47.38. In the pons, the leg fibers of the medial lemniscus swing laterally, but in the medulla, the "homunculus is held upright" by the inferior olive. Within the encircled medial lemniscus, place an "L" for leg fibers and a "T" for trunk fibers.

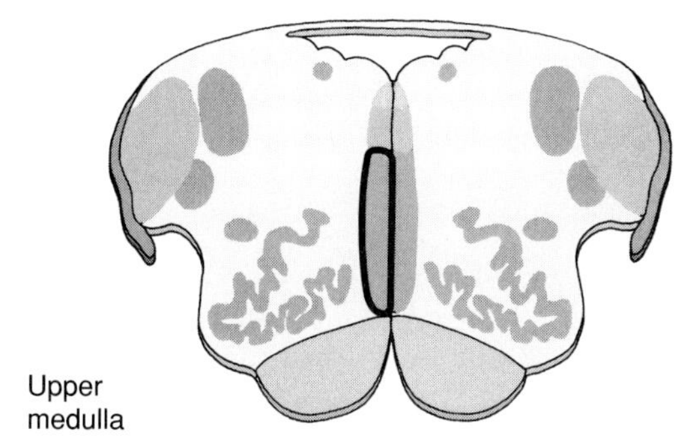

47.34A. inferior olive; thalamus

47.35A. kinesthetic; spinal ganglia; internal arcuate; gracilis; cuneatus; secondary; thalamus

47.36A. posterior; corticospinal; lateral corticospinal

47.37A. one; one

47.38A.

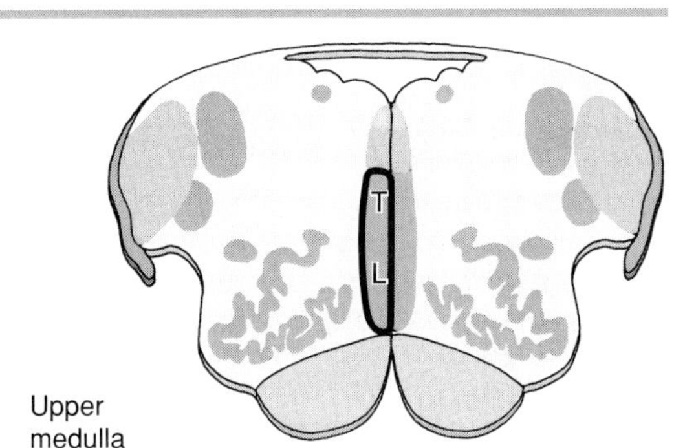

47.39. Label the sections with a "1," "2," and "3" from inferior to superior. Circle the medial lemniscus in all three images.

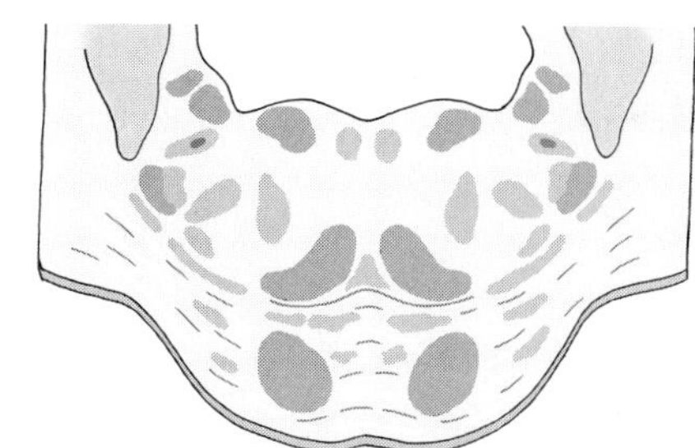

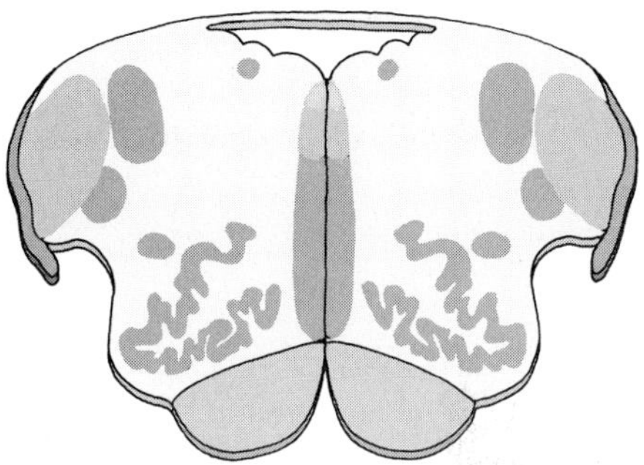

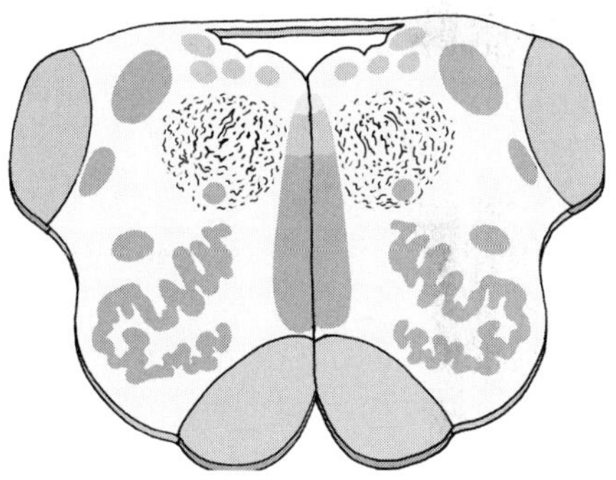

47.40. Complete the chart.

Function	**1st synapse in**	**2nd axon ascends in the**	**2nd axon terminates in the**
Temperature sense	Posterior horn of the cord	______________ ______________________ tract	______________ ______________
Joint sense	Nuclei ______________ and ______________	______________ ______________	______________
________ and ______________ senses	All the sites listed above	______________ ______________________ tracts and the ______________ ______________ ______________________ tracts	______________
Muscle tone	Nucleus ______________		______________________

47.39A.

3

2

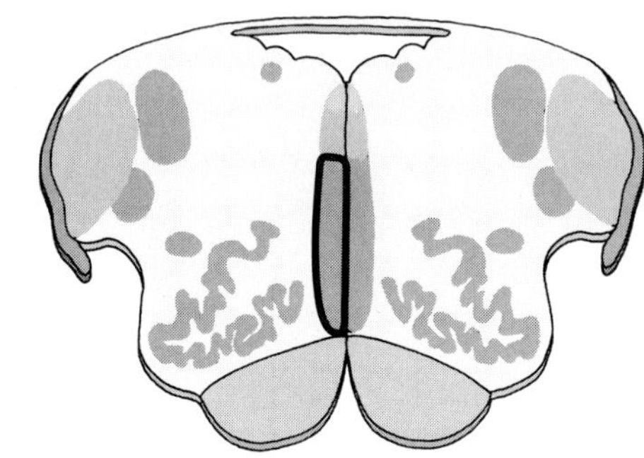

1

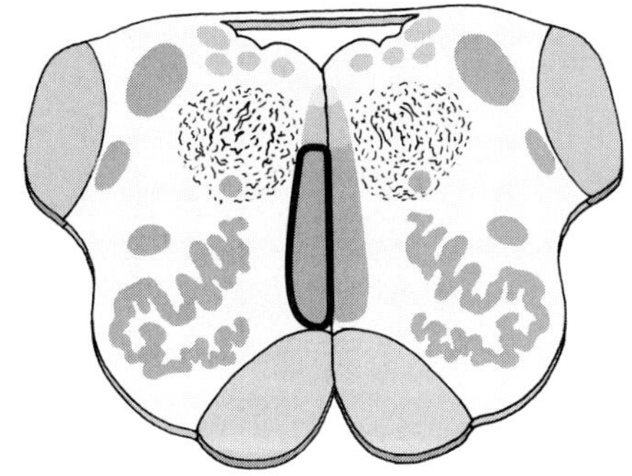

47.40A.

Function	**1st synapse in**	**2nd axon ascends in the**	**2nd axon terminates in the**
Temperature sense	Posterior horn of the cord	*Lateral spinothalamic* tract	*Thalamus*
Joint sense	Nuclei *gracilis* and *cuneatus* (in either order)	*Medial lemniscus*	*Thalamus*
touch and *pressure* senses	All the sites listed above	*Anterior spinothalamic* tracts and the *medial lemniscus*	*Thalamus*
Muscle tone	Nucleus *dorsalis*	*Spinocerebellar* tracts	*Cerebellum*

48 Brainstem: Spinal Trigeminal System in the Transition Zone from Spinal Cord to Medulla

48.1. Information about pain, temperature, touch, and pressure from the trunk and limbs is mediated by sensory ganglia on both sides of each spinal segment. With an arrow, indicate a spinal ganglion drawn on the diagram. No such series of segmental ganglia is found for the somesthetic senses of the head. Instead, the ________________ ganglion may be conceived of as several "fused" segmental ganglia containing all of the primary neurons for the head's ________________ senses.

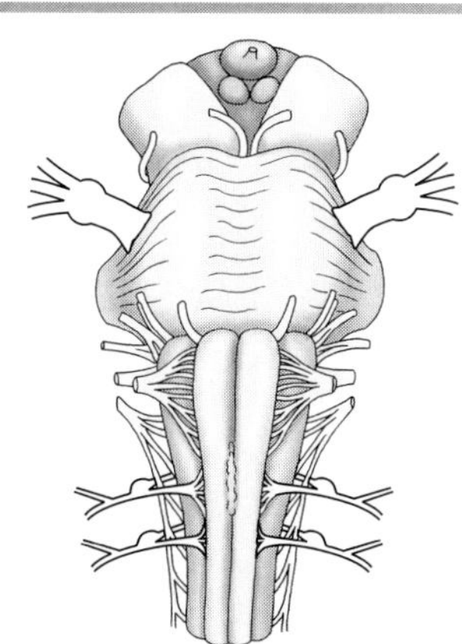

Anterior view of the brainstem

48.2. The nerve indicated by the arrow is called the trigeminal because the number of main nerve divisions peripheral to the ganglion is ______. The ______geminal ganglion is a cranial ganglion. Its cells are comparable to cells in the sensory ganglia, which lie outside the __________ ______.

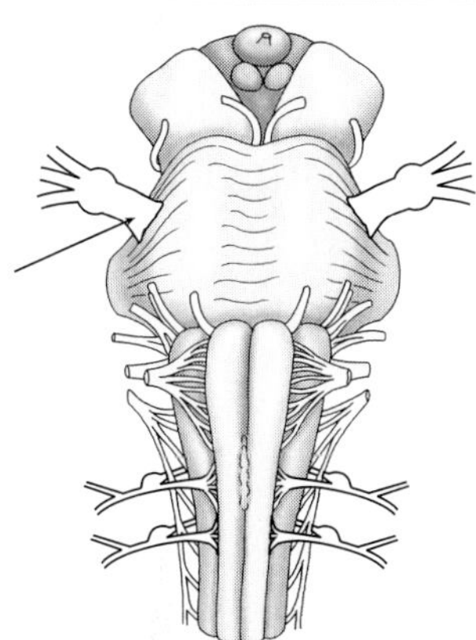

Anterior view of the brainstem

48.3. The trigeminal nerve has only one root between the ganglion and the pons. Indicate it on the diagram with an arrow. This root is the equivalent of the anterior plus posterior roots of spinal nerves. The trigeminal root contains both __________ and __________ fibers.

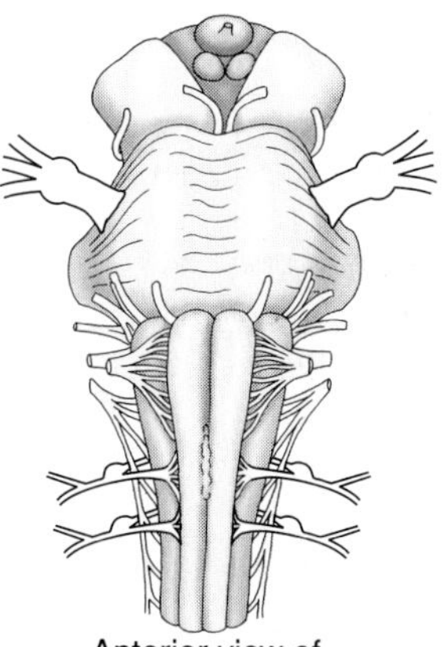

Anterior view of the brainstem

48.1A. trigeminal; somesthetic

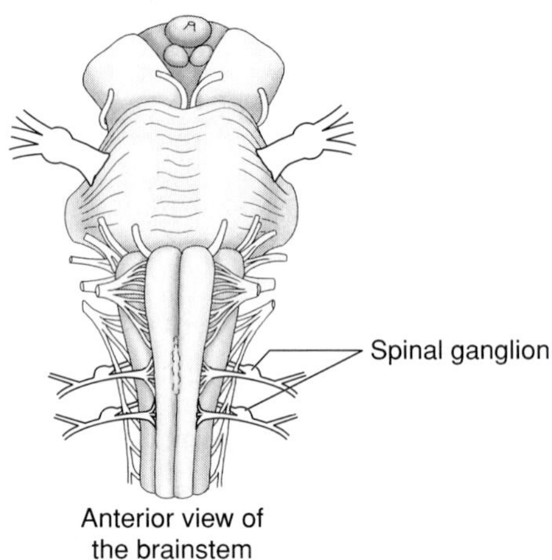

Anterior view of the brainstem

48.2A. 3; trigeminal; spinal cord

48.3A. afferent (or sensory); efferent (or motor)

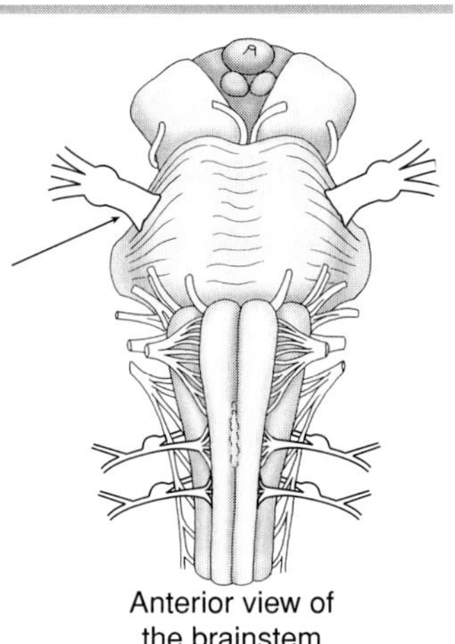
Anterior view of the brainstem

48.4. The trigeminal root enters the region of the brainstem called the ______. Fibers mediating pain, temperature, and (to some extent) touch and pressure then turn and descend (as illustrated) through the whole length of the ____________ into the upper ____________ segments of spinal cord.

Anterior view of the brainstem

48.5. The afferent trigeminal fibers that descend from the pons through the medulla and into the cervical cord have cell bodies ______side the brainstem in a cranial ____________. The descending trigeminal fibers collectively form the ____________ tract of the ____________________. Draw an arrow to indicate the direction of impulse conduction in the fibers passing through the medulla.

Anterior view of the brainstem

48.6. The abbreviated term *spinal tract of V* is commonly used because the ____________________ is cranial nerve number ______. Although impulses in this tract pass inferiorly into the spinal cord, the impulses are destined ultimately for the thalamus and cerebral cortex. The spinal (descending) tract of V contains axons of ______ary ______ferent neurons.

48.7. In the spinal portions of the pain, temperature, touch, and pressure pathways, the axon of the primary neuron bifurcates upon entering the spinal cord. The branches run a short distance up and down the cord in the dorsolateral fasciculus on the margin of the ____________ horn. Branches of the equivalent cranial fibers run downward in the brainstem as the ____________ ______ of ______.

48.8. The spinal tract of V, in the upper cervical cord and ____________, is comparable in structure and function to the ____________________ ____________________ in the ____________ ______.

48.4A. pons; medulla; cervical

48.5A. outside; ganglion; spinal; trigeminal

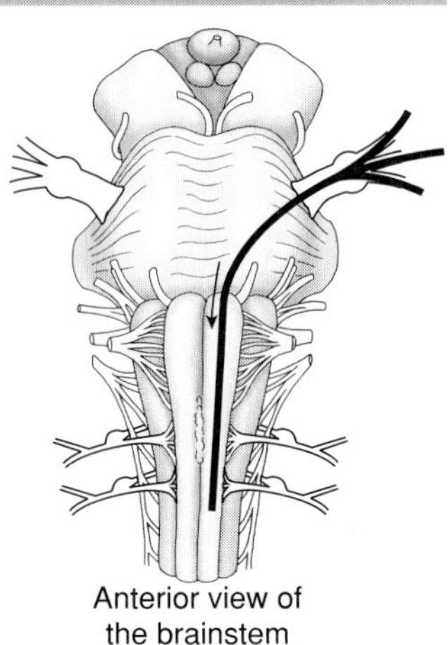

Anterior view of the brainstem

48.6A. trigeminal; V; primary; afferent

48.7A. posterior; spinal tract of V

48.8A. medulla; dorsolateral fasciculus; spinal cord

48.9. The encircled fibers in the cross section are afferent fibers whose cell bodies are located in ____________ ____________. Comparable fibers occupy the same position in all cord regions. Their central processes enter the dorsolateral fasciculus and pass up and down the cord for a segment or two.

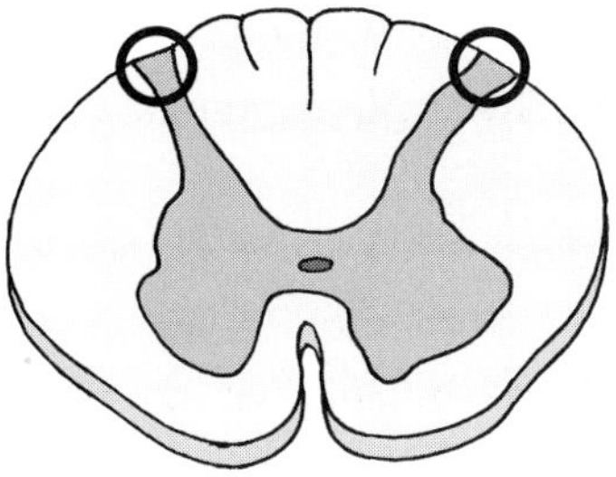

48.10. Like the short segmental fibers of the dorsolateral fasciculus in the spinal cord, the long fibers in the spinal tract of V in the medulla are ______ary axons.

48.11. Fibers of the spinal tract of V make synaptic contact with secondary cell bodies lying immediately medial to the fibers in the spinal ____________ of V.

48.12. Note the position of the spinal nucleus of V at the C2 level. Between approximately C4 and C2, the dorsolateral fasciculus is replaced by the corresponding ____________ ______ of ______, while the secondary afferent neurons of the posterior horn are replaced by the corresponding neurons of the ____________ ____________ of ______.

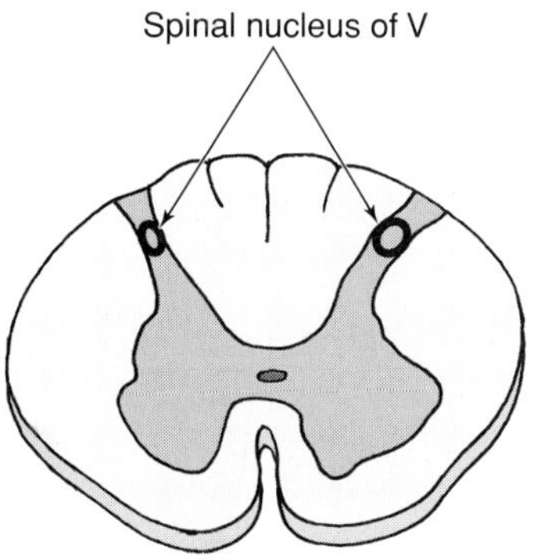

Spinal nucleus of V

48.13. Cells of the posterior horn of the spinal cord receive synaptic contacts from posterior root fibers entering in every spinal segment. The posterior horn is continuous with a homologous structure in the brainstem, where cells in the ____________ ____________ of V receive synaptic contacts from fibers of the ____________ ______ of V. In the medulla and pons, the expected series of segmental sensory nerves is largely replaced by one large nerve, the ________________.

48.9A. spinal ganglia

48.10A. primary

48.11A. nucleus

48.12A. spinal tract of V; spinal nucleus of V

48.13A. spinal nucleus; spinal tract; trigeminal

48.14. In the left picture, the cell bodies at "2" are ____________ary sensory neurons. The fibers at "1" belong to ________ary sensory neurons. The spinal tract of V on the right picture corresponds in position and function to number ______ on the left picture. On each side of the section at C2, place an "X" on the dilated part of the posterior horn, representing the spinal nucleus of V.

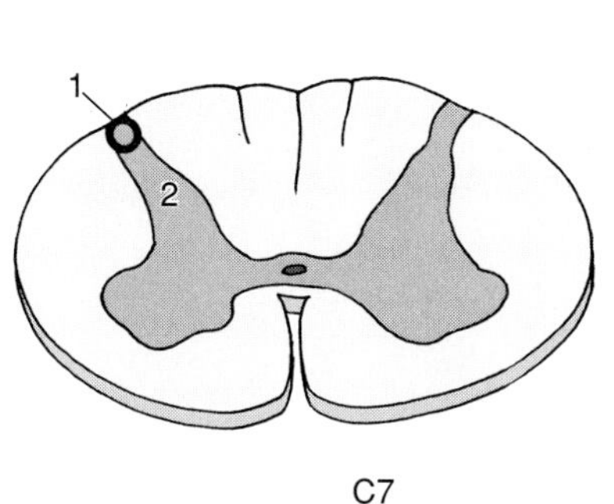

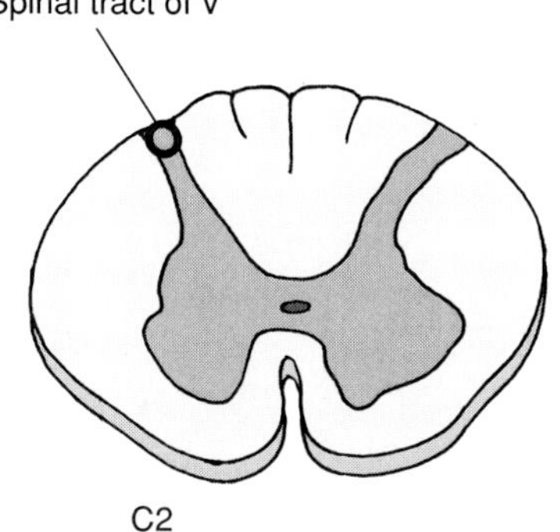

48.15. On the picture, label the circles drawn on the medulla section with a "G" and a "C" to represent the nuclei gracilis and cuneatus, and put an "N" on the spinal nucleus of V and a "T" on the spinal tract of V.

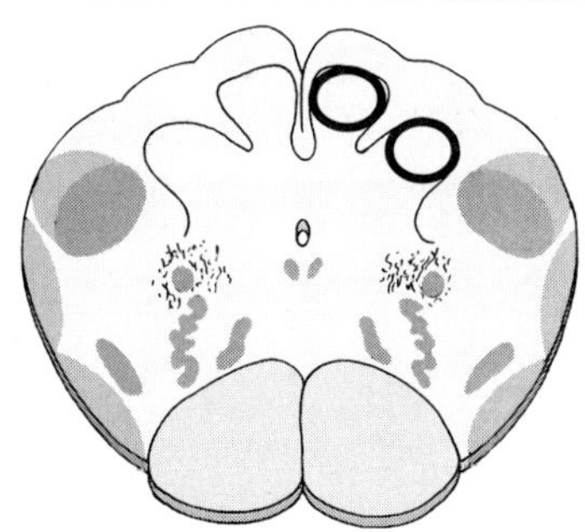

48.16. Fibers in the spinal ______ of V transmit impulses to neurons with cell bodies in the spinal ____________ of V; the latter neurons are ____________ary sensory neurons of the tri____________ system. They convey information about the ________________ senses.

48.17. On both sides of the appropriate picture, connect the dorso-lateral fasciculus and the nerve cell bodies of the posterior horn with an arrow to show the direction of impulse conduction across the synapses. Do the same for the spinal tract and spinal nucleus of V.

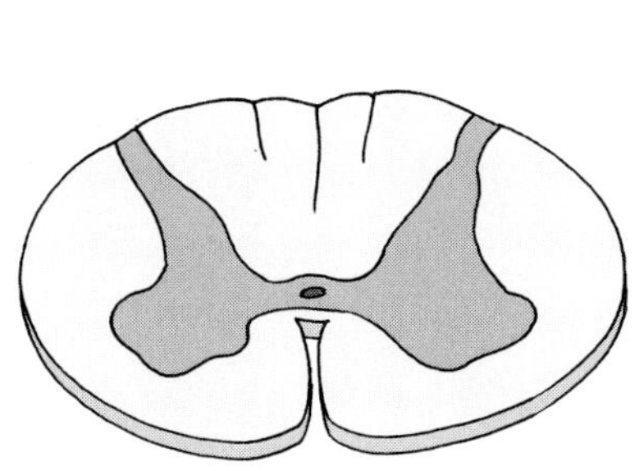

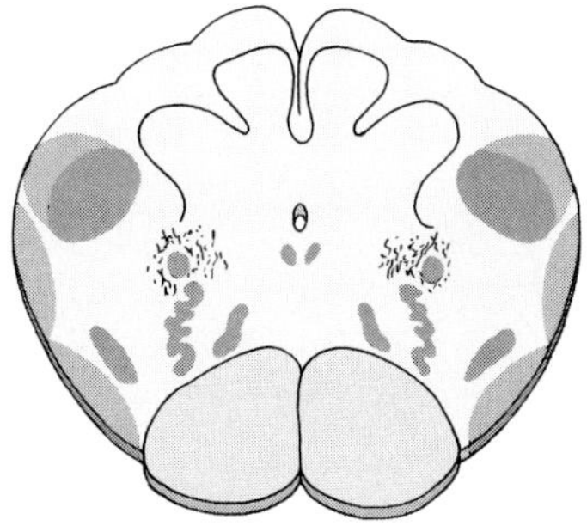

48.14A. secondary; primary; 1

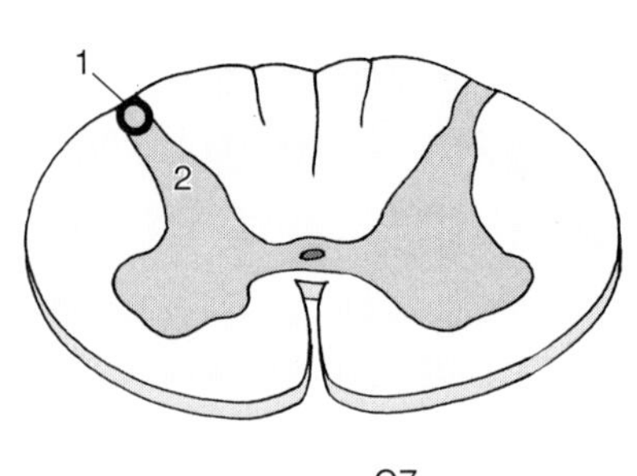

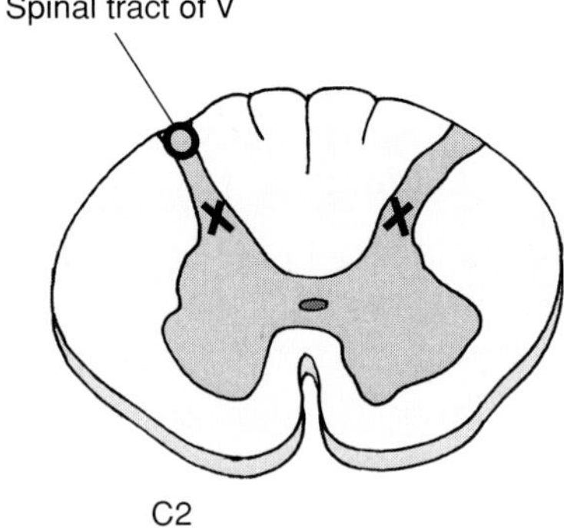

48.15A.

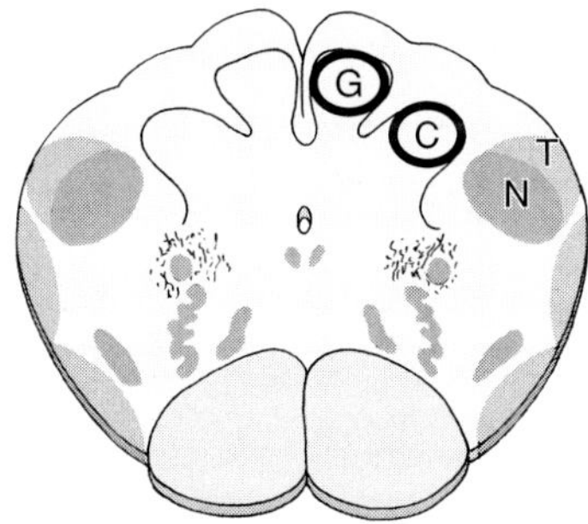

48.16A. tract; nucleus; secondary; trigeminal; somesthetic

48.17A.

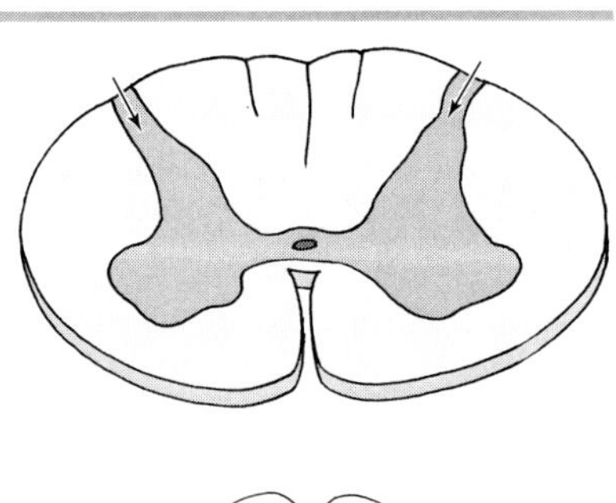

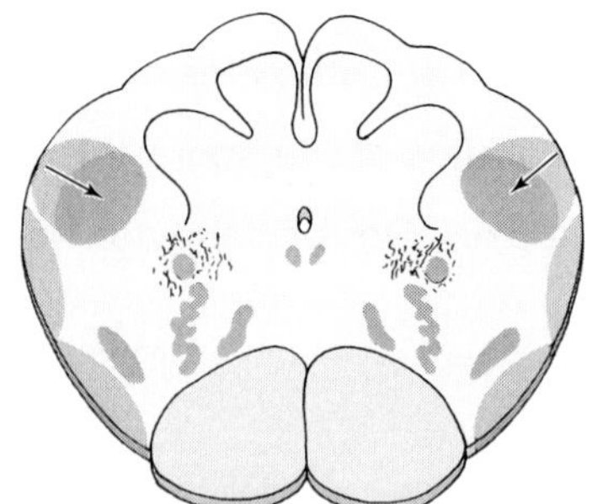

48.18. Place an "X" on the right poste-rior horn and right spinal nucleus of the trigeminal. Label the approximate level of each section.

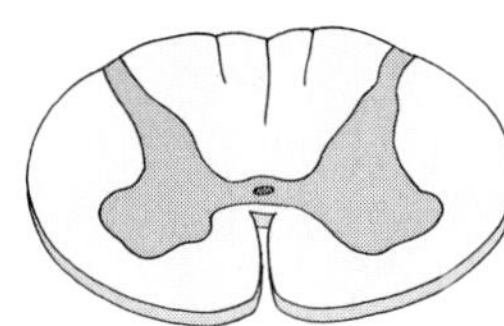

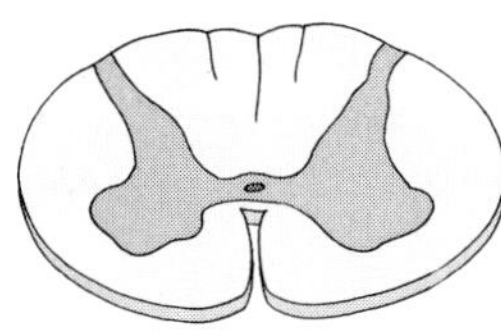

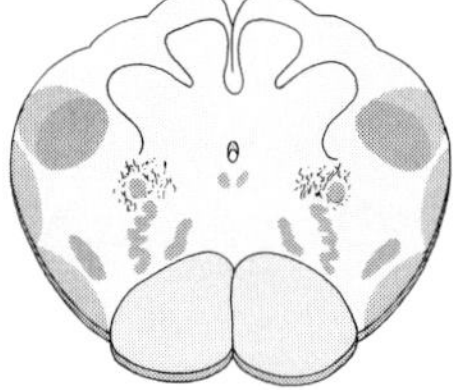

48.19. Nerve cell bodies in the posterior horn of the cord and spinal nucleus of V comprise virtually all of the secondary neurons in pathways for the senses of ______ and ________________ and a lesser percentage of the neurons for the senses of ______ and __________.

48.20. On both pictures, draw a fiber of the spinal tract of V all the way from the pons into the cervical cord. Indicate the direction of impulse conduction with an arrow.

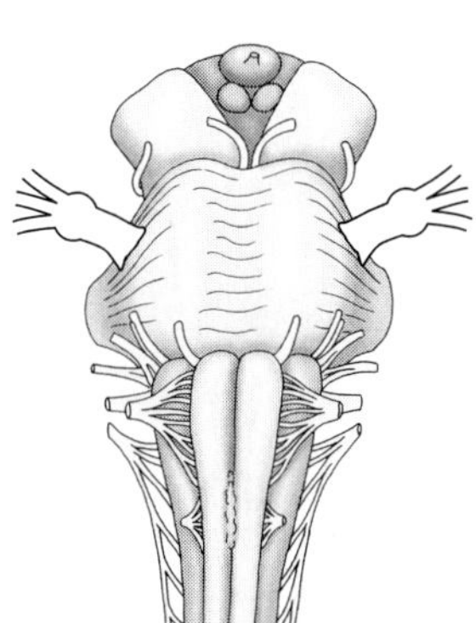

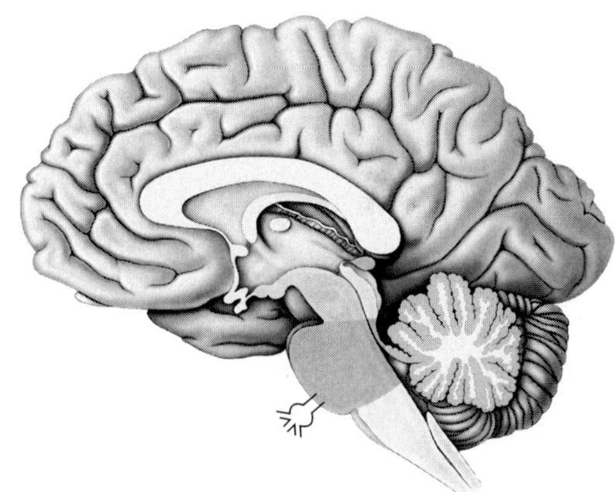

48.21. Trigeminal components mediate ______thetic sensation for the head. Like the spinal components, the axons of secondary trigeminal neurons terminate in the __________lateral __________.

48.18A.

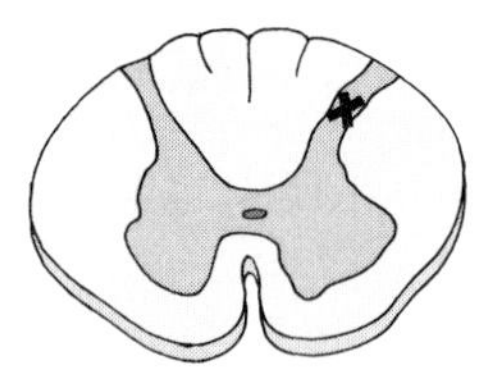

C3

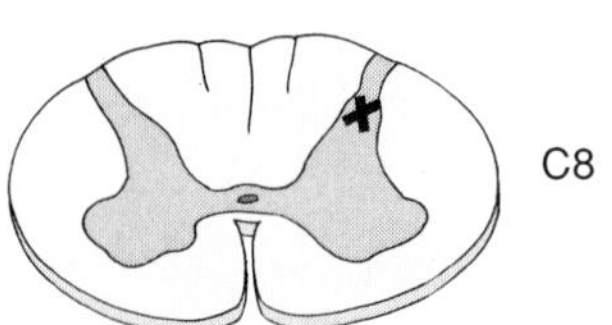

C8

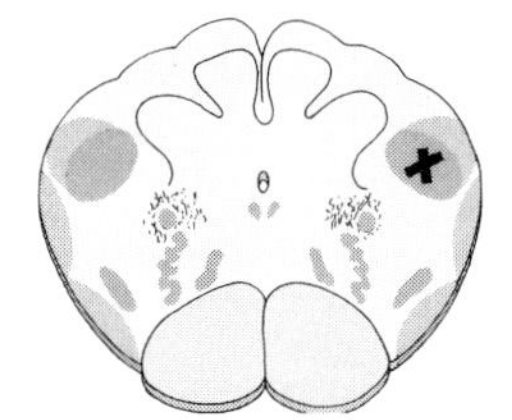

Medulla

48.19A. pain; temperature; touch; pressure

48.20A.

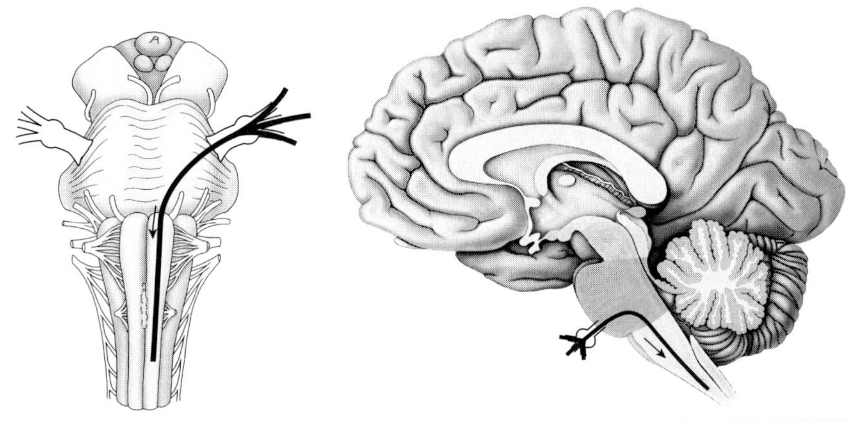

48.21A. somesthetic; contralateral; thalamus

48.22. The encircled cells send axons to terminate in the ____________________ ____________. They convey information about a ____________________ class of senses arising on the ______ side of the face and head.

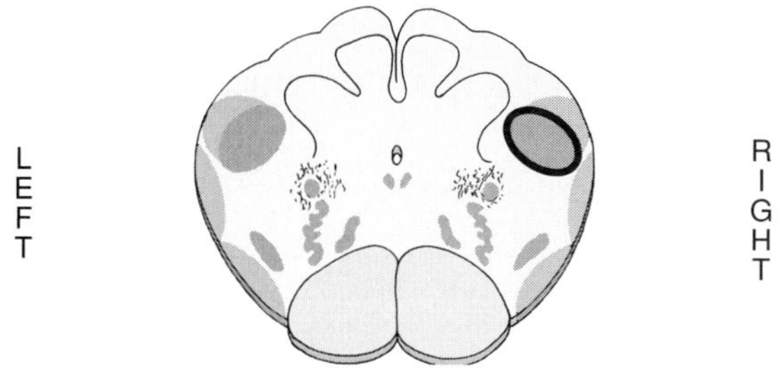

LEFT

RIGHT

48.23. A secondary "pain" axon is drawn at C7 and ascends into the brainstem. At C2, draw a corresponding axon emerging from a cell body in the spinal nucleus of V. Both axons will terminate in the ____________ on the ____________________ side.

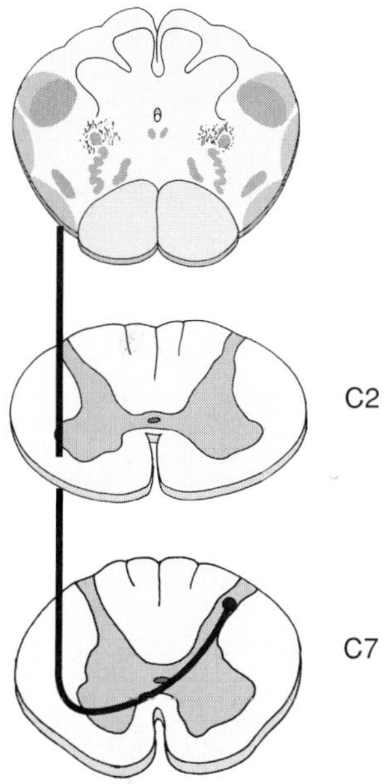

C2

C7

48.24. The encircled fibers collectively form the ____________ ____________________ tract. These are crossed axons of neuron number ______ in the afferent patway.

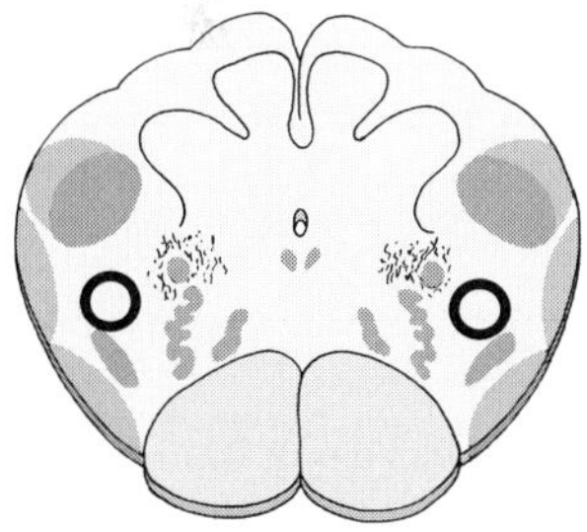

48.22A. contralateral thalamus; somesthetic; right

48.23A. thalamus; contralateral

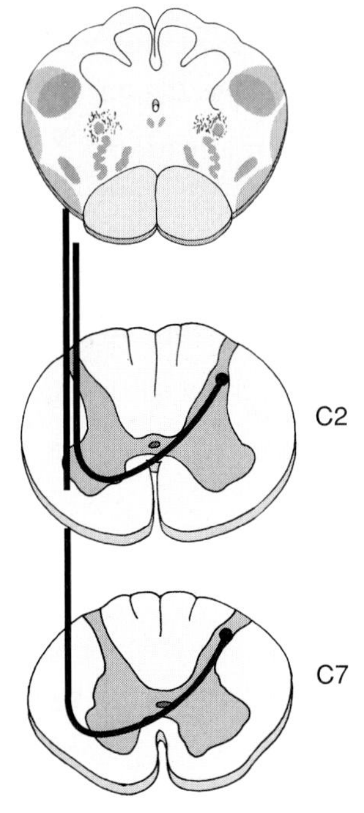

48.24A. anterior trigeminothalamic; 2

48.25. Axons in the lateral spinothalamic tract, axons in the medial lemniscus, and axons from nerve cell bodies in the spinal nucleus of V all make their highest synaptic contacts with neurons in the ____________ and convey information about various sensory modalities on the ________________ side of the body. The trunk and limbs are served by the lateral ________________ tracts the way the face and head are served by the anterior ________________ tracts.

48.26. The lesion indicated by the crosshatching would cause loss of pain and temperature senses in the limbs and trunks on the ______ side of the body because the lesion interrupts the lateral ________________ tract as it ascends in the ______ side of the medulla. The lesion also interrupts the descending primary axons in the spinal tract of V and causes loss of pain and temperature senses on the ______ side of the face. Thus, in this fairly common lesion in the lateral medulla, the sensory loss is on one side of the face and the ________________ side of the body.

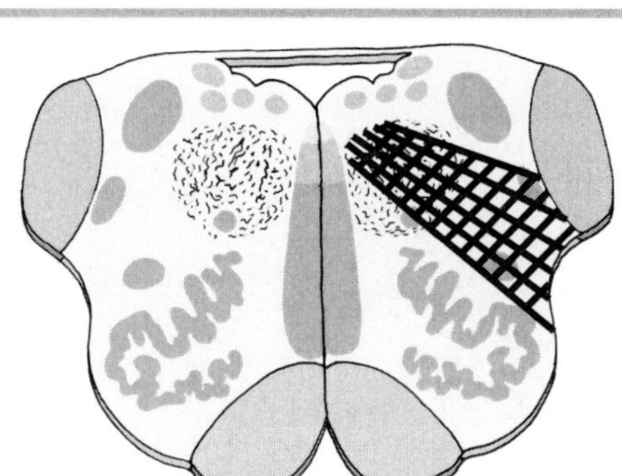

48.25A. thalamus; contralateral; spinothalamic; trigeminothalamic

48.26A. left; spinothalamic; right; right; contralateral

49 Introduction to Motor Nuclei of the Brainstem

49.1. The gray matter of the spinal cord is continuous with the gray matter of the medulla. In each picture on the right, the arrow points to the __________ ______, and the large area within the heavy outline is composed mainly of ______ matter.

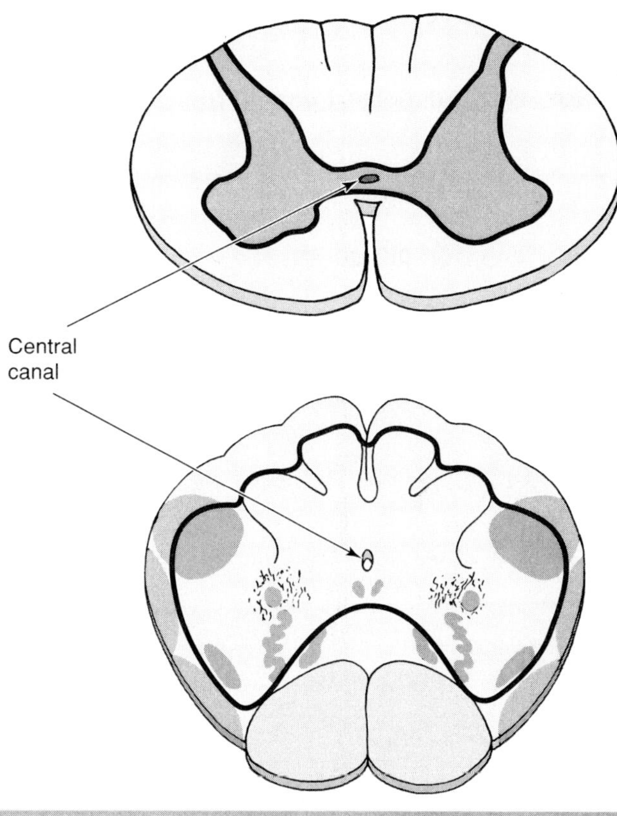

49.2. The spinal nucleus of V, located in the medulla and upper part of the __________ region of the spinal cord, is continuous with components of the __________ horns at lower levels of the spinal cord. In the same way, some of the motor components of the brainstem are continuous with components of the __________ horns of the cord.

49.3. Note the position of the central canal relative to the encircled nucleus on the right hand picture. The cells in this nucleus are similar in position and function to cells of the __________ horn of the spinal cord. The cell bodies in the encircled area are ______ in function.

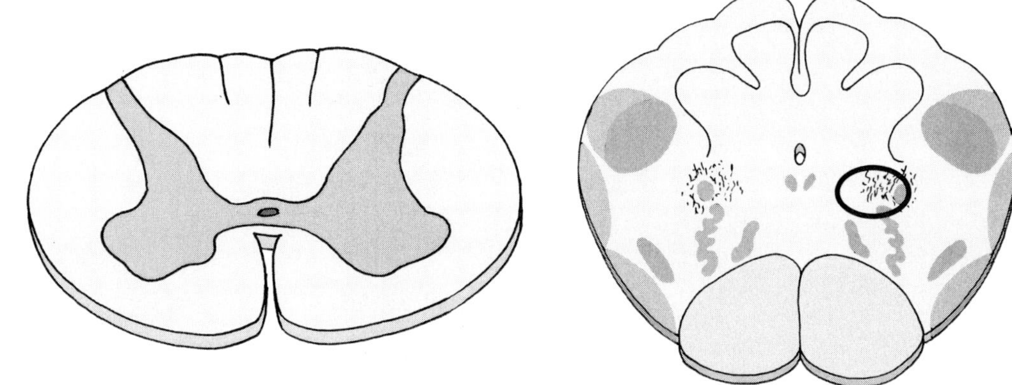

49.1A. central canal; gray

49.2A. cervical; posterior; anterior

49.3A. anterior; motor

49.4. In the spinal cord, motor neurons are anterior to the central canal, and sensory neurons are posterior. In the upper medulla, the ______ ventricle becomes wide. The motor nuclei remain in the same relative position, near the midline and ______ior to the ventricle. The sensory nuclei are displaced by the expanding ventricle to a more anterior and ____________ position.

49.5. There are three groups of motor nuclei in the brainstem: somatic, branchial, and visceral. They innervate two types of muscle; somatic motor nuclei and branchial motor nuclei both innervate skeletal muscle, whereas visceral motor nuclei innervate smooth muscle of viscera, vessels, and glands. ____________ and ____________ motor nuclei innervate ____________ muscle.

49.6. The two groups of brainstem motor nuclei that innervate skeletal muscles are distinguished on the basis of the embryonic origin of the muscles they innervate; one group innervates muscle derived from somites, whereas the other group innervates muscle derived from branchial (pharyngeal) arches. Which group of brainstem motor nuclei innervates skeletal muscle derived from embryonic somites? ____________ Skeletal muscles originating in branchial/pharyngeal arches of the embryo are innervated by the ____________ group of motor nuclei.

49.7. Smooth muscle, much of it found in the walls of blood vessels and in the viscera of the thorax and abdomen, is supplied by the ____________ motor nuclei of the brainstem.

49.8. In contrast to skeletal muscles, smooth muscles and glands are innervated by the ____________ motor nuclei. Skeletal muscles located in the head and neck are innervated by ____________ and ____________ nuclei of the brainstem.

49.9. Embryonic somites give rise to the extraocular muscles and the intrinsic muscles of the tongue. Somatic motor nuclei innervate muscles involved in movements of the ______ and ____________.

49.10. The extraocular muscles are attached to the ______side of the eye; their function is to ______ the eyeball. The intrinsic muscles of the tongue are located ______side the tongue; their function is to ______ the tongue.

49.11. Somites give rise to the intrinsic muscles of the ____________ and to the ____________________ muscles.

49.4A. 4th; anterior; lateral

49.5A. Somatic; branchial; skeletal

49.6A. Somatic; branchial

49.7A. visceral

49.8A. visceral; somatic; branchial

49.9A. eye; tongue

49.10A. outside; move; inside; move

49.11A. tongue; extraocular

49.12. The sternocleidomastoid and trapezius muscles arise from the branchial/pharyngeal arches. The ________________mastoid and __________ muscles are supplied by __________ motor nuclei.

49.13. Most skeletal muscles of the face and neck originate in pharyngeal arches. The most inferior of these are the sternocleido__________ and trapezius muscles.

49.14. The muscles of the throat also originate from pharyngeal arches; muscles of the larynx and _____rynx are innervated by __________ motor nuclei.

49.15. Branchial and somatic motor nuclei supply muscles used in vocalization. A branchial nucleus innervates the __________; a somatic nucleus innervates the __________.

49.16. Branchial motor nuclei innervate two neck muscles, the ________________ and __________, and also innervate skeletal muscles of the __________ and __________. Other pharyngeal arches give rise to the upper and lower jaws and related soft tissues of the face; branchial motor nuclei supply the muscles of mastication and the muscles of __________ expression.

49.17. Although the muscles supplied by the branchial motor nuclei are striated (skeletal), some of them are functionally associated with the alimentary system. These are the muscles of _____tication and the muscles of the __________.

49.18. Viscera, vessels, and glands of the head and the two major body cavities, the _____ax and _____men, are innervated by the __________ motor nuclei of the brainstem.

49.19. The pupillo-constrictor muscle of the iris is smooth muscle and is innervated by a __________ motor nucleus of the brainstem. The pupillo-constrictor muscle acts to make the pupil of the eye _____er in size.

49.20. A visceral motor nucleus innervates the pupillo-constrictor muscle of the iris _____side the eye; somatic motor nuclei innervate the ________________ muscles of the eye.

49.12A. sternocleidomastoid; trapezius; branchial

49.13A. sternocleidomastoid

49.14A. pharynx; branchial

49.15A. larynx; tongue

49.16A. sternocleidomastoid; trapezius; larynx; pharynx; facial

49.17A. mastication; pharynx

49.18A. thorax; abdomen; visceral

49.19A. visceral; smaller

49.20A. inside; extraocular

49.21. Visceral motor nuclei innervate the salivary ____________. The heart and involuntary (smooth) musculature of the respiratory passages, esophagus, stomach, and small intestines are all innervated by a single ____________ motor nucleus of the brainstem.

49.22. Use the letters "S," "B," and "V" to indicate which of the three groups of brainstem motor nuclei innervates each of the following:

Sternocleidomastoid and trapezius muscles: ______

Tongue muscles: ______

Smooth muscle of the thorax and abdomen: ______

Extraocular muscles: ______

Muscles of facial expression: ______

Salivary glands: ______

Muscles of mastication: ______

Striated muscles of the pharynx and larynx: ______

Pupillo-constrictor muscle: ______

49.21A. glands; visceral

49.22A. B; S; V; S; B; V; B; B; V

50 The Somatic Group of Brainstem Nuclei

50.1. Brainstem nuclei are collections of neuron cell bodies. The nuclei are part of the ______ matter. The cranial nerves and nuclei are designated by Roman numerals. The somatic group is made up of four nuclei associated with cranial nerves III, IV, VI, and XII. Nucleus XII, the most inferior in position, innervates the tongue, while ______, ______, and ______ innervate the ________________ muscles of the eye.

50.2. Of the four somatic brainstem nuclei, cranial nucleus IV supplies an ________________ muscle. Cranial nucleus III supplies several ________________ muscles. Cranial nucleus ______ supplies the tongue muscles. Cranial nucleus ______ supplies one extraocular muscle.

50.3. Since its axons constitute the hypoglossal nerve, the XIIth nucleus is also called the ________________ nucleus.

50.4. A major action of the tongue muscles is to push the tongue forward and allow it to protrude from the mouth. The musculature of the left side, if unopposed, would push the tongue __________ and to the right. Equal action of muscles of both sides causes the tongue to protrude __________ ahead.

50.5. A patient has a lesion affecting the right hypoglossal nucleus or nerve. He was asked to stick out his tongue. It protrudes forward and to his right side because the intact muscles of the ______ side push unopposed. Innervated tongue muscles of one side, if unopposed, push the tongue forward and toward the ________________ side.

50.6. A patient whose tongue protrudes to the left may have normally functioning muscle in the ______ side and impaired muscle in the ______ side of the tongue. The hypoglossal nerve or nucleus may be impaired on the ______ side. The protruded tongue "points __________ the side of the hypoglossal lesion."

50.7. The hypoglossal nucleus supplies the __________ muscles. Cranial nuclei VI, ______, and ______ supply the extraocular muscles. The extraocular muscles that contract and turn the eyes from left to right and right to left are the medial __________ and the __________ __________ muscles.

50.1A. gray; III; IV; VI; extraocular

50.2A. extraocular; extraocular; XII; VI

50.3A. hypoglossal

50.4A. forward; straight

50.5A. left; contralateral

50.6A. right; left; left; toward

50.7A. tongue; III; IV; rectus; lateral rectus

50.8. The eyeball is abducted (moved outward) by contraction of the ____________ rectus muscle. Contraction of the ____________ ____________ muscle adducts (moves inward) the eye.

50.9. In order to look towards the left with both eyes, the ______ lateral rectus and the ______ medial rectus both need to contract.

50.10. Cranial motor nuclei controlling the extraocular muscles have the same names as the corresponding cranial nerves. Cell bodies of the abducens nerve constitute the ____________ nucleus. The abducens nucleus and nerve supply the lateral rectus muscle. Right lateral gaze requires excitation of cranial nerve VI on the ______ side.

50.11. The lateral rectus is supplied by cranial nerve ______, named the ____________ nerve. Cranial nerve IV (the trochlear) supplies the superior oblique muscle. All of the other extraocular muscles are supplied by cranial nerve ______, the oculomotor nerve. How many extraocular muscles does the oculomotor nerve innervate? ______

50.12. Draw a line connecting the medial rectus muscle with its nucleus and another line connecting that nucleus with the appropriate cranial nerve number. Do the same for the superior oblique muscle.

	Oculomotor nucleus	VI
Medial rectus muscle		IV
	Abducens nucleus	III

In the same manner, connect the superior oblique muscle with its nucleus, and that nucleus with its number.

	Abducens nucleus	VI
Superior oblique muscle	Oculomotor nucleus	IV
	Trochlear nucleus	III

50.13. This eye is on the ______ side of the head. Place a Roman numeral on or beside each of the six extraocular muscles to indicate its source of innervation.

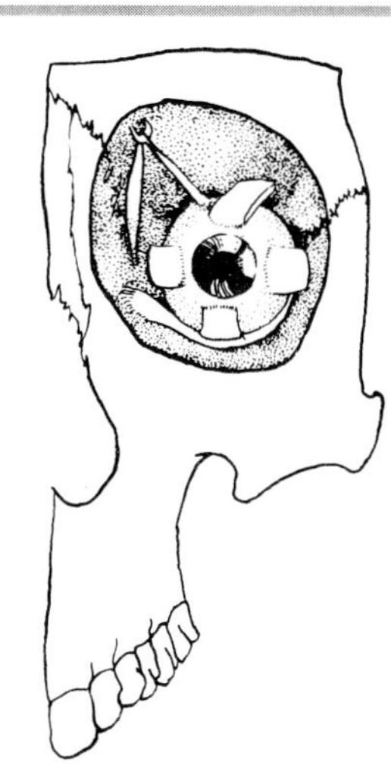

50.8A. lateral; medial rectus

50.9A. left; right

50.10A. abducens; right

50.11A. VI; abducens; III; four

50.12A.

	Oculomotor nucleus	VI
Medial rectus muscle		IV
	Abducens nucleus	III

(Medial rectus muscle — Oculomotor nucleus — III)

	Abducens nucleus	VI
Superior oblique muscle	Oculomotor nucleus	IV
	Trochlear nucleus	III

(Superior oblique muscle — Trochlear nucleus — IV)

50.13A. left

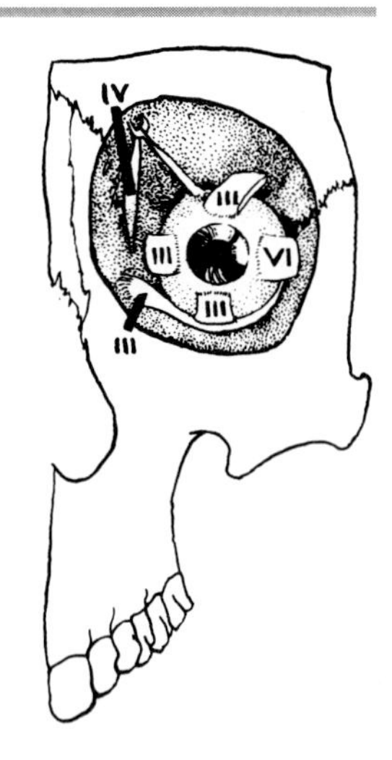

50.14. When the right eye moves outward, the ____________ rectus muscle of that eye contracts and the ____________ ____________ muscle of the same eye simultaneously relaxes. The simultaneous contraction and relaxation of extraocular muscles is accomplished by excitation and ____________________ of the appropriate cranial nerve nuclei in the brainstem.

50.15. Muscle action in both eyes must be integrated for focused vision. Right lateral gaze requires

contraction of the right ____________ ____________ muscle and left ____________ ____________ muscle. Simultaneously, there is relaxation of the lateral rectus on the ______ side and of the medial rectus on the ______ side.

50.16. The superior rectus pulls the eye up and rotates it slightly. An eye initially turned outward is pulled directly upward by contraction of the ____________ rectus.

50.17. In many situations, the rotating effect of the rectus muscles may be ignored. Upward gaze mainly involves simultaneous contraction of the ____________ rectus of each eye and relaxation of the ____________ rectus of each eye.

50.18. All of the extraocular muscles, except the superior oblique and the ____________ ____________, are supplied by cranial nerve ______. The three rectus muscles supplied by cranial nerve III are the ____________ rectus, the ____________ rectus, and the ____________ rectus. The extraocular muscle contracting most strongly in the diagram is innervated by cranial nerve ______.

50.19. Axons of cranial nerve VI arise from cell bodies in the brainstem nucleus named the ____________ nucleus. Downward gaze involves simultaneous contraction of the inferior rectus muscles and relaxation of the superior rectus muscles in both eyes. When the eyes move upward or downward, some neurons in the ____________________ nucleus are excited, and others are ____________. Both of these nuclei are classified among the ____________ motor nuclei of the brainstem.

50.14A. lateral; medial rectus; inhibition

50.15A. lateral rectus; medial rectus; left; right

50.16A. superior

50.17A. superior; inferior

50.18A. lateral rectus; III; medial; superior; inferior; VI

50.19A. abducens; oculomotor; inhibited; somatic

50.20. Cranial nerve IV arises from the IVth, or ____________, nucleus and supplies the superior ____________ muscle. The inferior oblique is supplied by cranial nerve ______.

50.21. With Roman numerals, designate which cranial nerves supply the following muscles:

Superior oblique: ______

Inferior oblique: ______

Inferior rectus: ______

Superior rectus: ______

Medial rectus: ______

Lateral rectus: ______

50.22. Provide the name for each numbered nucleus (and nerve):

XII: ____________________

IV: ____________________

VI: ____________________

III: ____________________

All are ____________ motor nuclei of the brainstem.

50.23. Name the muscles innervated by:

a. cranial nerve VI: ____________________

b. cranial nerve IV: ____________________

c. cranial nerve III: ____________________

d. cranial nerve XII: ____________________

50.24. If the lateral rectus muscle is paralyzed, then the eye will be pulled ______ward by the unopposed action of the ____________ ____________ muscle.

50.25. A patient who shows a right internal strabismus (a turning of the right eye toward the nose) may be suspected of having a weak ____________ ____________ muscle. He may have a lesion of the right ____________ nerve. If the left oculomotor nerve is diseased, then movement of the left eye upward, downward, and ____________ will be impaired.

50.20A. trochlear; oblique; III

50.21A. IV; III; III; III; III; VI

50.22A. hypoglossal; trochlear; abducens; oculomotor; somatic

50.23A. a. lateral rectus; b. superior oblique; c. medial, superior, and inferior recti; d. tongue muscles

50.24A. inward; medial rectus

50.25A. lateral rectus; abducens; inward

50.26. The remarkable coordination of several extraocular muscles of both eyes implies that there must be some rapidly conducting anatomical pathway that connects cranial nuclei ______, ______, and ______. Much of the coordination of the somatic motor nuclei is accomplished by a tract (fascicle) of nerve fibers that lies medially and runs longitudinally in the brainstem. It is called the m______ l________________ fasciculus.

50.27. Eye movements are coordinated with other movements of the face and neck. The __________ ________________ fasciculus interconnects nearly all motor nuclei of the cranial nerves.

50.28. When an individual is looking to the left and whistling, the __________ ________________ ________________ is coordinating almost simultaneous stimulation of the left __________ nucleus and the right ________________ nucleus, inhibition of the ______ oculomotor and ______ abducens nuclei, and stimulation bilaterally of somatic motor nucleus ______ (tongue movements for whistling) and of some __________ motor nuclei (facial expression and phonation).

50.26A. III; IV; VI; medial; longitudinal

50.27A. medial; longitudinal

50.28A. medial longitudinal fasciculus; abducens; oculomotor; left; right; XII; branchial

51 The Branchial and Visceral Groups of Brainstem Motor Nuclei

51.1. Embryonic pharyngeal arches give origin to the trapezius and ________________ muscles, to muscles of the __________ and __________, to muscles of ________________, and to muscles of __________ expression. Of cranial nerves III, IV, V, VI, VII, IX, X, XI, and XII, which five innervate branchial/pharyngeal musculature? _____, _____, _____, _____, and _____

51.2. Cranial nerve XI supplies the most inferior group of branchial muscles, the __________ and ________________ muscles of the neck. Cranial nerves IX and X innervate the __________ and __________.

51.3. The cranial nerves that innervate branchial muscles are V, VII, _____, _____, and _____. Which of the five nerves supply muscles of the face and jaws? _____ and _____ Cranial nerve VII supplies the muscles of __________ expression. Cranial nerve _____ supplies the muscles of mastication.

51.4. This patient has a common neurological disorder called Bell's palsy. One side of the face droops, as evidenced by a flattened eyebrow, diminished creasing of the cheek, and lowered corner of the mouth. The _____ cranial nerve is paralyzed on the drooping side of the face. In Bell's day, the term for paralysis was _____.

51.5. If a patient is unable to smile on one side, we may suspect injury to cranial nerve _____.

51.6. Match the following branchial muscles with the appropriate cranial nerves:

a. larynx and pharynx: cranial nerves _____, _____
b. sternocleidomastoid and trapezius: cranial nerve _____
c. muscles of mastication: cranial nerve _____
d. muscles of facial expression: cranial nerve _____

51.1A. sternocleidomastoid; larynx; pharynx; mastication; facial; V; VII; IX; X; XI

51.2A. trapezius; sternocleidomastoid; larynx; pharynx

51.3A. IX; X; XI; V; VII; facial; V

51.4A. VIIth; palsy

51.5A. VII

51.6A. IX; X; XI; V; VII

51.7. For the following cranial nerve numbers, list the appropriate skeletal muscles. Indicate whether the innervation is branchial motor or somatic motor.

III: __________ __________, __________
__________, __________ __________,
__________ __________; __________ motor
IV: __________ __________; __________ motor
V: _______________; __________ motor
VI: __________ __________; __________ motor
VII: __________ _______________; __________ motor
IX: __________, __________; __________ motor
X: __________, __________; __________ motor
XI: __________, _______________ motor
XII: __________; __________ motor

51.8. Branchial motor nuclei supply striated (skeletal) muscles, as do the __________ motor nuclei. Sympathetic and parasympathetic parts of the autonomic nervous system innervate __________ muscle of viscera throughout the body.

51.9. The presynaptic sympathetic nerve cell bodies are located in the thoracic and __________ segments of the spinal cord, where the cell bodies form a bulge named (according to its position) the _______________ cell column. Parasympathetic nerve cell bodies are located in the brainstem and sacral spinal cord. The sacral and cranial visceral components are classed as _____sympathetic.

51.10. Four cranial nerves carry the parasympathetic outflow from nuclei of the brainstem: III, VII, IX, and X. Together, they constitute the class of cranial __________ motor nuclei. Which of these nerves also have branchial motor components? _____, _____, and _____

51.11. The most widely distributed of the visceral motor nerves is cranial nerve X, which wanders (Latin vagus: wandering) from the head down through the chest and abdomen. The common name for nerve X is the v_____ nerve.

51.12. Smooth muscles of the thorax and abdomen are innervated by __________ motor components of cranial nerve number _____, named the _____ nerve. The larynx and pharynx are innervated by __________ components of the same cranial nerve. Other cranial nerves may also contain axons from more than one brainstem nucleus. For example, cranial nerve VII contains axons of neurons in visceral and __________ motor nuclei. CN III contains axons arising in visceral and __________ motor nuclei.

51.7A.

III:	Medial rectus, superior rectus, inferior rectus, inferior oblique; somatic
IV:	Superior oblique; somatic
V:	Mastication; branchial
VI:	Lateral rectus; somatic
VII:	Facial expression; branchial
IX:	Larynx, pharynx; branchial
X:	Larynx, pharynx; branchial
XI:	Trapezius, sternocleidomastoid; branchial
XII:	Tongue; somatic

51.8A. somatic; smooth

51.9A. lumbar; intermediolateral; parasympathetic

51.10A. visceral; VII; IX; X

51.11A. vagus

51.12A. visceral; X; vagus; branchial; branchial; somatic

51.13. The visceral motor nuclei are ______, IX, VII, and ______; they innervate glands and ____________ muscle. Cranial nerves VII and IX innervate salivary glands. The salivary glands are innervated by ____________ components of nerves VII and IX, and skeletal muscles are innervated by ____________ components.

51.14. If the VIIth nerve is cut as it emerges from the skull, then function of ____________ glands and muscles of ____________ ____________________ is impaired.

51.15. The visceral components of nerves ______ and IX innervate the salivary glands. Cranial nerve ______ innervates viscera of the thorax and abdomen. Cranial nerve III carries a visceral motor component in addition to its larger ____________ motor component. The pupil of the eye constricts under the influence of the visceral component of cranial nerve ______. The nerve innervates the pupillo-____________________ muscle of the iris.

51.16. Sympathetic and parasympathetic nerves both influence the size of the pupil. Dilation (enlargement) of the pupil results either from sympathetic nerve stimulation or from removal of ____________________ stimulation coming via cranial nerve ______.

51.17. This patient's left eye is turned outward, and his left pupil is ____________. He probably has a lesion affecting left cranial nerve ______ in both its ____________ and ____________ motor components.

51.18. Which cranial nerves innervate the following:

Smooth muscle of the thorax and abdomen: cranial nerve ______

Salivary glands: cranial nerves ______ and ______

Pupillo-constrictor muscle: cranial nerve ______

51.13A. X; III; smooth; visceral; branchial

51.14A. salivary; facial expression

51.15A. VII; X; somatic; III; pupillo-constrictor

51.16A. parasympathetic; III

51.17A. dilated; III; visceral; somatic

51.18A. X; VII; IX; III

51.19. Which nerves contain axons of neurons of the following nuclei?

Somatic motor nuclei: ______, ______, ______, ______

Branchial motor nuclei: ______, ______, ______, ______, ______

Visceral motor nuclei: ______, ______, ______, ______

51.20. Somatic components of cranial nerve XII are derived from the ________________ nucleus; somatic components of cranial nerve VI are derived from the ____________ nucleus; somatic components of cranial nerve IV are derived from the ____________ nucleus; and somatic components of cranial nerve III are derived from the ________________ nucleus.

51.21. Visceral and branchial motor nuclei occupy ____________ sites in the brainstem even though their neurons may send out axons in the ______ peripheral nerve. Visceral, branchial, and somatic motor functions may all be affected in peripheral nerve lesions if the nerve contains axons of all these types. The functional loss is likely to be more selective in ____________ lesions.

51.22. Similarly, sensory and motor functions may both be impaired in peripheral nerve disease but are less likely to be affected together in central nervous system (CNS) disease because the nerve cell bodies occupy ____________ sites centrally.

51.23. The spinal accessory nucleus innervates skeletal muscles of the neck; the nucleus ambiguus innervates skeletal muscles of the throat. Cranial nerve XI contains fibers of the ____________ motor class; these fibers arise from neuron cell bodies in the ____________ ____________ nucleus. Neurons innervating the throat are found in the ____________ ____________.

51.24. After each of the following cranial nerves, place an "S" for somatic, "B" for branchial, or "V" for visceral. More than one initial may be placed after a given nerve.

Spinal accessory nerve: ______

Trochlear nerve: ______

Hypoglossal nerve: ______

Oculomotor nerve: ______

51.19A.

III; IV; VI; XII

V; VII; IX; X; XI

III; VII; IX; X

51.20A. hypoglossal; abducens; trochlear; oculomotor

51.21A. different; same; brainstem

51.22A. different (or separate)

51.23A. branchial; spinal accessory; nucleus ambiguus

51.24A. B; S; S; S and V

52 Contributions of Brainstem Motor Nuclei to the Cranial Nerves

52.1. As indicated in the diagram, the ________ ________ nucleus is an aggregation of nerve cell bodies extending along the upper cervical spinal cord inferior to the foramen magnum. The nucleus ________ lies superior to this nucleus in the medulla; both are classified as branchial motor nuclei. Branchial refers to structures derived from the branchial/pharyngeal arch tissue of the embryo.

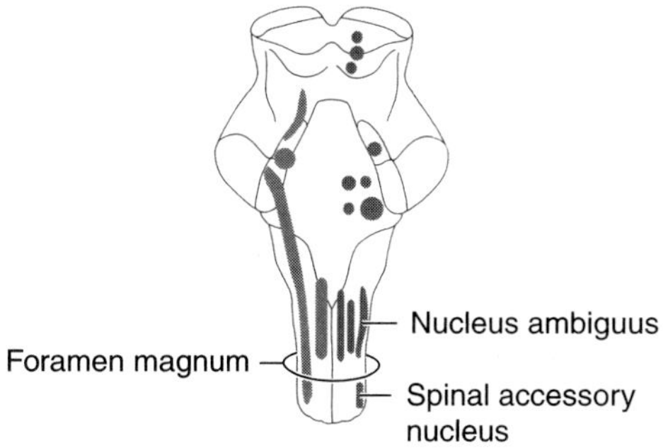

52.2. As labeled on the diagram, axons of neurons in the ________ ________ nucleus form the spinal root of the ________ nerve. This root ascends into the skull through the foramen magnum and then passes out again as cranial nerve XI to innervate the ________ and ________________ muscles of the neck.

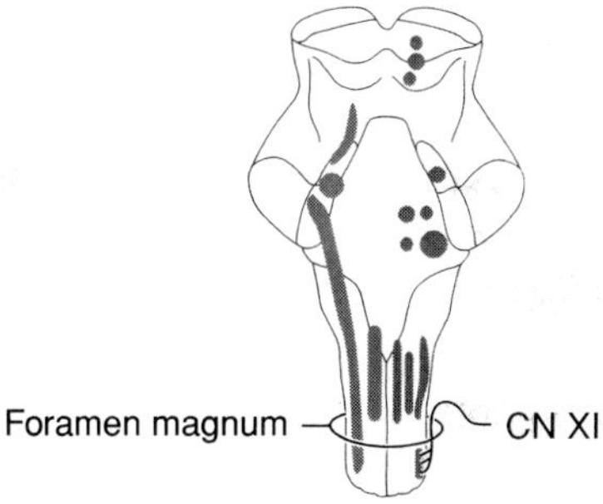

52.3. Axons from the nucleus ambiguus pass peripherally in cranial nerves ______ and ______. On the right side of the diagram, draw axons passing from cell bodies in the ambiguus and spinal accessory nuclei in cranial nerves IX, X, and XI.

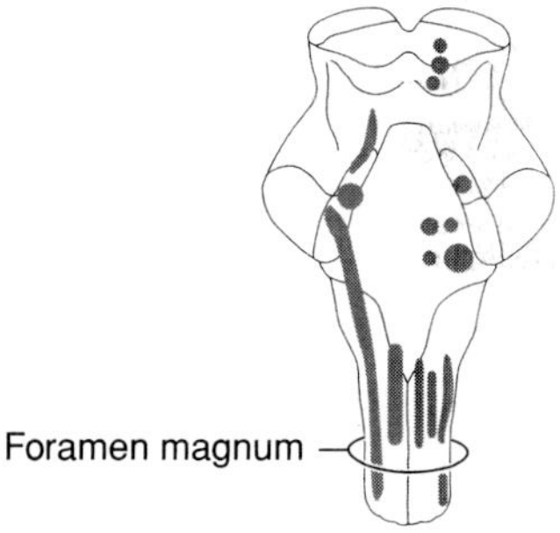

52.4. Label the spinal root of the accessory nerve (XI). Label nerves X and IX.

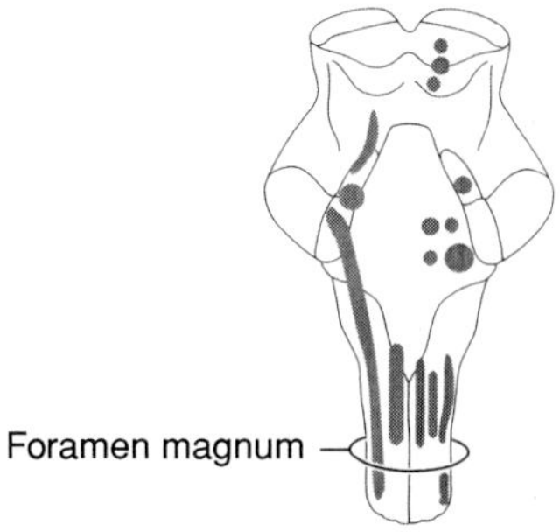

52.5. Of the two most inferior branchial motor nuclei, which one sends axons in cranial nerve XI to innervate the neck muscles? ________ ________ Branchial motor axons of cranial nerves IX and X arise in the ________ nucleus. Cranial nerves IX and X also contain axons of ________ motor nuclei.

52.1A. spinal accessory; ambiguus

52.2A. spinal accessory; accessory; trapezius; sternocleidomastoid

52.3A. IX; X

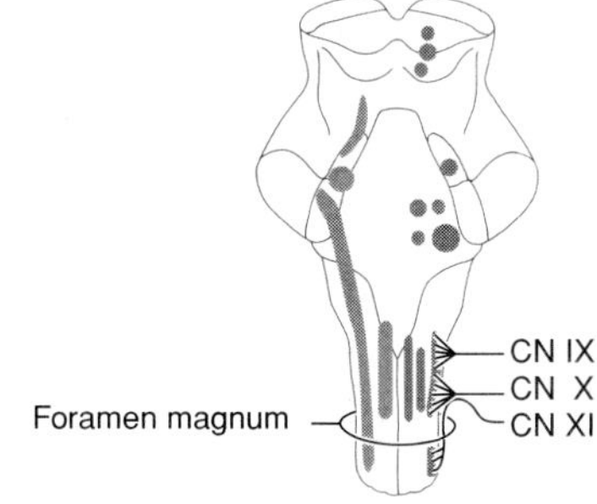

52.4A.

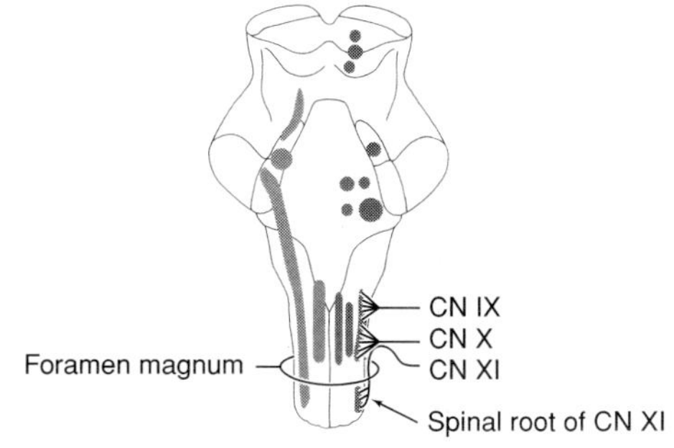

52.5A. spinal accessory; ambiguus; visceral

52.6. There are four branchial motor nuclei. Provide the numbers of the cranial nerves in which each sends its axons.

a. spinal accessory nucleus: cranial nerve ______
b. nucleus ambiguus: cranial nerves ______ and ______
c. facial nucleus: cranial nerve ______
d. trigeminal motor nucleus: cranial nerve ______

52.7. The ____________________ ______ nucleus innervates the jaw muscles used for chewing, called the muscles of ____________________. To distinguish it from the sensory part of V, the branchial component of V is called the trigeminal motor. The part of V concerned with pain and temperature has cell bodies in a cranial ____________ ganglion and root fibers that enter the brainstem and form the spinal tract of V.

52.8. Branchial muscles of the jaws and face are innervated, respectively, by the left and right motor ____________________ nuclei and by the ____________ nuclei.

52.9. List the cranial motor nerves (by Roman numeral) and nuclei (by name) that innervate the following branchial muscles:

a. facial expression: cranial nerve ______; ____________ nucleus
b. mastication: cranial nerve ______; ______ ____________________ nucleus
c. trapezius and sternocleidomastoid: cranial nerve ______; ____________ ____________ nucleus
d. larynx and pharynx: cranial nerves ______ and ______; nucleus ____________

52.10. The cranial portion of the parasympathetic nervous system is synonymous with the ____________ motor class of brainstem neurons. Its axons pass distally in cranial nerves ______, ______, ______, and ______.

52.11. The longest cranial parasympathetic nerve innervates glands, viscera, and vessels of the thorax and abdomen. Centuries before it was numbered as cranial nerve ______, this remarkably meandering nerve was named the ______ nerve.

52.6A. XI; IX and X; VII; V

52.7A. trigeminal motor; mastication; sensory

52.8A. trigeminal; facial

52.9A. VII; facial; V; motor trigeminal; XI; spinal accessory; IX and X; ambiguus

52.10A. visceral; III; VII; IX; X

52.11A. X; vagus

52.12. Cranial nerve X contains axons from a branchial motor nucleus (the __________ nucleus) and from a __________ motor nucleus. As cranial nerve X emerges from the medulla, it contains axons that will supply __________ muscle and glands of viscera and __________ muscle of the throat. Fibers destined for the throat muscles separate from the main trunk of nerve X, while others continue inferiorly into the thorax as the ______ nerve proper.

52.13. The branchial component of X has cell bodies in the __________ __________, and the visceral component of cranial nerve X has cell bodies in the __________ ______ nucleus of the vagus nerve.

52.14. The dorsal ______ nucleus of the ______ nerve contains neuron cell bodies of the __________ component of cranial nerve number ______.

52.15. The axons of the recurrent laryngeal nerve arise from neurons in the nucleus __________. Axons that innervate the heart and smooth muscle and glands of viscera originate in neurons of the __________ ______ nucleus of the ______ nerve. Both sets of axons travel together just outside the brainstem in cranial nerve ______.

52.16. The visceral motor nuclei are the dorsal motor nucleus of the vagus nerve, the two salivatory nuclei, and the accessory oculomotor (Edinger-Westphal) nucleus. Axons of the dorsal motor nucleus of the vagus pass distally in cranial nerve ______. Axons of nerves VII and IX arise from the ________________ nuclei. The sphincter pupillae is innervated by the __________ ________________ nucleus. The axons arising in this nucleus and the axons arising in the oculomotor nucleus travel together in cranial nerve ______.

52.17. Cranial nerve III contains axons of cell bodies in two distinct nuclei: the oculomotor nucleus, a __________ motor component, and the __________ oculomotor nucleus, a __________ motor component. Salivary glands are innervated by visceral motor nuclei, the two ________________ nuclei.

52.18. The cranial nerves are numbered from I to XII, beginning rostrally with I. The superior salivatory nucleus sends axons distally in cranial nerve VII, and the inferior ________________ nucleus projects axons in cranial nerve ______.

52.12A. ambiguus; visceral; smooth; skeletal; vagus

52.13A. nucleus ambiguus; dorsal motor

52.14A. motor; vagus; visceral; X

52.15A. ambiguus; dorsal motor; vagus; X

52.16A. X; salivatory; accessory oculomotor; III

52.17A. somatic; accessory; visceral; salivatory

52.18A. salivatory; IX

52.19. The facial nerve contains visceral and ____________ motor components. The facial and ____________ ____________________ nuclei give origin to motor fibers of cranial nerve ______. The inferior salivatory nucleus and the nucleus ____________ give origin to motor fibers of cranial nerve ______.

52.20. The axons of cranial nerve III arise in the ____________________ and ____________ ____________________ nuclei. Fibers of cranial nerve X arise from cell bodies in the nucleus ____________ and the ____________ ______nucleus of the vagus nerve.

52.21. List the four visceral motor nuclei and the numbers of the nerves in which their axons emerge.

____

____

____

____

52.22. Which cranial nerves are purely sensory, carrying no fibers from any of the brainstem motor nucleus? ______, ______, and _____

52.23. In the chart below, check all of the motor components of each cranial nerve.

	XII	XI	X	IX	VIII	VII	VI	V	IV	III	II	I
Somatic												
Branchial												
Visceral												

52.19A. branchial; superior salivatory; VII; ambiguus; IX

52.20A. oculomotor; accessory oculomotor; ambiguus; dorsal motor

52.21A. dorsal motor nucleus of the vagus nerve, X; inferior salivatory, IX; superior salivatory, VII; accessory oculomotor, III

52.22A. I; II; VIII

52.23A.

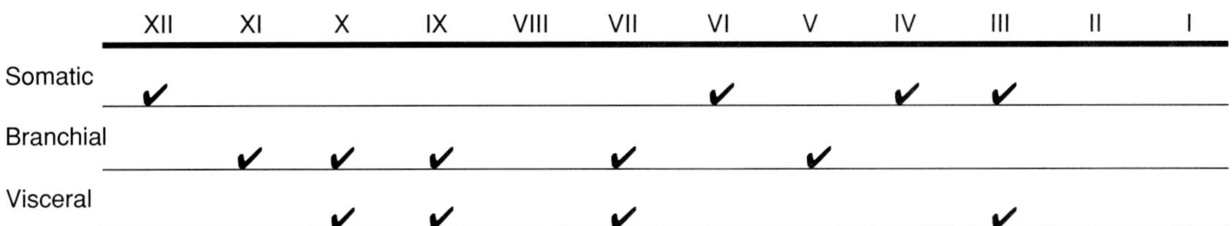

	XII	XI	X	IX	VIII	VII	VI	V	IV	III	II	I
Somatic	✔						✔		✔	✔		
Branchial		✔	✔	✔		✔		✔				
Visceral			✔	✔		✔				✔		

52.24. Name the nuclei that give rise to the motor components of each cranial nerve.

	XII	XI	X	IX	VIII	VII
Somatic						
Branchial						
Visceral						

	VI	V	IV	III	II	I
Somatic						
Branchial						
Visceral						

52.25. Name the muscles supplied by the following brainstem nuclei:

Nucleus ambiguus: ____________________

Accessory oculomotor nucleus: ____________________

Trochlear nucleus: ____________________

Spinal accessory nucleus: ____________________

52.26. In the chart below, write the names of the nuclei that innervate each structure.

	Tongue	Sternocleido-mastoid	Trapezius	Larynx & pharynx	Thorax & abdomen	Salivary glands
Somatic						
Branchial						
Visceral						

	Facial expression	Lateral rectus	Masti-cation	Superior oblique	Medial rectus	Sup. & inf. recti	Pupillo-constrictor
Somatic							
Branchial							
Visceral							

52.24A.

	XII	XI	X	IX	VIII	VII
Somatic	hypoglossal					
Branchial		spinal accessory	ambiguus	ambiguus		facial
Visceral			dorsal motor nucleus of the vagus nerve	inferior salivatory		superior salivatory

	VI	V	IV	III	II	I
Somatic	abducens		trochlear	oculomotor		
Branchial		trigeminal motor				
Visceral				accessory oculomotor		

52.25A. skeletal muscles of the larynx and pharynx; sphincter pupillae; superior oblique; sternocleidomastoid and trapezius

52.26A.

	Tongue	Sternocleido-mastoid	Trapezius	Larynx & pharynx	Thorax & abdomen	Salivary glands
Somatic	hypoglossal					
Branchial		spinal accessory	spinal accessory	ambiguus		
Visceral					dorsal motor nucleus of x	(superior & inferior) salivatory

	Facial expression	Lateral rectus	Masti-cation	Superior oblique	Medial rectus	Sup. & inf. recti	Pupillo-constrictor
Somatic		abducens		trochlear	oculomotor	oculomotor	
Branchial	facial		trigeminal motor				
Visceral							accessory oculomotor

53 Location of Motor Nuclei on Phantom Views of Brainstem

53.1. The most inferior somatic nucleus runs the length of the medulla. Label it with its name on the diagram. The only somatic motor nucleus lying in the pons is the abducens nucleus; label it. Label the two somatic motor nuclei in the midbrain.

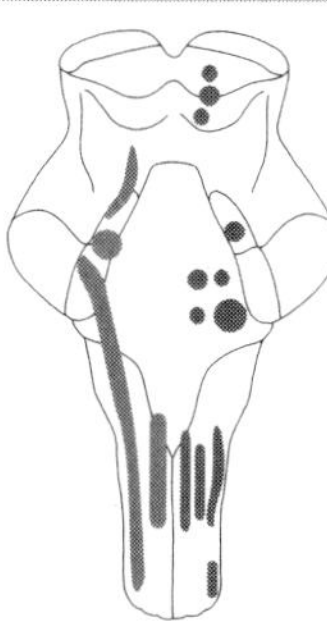

53.2. Which somatic motor nucleus lies entirely within the medulla? ________________ Which one lies within the pons? __________ Which one underlies the inferior colliculi? __________

53.3. The only cranial nerves that are completely crossed are the __________ nerves. Thus, the __________ __________ muscle of the left eye is innervated by the ______ __________ nucleus.

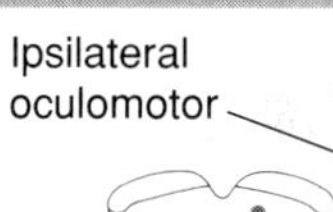

53.4. Clinical lesions of III, IV, or VI almost always affect the nerve and not the nucleus. Regardless of where the cell bodies lie, a lesion along the course of one of these cranial nerves on the right side will affect muscle function of the ______ eye.

53.5. The most inferior nucleus in the branchial motor column lies in the cervical spinal cord; this nucleus is the spinal __________ nucleus. Label it on the diagram.

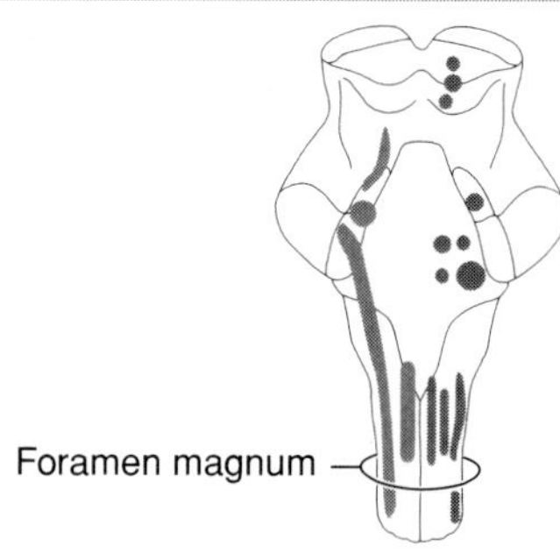

53.1A.

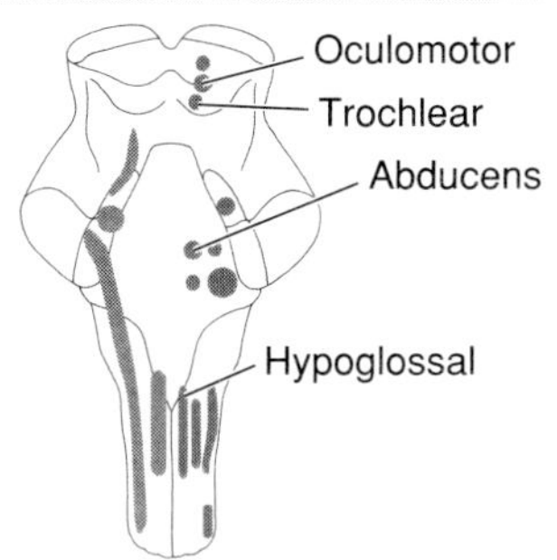

53.2A. Hypoglossal; Abducens; Trochlear

53.3A. trochlear; superior oblique; right trochlear

53.4A. right

53.5A. accessory

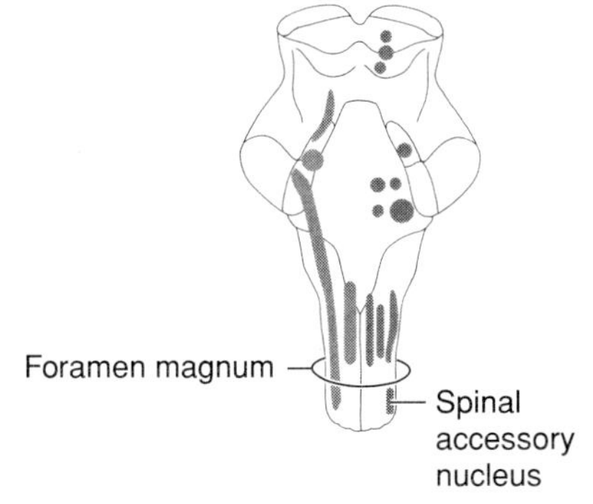

53.6. Immediately superior to the spinal accessory nucleus in the branchial motor column is the nucleus ____________. It parallels the ____________ ______ nucleus of the vagus. The facial nucleus lies just superior to the junction of the medulla and ______. Label the facial nucleus, spinal accessory nucleus, nucleus ambiguus, and the dorsal motor nucleus of the vagus.

53.7. Label the four nuclei of the branchial motor column. The most superior branchial motor nucleus, lying in the mid pons, supplies the muscles of ____________.

53.8. The two somatic nuclei in the midbrain are the ____________ nucleus (more inferiorly positioned) and the __________________ nucleus (more superiorly positioned).

53.9. Label each of the somatic and branchial motor nuclei. Place the numbers of the cranial motor nerves to which each gives rise. Label each of the four visceral motor nuclei.

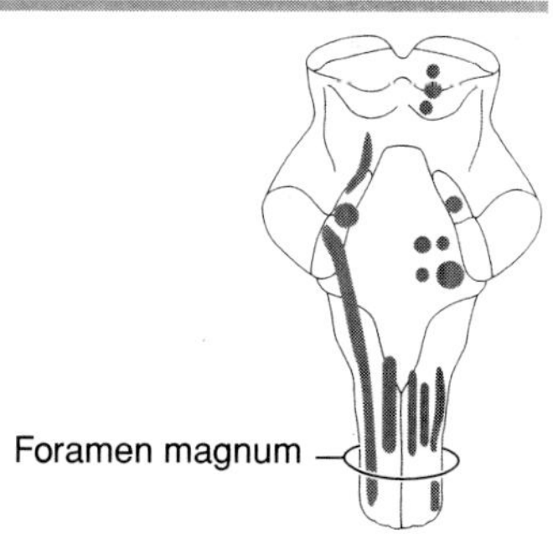

53.6A. ambiguus; dorsal motor; pons

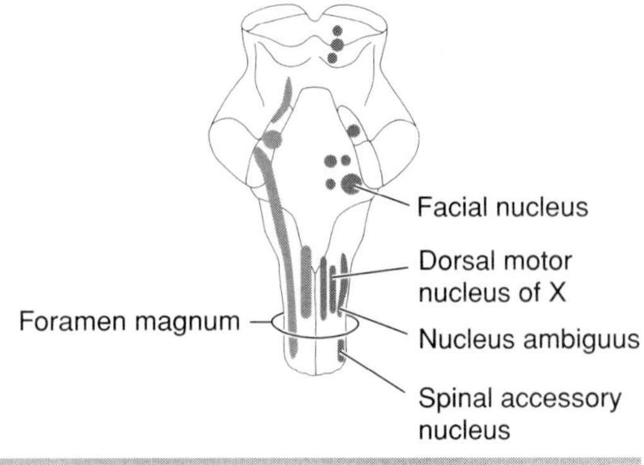

53.7A. mastication

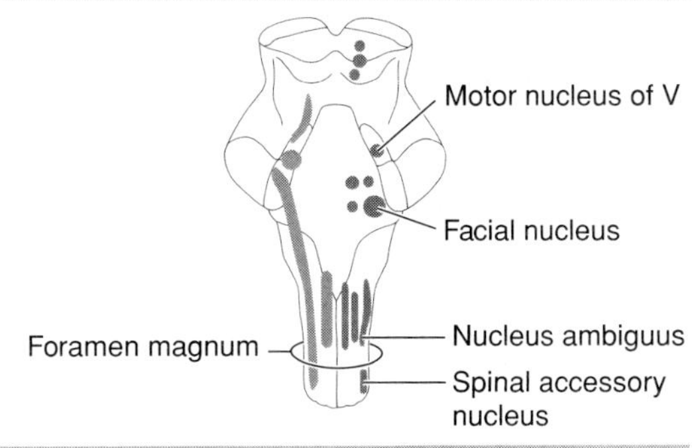

53.8A. trochlear; oculomotor

53.9A.

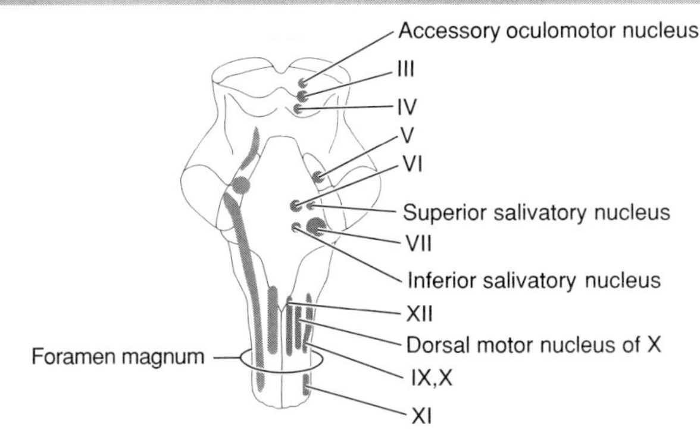

53.10. The dorsal motor nucleus of the vagus is a column of cells in the medulla, positioned between the ____________ nucleus (laterally) and the ____________________ nucleus (medially). Place an "X" on the dorsal motor nucleus of the vagus. Just superior to the dorsal motor nucleus of the vagus are two small visceral motor nuclei; label them. The most superior of the visceral motor nuclei is the accessory oculomotor nucleus, lying in the ____________. It forms a cap over the medial, posterior, and superior aspects of the superior portion of the ____________________ nucleus.

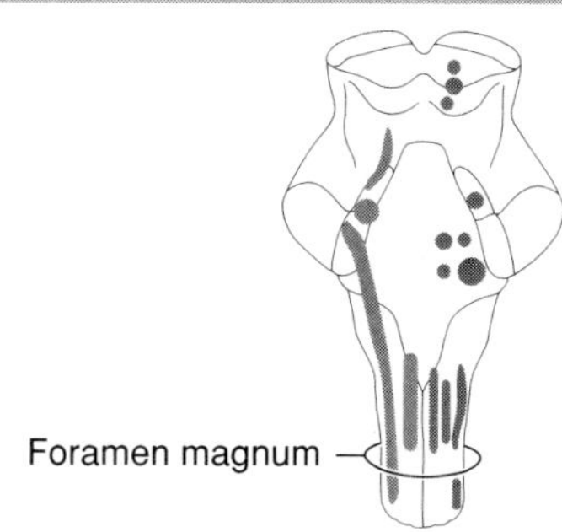

53.11. Place an "X" on the largest visceral motor nucleus, which runs the length of the ____________. Label the other three visceral motor nuclei with their names and indicate in which cranial nerve their fibers travel.

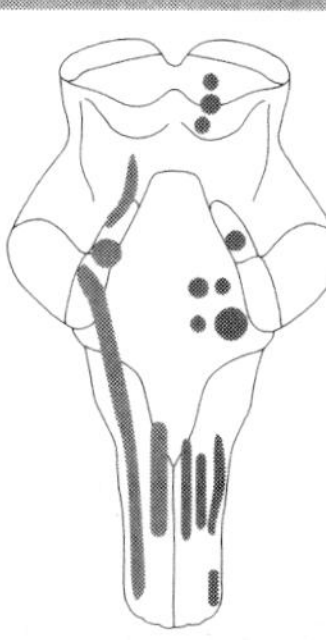

53.12. Label all of the branchial and somatic motor nuclei.

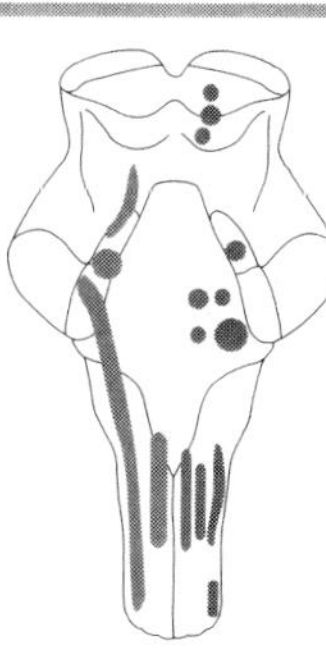

53.10A. ambiguus; hypoglossal; midbrain; oculomotor

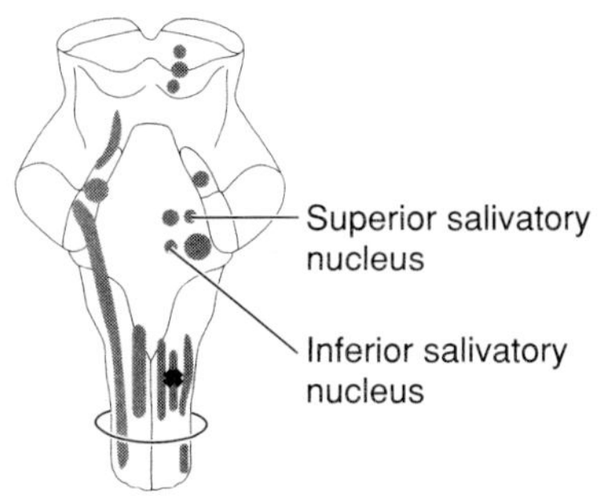

53.11A. medulla

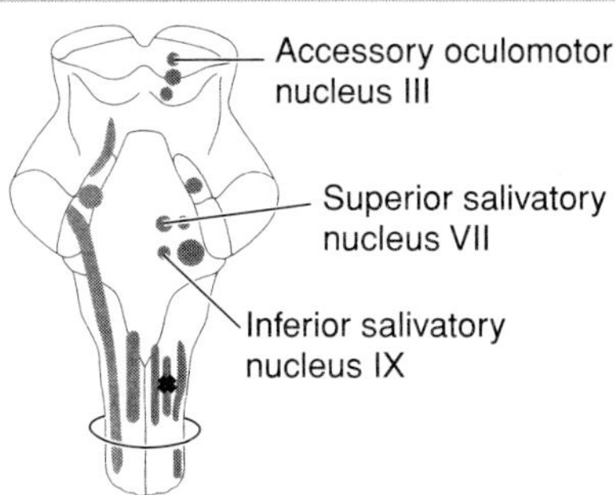

53.12A.

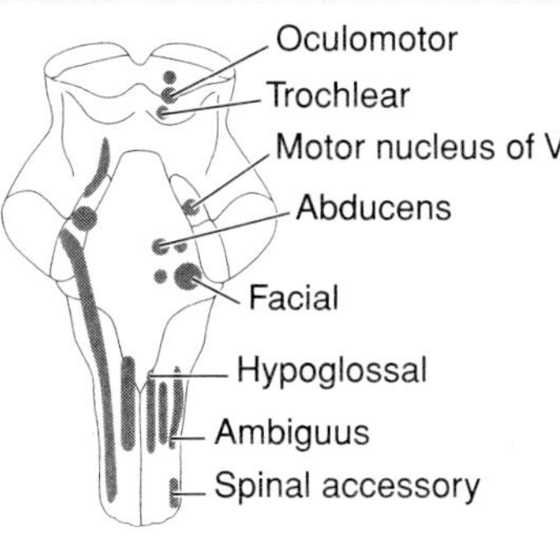

54 Motor Nuclei and Other Landmarks in Transverse Sections Through the Brainstem

54.1. On the upper picture, label the structures indicated. The presence of the most anterior of these structures indicates that this section passes through the region of the brainstem called the ___________. On the lower section, the encircled tract contains afferent axons from ___________ary neuron cell bodies in the nucleus dorsalis on the _____ side. At this level of the brainstem, the axons of the encircled tracts are just beginning to enter the inferior ________________ ___________.

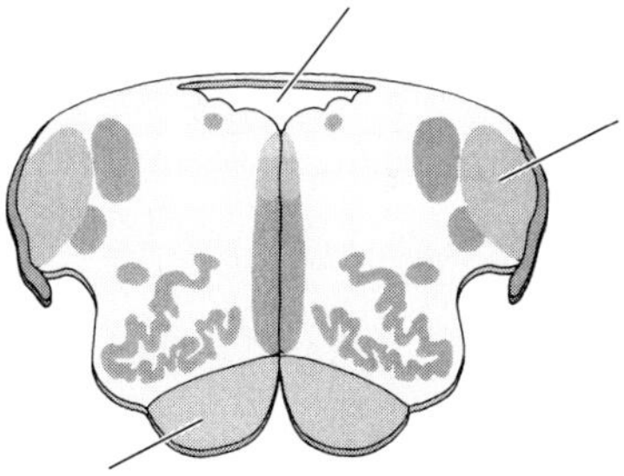

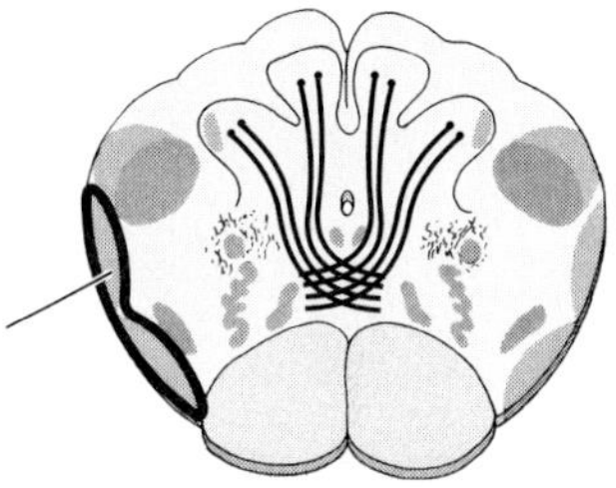

Spinocerebellar tracts

54.2. The ___________ cerebellar peduncle conveys information about muscle tone to the ________________ from the lower medulla and from the ________________ tracts of the spinal cord. Place an "X" on this peduncle bilaterally on both pictures.

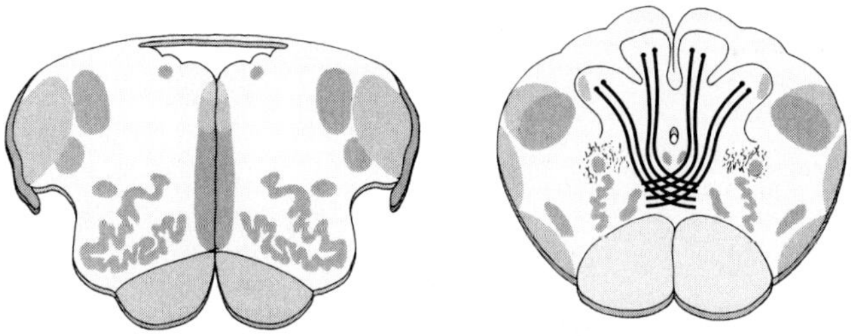

54.3. The nucleus dorsalis, located mainly in ___________ segments of the spinal cord, is analogous to the external ___________ nucleus of the lower medulla. Both send axons into the ___________ ________________ ___________ of the _____ side.

54.4. Place an "X" on the external cuneate nucleus. It is enveloped by fibers of the fasciculus ___________.

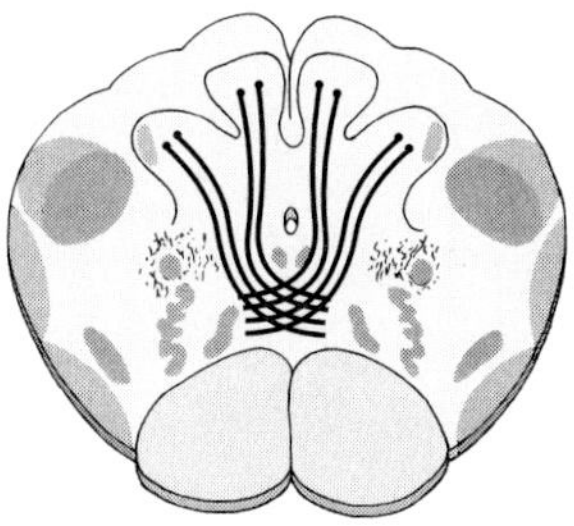

54.1A. medulla; secondary; same; cerebellar peduncle

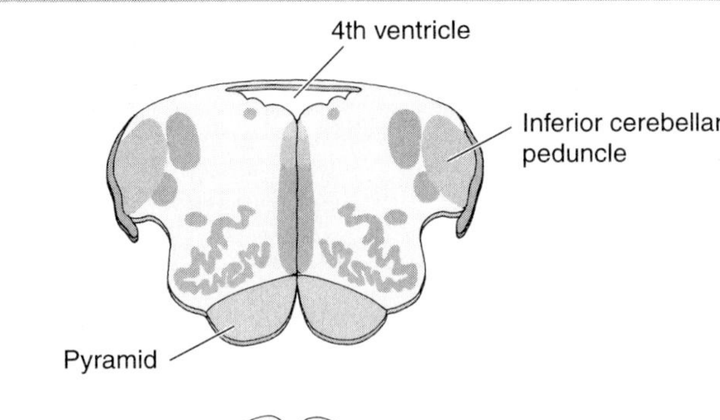

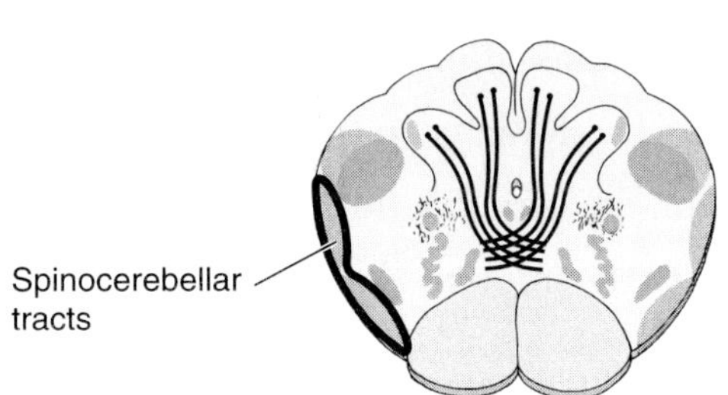

54.2A. inferior; cerebellum; spinocerebellar

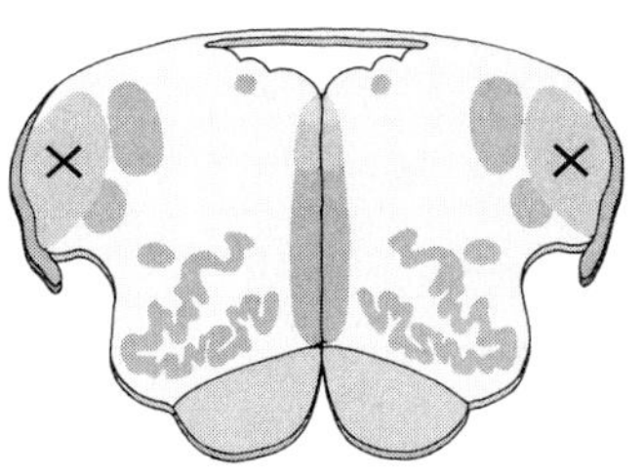

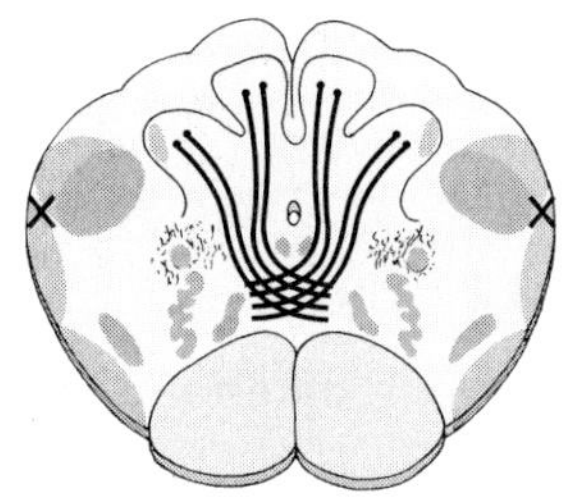

54.3A. thoracic; cuneate; inferior cerebellar peduncle; same

54.4A. cuneatus

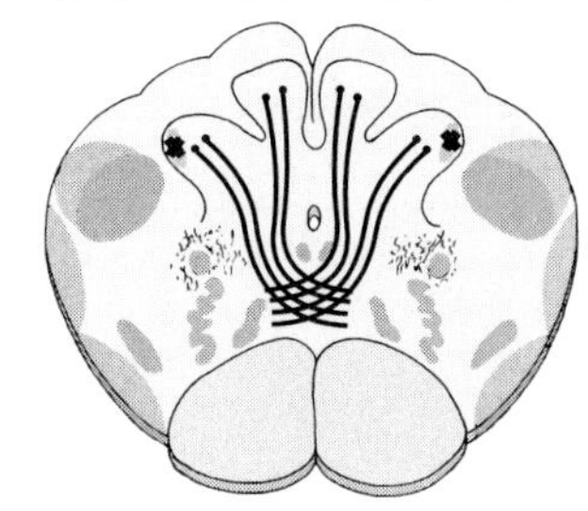

54.5. Cell bodies of secondary neurons in the kinesthetic pathway lie in the nuclei ________ and ________. As axons of these neurons curve anteriorly, the axons collectively are named ________ ________ fibers; they cross the midline and ascend all the way to the ________ in the ________ ________.

54.6. On the diagram, label each of the following structures with its number:

1. Left nucleus gracilis
2. Right nucleus cuneatus
3. Right fasciculus cuneatus
4. Right external cuneate nucleus
5. Central canal
6. Left internal arcuate fibers
7. Decussation of the medial lemniscus

54.7. The posterior gray columns of the spinal cord contain many neuronal cell bodies that convey information about pain and temperature senses. The medulla and pons contain analogous ________ary sensory nerve cell bodies, which are located in the spinal ________ of the trigeminal. In the pain and temperature pathways of both the spinal cord and brainstem, the primary and secondary cell bodies lie on the ____ side.

54.8. The nucleus encircled on both pictures, which is concerned with pain and temperature senses on the ____ side of the face, is the ________ ________ of ____. Encircle the same nucleus on the other side of each section.

54.9. Place an "X" on the areas containing secondary sensory cell bodies concerned with pain sensation in the left side of the body, neck, or face.

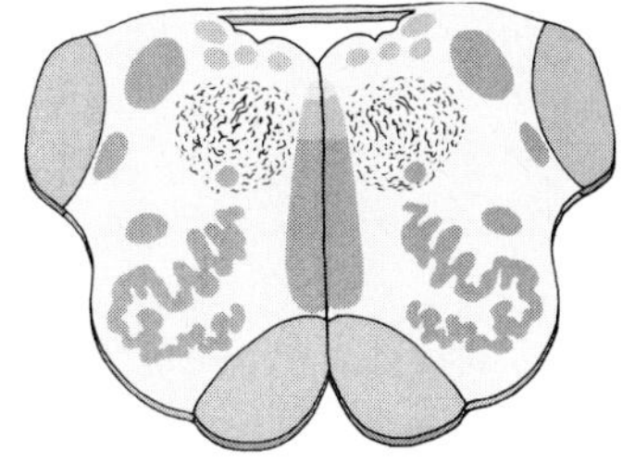

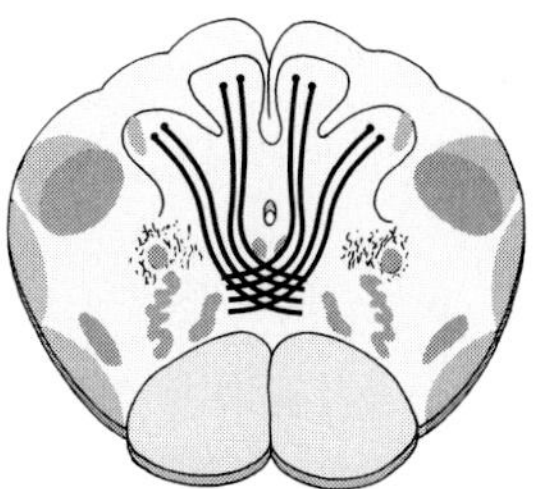

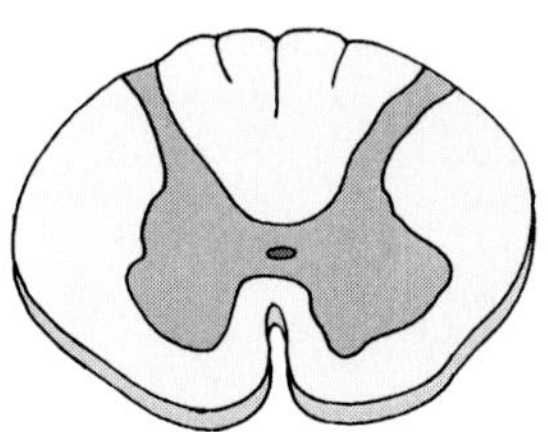

54.5A. gracilis; cuneatus; internal arcuate; thalamus; medial lemniscus

54.6A.

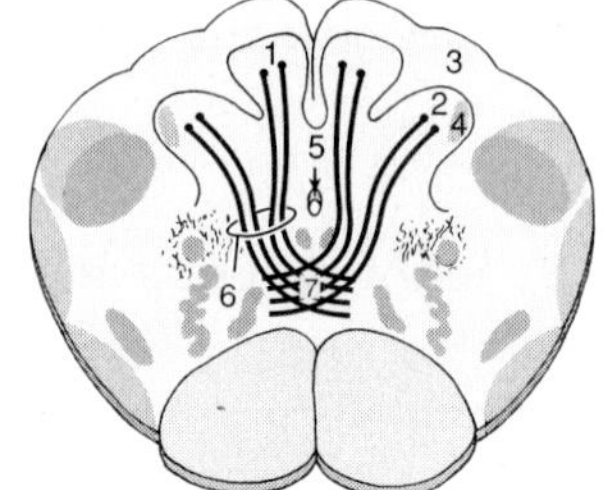

54.7A. secondary; nucleus; same

54.8A. same; spinal nucleus of V

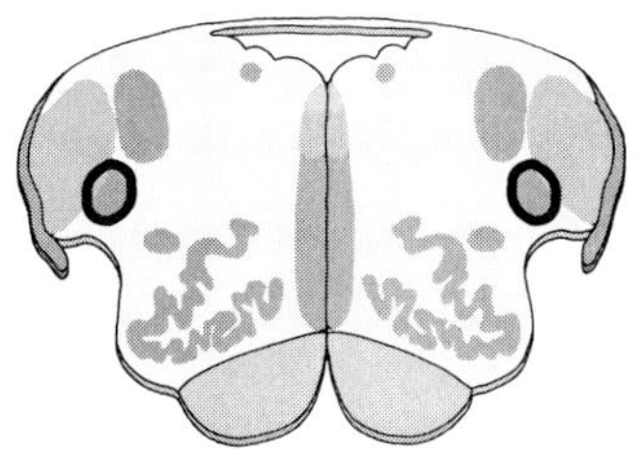

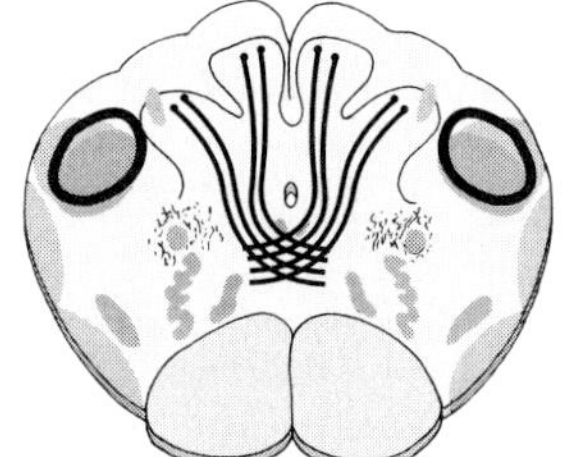

54.9A.

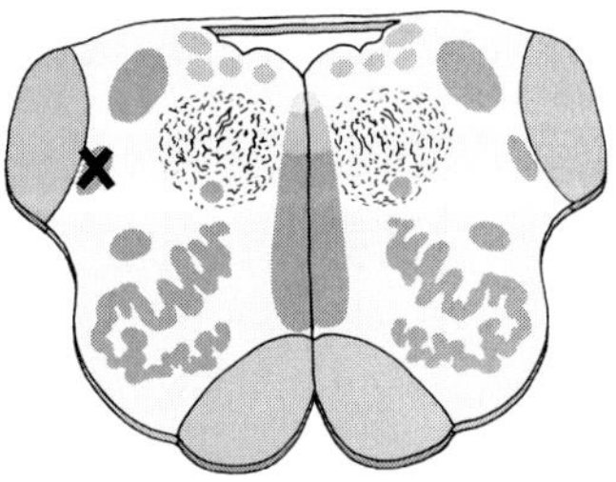

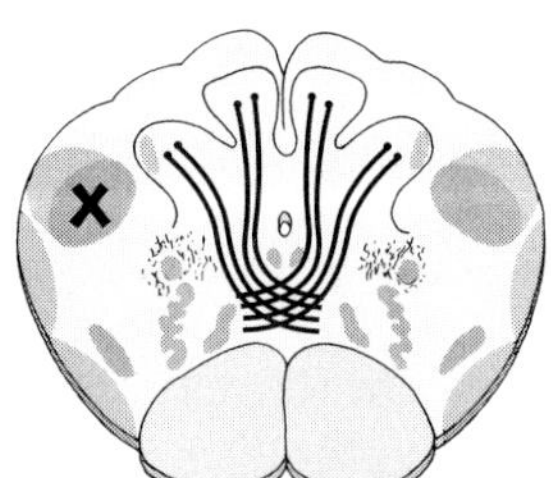

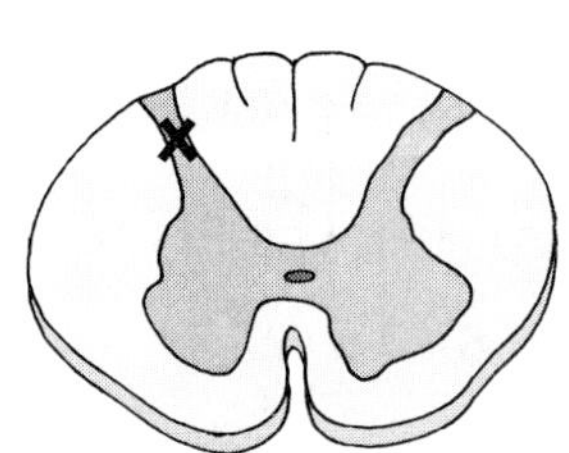

54.10. Posterior root fibers for pain and temperature in the right foot enter the cord, bifurcate, ascend, and descend short distances in the ________________ fasciculus and then make synaptic contact with secondary neurons. Draw a small arrow in the area of such a synapse; point the arrow to indicate the direction of impulse conduction. Impulses cross a synapse in how many directions? ______

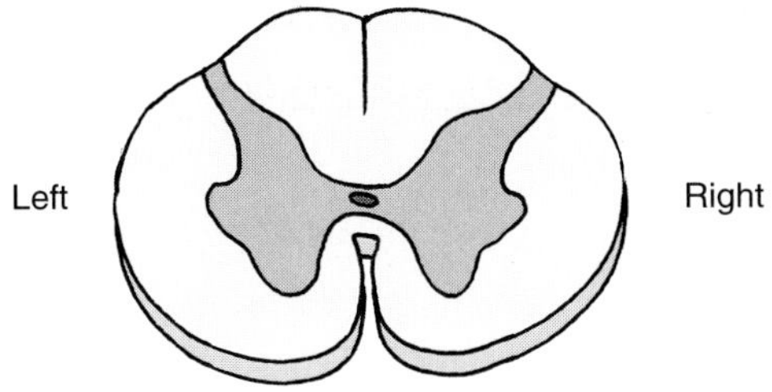

Left

Right

54.11. The primary neuronal cell bodies for pain sensation on the face lie in the cranial sensory ganglion named the ________________ ganglion. The root fibers descend in the __________ ______ of V. Label the components of this sensory system indicated in the diagram, and with a small arrow, indicate the direction of impulse conduction from one to the other.

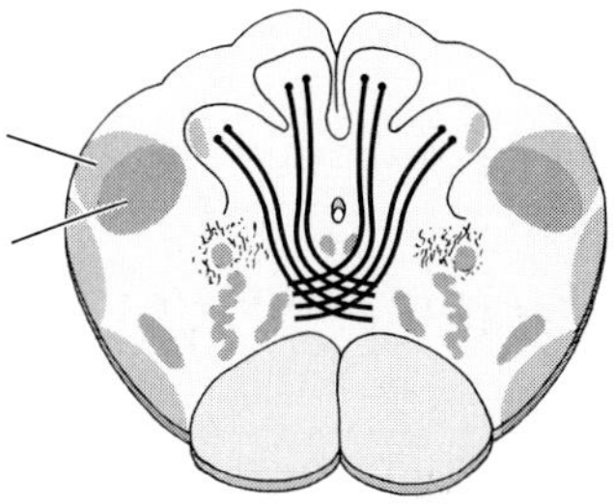

54.12. Synaptic zones in two different sensory systems are circled. In each case, label the tract containing the presynaptic axons, and draw an arrow to indicate the direction of impulse conduction.

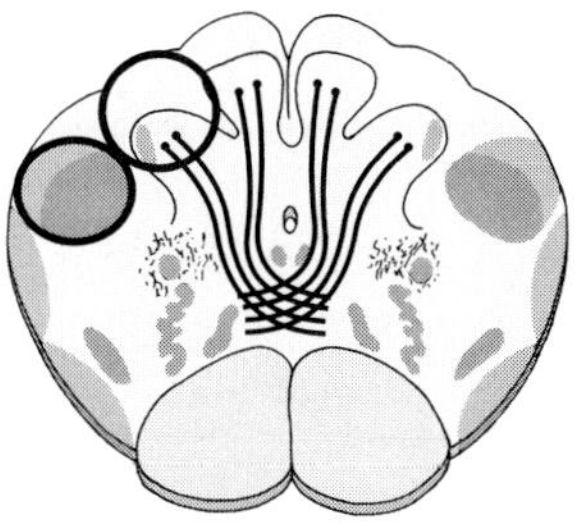

54.13. The prominent, wormy-looking mass of gray matter appearing on each side of the image is called the __________ __________ nucleus.

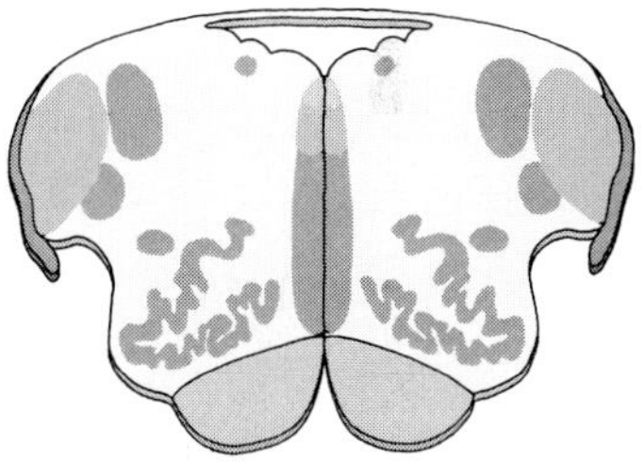

54.14. Neurons of the "inferior olives" (the nuclei are sometimes abbreviated) send axons out the medial, open end of each complex and into the inferior cerebellar peduncle of the __________ side.

54.15. The inferior olives relay impulses that reach the ________________ via the __________ ________________ peduncle of the opposite side. The axons of olivary neurons thus form a tract named for their origin and termination: the ______vo-________________ tract.

54.10A. dorsolateral; One

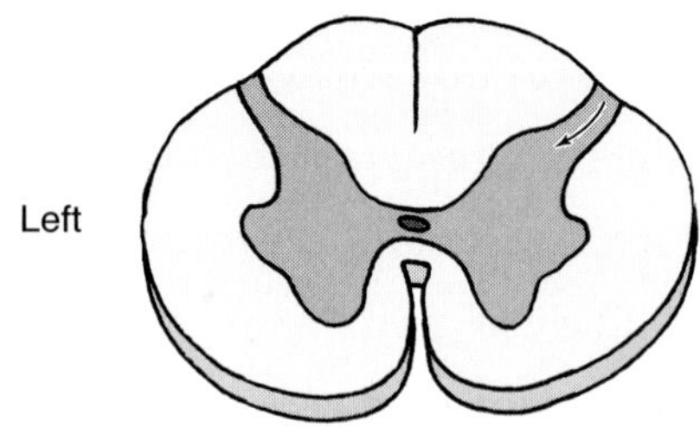

54.11A. trigeminal; spinal tract

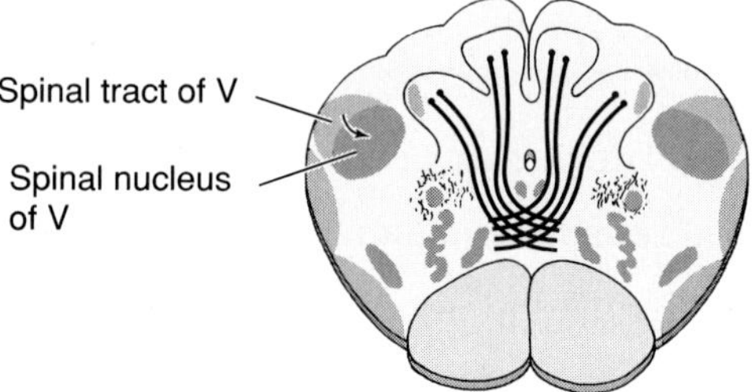

54.12A.

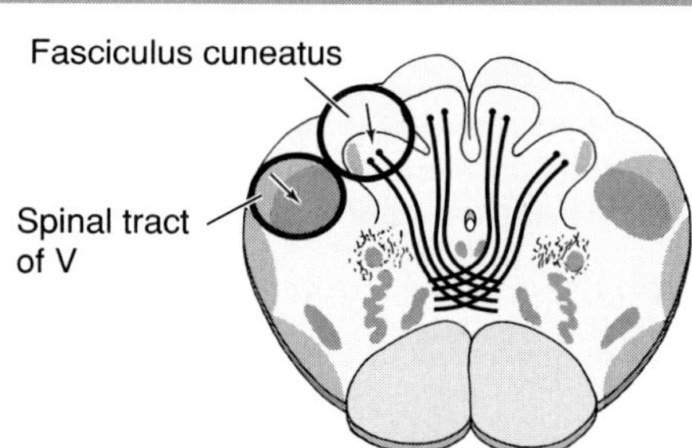

54.13A. inferior olivary

54.14A. opposite

54.15A. cerebellum; inferior cerebellar; olivo-cerebellar

54.16. The inferior cerebellar peduncles receive fibers from three sources:

a. uncrossed secondary neurons from the spinal cord, originating in the nucleus __________ (__________'s column)

b. analogous axons but carrying afferent information from neck muscles and originating in the __________ __________ nucleus.

c. crossed fibers of the ______ - ________________ tract.

54.17. A dense band of white matter is closely applied to the outside of the olive. These fibers descend from the upper brainstem to the inferior olive in the central __________ tract. On the left side, indicate with an arrow the direction of impulse conduction between the central tegmental tract and nerve cell bodies of the inferior olive. Draw several axons passing from this olive to the cerebellum.

Central tegmental tract

54.18. Impulses descending to the olive in the __________ __________ tract cross a synapse and are relayed via olivary neurons to the ________________ side of the cerebellum.

54.19. Label the three motor nuclei that extend most of the length of the medulla. Beside each name, place a "V," "S," or "B" in parentheses to indicate the class to which each belongs.

54.20. Use specific names on the right side of the diagram to label the nuclei that have been marked on the left with their class names.

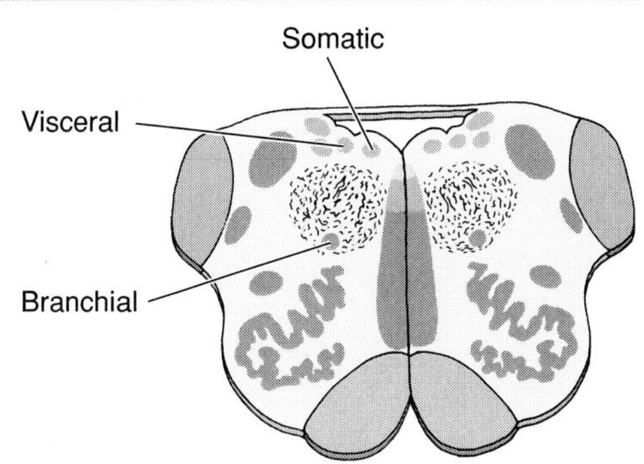

54.16A. dorsalis; Clarke's; external cuneate; olivo-cerebellar

54.17A. tegmental

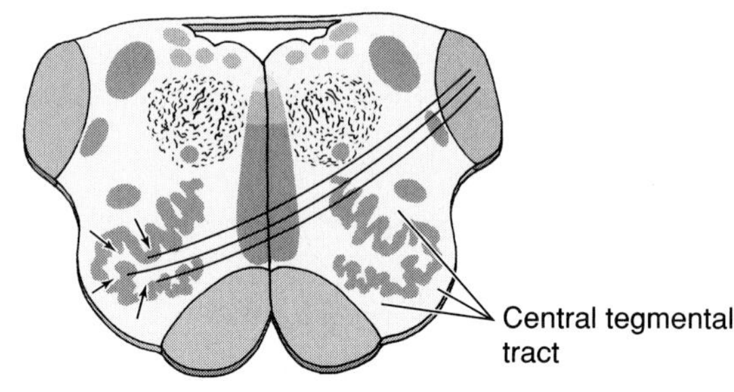

54.18A. central tegmental; contralateral

54.19A.

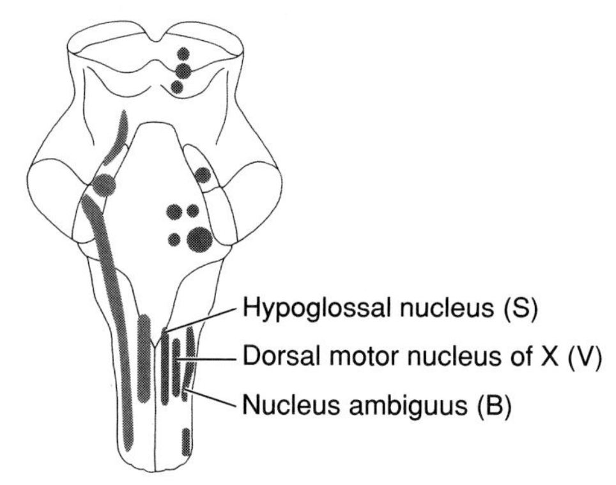

54.20A.

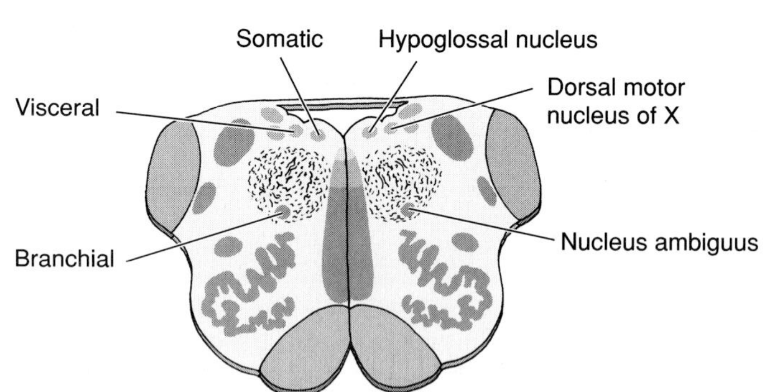

54.21. In the early embryo, all motor neuron cell bodies lie near the midline just below (anterior to) the ventricle. Subsequently, cell bodies of the class of __________ motor nuclei migrate to new positions, as illustrated. Encircle these neurons on the contralateral side.

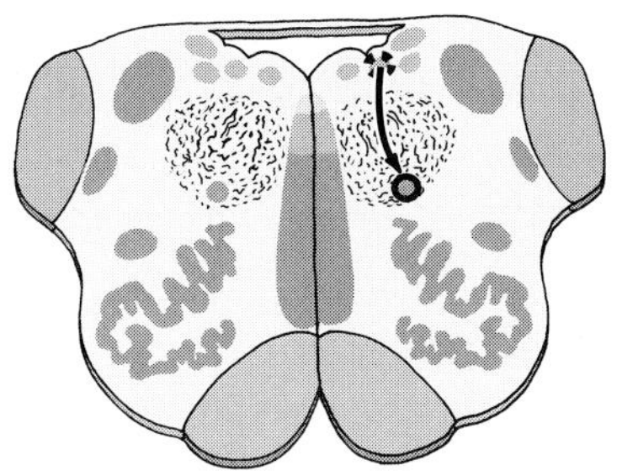

54.22. Encircle the position of the nucleus ambiguus on both sides.

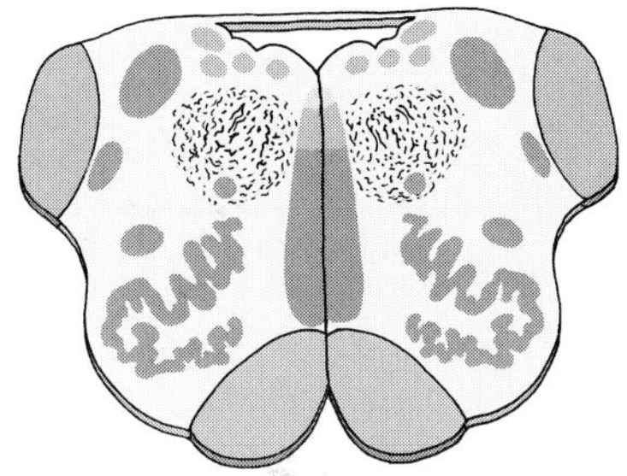

54.23. The inferior olivary nucleus is outlined by myelinated fibers of the __________ __________ tract (around the outside of the nucleus) and fibers of the ______-________________ tract (on the inside).

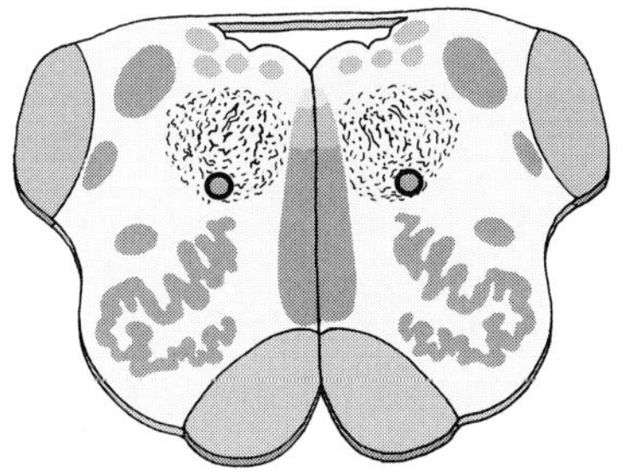

54.24. The nucleus ambiguus really is ambiguous. Its side is obscured by ______-________________ fibers coming from cell bodies of the __________ ______ of the ________________ side and crossing toward the __________ ________________ __________. All somatic and __________ motor nuclei lie close to the ventricle. Because of cell migration in embryonic development, there has been displacement of the __________ motor nuclei in an __________ and __________ direction.

54.25. In the early embryo, neurons of the nucleus ambiguus send axons to enter the cranial nerves numbered ______ and ______. The cell bodies migrate anteriorly during development, returning toward their original position. Draw several of these axons on the section of the adult medulla, and label the nucleus ambiguus on the opposite side.

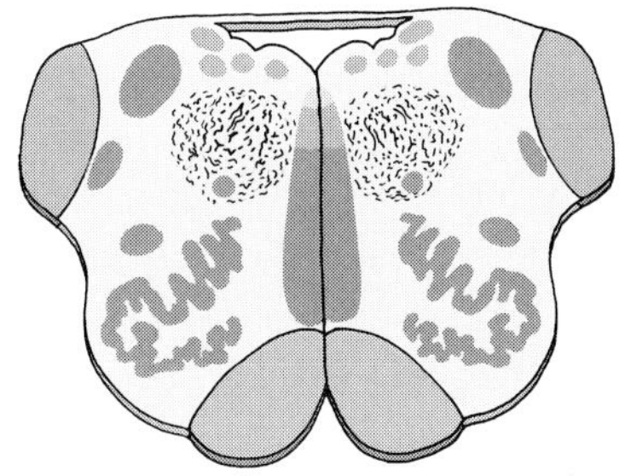

54.21A. branchial

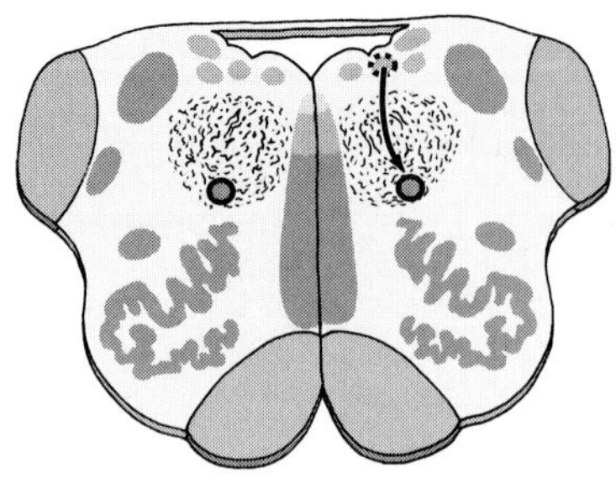

54.22A.

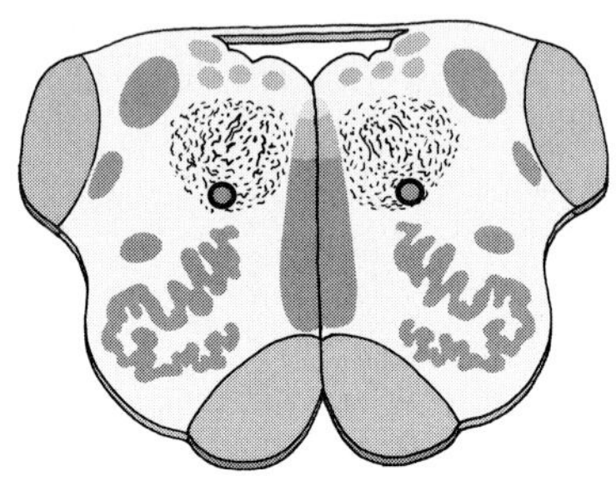

54.23A. central tegmental; olivo-cerebellar

54.24A. olivo-cerebellar; inferior olive; contralateral; inferior cerebellar peduncle; visceral; branchial; anterior; lateral

54.25A. IX; X

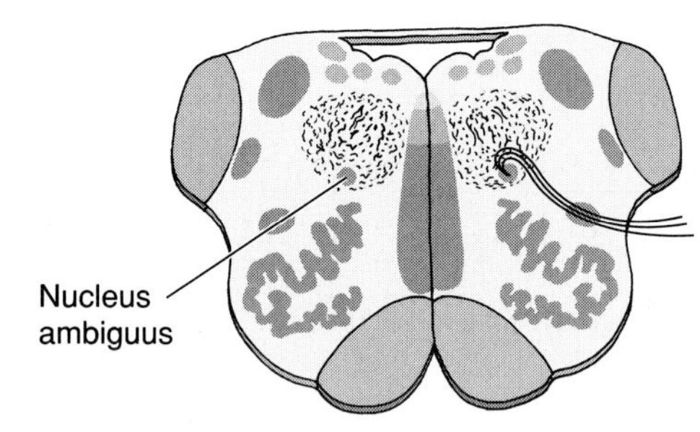

54.26. Label cranial nerves XII and X with Roman numerals as they emerge from the medulla. Nerve XII emerges between the ____________ ______ and the ____________.

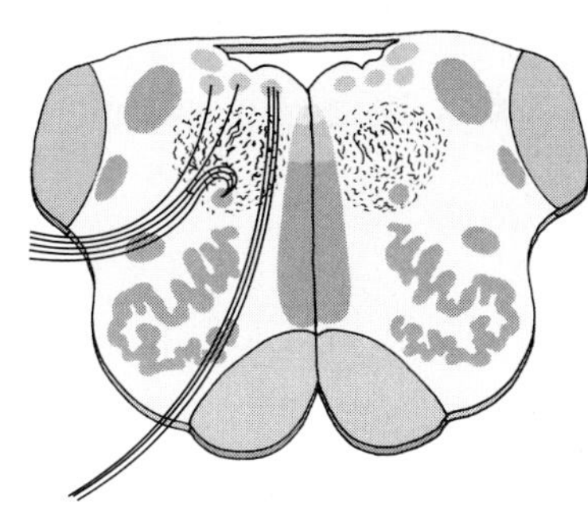

54.27. The visceral motor nuclei lie lateral to the ____________ motor nuclei. On both sides of the picture, encircle and label the nuclei of both classes with their Roman numerals.

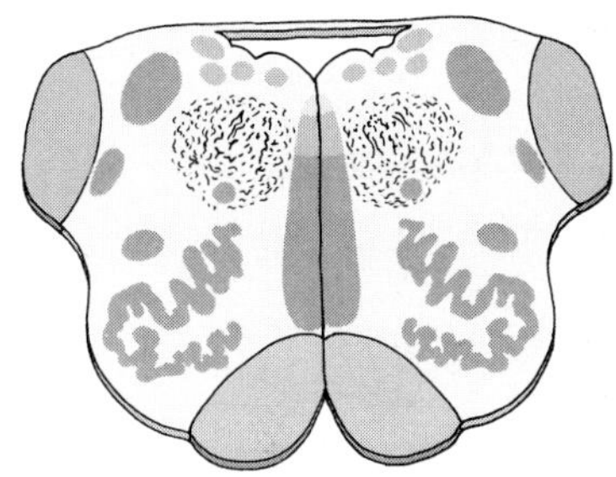

54.28. Both the dorsal motor nucleus of the vagus and the ambiguus nucleus contribute axons that emerge together in cranial nerve X. The hypoglossal nerve is separate and emerges more anteriorly. Draw a few axons from cell bodies in the visceral, branchial, and somatic motor nuclei on the right side of the image to the point of emergence of the cranial nerves.

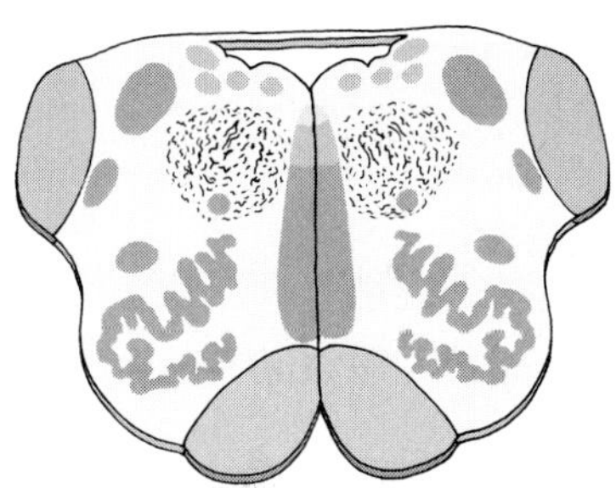

54.29. On the left side of the figure, draw the course of cranial nerves XII and X from the nuclei of origin to the points of emergence from the brainstem. On the right side of the figure, write "P" on the pyramid, "ML" on the medial lemniscus, and "ICP" on the inferior cerebellar peduncle.

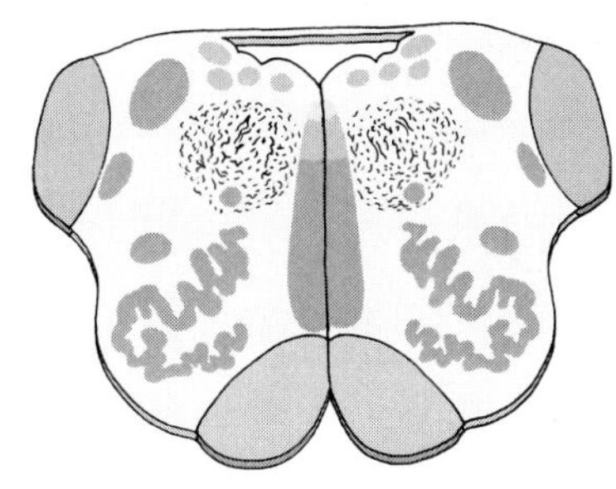

54.30. The nucleus ambiguus, like all the branchial motor nuclei, sends its axons in nerves that emerge from the ______al surface of the brainstem. Thus, cranial nerves XI, X, IX, ______, and ______ all emerge from the ____________ surface of the brainstem.

54.26A. <u>inferior</u> <u>olive</u>; <u>pyramid</u>

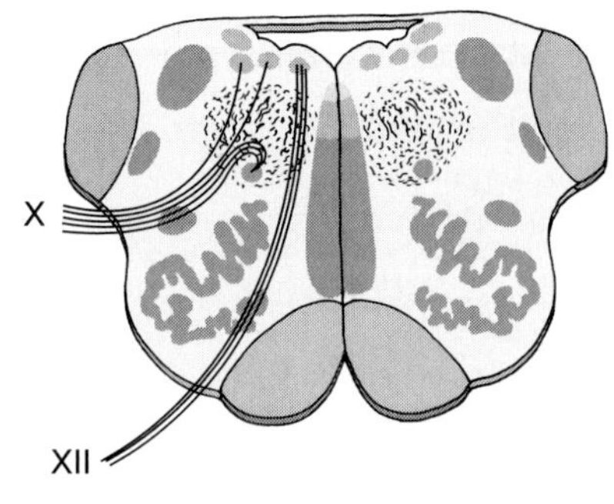

54.27A. <u>somatic</u>

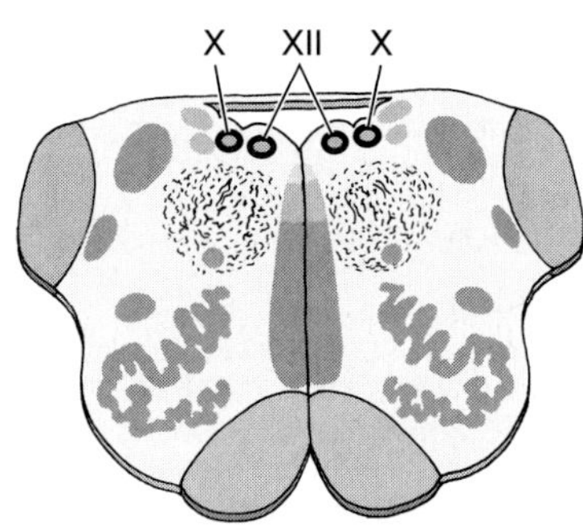

54.28A.

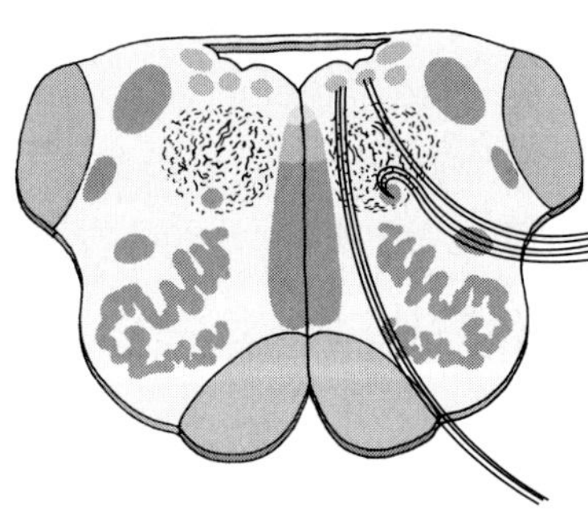

54.29A.

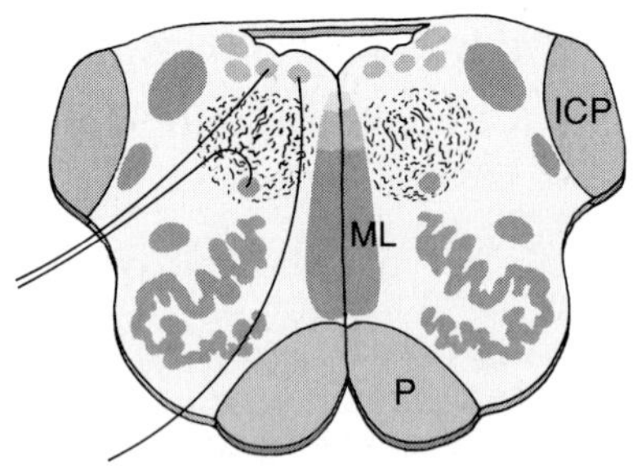

54.30A. <u>later</u>al; <u>VII</u>; <u>V</u>; <u>lateral</u>

54.31. Observe the only somatic motor nucleus in the pons and the branchial motor nucleus located in the pons near the pontomedullary junction. Label the two nuclei with their Roman numerals and names.

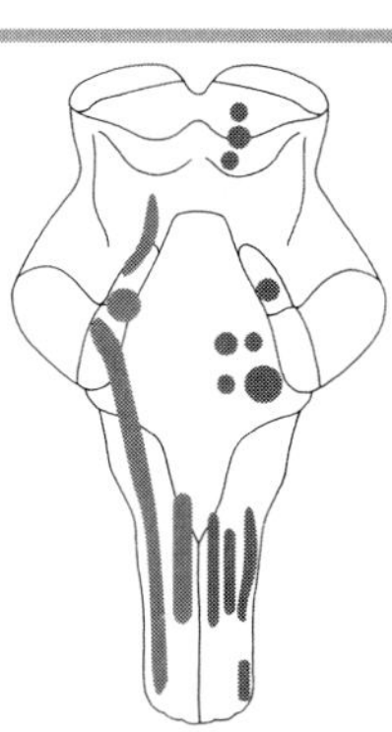

54.32. The axons of branchial motor neurons in cranial nerve VII retrace the path of the embryonic migration of their cell. The axons collectively form a bent "knee." The "knee" is called, in Latin, the ______ of the facial nerve and bends around the ____________ nucleus.

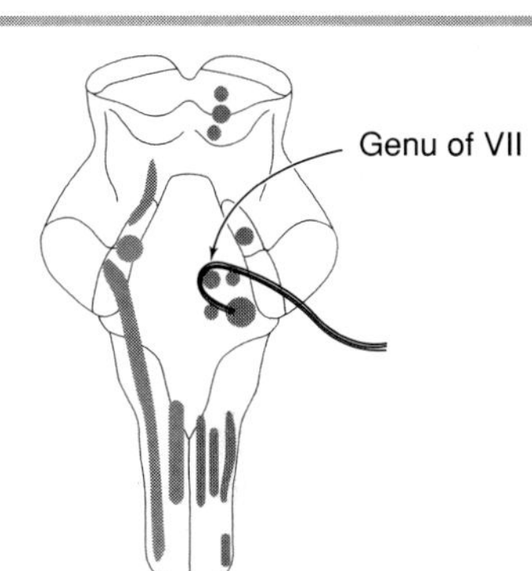

54.33. The fibers of nerve VII run a complex course. The fibers leave the facial nucleus and form the genu by passing superiorly and medially to the abducens nucleus, and then turn laterally and inferiorly around thc abducens nucleus. They then return almost to their starting point before emerging laterally at the junction of the medulla and pons. Place arrows indicating the direction of impulse conduction near the point of origin of the VIIth nerve fibers, around the genu, and at their point of emergence.

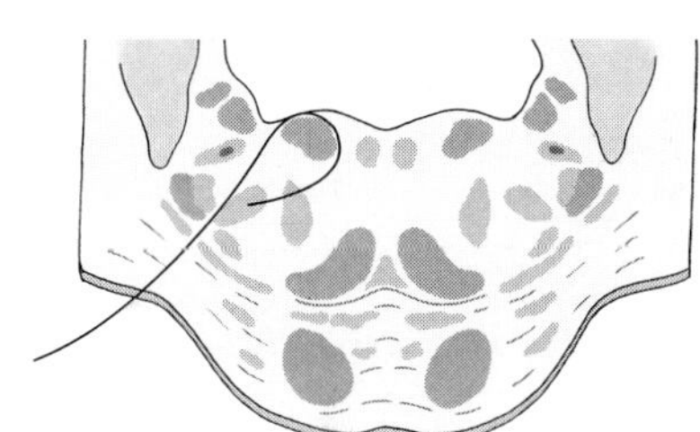

54.34. The abducens nucleus, like its somatic motor counter part in the medulla, the ____________________ nucleus, sends its axons out the anterior side of the medulla. On the right side of the brainstem, label the facial and abducens nuclei, and draw the courses of nerves VI and VII.

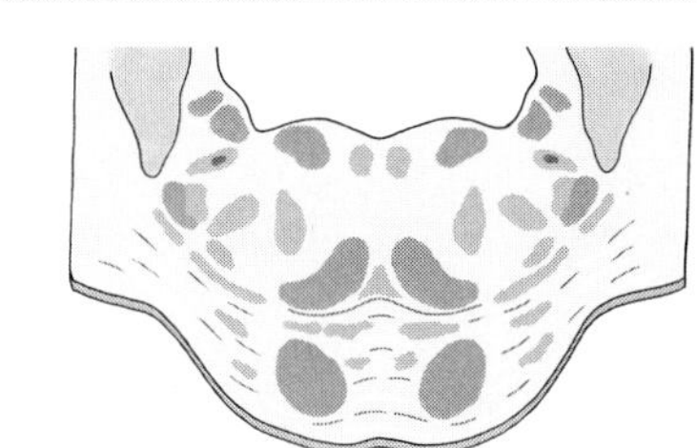

54.35. A transverse section at "A" will not include the facial nucleus but will pass through fibers in the ______ of the facial nerve. A transverse section at "B" misses the abducens nucleus but includes the ____________ nucleus and both the abducens and ____________ nerves just prior to their emergence from the brainstem.

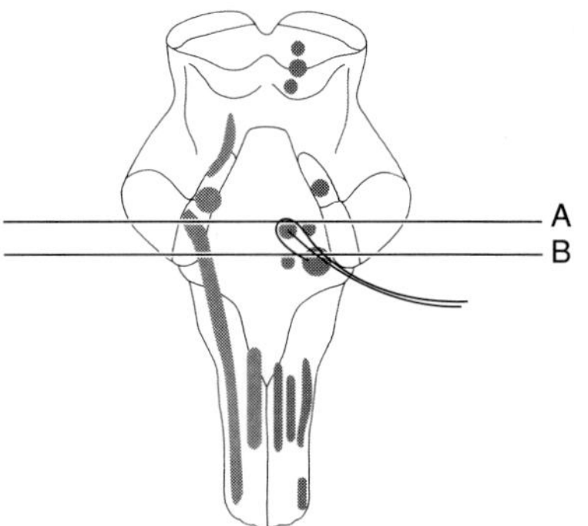

54.31A.

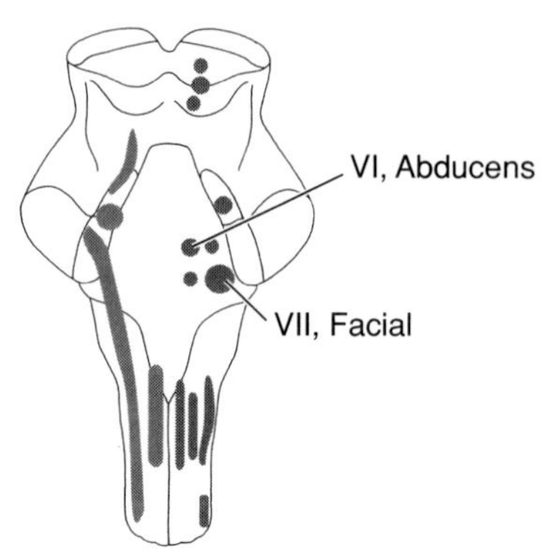

54.32A. genu; abducens

54.33A.

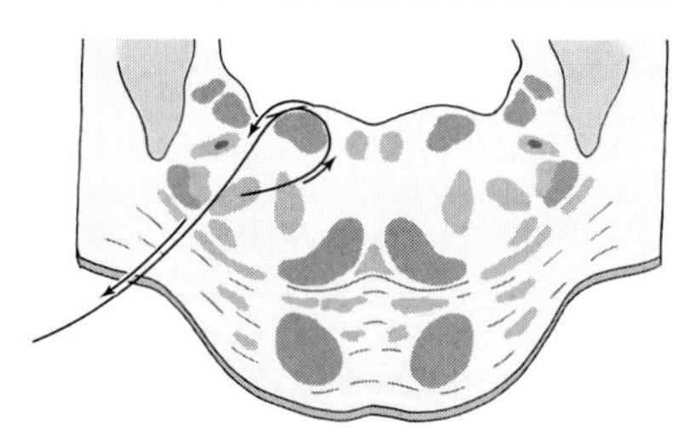

54.34A. hypoglossal

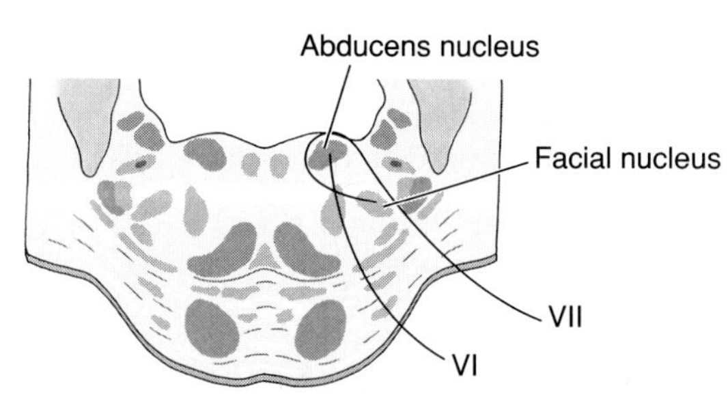

54.35A. genu; facial; facial

54.36. On the left side of the picture, place a "VI" on the abducens nucleus and a "G" on the myelinated fibers forming the genu of the facial nerve.

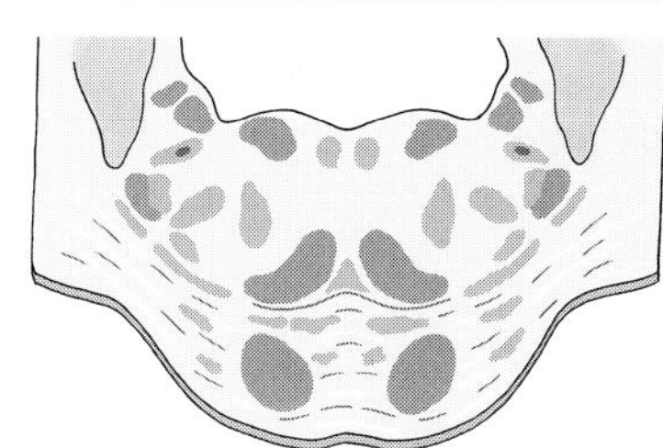

54.37. More superiorly in the pons is another branchial motor nucleus. Label it with its specific name on the diagram.

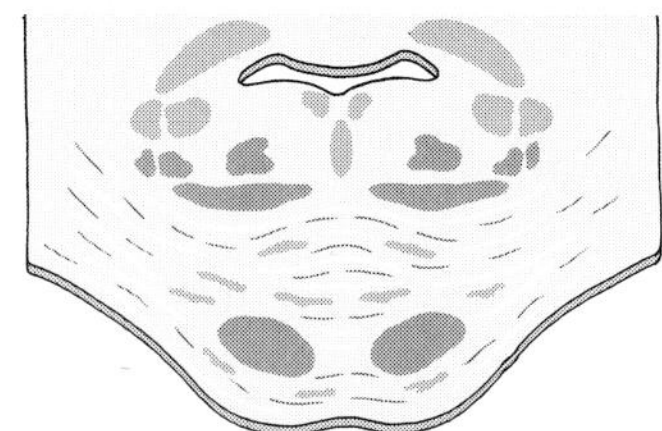

54.38. This section passes through the __________ region of the brainstem. Of the two nuclei of the somatic column in this region of the brainstem, the encircled one is the more ______ior in position (note the colliculi). Its name is the __________ nucleus.

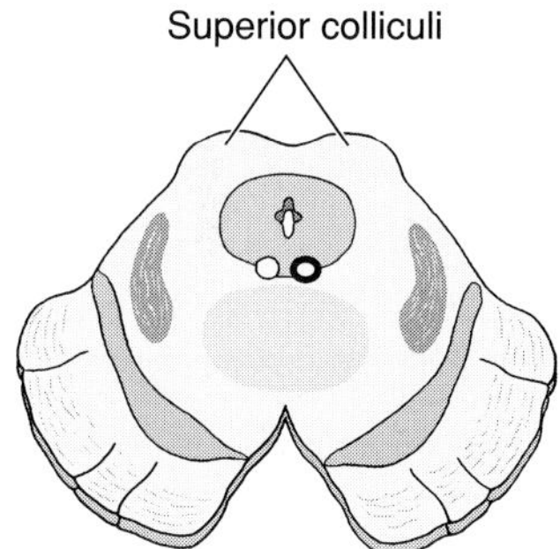

54.39. The trochlear nerve is the only cranial nerve that exits from the __________ ior side of the brainstem. Cell bodies in the trochlear nucleus on the right side of the midbrain send axons looping around the aqueduct to cross the midline and emerge just inferior to the inferior colliculi. These axons then pass forward to reach the __________ __________ muscle of the __________ eye. Draw an axon from its point of origin in the trochlear nucleus on the left side of the image to its point of emergence from the brainstem.

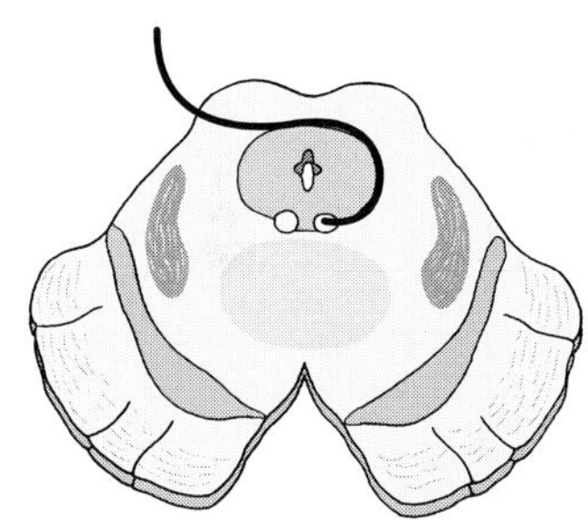

54.36A.

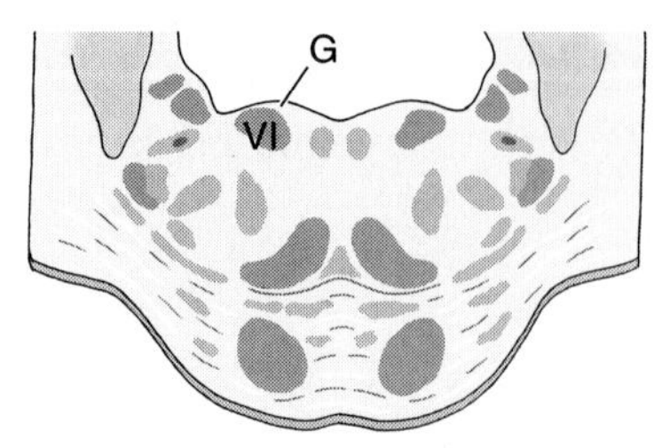

54.37A.

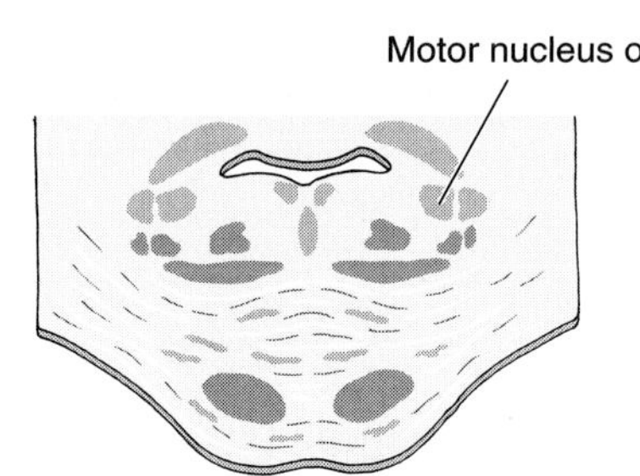

54.38A. midbrain; inferior; trochlear

54.39A. posterior; superior oblique; left

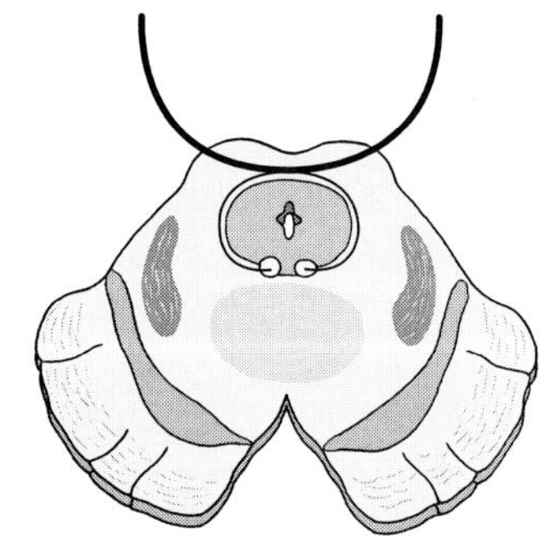

54.40. Two motor nuclei lie at the level of the superior colliculus. Of the two, the somatic motor nucleus lies near the midline, and the nucleus in the ___________ motor class forms a "cap" immediately over it. Label each with its specific name.

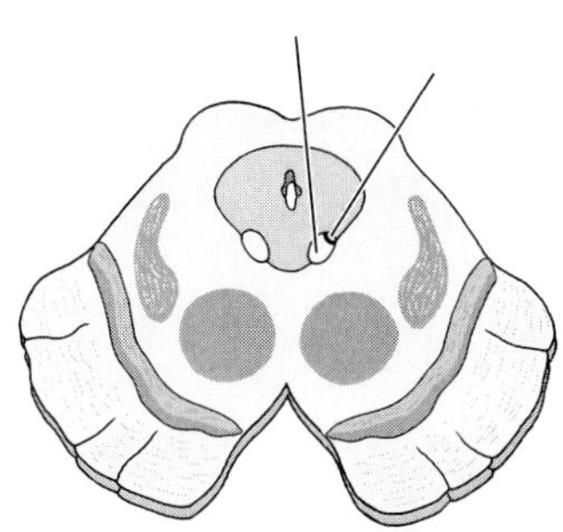

54.41. After each item, write "S," "B," or "V" for somatic, branchial, and visceral motor class, respectively, and write "A," "L," or "P" depending on whether the axons emerge from the anterior, lateral, or posterior sides of the brainstem, respectively. Axons innervating:

facial muscles	___ ___	lateral rectus muscle	___ ___
four extraocular muscles	___ ___	pupillo-constrictor muscles	___ ___
intrinsic tongue muscles	___ ___	smooth muscle of chest and abdomen	___ ___
muscles of larynx and pharynx	___ ___	superior oblique muscle	___ ___
muscles of mastication	___ ___	sternocleidomastoid and trapezius muscles	___ ___

54.40A. visceral

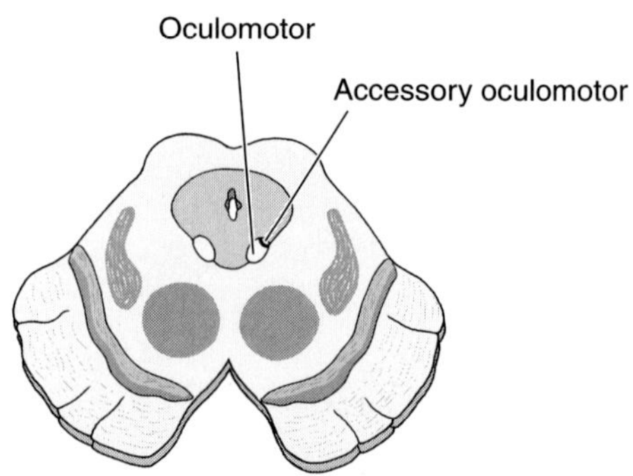

54.41A.

facial muscles	B L	lateral rectus muscle	S A
four extraocular muscles	S A	pupillo-constrictor muscles	V A
intrinsic tongue muscles	S A	smooth muscle of chest and abdomen	V L
muscles of larynx and pharynx	B L	superior oblique muscle	S P
muscles of mastication	B L	sternocleidomastoid and trapezius muscles	B L

55 Somatic and Visceral Sensory Components of the Brainstem: Trigeminal System

55.1. Draw lines between the corresponding items in the two columns.

Classification	Description
somatic sensory	somesthetic senses
special (somatic) sensory	nerve endings in walls of viscera
general visceral sensory	taste and smell
special visceral sensory	hearing, vestibular, and visual senses

55.2. A touch on the skin of the nose may evoke both conscious and reflex responses. The afferent component is classified as a somesthetic or (in more general terms) as a ____________ sensory stimulus. Stimulation of the mucosa lining the inner surface of the nose is likely to evoke a sneeze—a complex, stereotyped reflex. The afferent component of this reflex is in the general ____________ sensory class.

55.3. Apart from the special somatic senses, the brainstem uses only two anatomical systems to process sensory information. Draw lines between the corresponding items in the two columns.

somatic sensory	trigeminal system
visceral sensory	solitarius system

55.4. Impulses enter the trigeminal system via cranial nerve number ______. Cranial nerves VII, IX, and X carry afferent impulses to another sensory system of the medulla, the visceral sensory system, which is named the ____________________ system.

55.5. The trigeminal system will be considered now and the solitarius system later. The trigeminal system, by itself, serves all the sensory functions for the head that are served at the spinal level by several afferent pathways: fasciculi ____________ and ____________, lateral and anterior ____________________ tracts, and the spino____________________ tracts.

55.1A.

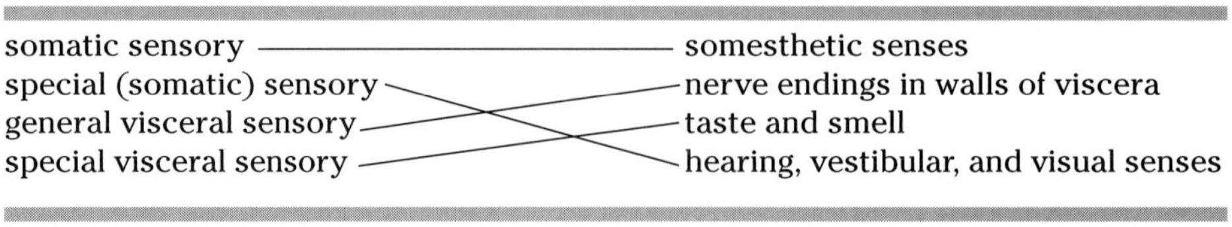

somatic sensory	somesthetic senses
special (somatic) sensory	hearing, vestibular, and visual senses
general visceral sensory	nerve endings in walls of viscera
special visceral sensory	taste and smell

55.2A. somatic; visceral

55.3A.

somatic sensory	trigeminal system
visceral sensory	solitarius system

55.4A. V; solitarius

55.5A. gracilis; cuneatus; spinothalamic; spinocerebellar

55.6. Primary afferent fibers descend in the spinal tract of V and synapse with secondary neurons in the ______ ______ of ______, just as primary afferent fibers at spinal levels ascend and descend short distances in the ______ fasciculus and synapse with secondary neurons in the ______ ______ of the spinal gray matter.

55.7. Secondary afferent neurons in a posterior horn of the spinal cord send axons into the anterior spinothalamic tracts of both sides (these convey information about the senses of ______ and ______) and into the ______ spinothalamic tract of the ______ side (for the senses of ______ and ______).

55.8. Axons of the spinal nucleus of V, like their spinal cord counterparts, convey information about the senses of ______, ______, ______, and ______ to the ______ on the ______ side of the brain.

55.9. The arrow points to a lesion that affects pain and temperature sensibility on the ______ side of the face.

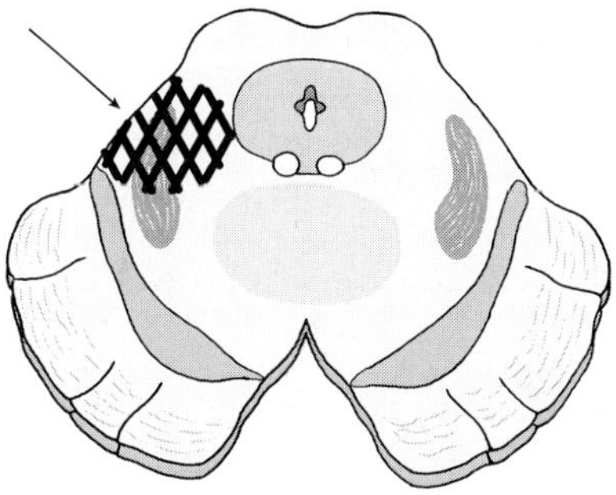

55.10. Axons of the anterior trigeminothalamic pathway (carrying pain and temperature) ascend in a poorly delineated tract in the anterior part of the medulla and pons. The complete name of this tract is the anterior trigeminothalamic tract. Impulses for pain and temperature from spinal and cranial parts of the body ascend the brainstem more or less together—spinal impulses in the ______ ______ tract and cranial impulses in the ______ ______ tract. Relative to the side stimulated, both tracts are ______lateral.

55.11. The secondary pain and temperature tracts are named in part for their destination, the ______. However, it should be recognized that many of the fibers terminate or give off collateral branches for reflex connections within the brainstem. The afferent fibers contribute to brainstem reflexes by making synaptic contact with internuncial neurons and with ______ neurons.

55.6A. spinal nucleus; V; dorsolateral; posterior horn

55.7A. touch; pressure; lateral; contralateral; pain; temperature

55.8A. touch; pressure; pain; temperature; thalamus; contralateral

55.9A. contralateral

55.10A. lateral spinothalamic; anterior trigeminothalamic; contralateral

55.11A. thalamus; efferent

55.12. All three encircled tracts contain axons of ____________ary afferent neurons. All convey information arising in sense organs on the ____________lateral side. The tract carrying information about pain and temperature senses on the face lies in a position just ____________ to the encircled ____________ ________________ tract. The medial lemniscus lies immediately ____________ to the other two encircled tracts.

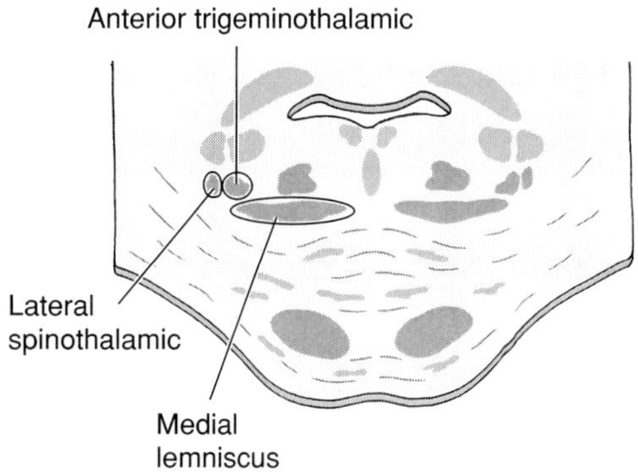

55.13. Information about touch and pressure on the face is transmitted from primary trigeminal fibers to two sets of secondary neurons—the spinal nucleus (extending the length of the ____________) and the main/chief/principal sensory nucleus located in the ______. On the left side of the brainstem, encircle the main sensory nucleus of V.

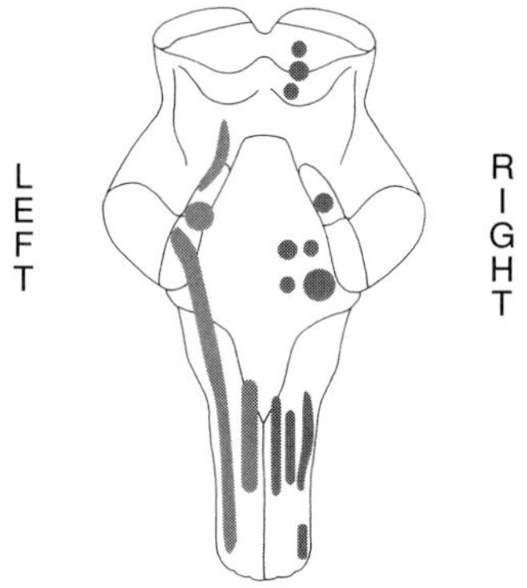

55.14. Secondary afferent neurons form a continuous column of cells from the sacral spinal cord to the middle of the pons. Label this column of cells with its different names on each of the diagrams.

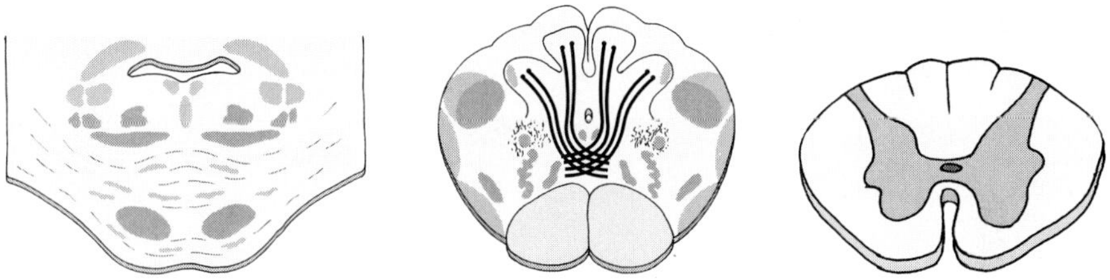

55.15. The spinal nucleus of V is not uniform in structure or function along its length. Pain and temperature information for the entire face and head is transmitted through the inferior one-third of the nucleus, lying ____________ to the level of the Xth cranial nerve and reaching to about the C4 level of the ____________ ______. The more superior parts of the spinal nucleus transmit information about ______ and ____________.

55.12A. secondary; contralateral; medial; lateral spinothalamic; anterior

55.13A. medulla; pons

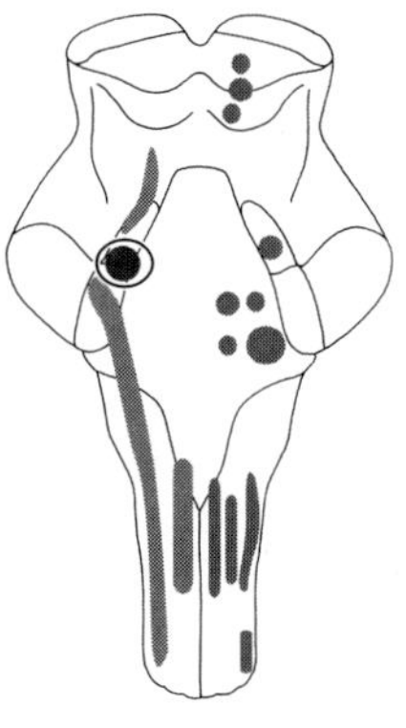

55.14A.

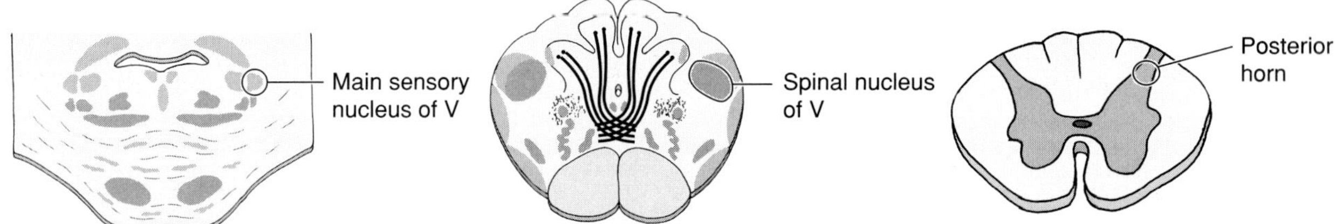

55.15A. inferior; spinal cord; touch; pressure

55.16. Two primary trigeminal neurons and their axons are drawn, one transmitting to both the spinal and main sensory nuclei of V and the other transmitting only to the spinal nucleus. The cell with the branched central axon is concerned with the modalities of ______ and ____________. Blacken the portion of the spinal nucleus containing secondary neurons mediating pain in the face.

55.17. The main sensory nucleus is small and lies just lateral to the motor nucleus of V. The fibers of the Vth nerve separate the two nuclei. Label the nuclei "S" and "M," respectively, on the right side of the section, which is through the mid ______. Draw arrows to indicate the direction of impulse conduction in each of the two diagrammed Vth nerve fibers.

Trigeminal nerve

55.18. Like the pain and temperature neurons, most of the touch and pressure neurons throughout the spinal nucleus of V send axons across the midline into the ____________ ____________________ tract. Neurons in the main sensory nucleus of V send axons up both sides of the brainstem in tracts lying in a more posterior position. These fibers form the left and right ____________ior trigeminothalamic tracts.

55.19. Information about touch and pressure on the left leg is transmitted up the spinal cord along widely separated tracts, the left and right ____________ ____________________ tracts and the ____________________ fasciculus ____________. Of these, the latter conveys information particularly about more refined aspects of touch and pressure and about the related __________________ sense arising in tendons and joints.

55.20. In the trigeminal system, information about the more refined aspects of touch and pressure sense (the abilities to recognize the location and other qualities of the stimulus) are transmitted via the more superior secondary neurons, particularly those in the ______ sensory nucleus of V. However, the analogy with functionally similar spinal components is weak: the fasciculi gracilis and cuneatus carry information arising ______laterally, and the axons of secondary neurons cross the midline and ascend in the ____________ ____________; the secondary trigeminal neurons send axons up ______ sides in the ____________ ____________________ tracts.

55.16A. touch; pressure

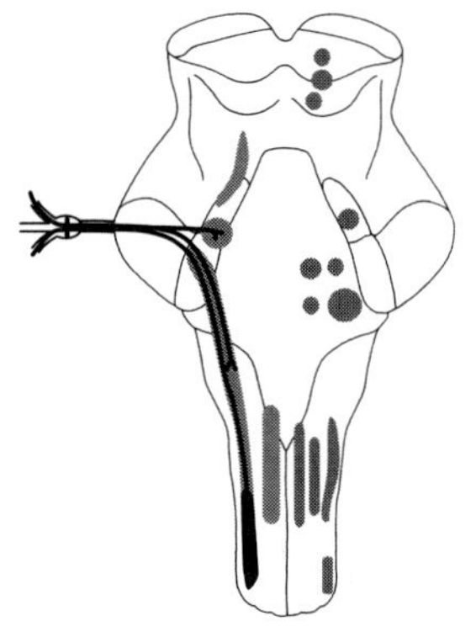

55.17A. pons

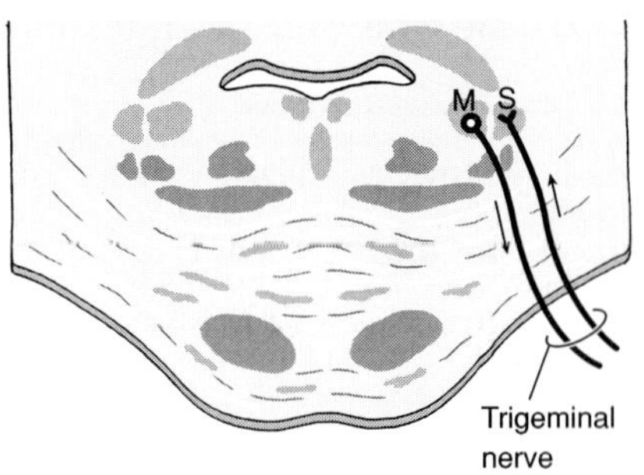

55.18A. anterior trigeminothalamic; posterior

55.19A. anterior spinothalamic; ipsilateral; gracilis; kinesthetic

55.20A. main; ipsilaterally; medial lemniscus; both; posterior trigeminothalamic

55.21. Most of the axons in the encircled tracts arise in the ______ ____________ nuclei. A lesion in one of these tracts, sparing the other, would not impair sensation on either side of the face because the intact tract ____ (complete statement).

Posterior trigeminothalamic tracts

55.22. Label the indicated tracts. The outlined tracts all convey information arising on the left side of the face. Explain briefly.

____

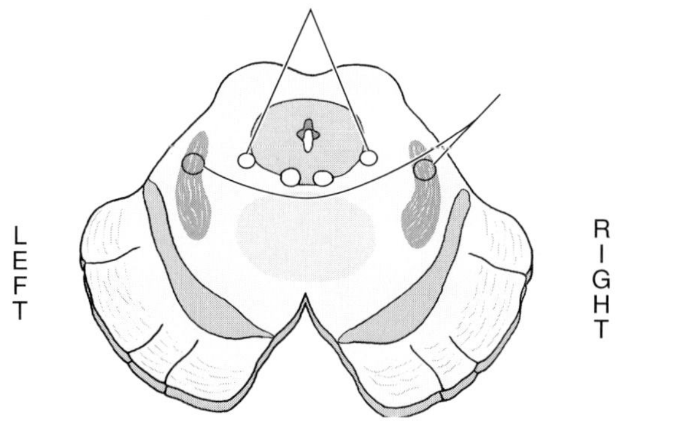

55.23. Touch and pressure sensibility for any given part of the body or head may be altered but is unlikely to be destroyed completely by any focal CNS lesion because the pathways are too ____________.

55.21A. main sensory; contains fibers arising in both left and right nuclei

55.22A. The posterior tracts contain both crossed and uncrossed fibers. The anterior tracts contain only crossed fibers.

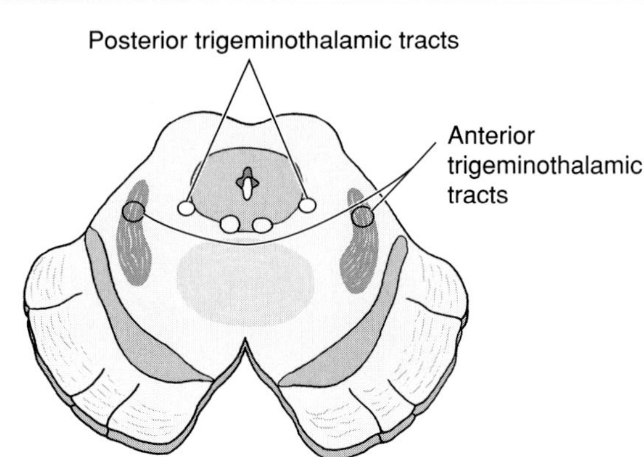

55.23A. separate

55.24. Fill in the chart comparing spinal and cranial pain-temperature pathways.

	Limbs and Trunk	**Face**
Primary neuron cells bodies are in the	spinal sensory ganglia	____________
Primary nerve fibers travel within the CNS in the	____________ fasciculus	________ ________
Secondary neuron cell bodies are in the	________ horn	____ ____ ____ ________
Secondary axons ascend in the	________ ____________ ____	________ ____ ____ ________ ____________ ____
on the	____________ side	____________ side

55.25. Fill in this chart comparing spinal and cranial touch-pressure pathways.

	Limbs and Trunk	**Face**
Location of first synapse	________ ____ and in the nuclei ________ and ________	________ ________ ____ ____ and in the ____ ________ ________ ____ ____
Secondary axons from the *nuclei* gracilis and cuneatus ascend in the	________ ________ on the ________ side(s)	
Secondary axons from other secondary cell bodies ascend in the	________ ____________ ________ on ____ side(s)	________ ________ on ____ side(s) and in the ________ ____________ ________ on the ________ side

55.26. Sensation over the entire face, eye, and forehead is mediated by the trigeminal system. An ill first-year student, familiar with neurological terminology, reported analgesia and numbness around the lips and nose with normal sensation elsewhere. Another patient reported anesthesia localized to the cornea of one eye. Is it likely that the nerve fibers innervating widely different regions of the face belong to the same trigeminal ganglion cell? ________

55.24A.

	Limbs and Trunk	**Face**
Primary neuron cells bodies are in the	spinal sensory ganglia	trigeminal ganglion (or V, semilunar)
Primary nerve fibers travel within the CNS in the	dorsolateral fasciculus	spinal tract of V
Secondary neuron cell bodies are in the	posterior horn	spinal nucleus of V
Secondary axons ascend in the	lateral spinothalamic tract	anterior trigeminothalamic tract
on the	contralateral side	contralateral side

55.25A

	Limbs and Trunk	**Face**
Location of first synapse	posterior horns and in the nuclei gracilis and cuneatus	spinal nucleus of V and in the main sensory nucleus of V
Secondary axons from the *nuclei* gracilis and cuneatus ascend in the	medial lemniscus on the opposite side(s)	
Secondary axons from other secondary cell bodies ascend in the	anterior spinothalamic tracts on both sides	posterior trigeminothalamic tracts on both sides and in the anterior trigeminothalamic tracts on the opposite side

55.26A. No

55.27. As the name trigeminal indicates, the Vth nerve has ______ peripheral branches: one to the eye and forehead region (________________ branch), one to the upper jaw (____________ branch), and one to the lower jaw (________________ branch). All three branches contain afferent fibers, but only the ________________ branch contains efferent fibers.

55.28. In the spinal tract and nucleus, the ______ peripheral divisions of V have somewhat distinct representations. The division that is most anterior and seems to be represented furthest down into the cervical cord is the ophthalmic division.

55.29. Consider a lesion affecting primary fibers in the spinal tract of V on one side of the medulla. On the side of the lesion, impulses from the face fail to reach the ______ synapse in the afferent pathway, and therefore, pain and temperature senses are impaired on the ________________ side of the face.

55.30. Pain over the face and head is transmitted mainly via fibers of the spinal tract of V terminating in the cervical spinal cord, apparently intermingling there with the fibers of nerves C2–C4. There is a concentric, "onion skin" arrangement of "pain dermatomes" on the face. The midline portions of the face, including the lips, are furthest from the cervical dermatomes and therefore are represented in the most ____________ part of the "pain" portion of the spinal nucleus of V.

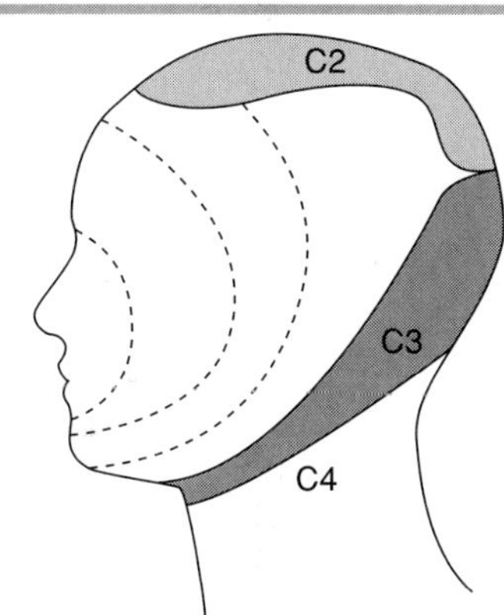

55.31. On the appropriate section, indicate a lesion "A" in the spinal tract of V that would cause analgesia on the entire ipsilateral side of the face. On another section, draw and label a lesion "B" that would have the same effect except to spare the sense of pain on the lips. The lip region is spared with lesion "B" because primary pain fibers already have made synaptic contact with secondary neurons at a ______er level of the ____________ ____________ of V.

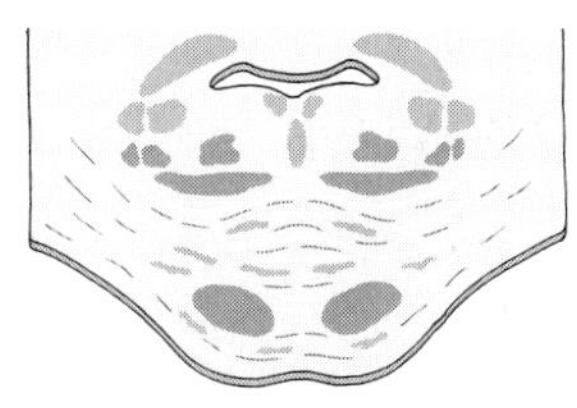

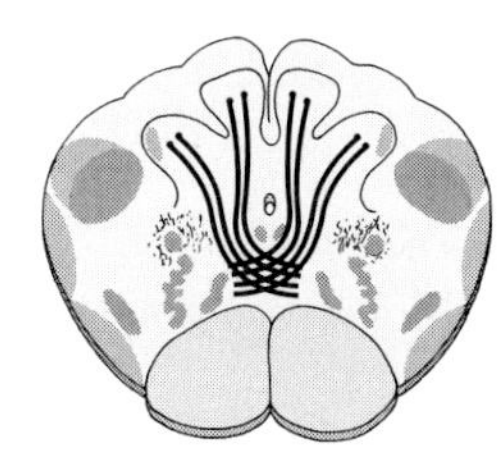

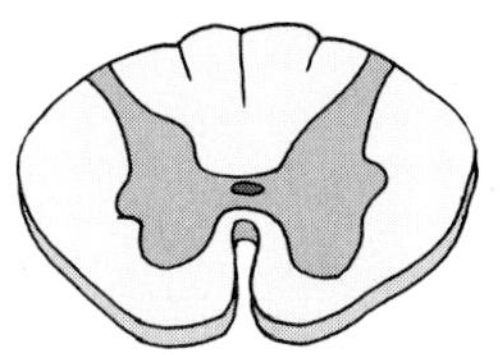

55.27A. 3; ophthalmic; maxillary; mandibular; mandibular

55.28A. 3

55.29A. first; ipsilateral

55.30A. superior

55.31A. higher; spinal nucleus

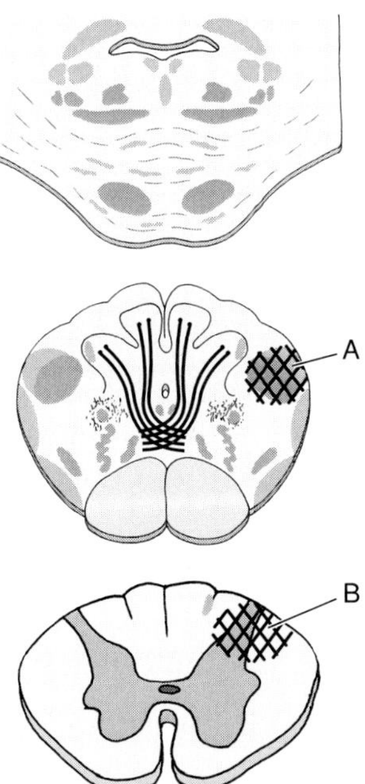

55.32. Pain pathways are not identical to temperature pathways. The surgical lesion indicated on the diagram was made deliberately to relieve intractable pain on the ______________ side of the face. Temperature sense was not lost, which is evidence that, in the spinal tract of V, "temperature" fibers lie a bit ______al to "pain" fibers.

55.33. Trigeminal pain and temperature axons ascend considerably as they cross the midline en route to the anterior ______________ tract, much more than their spinal counterparts did while crossing in the __________ ______________ of the cord en route to the __________ ______________ tract.

55.34. The anterior trigeminothalamic tract carries pain and temperature information. Some of these fibers, and their spinal counterparts, appear to join the medial lemniscus, which reaches as high as the __________.

55.35. A lesion at "B" impairs pain and temperature sensation on the ______________ side of the body and face because it interrupts the crossed lateral spinothalamic and __________ trigeminothalamic fibers. A lesion at "A" impairs pain and temperature sensation on the ______________ side of the body. Lesion "A" also destroys the descending fibers of the right spinal tract of V and therefore affects pain and temperature sensation on the ______________ side of the face. Thus, a lesion in the lateral medulla affects pain on the ipsilateral side of the face and on the ______________ side of the body, whereas the contralateral side of the face and body are affected if the lesion is at more ______ior levels of the brainstem.

B

A

55.36. Since the three labeled tracts lie very close to each other, a lesion causing loss of pain is also likely to cause altered sensibility to touch (although not complete anesthesia). Draw a lesion causing analgesia and hypesthesia on the entire left side of the face and body.

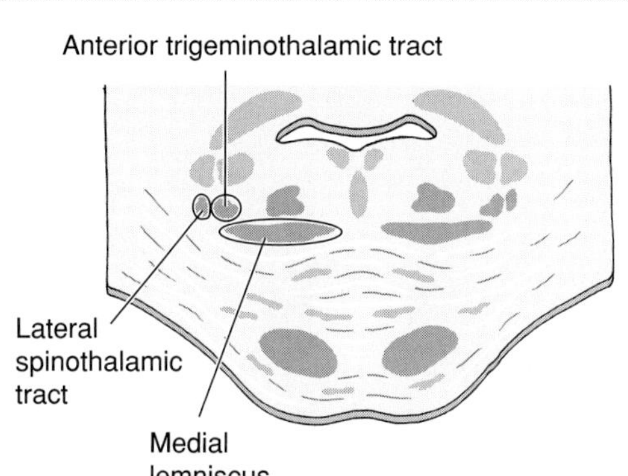

55.32A. ipsilateral; medial

55.33A. trigeminothalamic; anterior commissure; lateral spinothalamic

55.34A. thalamus

55.35A. contralateral; anterior; contralateral; ipsilateral; contralateral; superior

55.36A.

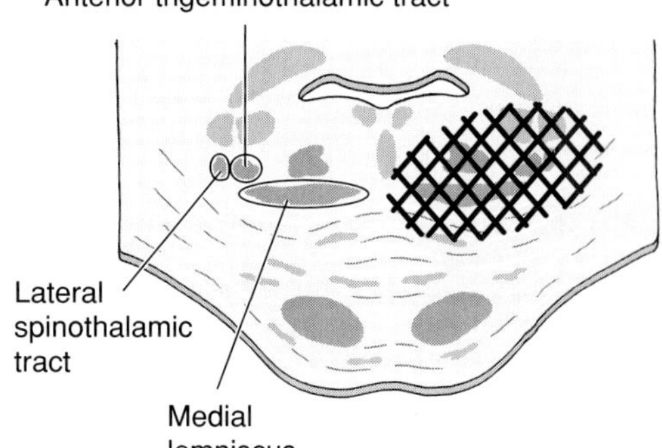

56 Somatic and Visceral Sensory Components of the Brainstem, Concluded: Mesencephalic V and Solitarius Systems

56.1. In the afferent system conveying information about muscle ______, there is a minimum of ______ neurons between muscle and cerebellum.

56.2. What happens to afferent impulses arising in skeletal muscles of the face? For example, what becomes of the impulses recording muscle tone and helping to control movements of the jaws? First, review the counterparts of these afferent impulses that arise in skeletal muscle of the limbs or neck.

	Limb Muscles	**Neck Muscles**
Primary neuron cell body is in	______	______
Secondary neuron cell body is in	______	______ nucleus
located in the	______	______
Secondary axons ascend to the	______	______
on the	______ side	______ side

56.3. Afferents from jaw and extraocular muscles have a most unusual course. Like the somesthetic afferents of the face, they reach the CNS via the ______ nerve, but, as the diagram shows, the primary neuron cell body is unique in lying ______side the CNS.

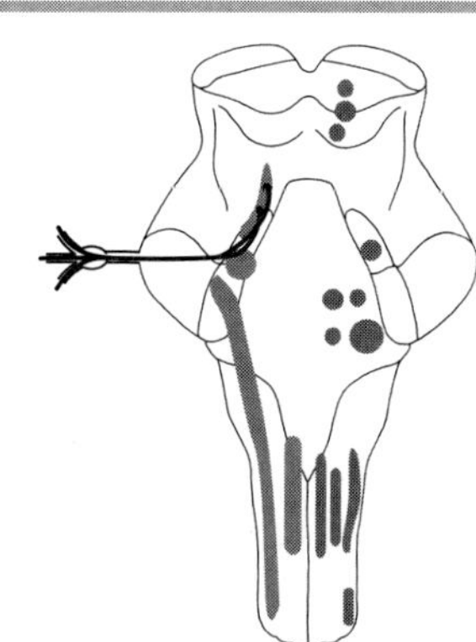

56.4. The only nucleus inside the brain that is the equivalent of a sensory ganglion (see diagram) is the ______ nucleus of V. Draw fibers connecting skeletal muscle and the labeled neuron cell bodies. Draw an arrow to indicate the direction of impulse conduction. The mesencephalic nucleus of V and the trigeminal ganglion both contain ______ary neuronal cell bodies.

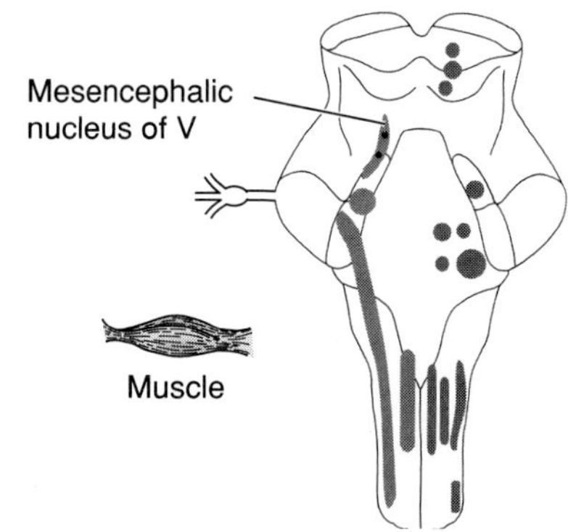

56.1A. tone; two

56.2A.

	Limb Muscles	**Neck Muscles**
Primary neuron cell body is in	spinal ganglia	spinal ganglia
Secondary neuron cell body is in	posterior horn	external cuneate nucleus
located in the	thoracic (also upper lumbar and lower cervical) cord	medulla
Secondary axons ascend to the	cerebellum	cerebellum
on the	ipsilateral side	ipsilateral side

56.3A. trigeminal; inside

56.4A. mesencephalic; primary

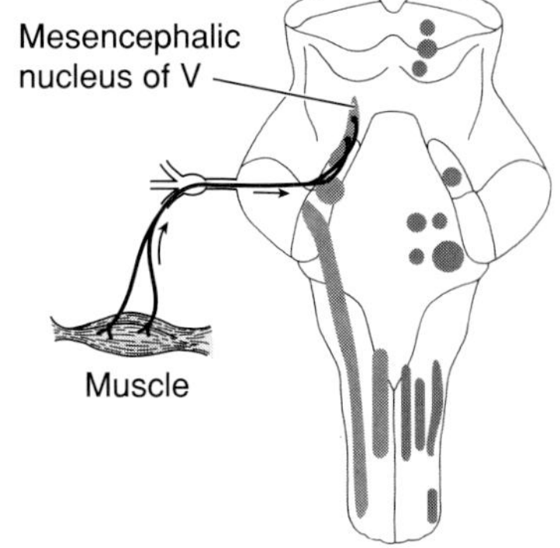

56.5. Impulses routed through the mesencephalic nucleus of V give "unconscious" information about ________ ______. Some of these impulses probably reach the ________________. Other impulses are relayed from the mesencephalic nucleus to the main sensory nucleus of V, which suggests that other information, in addition to that referred to in the first sentence above, may be transmitted from skeletal muscles via the ________________ nucleus of V.

56.6. Mesencephalon is another name for midbrain. The trigeminal system has one set of primary neurons in a cranial sensory __________ and another set broadly distributed in the pons and __________ regions of the brainstem. Secondary neuronal cell bodies of the trigeminal system lie in the ______ and __________ regions of the brainstem and in the __________ region of the spinal cord, down to about segment number ______.

56.7. On the picture, draw the relationship between the trigeminal ganglia, the Vth nerve, and the three trigeminal nuclei illustrated. Use arrows to indicate a fiber emerging from a cell body and an "X" to indicate a synaptic ending. Draw an arrow on the mesencephalic root of V to indicate the direction of impulse conduction.

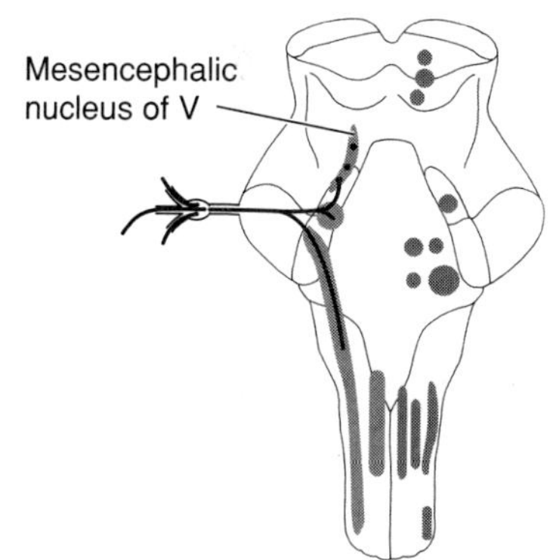

56.8. Arrows point to the mesencephalic root of V, distributed through the superior part of the pons and the inferior part of the midbrain. All neurons of the mesencephalic nucleus of V connect peripherally to __________ via the ______ nerve.

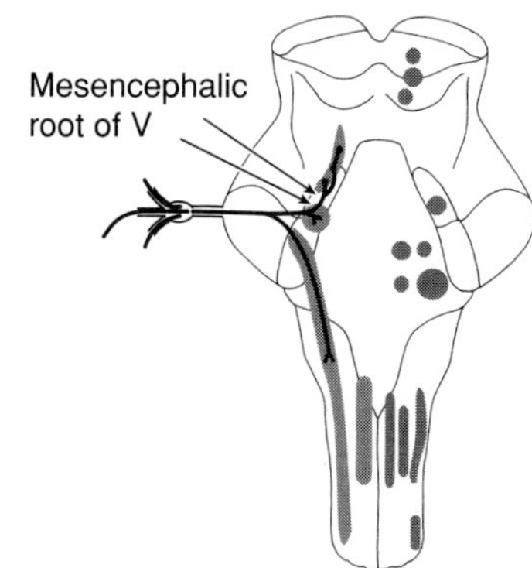

56.5A. muscle tone; cerebellum; mesencephalic

56.6A. ganglion; midbrain; pons; medulla; cervical; C4

56.7A.

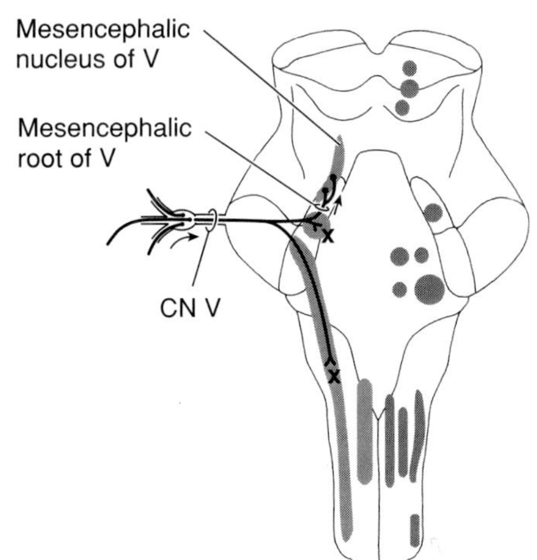

56.8A. muscle; Vth

56.9. The trigeminal nerve contains efferent fibers terminating in muscles that we use to ______. The nerve also carries afferent fibers. Those fibers mediating pain and temperature synapse in the __________ __________ of ______. Those fibers mediating touch and pressure send branches both to the ______ __________ and the __________ __________. Those fibers mediating tone and possibly other information from muscles have primary cell bodies in the ______________ nucleus.

56.10. The trigeminal system is concerned with somatic sensory functions. The solitarius system is concerned with general and special __________ sensory functions.

56.11. Begin at the geniculate and nodose (inferior ganglion of the vagus nerve) ganglia on the diagram and draw afferent roots (like the one from the inferior ganglion of the glossopharyngeal nerve [petrosal]) entering the lateral medulla and descending a bit in the tractus solitarius. Number the roots VII, IX, and X. Sensory fibers descending in the tractus solitarius follow a course reminiscent of the fiber arrangement in the __________ ______ of ______.

Geniculate ganglion

Petrosal ganglion

Nodose ganglion

56.12. Both the spinal tract of V and the tractus solitarius run lengthwise in the medulla and are composed of the central fibers of ______ary afferent neurons. Of the two brainstem sensory systems, the ______________ is more segmentally arranged and receives many impulses via the ganglia of nerves ______, ______, ______, and ______.

56.13. The fibers of the tractus solitarius run lengthwise in the medulla and are surrounded by nerve cells with which they synapse. These nerve cells, collectively named the nucleus of the tractus solitarius, are the __________ary afferent cells. In a transverse section, the solitarius system appears thus:

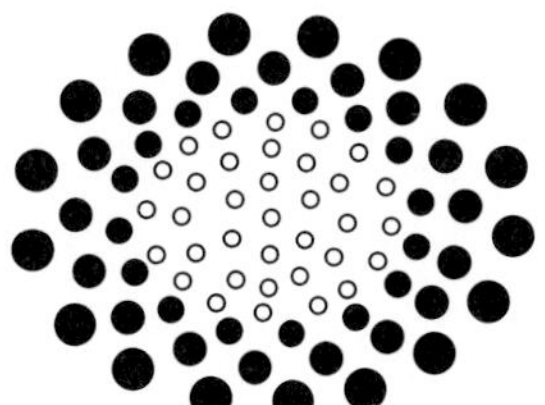

Draw lines from the labels to the appropriate parts of the diagram.

56.9A. chew; spinal nucleus of V; main sensory; spinal nucleus; mesencephalic

56.10A. visceral

56.11A. spinal tract of V

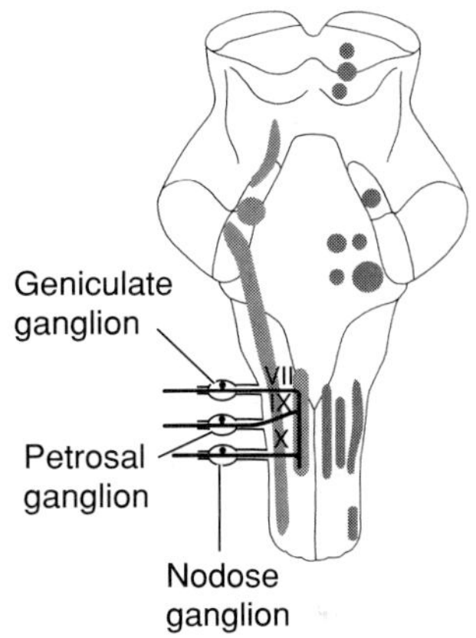

56.12A. primary; trigeminal; V; VII; IX; X

56.13A. secondary

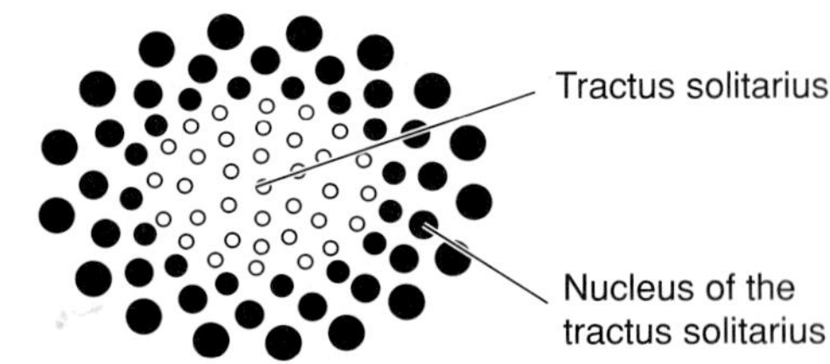

56.14. In this section through the ____________, the tractus solitarius stands out because it is surrounded by cell bodies of the ____________ of the tractus ____________________, which tend to stain poorly. Use the arrow on the left side of the figure as a guide and encircle the nucleus and tract on the other side.

56.15. The solitarius runs an oblique course through the medulla. The nuclei of the two sides fuse in the midline at more ____________ior levels of the medulla, supplied mainly by cranial nerve ______. Because of its oblique position, the solitarius appears about the same in sagittal as in transverse sections. The centrally positioned fibers belong to the ____________ ____________________, and the surrounding cells make up the ____________ of the ____________ ____________________.

56.16. The picture illustrates the four main components of cranial nerve X: efferent components from the ____________ ______ and ____________ nuclei, and afferent components to the ____________________ and ____________________ systems.

56.17. In general, somatic sensory information enters the ____________________ system, and visceral sensory information enters the ____________________ system. Components in the CNS appear to be more rationally arranged than in the peripheral nerves, where disparate elements may travel together. For example, cranial nerve X contains a few fibers mediating cutaneous sensation on a portion of the external ear, whereas most facial cutaneous sensation is mediated by nerve ______. Centrally, however (as diagrammed), the impulses arising from the skin of the ear and travelling along nerve ______ do find their way properly to the ____________ ______ and nucleus of ______.

56.14A. medulla; nucleus; solitarius

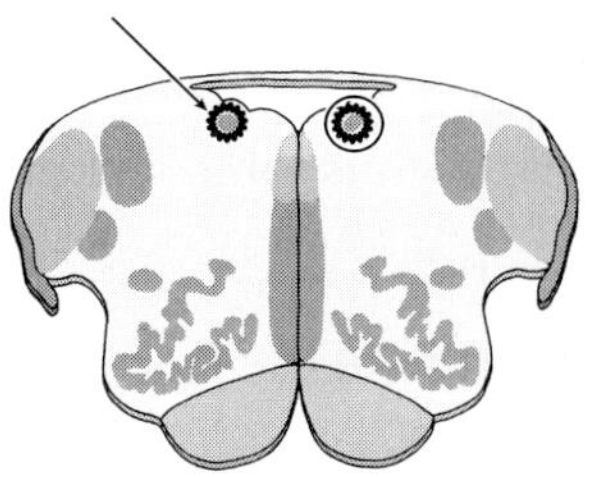

56.15A. inferior; X; tractus solitarius; nucleus; tractus solitarius

56.16A. dorsal vagal; ambiguus; solitarius; trigeminal

56.17A. trigeminal; solitarius; V; X; spinal tract; V

56.18. The inferior parts of the solitarius system are more concerned with general visceral sensation, and the superior parts are more concerned with the special visceral category of taste. The afferent impulses in nerve VII are almost entirely in the __________ visceral category. Two other cranial nerves, conveying most impulses in the general visceral category, are numbers ______ and ______. In keeping with its intermediate location, both general and special visceral impulses are carried in nerve ______.

56.19. General visceral afferent fibers make synaptic contact with neurons of the __________ of the __________ ______________. These, in turn, transmit mainly to local internuncial and motor neurons to mediate a series of complex but stereotyped __________. For example, a small bone lodging in the pharynx stimulates a gag reflex. Afferent impulses from the pharynx travel predominantly along cranial nerve ______ and reach internuncial neurons. From these internuncials, impulses reach cell bodies in the anterior horn at C4, and then efferent impulses cause contraction of the diaphragm (via the phrenic nerve). Other impulses cause contraction of pharyngeal muscles (via cranial nerve fibers arising in cell bodies of the nucleus __________).

56.20. In nerves IX and X, the afferent and efferent components innervate the same regions of the body. Afferent impulses transmitted via the petrosal ganglion of nerve IX arise mainly from taste buds on the back of the tongue and from mucosal surfaces of the __________ and __________. Afferent impulses transmitted via the nodose ganglion of nerve ______ arise mainly in the viscera of the abdomen and __________. Efferent impulses in these two nerves arise from the nucleus ambiguus and __________ ______ nuclei, classified as __________ motor and __________ motor, respectively. These afferent and efferent systems are connected by ______________ neurons.

56.21. The general term *reticular formation* is used to encompass many different groups of internuncial neurons. Much of the unlabeled territory in the gray matter at all levels of the brainstem may be considered to be part of the __________ formation.

56.22. The term __________ __________ encompasses a variety of anatomical structures: nerve cell bodies in large nuclei and in scattered small groups, short and long axons with varied patterns of branching, fibers intrinsic to the brainstem, and fibers passing between the brainstem, spinal cord, and cerebellum.

56.18A. special; X; IX; IX

56.19A. nucleus; tractus solitarius; reflexes; IX; ambiguus

56.20A. larynx; pharynx; X; thorax; dorsal vagal; branchial; visceral; internuncial

56.21A. reticular

56.22A. reticular formation

56.23. Several stereotyped visceral reflexes are mediated in the reticular formation. For example, the glossopharyngeal nerve transmits afferent impulses from the carotid sinus in the neck (as well as from taste buds and mucosal surfaces), and the vagus nerve transmits efferent impulses that slow the heart rate. When pressure rises in the carotid artery, the carotid sinus sends more impulses along cranial nerve ______. Other neurons of this reflex pathway, in sequence, are: the nucleus of the ____________ ____________________, internuncials of the ____________ ____________, and efferent neurons with cell bodies in the ____________ ______ nucleus. The usual reflex response to a rise in carotid artery pressure is a ____________ of the heart rate.

56.24. Impulses in the CNS conveying information for control of visceral functions often cross back and forth freely from side to side in the medial parts of the reticular formation. Even the ____________ ____________________ is fused in the midline in its most inferior levels where the vagus nerve feeds into it.

56.25. Draw lines between appropriate items in the two columns:
The central fibers of all primary visceral afferent neurons enter the medulla and collectively form the ____________ ____________________.

General visceral sensory	VII
	IX
Special visceral sensory	X

56.26. Glossopharyngeal means tongue pharynx. It is logical to reason that most taste impulses from the back of the tongue, near the pharynx, are transmitted along cranial nerve ______. The remainder of the tongue is innervated differently. A lesion involving the geniculate ganglion of the facial nerve impairs taste mainly in the ____________ part of the tongue.

56.27. Secondary neuron cell bodies in the taste pathway lie in the most superior one-third of the ____________ of the ____________ ____________________. From your experience with other sensory systems, you might guess that tertiary neuron cell bodies lie in the ____________.

56.28. Ascending pathways of secondary "taste" axons join secondary "kinesthetic" and other axons and travel to the thalamus in the ____________ ____________. Branches of these "taste" axons make many synaptic connections with neurons of the ____________ formation, and some branches are thought to reach the region anterior to the thalamus, called the ______thalamus.

56.23A. IX; tractus solitarius; reticular formation; dorsal vagal; decrease

56.24A. nucleus solitarius

56.25A. tractus solitarius

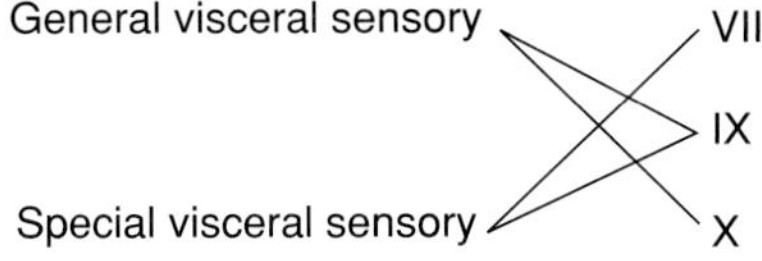

56.26A. IX; anterior

56.27A. nucleus; tractus solitarius; thalamus

56.28A. medial lemniscus; reticular; hypothalamus

56.29. Number the following as 1 to 5 in the order of their basic position in the brainstem from medial to lateral:

Branchial motor: ______

Somatic sensory: ______

Somatic motor: ______

Visceral sensory: ______

Visceral motor: ______

56.30. Place a checkmark in each appropriate box:

	XII	XI	X	IX	VII	VI	V	IV	III
Somatic motor									
Branchial motor									
Visceral motor									
General visceral sensory									
Special visceral sensory									
Somatic sensory									

56.31. A practical clinical-anatomical correlation is that focal lesions in the brainstem commonly cause cranial nerve symptoms by involving the central course of nerves rather than by destroying nuclei. The lesion illustrated caused paralysis of the right vocal cord. The right side of the soft palate was paralyzed and insensitive. The lesion, which extended for some distance along the length of the medulla, spared the three circled nuclei, named the __________, __________ ______, and ________________, but interrupted their fibers in cranial nerves ______ and ______.

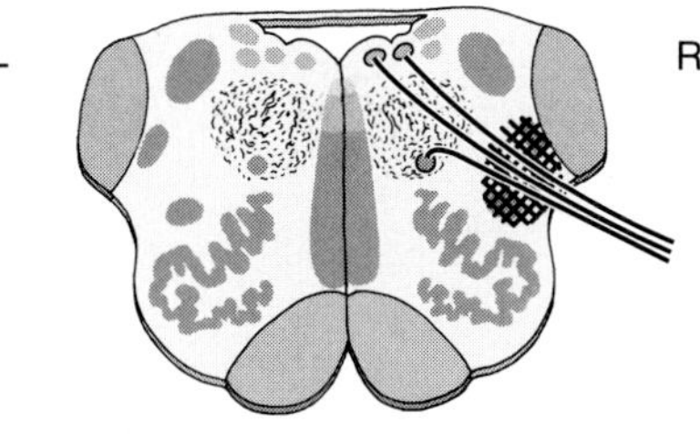

56.32. The same lesion interrupted the spinal tract of V and the lateral spinothalamic tract on the right side of the medulla. Pain and temperature sensibility were impaired on the ________________ side of the face and on the ________________ side of the body. Pain on the other side of the face was unaffected because the secondary pain axons ascend as they cross and, at this level, have not yet formed the __________ ________________ tract.

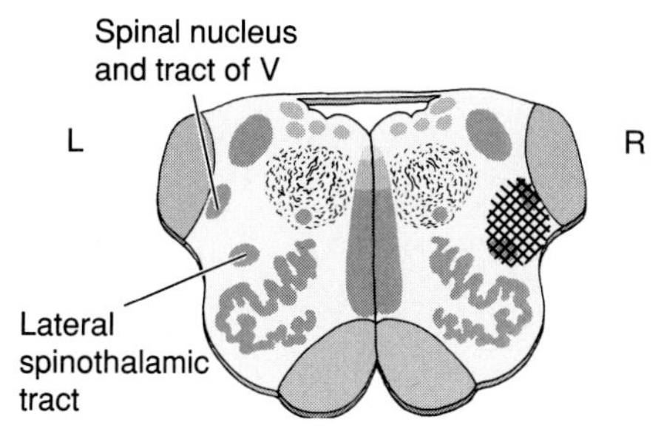

56.29A. 2; 5; 1; 4; 3

56.30A.

	XII	XI	X	IX	VII	VI	V	IV	III
Somatic motor	✓					✓		✓	✓
Branchial motor		✓	✓	✓	✓		✓		
Visceral motor			✓	✓	✓				✓
General visceral sensory			✓	✓					
Special visceral sensory			✓	✓	✓				
Somatic sensory			✓	✓	✓		✓		

56.31A. ambiguus; dorsal vagal; solitarius; IX; X

56.32A. ipsilateral; contralateral; anterior trigeminothalamic

57 Review of Cranial Nerve Components

57.1. Each of the __________ pairs of cranial nerves contains some combination of somatic afferent, somatic efferent, visceral efferent, special sense, or visceral afferent fibers. Peripheral pathways are considered in human anatomy courses and texts, while the central connections are learned in neuroanatomy.

57.2. Cranial nerve I, the __________ nerve, mediates the sense of ______.

57.3. The olfactory nerve is actually composed of a group of bipolar neurons located in the superior aspect of the nasal cavity. The __________ nerve contains the only sensory information that reaches the cerebral cortex without first synapsing in the __________.

57.4. The ______polar neurons—the olfactory cells, the neurons of the olfactory nerve, synapse directly on the mitral cells of the olfactory bulb (an extension of the telencephalon).

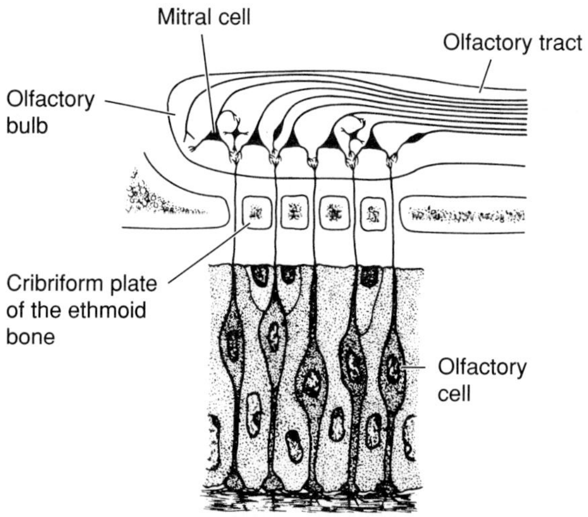

Mitral cell
Olfactory tract
Olfactory bulb
Cribriform plate of the ethmoid bone
Olfactory cell

57.5. Cranial nerve II, the ______ nerve, conveys visual information. The optic nerve is composed of the fibers of ganglion cells exiting the retina. The ganglion cell axons course posteriorly to the optic chiasm, where fibers carrying information from the nasal side of the retina decussate to run in the contralateral optic tract. The result of this decussation is that information from the left visual field of both eyes is carried together in one tract and visa versa. The ______ synapse does not occur until the lateral geniculate nucleus of the __________.

57.1A. twelve

57.2A. olfactory; smell

57.3A. olfactory; thalamus

57.4A. bipolar

57.5A. optic; first; thalamus

57.6. Afferents from the lateral ________________ nucleus pass posteriorly via the optic radiations to the primary __________ cortex (Brodmann's area 17) on the banks of the calcarine sulcus.

57.7. Label the primary visual cortex, lateral geniculate nucleus, optic tract, optic chiasm, optic radiations, and optic nerve on the following diagram.

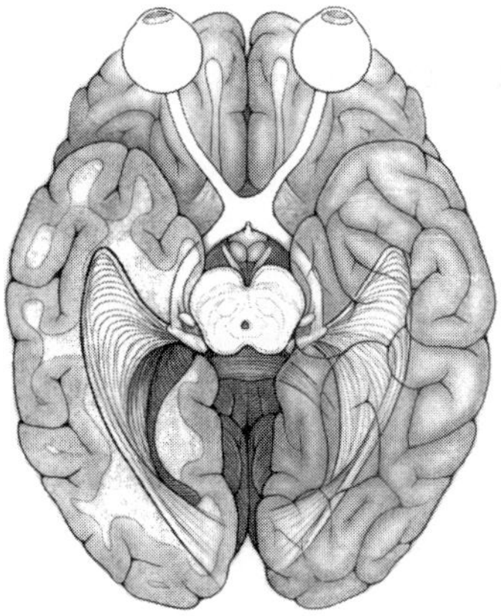

57.8. The oculomotor nerve, cranial nerve _____, carries motor fibers to five of the seven extraocular muscles and conveys presynaptic parasympathetic fibers from the __________-__________ nucleus of the midbrain to synapse in the ciliary ganglion. The parasympathetic fibers cause contraction of the ciliaris muscle, which allows the lens to "round up" (accommodation), and contraction of the sphincter pupillae, which causes pupillary ________________.

57.9. Draw in and label the fibers of CN III originating from the oculomotor and accessory oculomotor nuclei on both sides of the diagram of the midbrain.

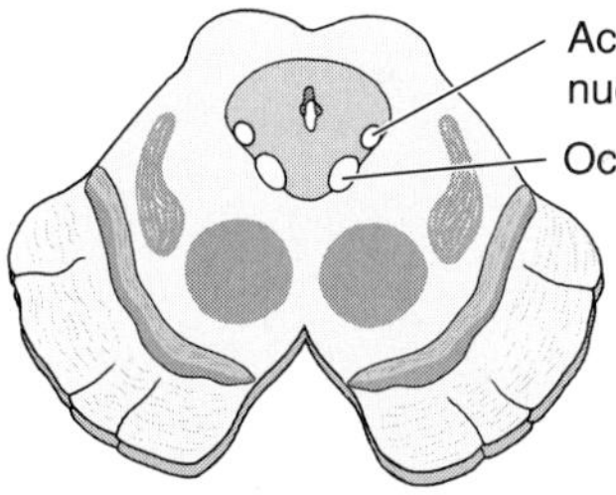

Accessory oculomotor nucleus

Oculomotor nucleus

57.10. The _____lear nerve, cranial nerve IV, is only associated with one central nervous system nucleus—the trochlear. The trochlear nerve has the unique distinction of being the only cranial nerve to emerge from the posterior aspect of the brainstem and the only nerve to innervate its target __________laterally.

57.6A. geniculate; visual

57.7A.

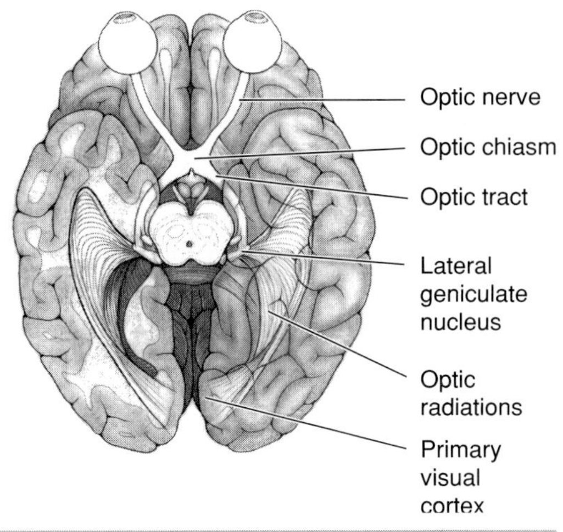

57.8A. III; Edinger-Westphal (or accessory oculomotor); constriction

57.9A.

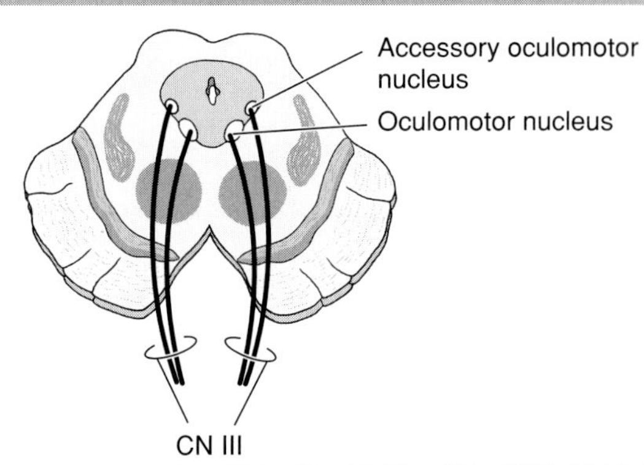

57.10A. trochlear; contralaterally

57.11. Label the trochlear nucleus and CN IV on the midbrain pictured.

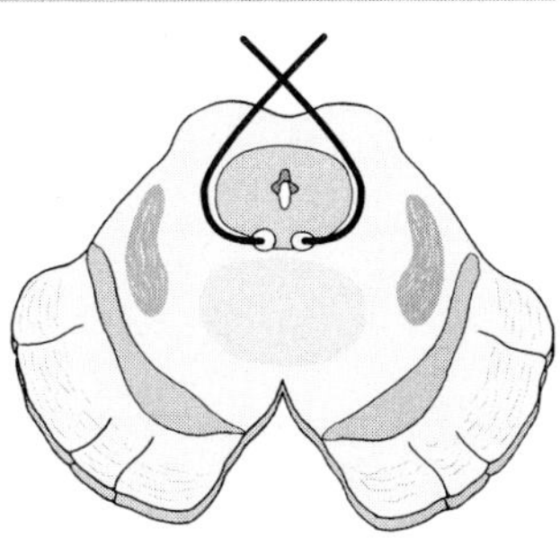

57.12. The fifth cranial nerve, the trigeminal, has ______ major divisions (trigeminal = three twins): the ophthalmic (V_1), maxillary (V_2), and mandibular (V_3) divisions.

57.13. Label the trigeminal ganglion and the three divisions of the trigeminal nerve on the diagram.

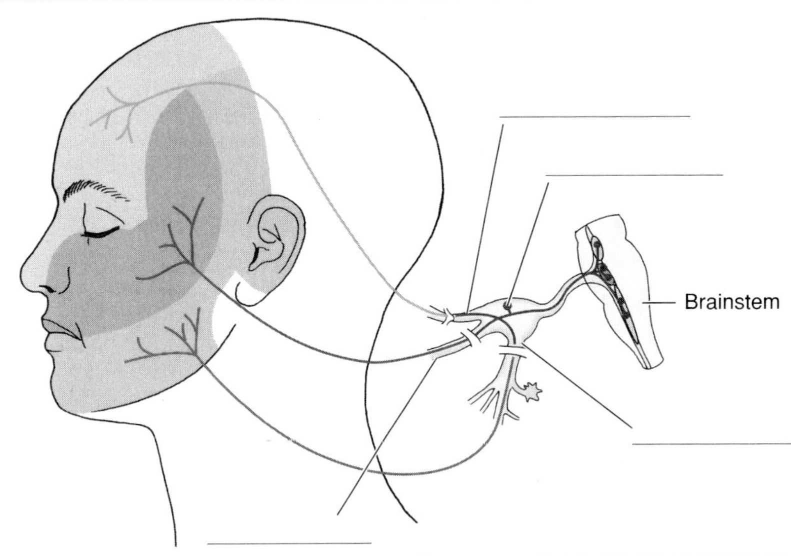

57.14. The trigeminal nerve is the major sensory nerve of the face. As such, the trigeminal ganglion contains pseudounipolar, primary afferent neurons and is analogous to the ____________ ganglia associated with the spinal cord.

57.15. Sensory information from the face enters the pons via the trigeminal nerve. Pain and temperature information descends in the spinal tri____________ tract to cervical spinal cord levels before synapsing on the spinal trigeminal nucleus. The spinal cord homologue of the spinal trigeminal nucleus is the ________________ ________________.

57.11A.

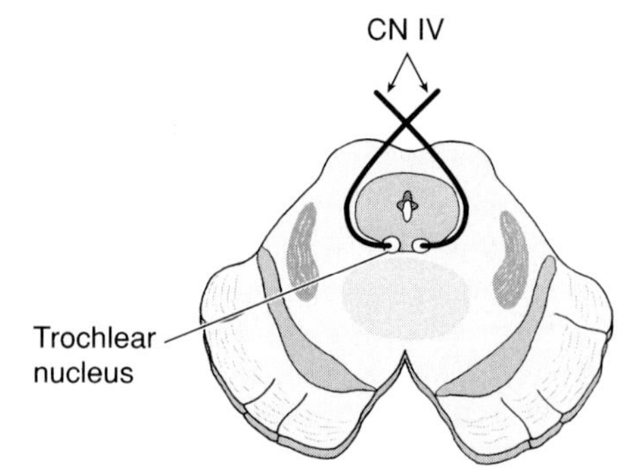

57.12A. <u>three</u>

57.13A.

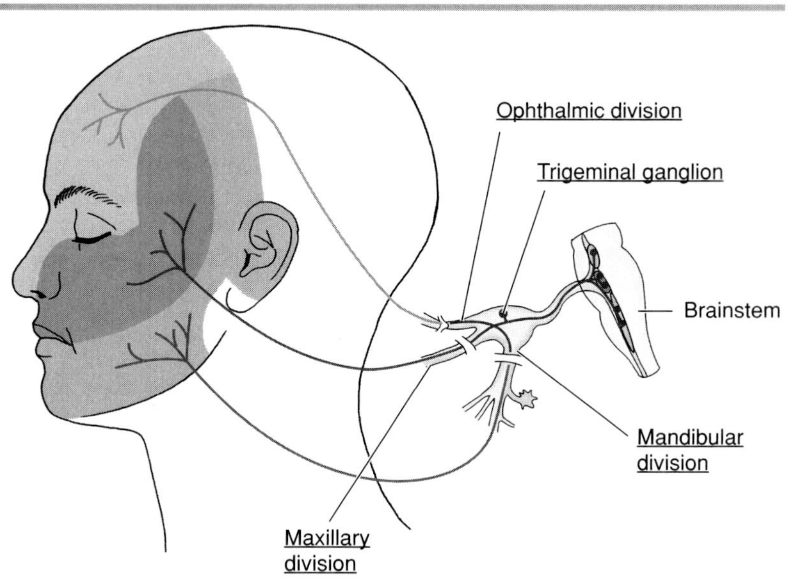

57.14A. <u>spinal</u> (or dorsal root)

57.15A. trigeminal; substantia gelatinosa

57.16. Crude touch information from the face also descends in the __________ trigeminal ______ but only to the medullary levels of the spinal trigeminal nucleus. Posterior/dorsal column modalities conveyed to the pons via CN V synapse in the chief sensory nucleus of the pons. The chief sensory and spinal trigeminal nuclei give rise to the ventral trigeminothalamic tract, which is a crossed tract that terminates in the ventral posterior medial nucleus of the __________.

57.17. There is only one moveable joint in the head—the temporo__________ular joint or TMJ. The presence of the joint necessitates the need for proprioceptive information regarding the position of the mandible. Some fibers of the ______geminal nerve enter the pons and ascend to the mesencephalic nucleus, which mediates proprioceptive information.

57.18. Cranial nerves VII, IX, and X also send fibers into the spinal trigeminal system, as they also convey __________ information from the ______lateral face.

57.19. Eight muscles receive motor innervation from the mandibular division of the ______________ nerve, including the muscles of mastication. Motor fibers found in the trigeminal nerve originate in the trigeminal motor nucleus of the ______.

57.20. The abducens nerve provides innervation to the lateral rectus. The cell bodies responsible for this motor innervation originate in the appropriately named ______ens nucleus.

57.21. We have now discussed three cranial nerves responsible for innervating the extraocular muscles of the orbit. Next to each muscle listed below, write the number of the cranial nerve responsible for its innervation.

Superior oblique –
Superior rectus –
Inferior oblique –
Inferior rectus –
Medial rectus –
Lateral rectus –
Levator palpebrae superioris –

57.16A. spinal; tract; thalamus

57.17A. temporomandibular; trigeminal

57.18A. sensory; ipsilateral

57.19A. trigeminal; pons

57.20A. abducens

57.21A.

Superior oblique – IV

Superior rectus – III

Inferior oblique – III

Inferior rectus – III

Medial rectus – III

Lateral rectus – VI

Levator palpebrae superioris – III

57.22. As you have learned, all but two of the seven extraocular muscles are innervated by the ______ motor nerve. A useful "chemical" symbol to help remember this pattern of innervation is $[SO_4LR_6]^3$—that is, the superior oblique is innervated by CN IV (SO_4), the lateral rectus by CN VI (LR_6), and all of the rest by CN III.

57.23. The facial nerve (CN ______) is a complicated cranial nerve. As its name indicates, it supplies motor innervation to all of the muscles of __________ expression with fibers that originate in the facial motor nucleus.

57.24. The facial nerve also conveys presynaptic parasympathetic fibers originating in the superior salivary nucleus to the pterygopalatine and submandibular ganglia. As the name indicates, the submandibular ganglion supplies the ________________ and sublingual glands with secretomotor innervation. Postsynaptic fibers from the pterygopalatine ganglion innervate the lacrimal gland, palatal glands, and mucous glands of the oral and nasal mucosa.

57.25. Like the motor component of the facial nerve, which has two parts (brachial and visceral), the __________ component has two central target nuclei. Sensation from the external ear is conveyed to the __________ ________________ nucleus as would be expected, and taste from the anterior two-thirds of the tongue is sent to the nucleus solitarius.

57.26. CN VIII, the __________ cochlear nerve is really two sensory nerves in one; the vestibular component is composed of fibers from cells of the vestibular (Scarpa's) ganglion that respond to changes in the position of the head that stimulate hair cells in the inner ear, while the cell bodies of the __________ component are located in the spiral ganglion and convey information on hearing to the cochlear nuclei of the pons.

57.27. The name glossopharyngeal nerve gives clear indication of the distribution of the fibers of CN ______. __________ fibers in the glossopharyngeal nerve are conveyed from the pharynx (general sensation) to the spinal trigeminal nucleus, and taste fibers are conveyed from the posterior one-third of the tongue to the nucleus ________________ to join with taste conveyed by the facial and vagus nerves. Other fibers from CN IX conveyed to the nucleus solitarius include those from the carotid body and sinus, which mediate the monitoring of the CO_2 concentration and the pressure of the blood.

57.22A. oculomotor

57.23A. VII; facial

57.24A. submandibular

57.25A. sensory; spinal trigeminal

57.26A. vestibulocochlear; cochlear

57.27A. IX; Sensory; solitarius

57.28. Other components of the glossopharyngeal nerve include sensation from the middle ear, which is conveyed to the ____________ trigeminal nucleus and motor fibers originating in the nucleus ambiguus and the inferior salivary nucleus. The nucleus ambiguus supplies motor fibers to the stylopharyngeus muscle, while the inferior salivary nucleus supplies presynaptic para________________ innervation to the otic ganglion for secretomotor supply to the parotid gland.

57.29. The fourth and final parasympathetic nucleus, the dorsal motor nucleus of the vagus, sends fibers into CN X, the ______. These fibers innervate numerous ganglia in the walls of the thoracic and abdominal viscera.

57.30. Match the presynaptic nucleus on the left with the correct cranial nerve into which it sends fibers listed on the right by drawing lines between the two columns.

dorsal motor nucleus of X	III
accessory oculomotor	VII
	IX
	X

57.31. Like the ________________ nerve, the vagus has fibers originating in the nucleus ambiguus that innervate the pharynx and larynx. A small somatic sensory component from the external ear projects to the spinal trigeminal nucleus, as do fibers in the ________________, ____________, and ________________ nerves. Taste from the epiglottis travels in the vagus to the nucleus ________________, as does taste in the ____________ and ________________ nerves.

57.32. The spinal accessory nerve has traditionally been described as having fibers originating in the nucleus ambiguus, as have the ________________ and ______ nerves, as well as a spinal component that innervates the sternocleidomastoid and trapezius muscles. Recent evidence ascribes the nucleus ambiguus component of CN XI to the vagus nerve, which innervates the pharyngeal musculature.

57.33. The last cranial nerve, the hypoglossal, is a simple ______ic motor nerve. Fibers originate in the aptly named ________________ nucleus, which innervates the tongue.

57.28A. spinal; parasympathetic

57.29A. vagus

57.30A.

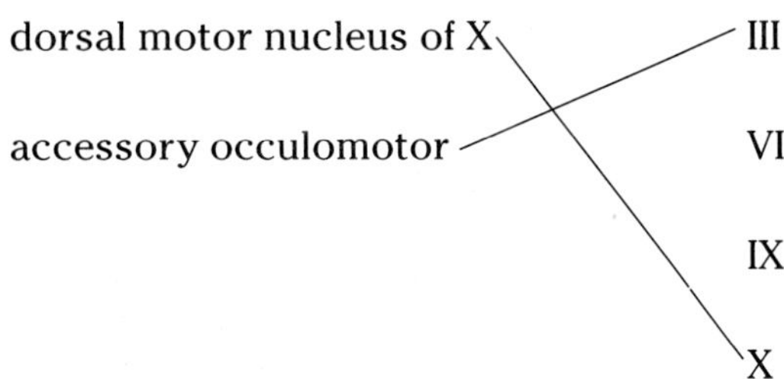

57.31A. glossopharyngeal; trigeminal; facial; glossopharyngeal; solitarius; facial; glossopharyngeal

57.32A. glossopharyngeal; vagus

57.33A. somatic; hypoglossal

58 Lesions of the Brainstem

58.1. Lesions of the brainstem are characterized by a lack of function(s) associated with multiple cranial nerves. Brainstem lesions are often a result of decreased __________ blood supply. We describe the results of vascular (arterial) insufficiency at all three levels of the brainstem. For purposes of brevity, we will limit our examination to two representative vascular lesions per level.

58.2. Medullary lesions typically manifest themselves in one of two classic syndromes: medial and lateral medullary syndromes. Both __________ are a result of occlusion of branches of the __________ arterial system. Functional loss relates to the nuclei and tracts that are deprived of arterial blood.

58.3. The vertebral arteries give rise to the anterior spinal artery. Lesion or blockage of the anterior __________artery leads to medial medullary syndrome. The area affected is shaded.

58.4. Label the structures affected by blockage of the anterior spinal artery on the unshaded side of the diagram.

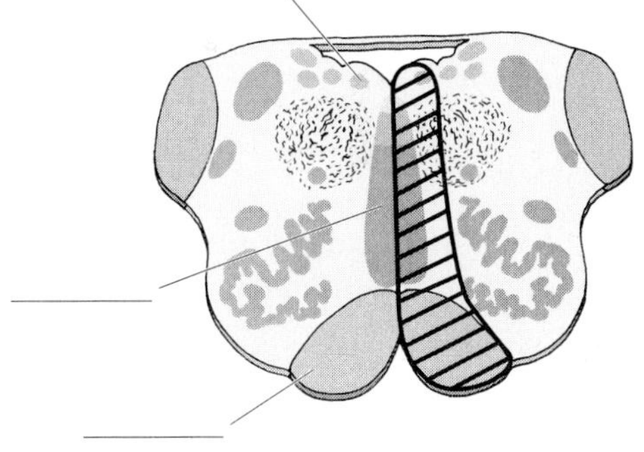

58.5. Next to each of the three structures you have identified, note the functional loss that is part of __________ medullary syndrome.

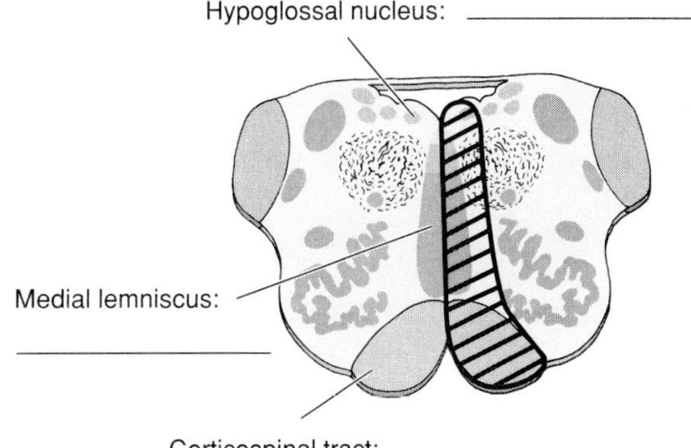

58.1A. arterial

58.2A. syndromes; vertebral

58.3A. spinal

58.4A.

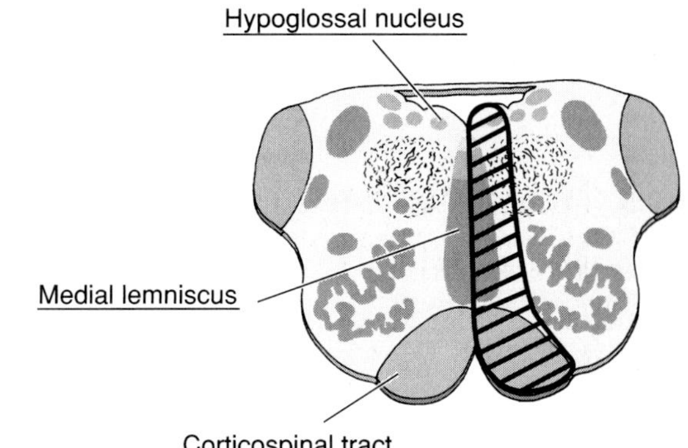

58.5A. medial

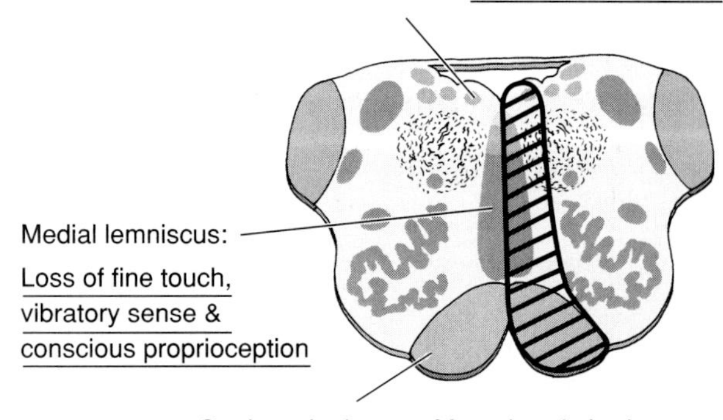

58.6. Indicate whether the loss is contralateral, ipsilateral, or bilateral.

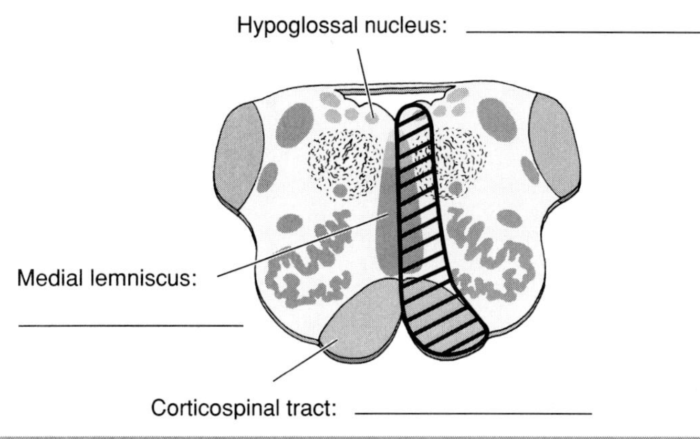

58.7. Lateral medullary syndrome often results from blockage of the posterior inferior cerebellar artery, a branch of the ________ arteries.

58.8. On the following diagram, the structures in the shaded area are affected in lateral medullary syndrome. On the unshaded side, label the structures indicated.

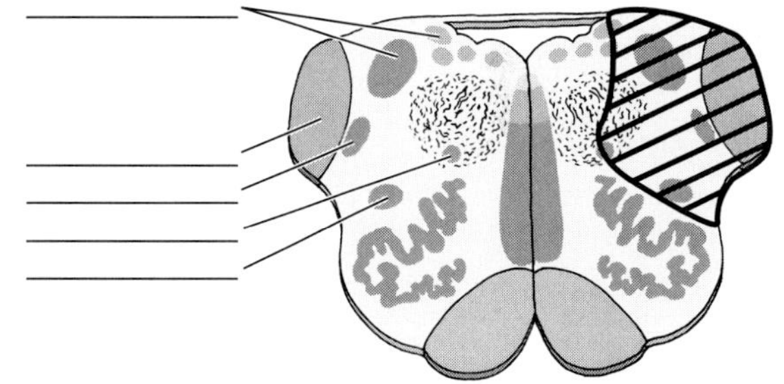

58.9. Next to each of the five items identified as being involved in lateral medullary syndrome, note the functional loss or effect.

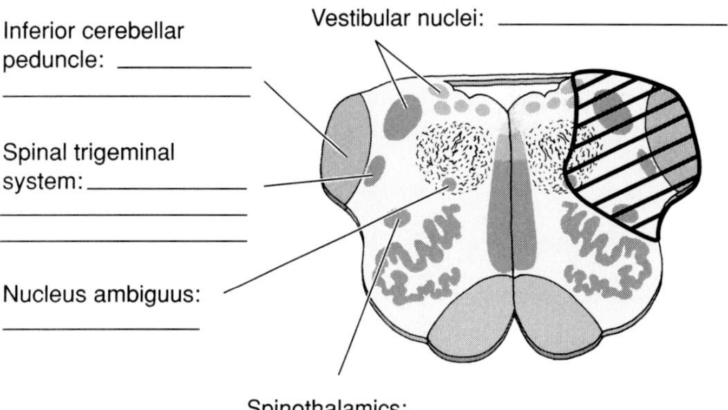

58.10. Lesion of the paramedian branches of the ________ artery—the artery supplying the pons—leads to characteristic deficits based on the structures deprived of blood shaded in the diagram.

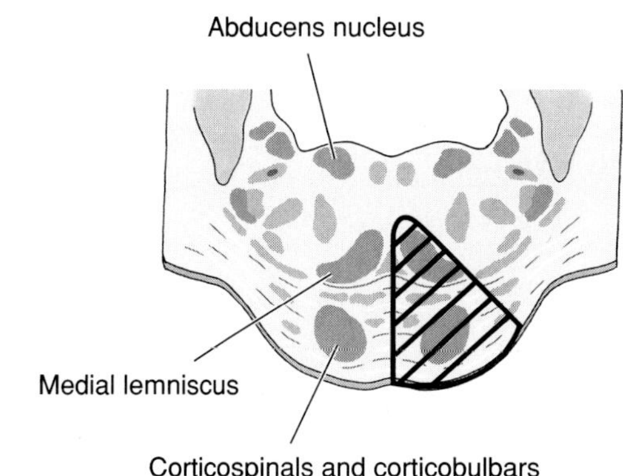

58.6A.

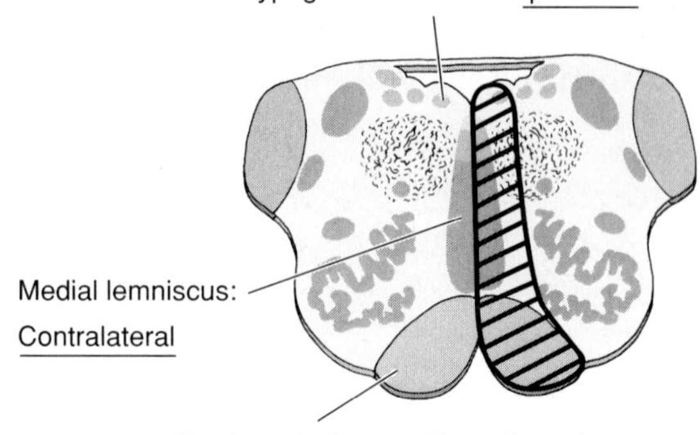

58.7A. vertebral

58.8A.

Vestibular nuclei

Inferior cerebellar peduncle

Spinal trigeminal nucleus & tract

Nucleus ambiguus

Spinothalamics

58.9A.

Vestibular nuclei: nausea, vertigo, nystagmus

Inferior cerebellar peduncle: cerebellar dysfunction

Spinal trigeminal system: ipsilateral loss of pain and temperature from the face

Nucleus ambiguus: paralysis of the larynx and pharynx

Spinothalamics: contralateral loss of pain and temperature from the body

58.10A. basilar

58.11. Medial strabismus (medial deviation of the eye) results from paralysis of the ____________ rectus muscle due to destruction of the fibers of the abducens nerve. In the diagram, draw in the abducens fibers as they pass through the lesioned (shaded) area. Label CN VI.

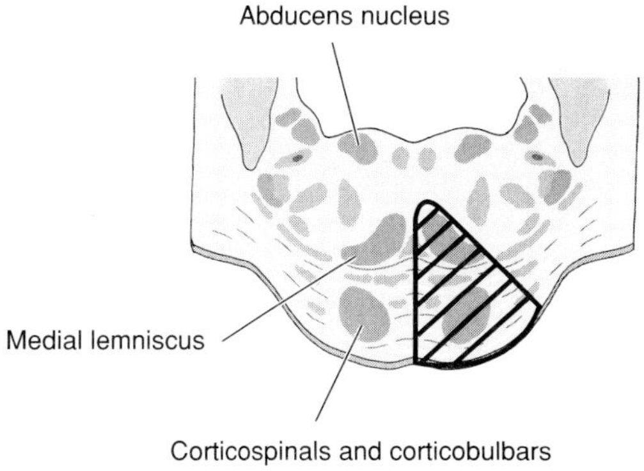

Abducens nucleus

Medial lemniscus

Corticospinals and corticobulbars

58.12. Descending tracts, including cortico____________ and cortico____________ are lost, leading to weakness of the facial musculature ______lateral to the lesion and paralysis of the ____________________ side of the body.

58.13. Damage to the ____________ ____________ causes a ____________lateral loss of the posterior/dorsal column modalities.

58.14. A blockage of the anterior inferior cerebellar artery—a branch of the ____________ artery—affects structures in the shaded region.

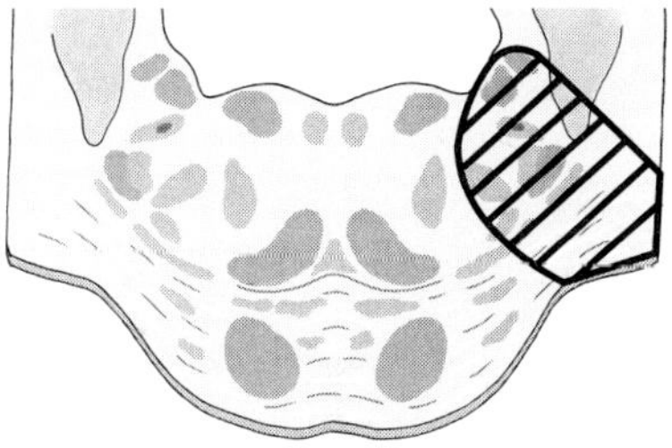

58.15. On the following diagram, label the affected structures on the side that is not shaded.

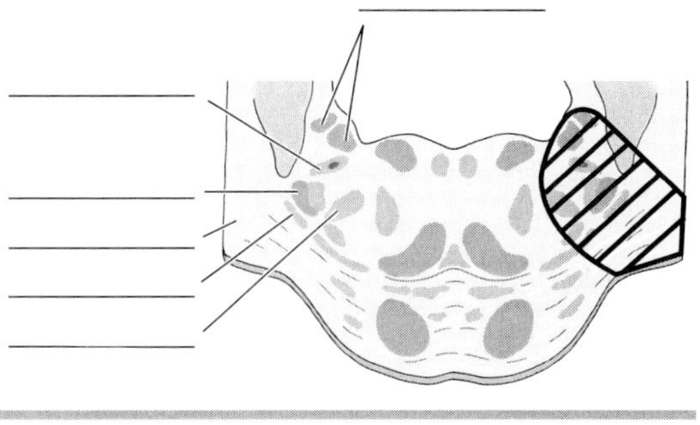

58.16. Next to each identified structure, indicate the major functional loss(es) or effects experienced in the lesion and, if applicable, whether the deficit is ipsilateral or contralateral.

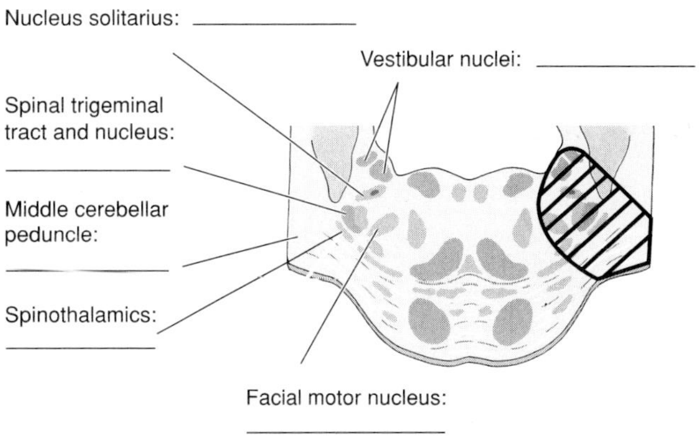

Nucleus solitarius: ____________

Vestibular nuclei: ____________

Spinal trigeminal tract and nucleus: ____________

Middle cerebellar peduncle: ____________

Spinothalamics: ____________

Facial motor nucleus: ____________

58.11A. lateral

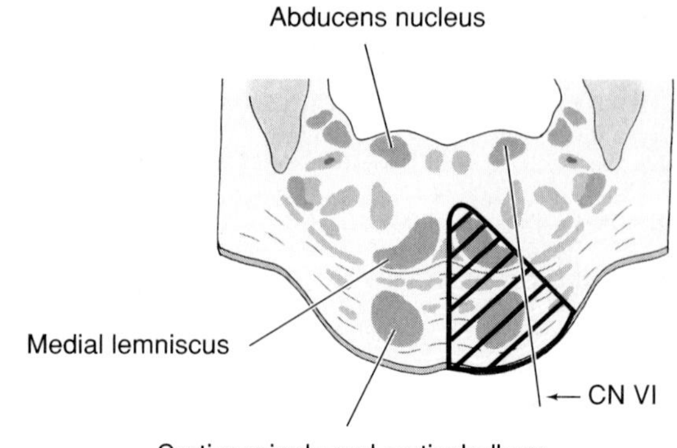

58.12A. corticobulbar; corticospinal; ipsilateral; contralateral

58.13A. medial lemniscus; contralateral

58.14A. basilar

58.15A.

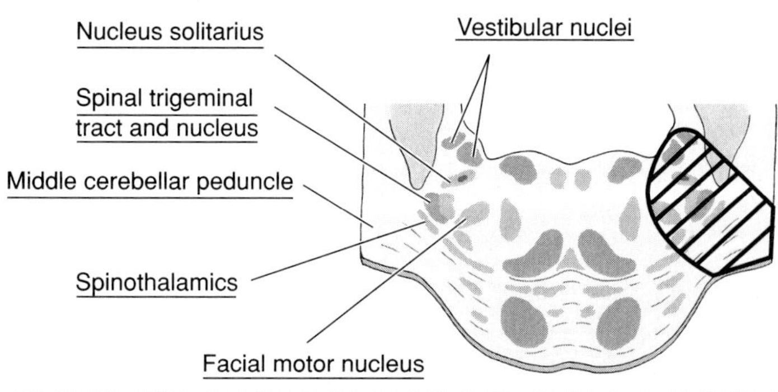

58.16A.

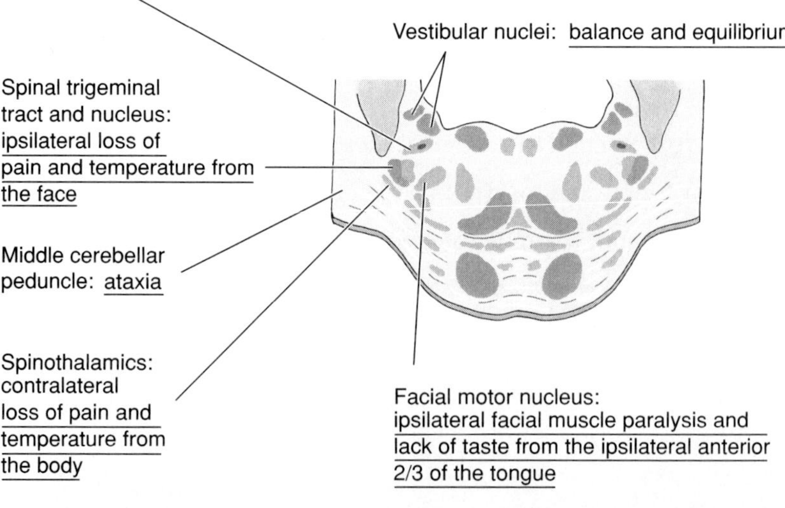

58.17. Also in the lesion shown in the previous question is damage to the descending hypothalamic tracts, leading to ______lateral Horner's syndrome, characterized by ptosis, miosis, and anhydrosis, as the upper motoneurons of the sympathetic system are lost.

58.18. Two well-described lesions associated with the midbrain include Weber's syndrome and Benedikt's syndrome. Both syndromes are associated with __________ insufficiency.

58.19. The __________ receives its blood from branches of the posterior cerebral arteries, the terminal branches of the __________ artery.

58.20. In Weber's syndrome, the oculomotor nerve fibers pass through the affected area and are compromised, as are the descending tracts discussed earlier—the corticobulbars and corticospinals. In the following diagram, draw the oculomotor fibers that pass through the lesioned (shaded) area that begin in the oculomotor and accessory oculomotor (Edinger-Westphal) nuclei.

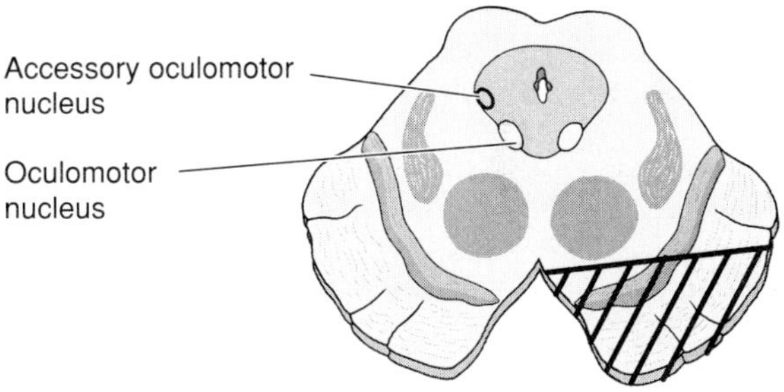

Accessory oculomotor nucleus

Oculomotor nucleus

58.21. Damage of the oculomotor fibers leaves the eye abducted and __________ due to the unopposed actions of the superior oblique and __________ __________ muscles. The eyelid droops (ptosis), and the pupil is __________.

58.22. Benedikt's syndrome also results from occlusion of branches of the posterior cerebral arteries and also affects the oculomotor fibers as seen in __________ syndrome.

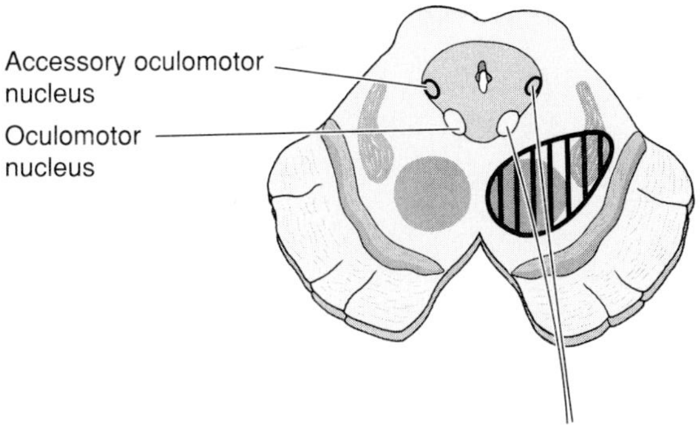

Accessory oculomotor nucleus

Oculomotor nucleus

58.17A. ipsilateral

58.18A. vascular

58.19A. midbrain; basilar

58.20A.

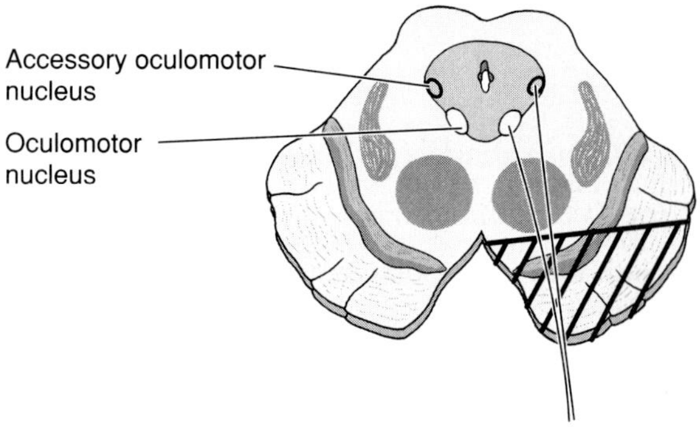

58.21A. depressed; lateral rectus; dilated

58.22A. Weber's

58.23. In addition to the above, the red nucleus and __________ lemniscus are compromised in Benedikt's syndrome. Label the red nucleus and medial lemniscus in the affected (shaded) area on the diagram.

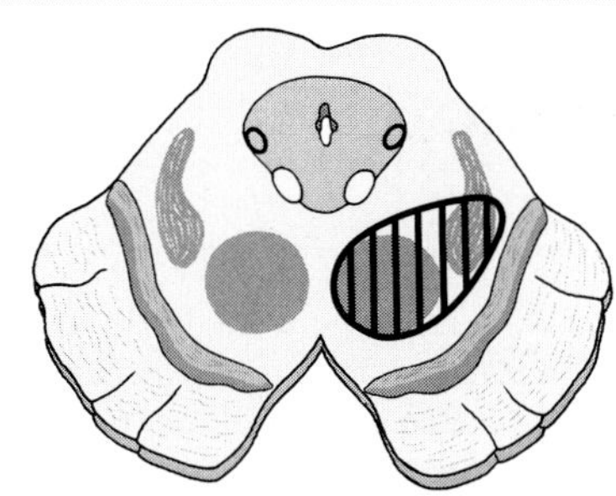

58.24. Damage to the red nucleus, a motor relay nucleus of the ______________, causes ataxia. Medial lemniscus damage causes a __________lateral loss of posterior/dorsal __________ modalities from the body.

58.23A. medial

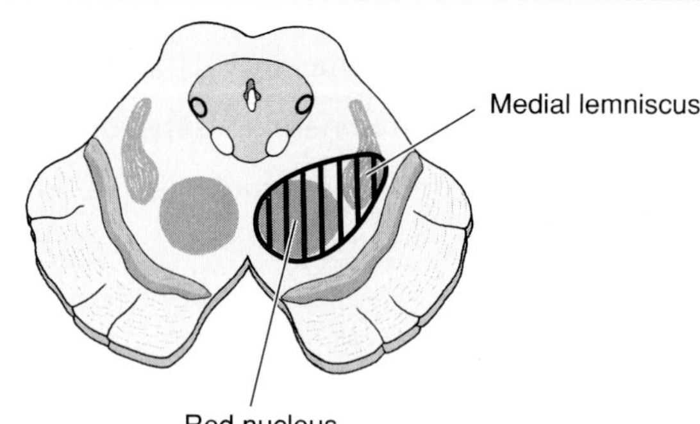

58.24A. cerebellum; contralateral; column

59 Peripheral Lesions of the Cranial Nerves

59.1. Functional loss resulting from peripheral lesions of the cranial nerves depends on the location of the ____________. For the purpose of emphasizing the function of each nerve, we will assume that the nerves are damaged near the brainstem and that the deficits will only affect one nerve.

59.2. Lesions of the ____________ nerve, such as may occur in fracture of the ethmoid bone, lead to anosmia (loss of smell); because these neurons are capable of regeneration, smell often returns over time. Lesions of the ______ nerve lead to ipsilateral loss of vision.

59.3. Lesions of the ____________________, ____________, and/or ____________ nerves affect eye movement. Damage to the oculomotor nerve results in a laterally deviated (lateral strabismus) depressed eye, diplopia (double vision) from the unopposed actions of the lateral rectus and superior oblique muscles, a dilated pupil, ptosis, and a loss of accommodation (close-up focus) from compromised parasympathetics. Lesion of the trochlear nerve leads to paralysis of the ____________ oblique muscle. The abducens nerve innervates the lateral rectus; lesion of CN VI leads to ____________ ____________________ (medial deviation of the eye).

59.4. Trigeminal nerve lesions lead to specific and predictable sensory deficits from the ______lateral face, dependent upon which division is lesioned. Furthermore, lesion of the ____________________ division affects the muscles of mastication as well as ____________ over the mandible. The trigeminal nerve also serves as the ______fferent limb of the corneal blink reflex, and so a failure in blinking may indicate ophthalmic division damage.

59.5. Characteristics of facial nerve lesions such as that may occur during trauma or childbirth include paralysis of the facial ____________________, loss of the efferent limb of the corneal blink reflex, decreased ____________ and tear production, and loss of taste from the anterior two-thirds of the tongue.

59.6. Lesion of cranial nerve VIII, the vestibulo____________ nerve, leads to ipsilateral deafness and problems with ____________ and equilibrium.

59.1A. lesion

59.2A. olfactory; optic

59.3A. oculomotor; trochlear; abducens; superior; medial strabismus

59.4A. ipsilateral; mandibular; sensation; afferent

59.5A. musculature; saliva

59.6A. vestibulocochlear; balance

59.7. The glosso________________ nerve conveys sensation from the pharynx; lesions manifest themselves most obviously as a decreased gag reflex, the motor aspect of which is mediated by cranial nerve ____.

59.8. Lesions of the vagus nerve produce dramatic and widespread results. Place a check next to some of the possible results of a lesion of the vagus nerve near its origin.

_____ increased heart rate

_____ decreased heart rate

_____ increased gastric motility

_____ decreased gastric motility

_____ dilated pupil

_____ constricted pupil

_____ bronchodilation

_____ bronchoconstriction

59.9. Many of the results of the vagal nerve lesion checked in the previous item are the result of the unopposed actions of the ________________ nervous system.

59.10. Other obvious effects of vagal nerve damage include a lack of the motor component of the _____ reflex and a horse voice due to paralysis of the ipsilateral vocal cord.

59.11. The __________ __________ nerve provides motor innervation to the trapezius and ________________ muscles. Damage to this nerve causes _____lateral paralysis of these muscles.

59.12. A lesion of the hypoglossal nerve causes ipsilateral paralysis of the __________. The tongue deviates towards the side of the lesioned nerve upon protrusion.

59.7A. glossopharyngeal; X

59.8A.

__✓__ increased heart rate

_____ decreased heart rate

_____ increased gastric motility

__✓__ decreased gastric motility

_____ dilated pupil

_____ constricted pupil

__✓__ bronchodilation

_____ bronchoconstriction

59.9A. sympathetic

59.10A. gag

59.11A. spinal accessory; sternocleidomastoid; ipsilateral

59.12A. tongue

59.13. Write the number of the cranial nerve next to the condition with which it is associated.

Anosmia –

Tongue paralysis –

Paralysis of the lateral rectus –

Loss of the afferent limb of the gag reflex –

Blindness –

Paralysis of the levator palpebrae superioris –

Decreased lacrimation –

Paralysis of the muscles of mastication –

Loss of sensation over the cheek –

Loss of taste from the anterior two-thirds of the tongue –

Paralysis of the vocal cords –

Inability to constrict the pupil –

Deafness –

Loss of gastric motility –

Decreased saliva from parotid gland –

Loss balance and equilibrium –

Lateral strabismus –

Loss of the afferent limb of the corneal blink reflex –

Loss of the efferent limb of the corneal blink reflex –

59.13A.

Anosmia – I

Tongue paralysis – XII

Paralysis of the lateral rectus – VI

Loss of the afferent limb of the gag reflex – IX

Blindness – II

Paralysis of the levator palpebrae superioris – III

Decreased lacrimation – VII

Paralysis of the muscles of mastication – V

Loss of sensation over the cheek – V

Loss of taste from the anterior two-thirds of the tongue – VII

Paralysis of the vocal cords – X

Inability to constrict the pupil – III

Deafness – VIII

Loss of gastric motility – X

Decreased saliva from parotid gland – IX

Loss balance and equilibrium – VIII

Lateral strabismus – III

Loss of the afferent limb of the corneal blink reflex – V

Loss of the efferent limb of the corneal blink reflex – VII

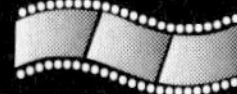

Animations

8. Fascial Movement (Chapters 49, 50, 51, 52, 54, 57)
9. Head Turning (Chapters 49, 50, 52, 54, 57)
10. Crude Movement (Chapter 50)
11. Postural Movement (Chapter 50)
12. Pain and Temperature Head (Chapters 48, 55, 57)
13. Crude Touch Head (Chapters 48, 55, 57)
14. Fine Touch Head (Chapters 48, 55, 57)
15. Reflex Proprioception Head (Chapters 48, 54, 55, 56, 57)
17. Visceral Head (Chapters 48, 51, 54, 55, 56, 57)
19. ANS Oculomotor (Chapters 49 and 57)
20. ANS Facial (Chapters 49 and 57)
21. ANS Glossopharyngeal (Chapters 49 and 57)
22. Vagus (Chapters 49 and 57)

VI SPINAL CORD

60 Spinal Cord: Relations Between Spine and Spinal Cord

60.1. The brainstem passes inferiorly into the spine through a great hole in the base of the skull, the foramen ____________, and becomes the ____________ spinal ______.

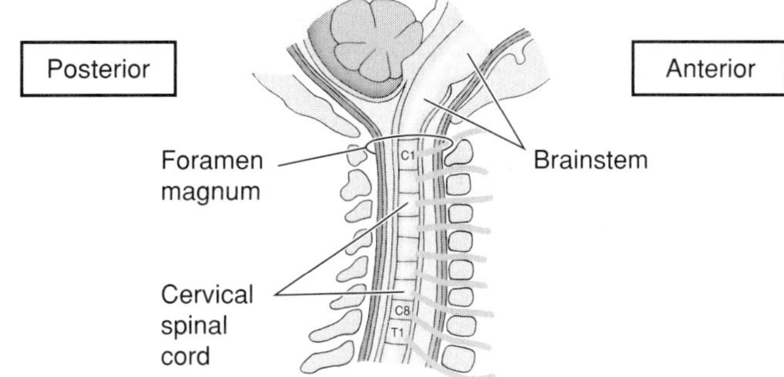

60.2. The spinal cord passes inferiorly within the vertebrae. The term "spine" refers to the column of bones, or vertebrae. The term "spinal cord" refers to the collection of ______ cells and fibers enclosed within the ______.

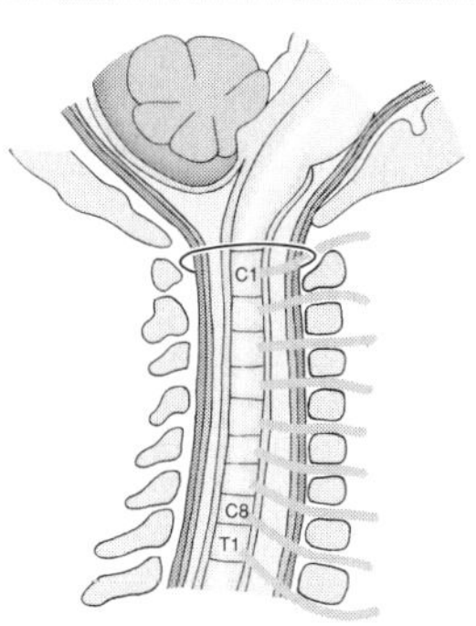

60.3. During postnatal growth, the vertebral column elongates much more than the spinal cord. Label the diagrams "A" for adult and "E" for embryonic.

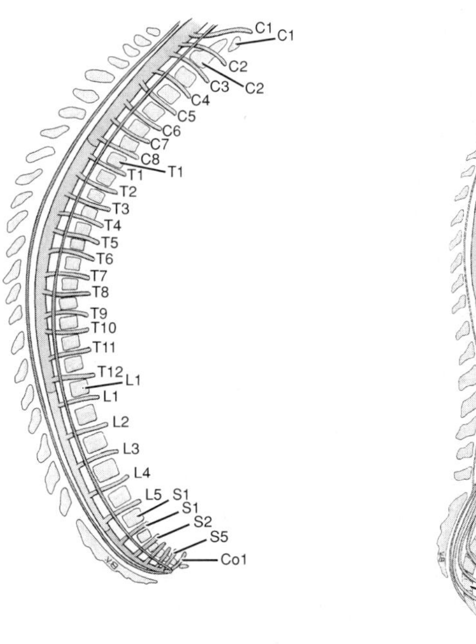

________ ________

60.1A. magnum; cervical; cord

60.2A. nerve; spine

60.3A.

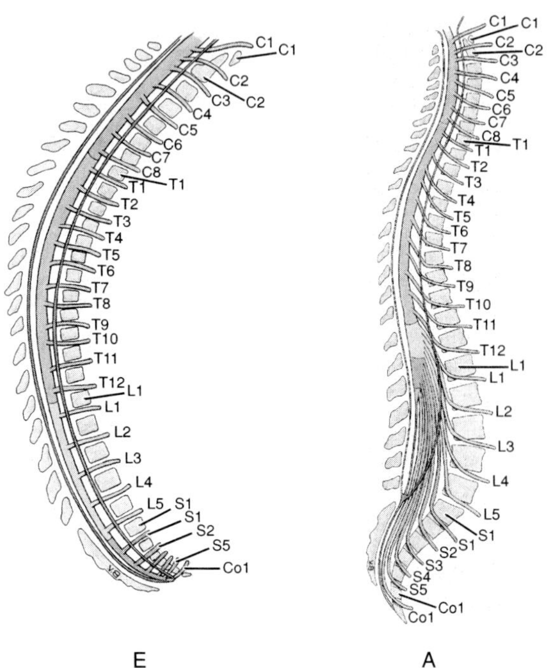

60.4. The adult spinal cord is ______er in length than the vertebral column.

60.5. The Latin word for neck is *cervix* (adjective, cervic______). The neck contains the __________ vertebrae and spinal cord. The thorax contains the __________ vertebrae and spinal cord. In adults, the spinal cord terminates at the level of the first or second __________ vertebrae. There is no spinal cord within the __________ vertebrae. Fill in the label on the diagram

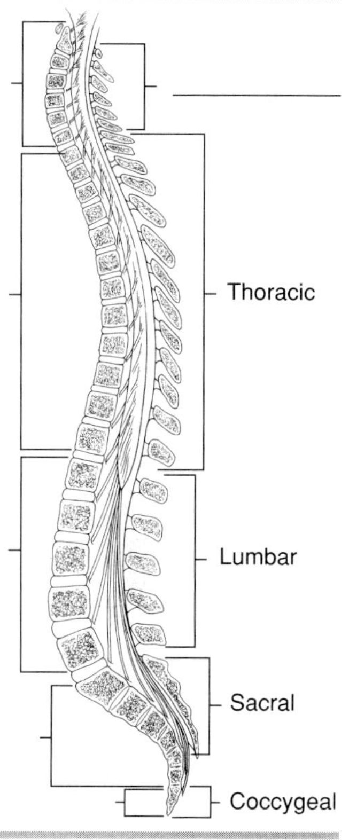

60.6. Spinal cord segments and vertebrae are labeled with their initial letters and with numbers to indicate their relative positions. There is *no* spinal cord within the __________ vertebrae and most of the __________ vertebrae. Thoracic, lumbar, and superior sacral segments of the spinal cord are all enclosed within the __________ region of spinal vertebrae.

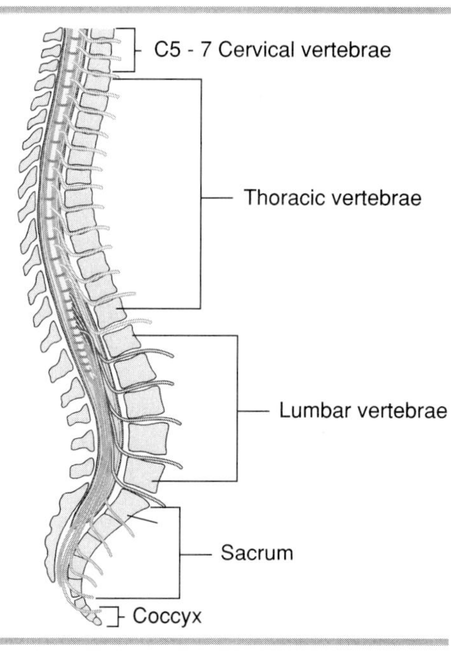

60.7. The lowest part of the spinal cord, the __________ spinal cord, terminates in the upper part of the __________ region of the vertebral column.

60.4A. shorter

60.5A. cervical; cervical; thoracic; lumbar; sacral

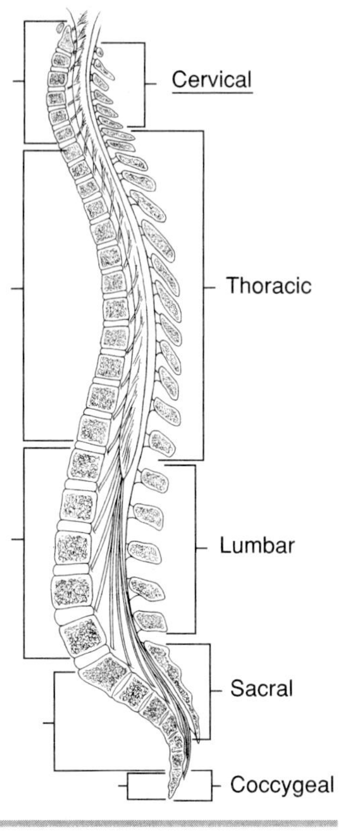

60.6A. sacral; lumbar; thoracic

60.7A. sacral; lumbar

60.8. The number of cervical spinal cord segments is ______. There are ______ thoracic spinal cord segments, ______ lumbar spinal cord segments, and ______ sacral spinal cord segments. (The most caudal portion, "CO," is the coccygeal remnant, not one of the sacral segments).

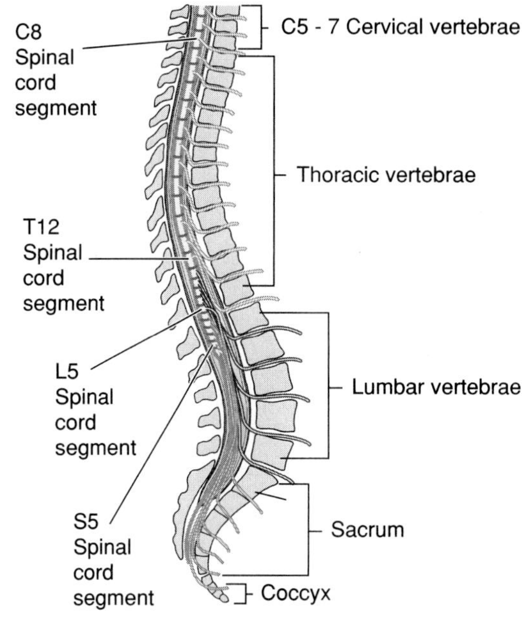

60.9. The total number of spinal cord segments is ______.

60.10. Labels on the left side pertain to ______ segments; labels on the right side pertain to ____________. Label each bracket with the full name of the segment it encloses.

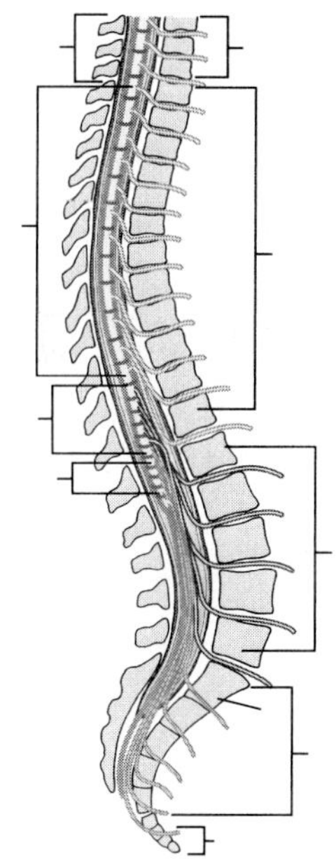

60.8A. 8; 12; 5; 5

60.9A. 31

60.10A. cord; vertebrae

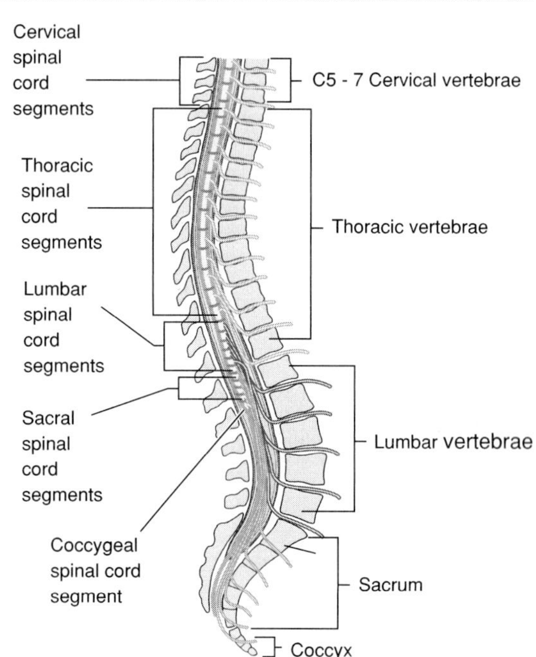

60.11. A neurosurgeon who has made a diagnosis of spinal cord tumor at L4 knows that he will operate at about the level of vertebra ______.

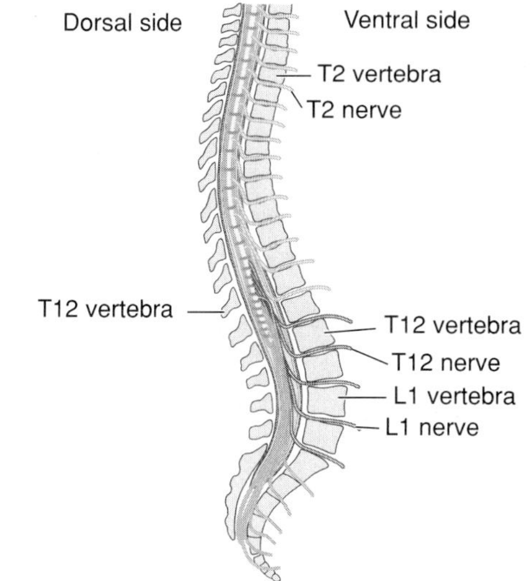

60.12. Nerves emerge from each segment of the spinal cord early in embryonic life and pass anteriorly outward between each pair of developing vertebrae. On this lateral view, draw the right 4th lumbar nerve passing out from the cord between vertebrae L4 and L5.

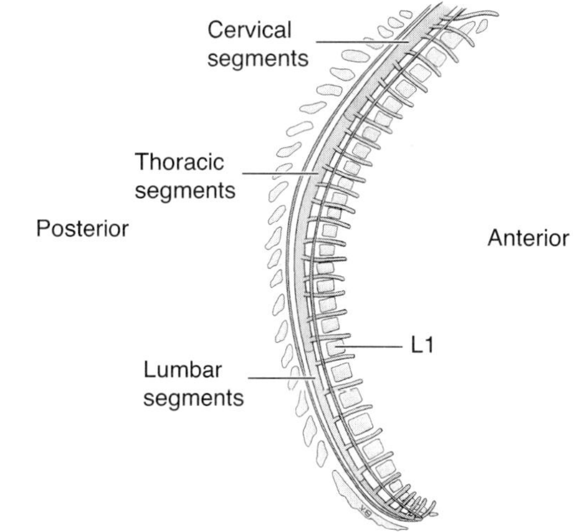

60.13. The portion of a spinal nerve within the vertebral column elongates as the vertebral column elongates. On the right hand diagram, draw the 4th lumbar nerve and complete the labels on the pair of vertebrae between which it passes.

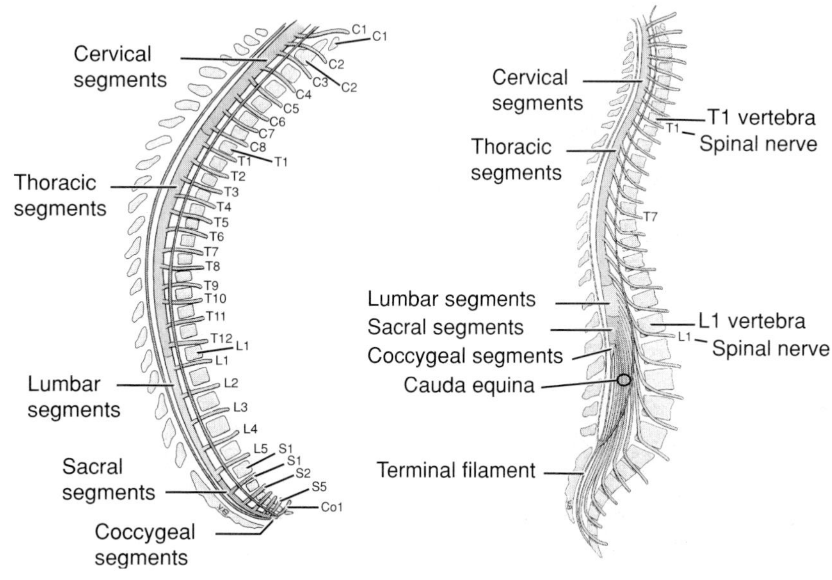

60.11A. T12

60.12A.

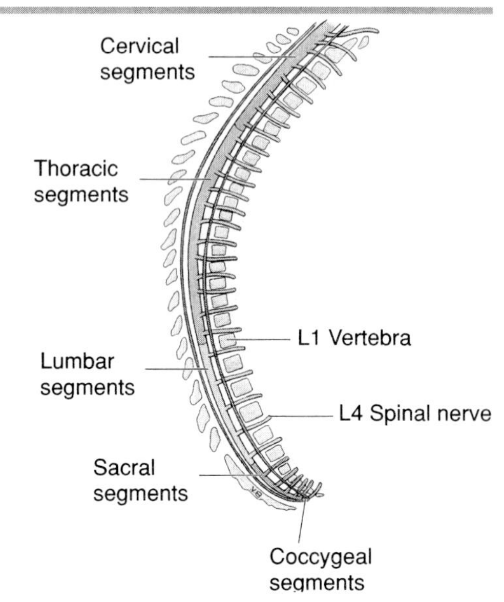
Cervical segments
Thoracic segments
L1 Vertebra
Lumbar segments
L4 Spinal nerve
Sacral segments
Coccygeal segments

60.13A.

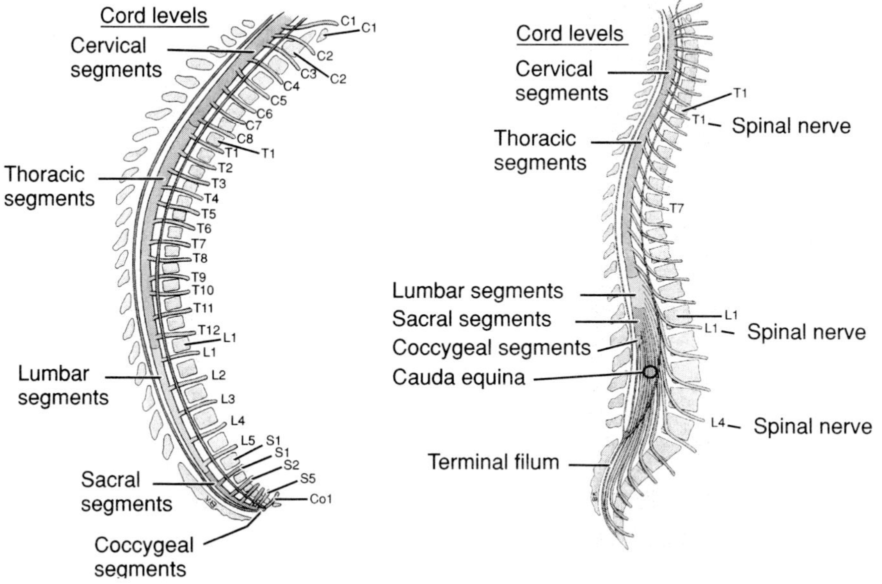
Cord levels
Cervical segments
Thoracic segments
Lumbar segments
Sacral segments
Coccygeal segments
C1
C2
C3
C4
C5
C6
C7
C8
T1
T2
T3
T4
T5
T6
T7
T8
T9
T10
T11
T12
L1
L2
L3
L4
L5
S1
S2
S5
Co1
Cord levels
Cervical segments
Thoracic segments
T1
Spinal nerve
T7
Lumbar segments
Sacral segments
Coccygeal segments
Cauda equina
L1
Spinal nerve
L4
Spinal nerve
Terminal filum

60.14. A nerve root is the portion of a nerve that extends from the spinal cord to the exit point between two vertebrae. It is numbered according to its corresponding cord segment. Encircle the nerve roots C6 and C8.

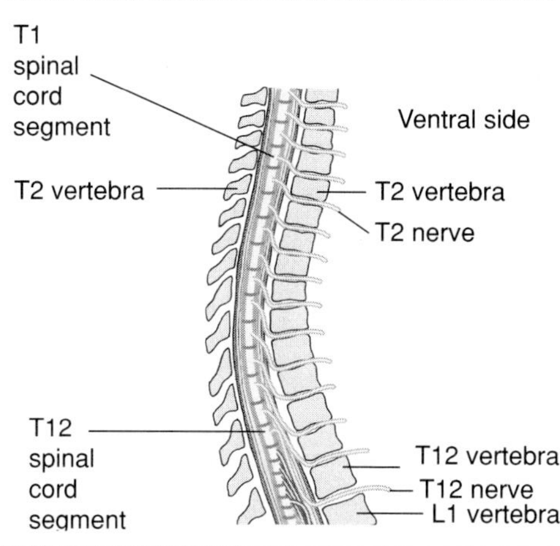

60.15. There are 8 cervical spinal cord segments but only ______ cervical vertebrae. Nerve C8 emerges between vertebrae ______ and ______. Nerve C5 would emerge between vertebrae C______ and C______; nerve C7 emerges between vertebrae C______ and C______.

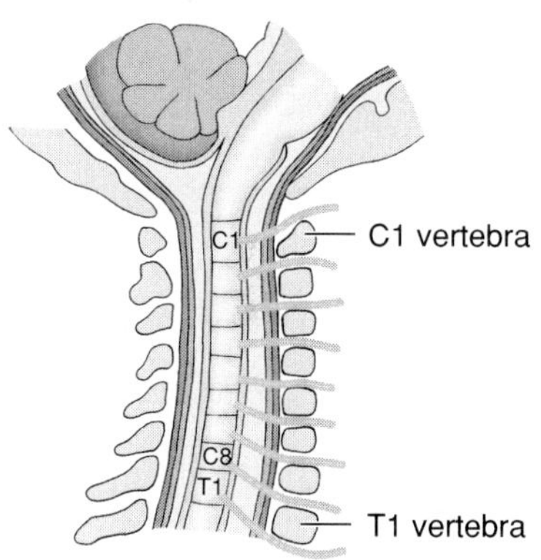

60.16. Most lumbar and all sacral vertebrae enclose no segments of ____________ ______ but enclose many nerve ______. Those bear some resemblance to a horse's tail and hence were named the ______ equina.

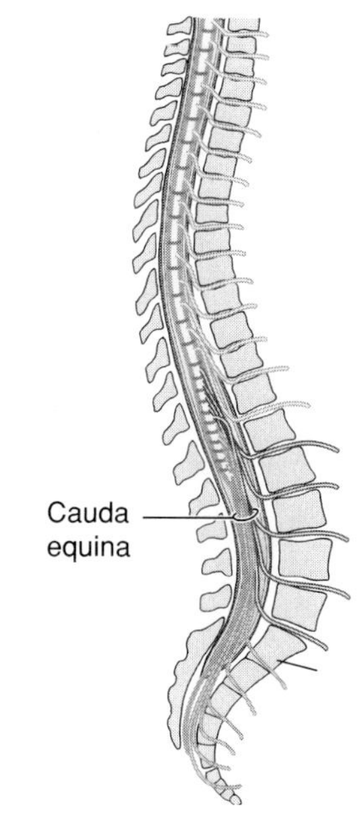

60.14.

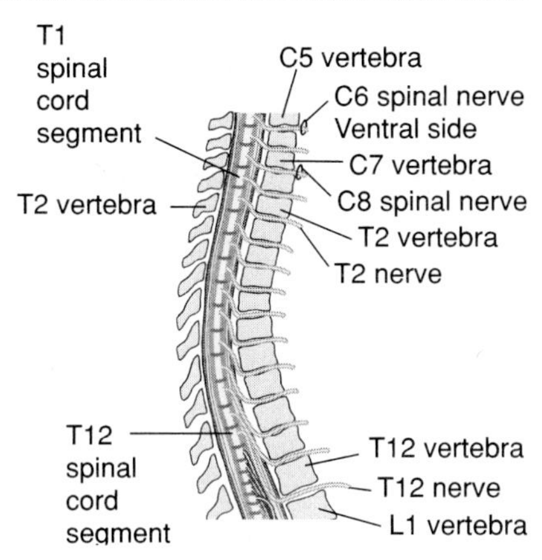

60.15A. 7; C7; T1; C4; C5; C6; C7

60.16A. spinal cord; roots; cauda

60.17. A transverse section between vertebrae T11 and T12 cuts across spinal cord segment ______, as well as across many roots. More inferiorly, these roots make up the ______ ____________.

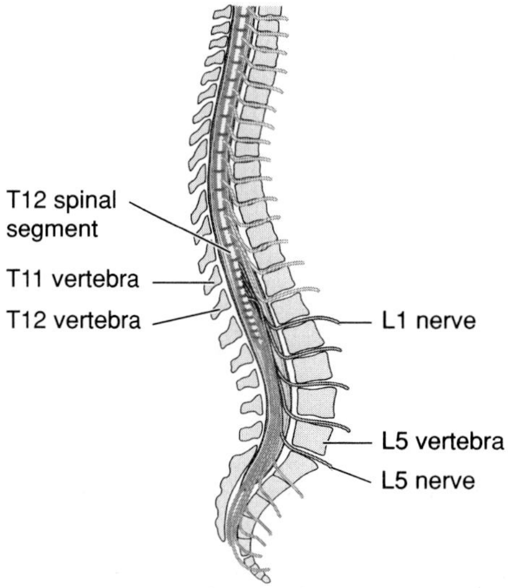

T12 spinal segment
T11 vertebra
T12 vertebra
L1 nerve
L5 vertebra
L5 nerve

60.18. Each thoracic, lumbar, and ____________ nerve emerges between the vertebrae of the same number and the next one caudal. For example, nerve T6 emerges between vertebrae T6 and ______.

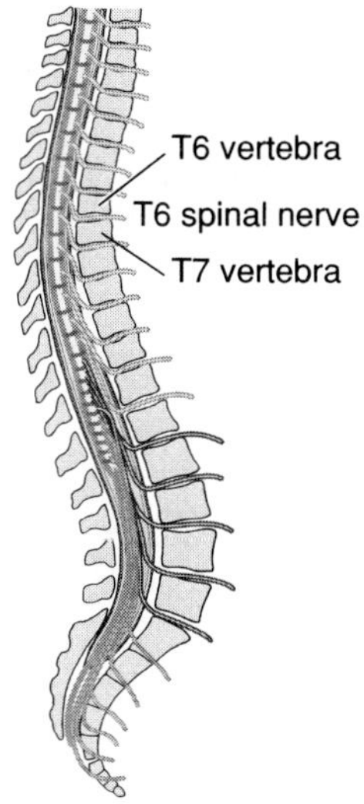

T6 vertebra
T6 spinal nerve
T7 vertebra

60.19. Nerve L5 has a long root that emerges between vertebrae ______ and ______. Draw this root on the diagram.

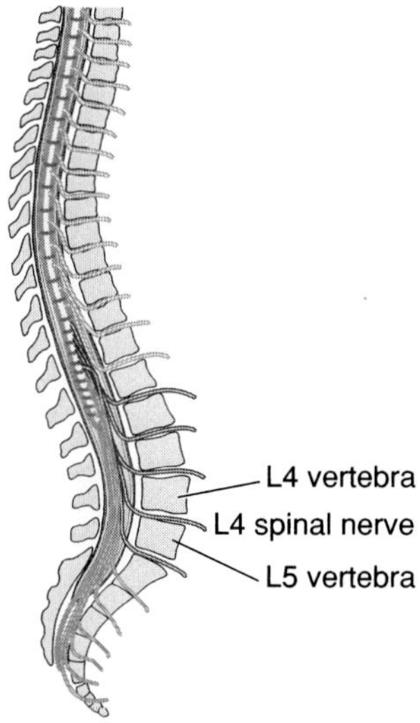

L4 vertebra
L4 spinal nerve
L5 vertebra

60.17A. L2/L3; cauda equina

60.18A. sacral; T7

60.19A. L5; S1

60.20. Since the spine runs down the back, most peripheral nerves must extend from the spinal cord in an anterior direction. Label the indicated sides as anterior and posterior.

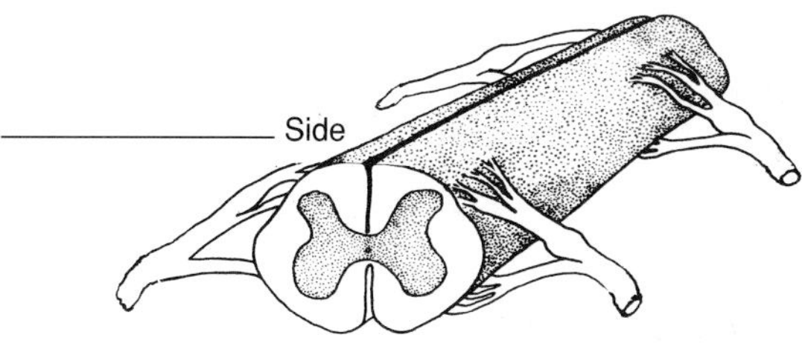

60.21. Most peripheral nerves contain both afferent and efferent fibers, as illustrated and labeled. Such a nerve is called a mixed _______________ nerve. It divides near the spinal cord, within the vertebral column, into a posterior __________ root and an anterior __________ _____.

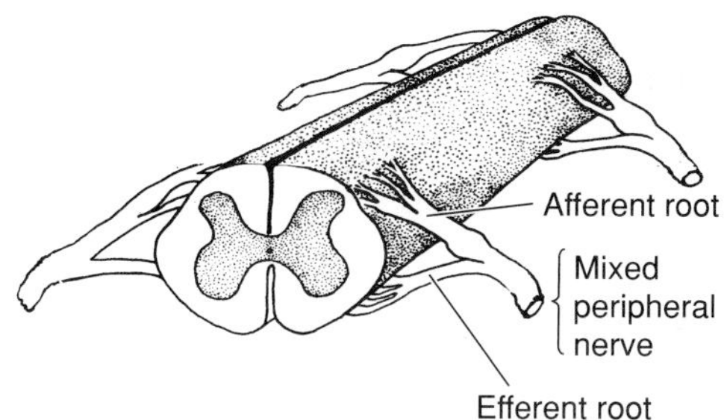

60.22. Efferent fibers emerge from the spinal cord via the _____ior root.

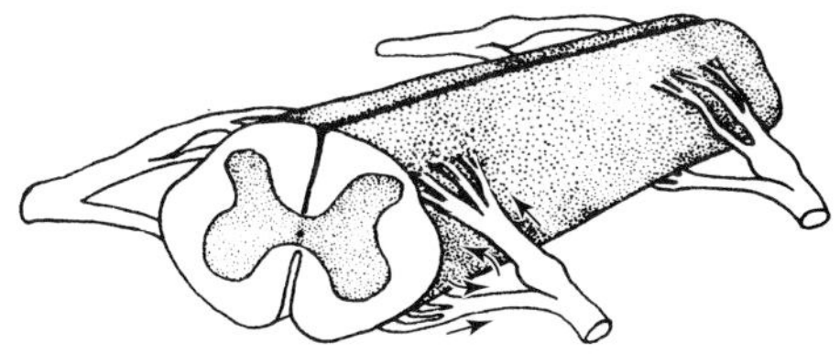

60.23. A nerve is composed of many individual fibers. A _____ peripheral nerve divides into posterior and anterior roots. The axon of a given cell is found in one or the other _____, not in both.

60.24. Many texts use other terms for anterior and posterior roots. For convenience, we shall maintain a consistent terminology, equating afferent or sensory with the __________ root and efferent or motor with the __________ root.

60.25. Fibers in the anterior root have cell bodies located within the gray matter of the __________ _____. Fibers of the posterior root emerge from cell bodies outside the cord, in the sensory spinal __________.

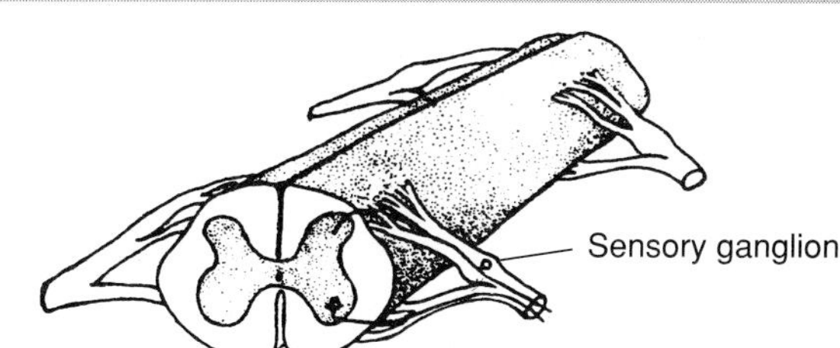

60.20A.

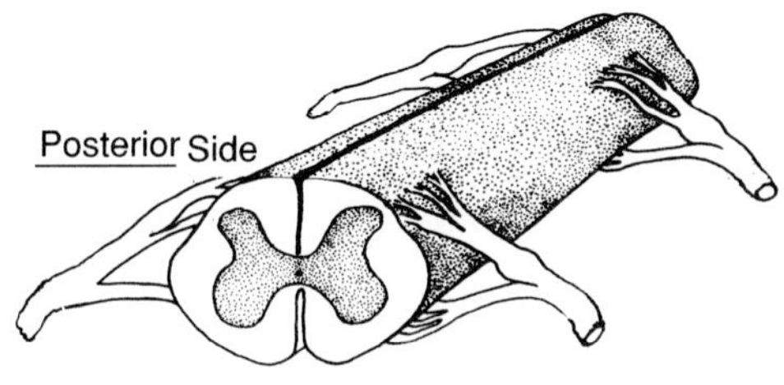

60.21A. peripheral; afferent; efferent root

60.22A. anterior

60.23A. mixed; root

60.24A. posterior; anterior

60.25A. spinal cord; ganglion

60.26. Nerve impulses descend from the precentral gyrus and reach the cell labeled ______ in the diagram.

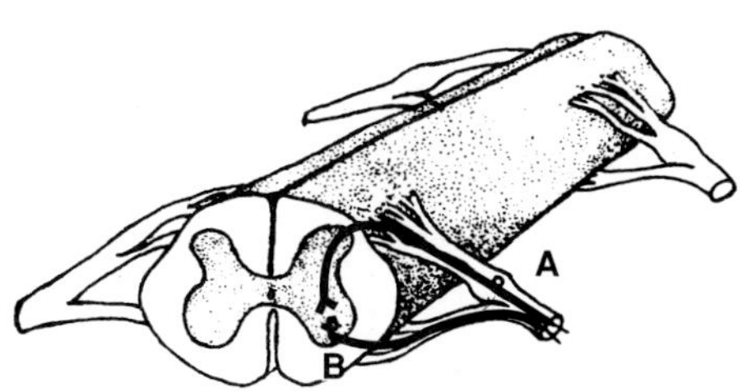

60.27. In the peripheral nervous system, a discrete mass of cell bodies is called a ______lion.

60.28. Peripheral sensory nerves have cell bodies ______side the central nervous system, in the ____________ lying in the ____________ roots.

60.29. Cell bodies in the gray matter of the central nervous system often are gathered into discrete masses called ______lei; for example, the red ____________ in the ____________ region of the brainstem. In one instance, the term "ganglion" has been used inaccurately to indicate the cell masses in gray matter of the central nervous system. These masses deep in the cerebral hemispheres were called the ______ ____________. They are now termed the ______ nuclei.

60.30. On the diagram, label posterior root (PR), sensory spinal ganglion (SG), anterior root (AR), and mixed peripheral nerve (MPN).

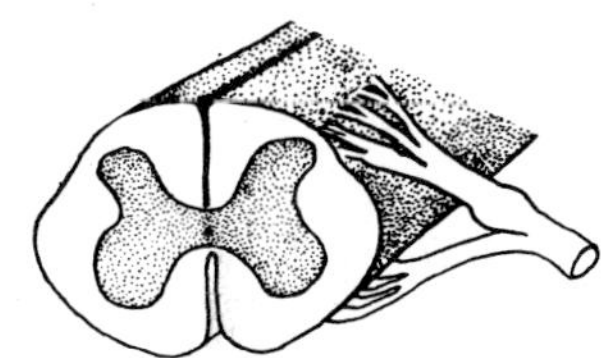

60.26A. B

60.27A. ganglion

60.28A. outside; ganglia; posterior

60.29A. nuclei; nucleus; midbrain; basal ganglia; basal

60.30A.

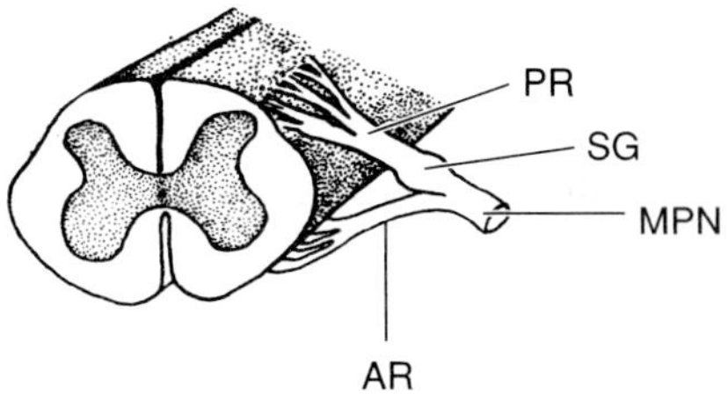

61 Blood Supply to the Spinal Cord

61.1. There are large, longitudinally oriented arteries on both the anterior and posterior aspects of the spinal cord. These arteries are particularly consistent at more cranial levels of the spinal cord and are supplemented at more ___________ levels by segmental branches originating from the descending aorta.

61.2. The unpaired anterior spinal artery is formed by a contribution from each vertebral artery. The anterior spinal artery supplies the ___________ two-thirds of the cord.

61.3. The anterior ___________ artery supplies the anterior, lateral, and part of the posterior horns of ______ matter and the anterior and lateral ___________ of white matter. In the following C8 spinal cord section, shade the areas that receive blood from the anterior spinal artery.

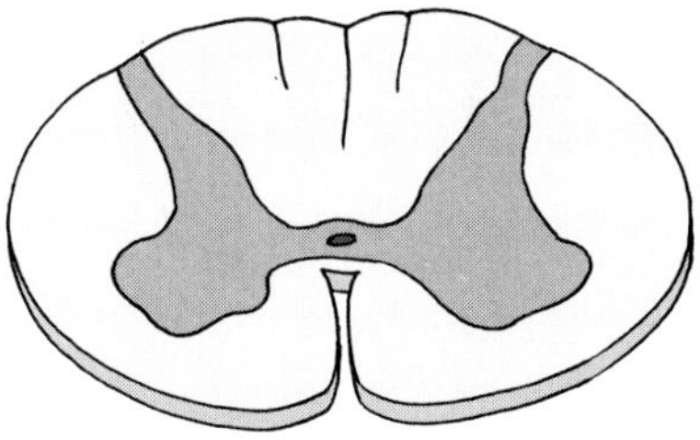

61.4. A pair of posterior spinal arteries supply the remaining aspects of the cord. The posterior spinal arteries are mainly responsible for the ___________ funiculus and portions of the ___________ horns of gray matter not supplied by the anterior spinal artery. In the following diagram, shade the areas that receive blood from the posterior spinal arteries.

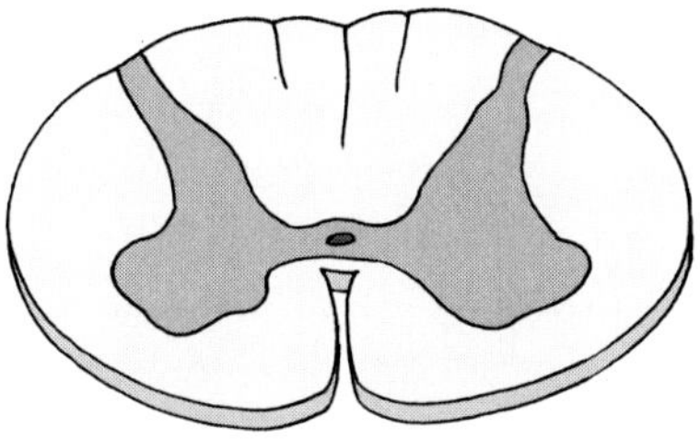

61.5. Although the segmental arteries give rise to branches that supply a great deal of the spinal cord, they mainly supply blood to the ___________ and ___________ spinal arteries at lower cord levels, and because they are segmental, they form significant anastamoses.

61.1A. caudal

61.2A. anterior

61.3A. spinal; gray; funiculi

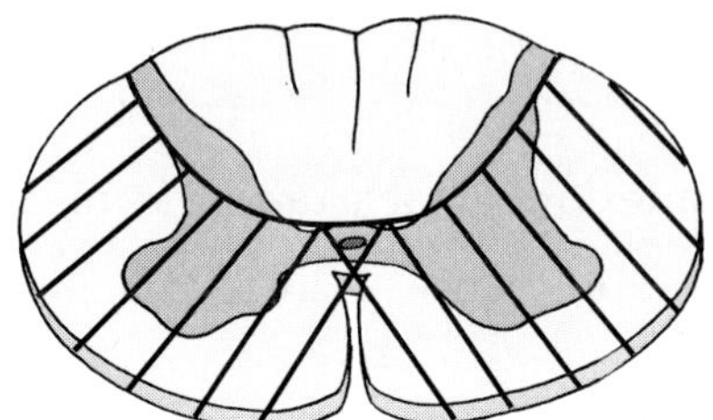

61.4A. posterior; posterior

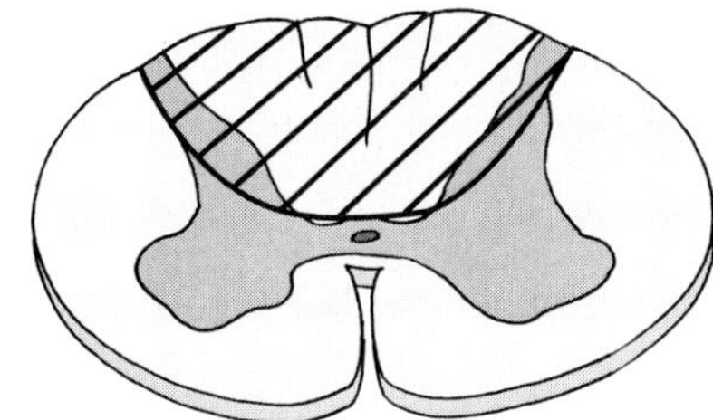

61.5A. anterior; posterior

62 Identification of Cord Levels

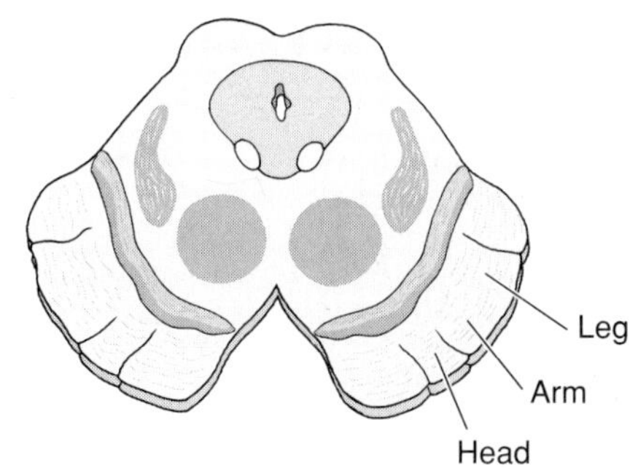

62.1. In almost all fiber bundles that have a somatotopic organization, upper parts of the body are represented medially, and lower parts are represented laterally. Check the labels that indicate corticospinal fibers in the basis ___________. However, the posterior columns are a special case; lower limbs are represented ___________ly, in the fasciculus ___________.

62.2. The posterior white columns are commonly referred to simply as the "posterior or dorsal columns." In this terminology, the posterior columns are _____ matter, and the posterior horns are _____ matter. In the posterior columns, the lower limbs are represented in a _____al position. In most other tracts, for example the lateral spinothalamic tract, axons representing the lower limb occupy a _____al position.

62.3. On the diagram, write "L," "A," and "H" for leg, arm, and head on the left basis pedunculi. On the left posterior column of the section at an upper cervical cord level, write "L," "T," and "A" for leg, trunk, and arm.

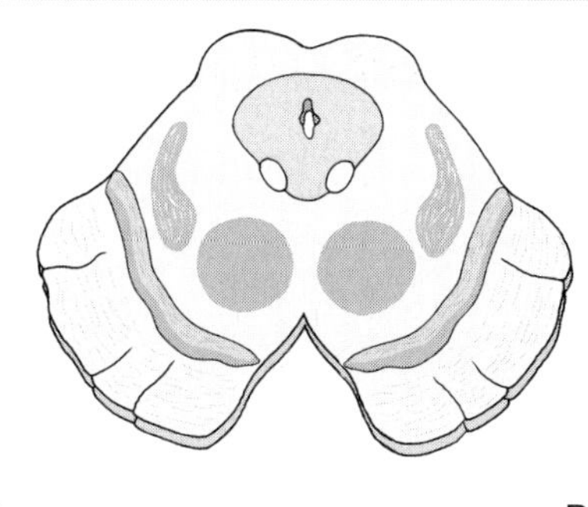

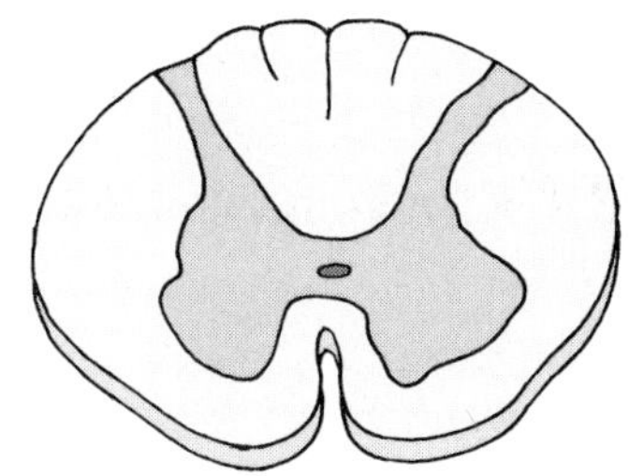

62.1A. pedunculi; medially; gracilis

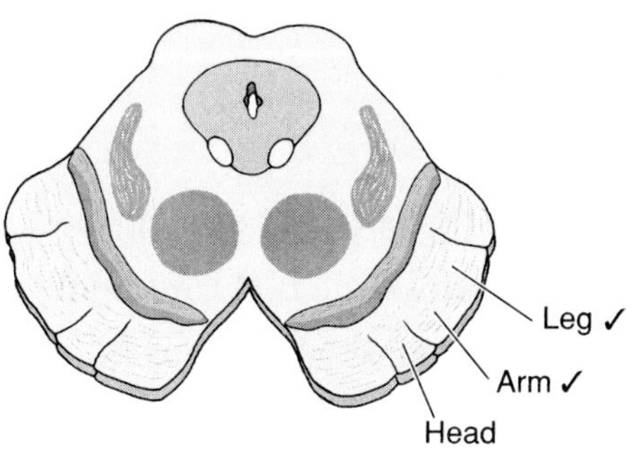

62.2A. white; gray; medial; lateral

62.3A.

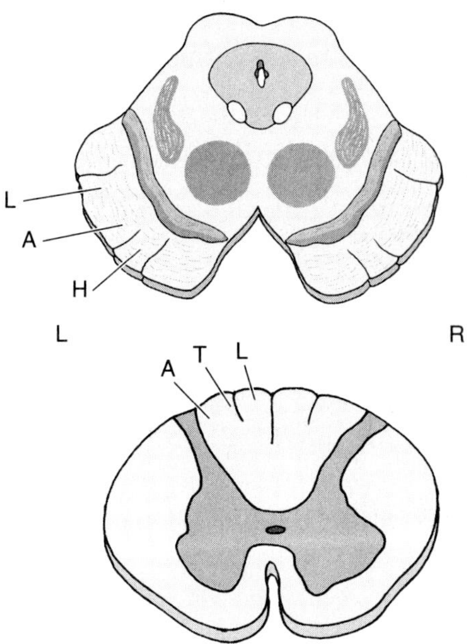

62.4. As the lateral corticospinal tract passes down the spinal cord, it gives off fibers that may make synaptic contact with lower motor neurons in the gray matter of the ____________ ______ of the spinal cord. The cervical plexus emerges mainly from lower cervical segments; therefore, the anterior horns are ______er in size in lower cervical segments. Sensory tracts become larger in size as they ______ scend the cord. Label the two sections appropriately as high (H) or low (L) cervical.

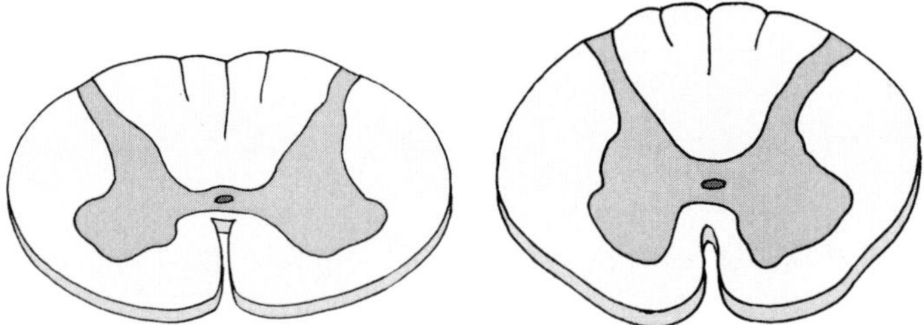

62.5. The sympathetic nervous system is sometimes called the thoracolumbar system. The intermediolateral cell column is absent at the ____________ and ____________ cord levels.

62.6. The thoracic and upper lumbar segments of the cord are distinguished from all other levels by the presence of ____________________ cell columns.

62.7. Although these two sections look similar in some respects, the ratio of white to gray matter and the intermediolateral cell column indicate that the ______ hand section is high cervical, and the other section is at a ____________ level.

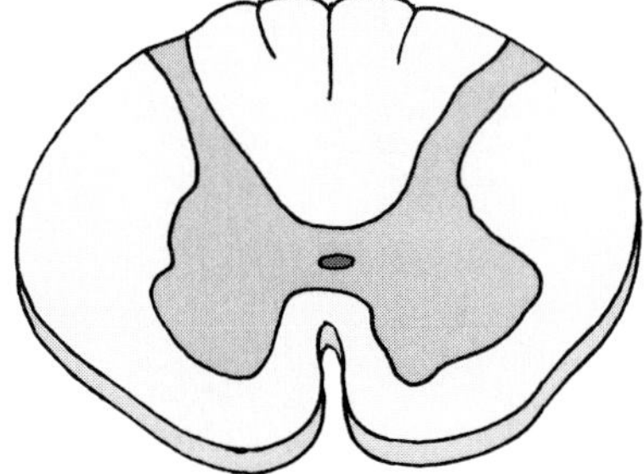

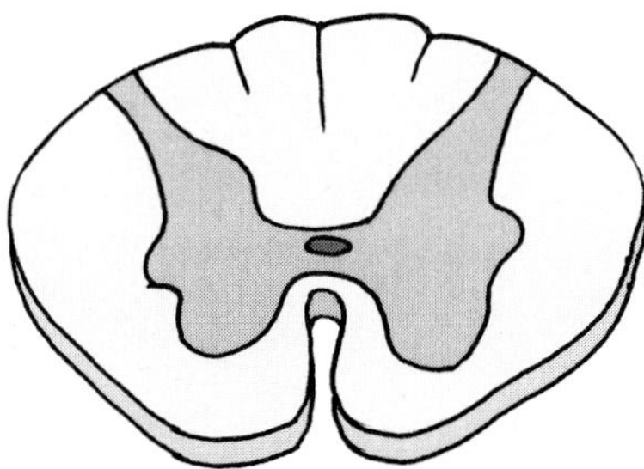

62.8. Check the following features that are characteristic of the C7 cord segment: large efferent and afferent white matter tracts ______; large anterior horns ______; intermediolateral cell column ______.

62.4A. anterior horn; larger; ascend

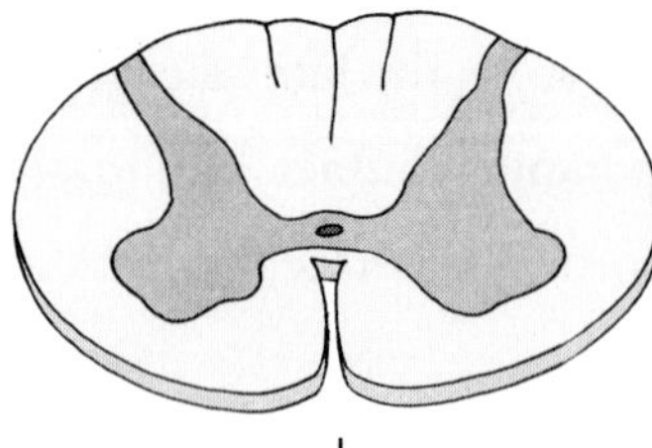

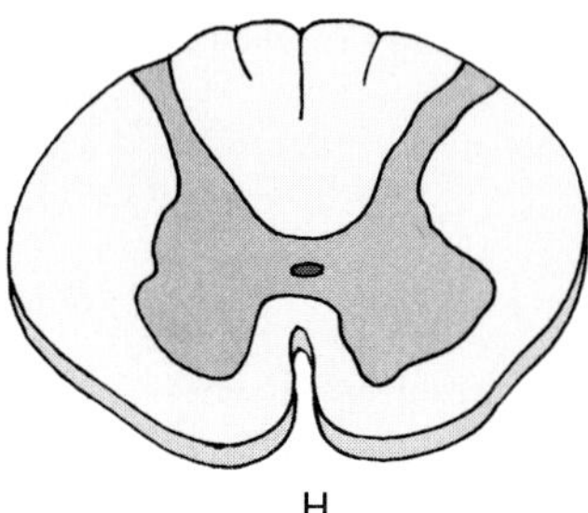

62.5A. cervical; sacral

62.6A. intermediolateral

62.7A. left; thoracic

62.8A. Check the first two; the last blank remains unchecked

62.9. The cauda equina consists of nerve roots from the lumbar and sacral regions of the cord; these names may be joined and the roots collectively called the l______os______l nerve roots.

62.10. Of the following transverse sections, label the appropriate one as S3.

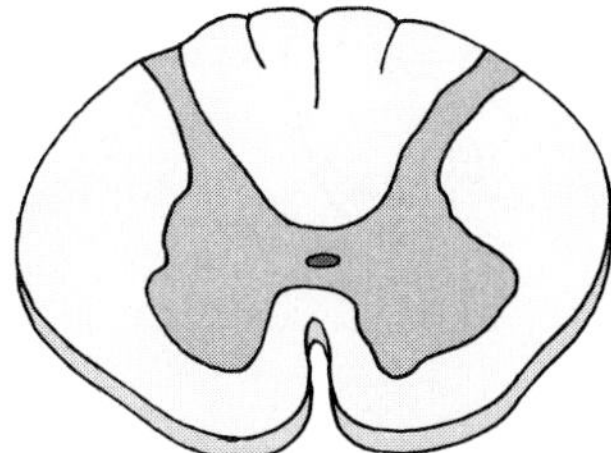
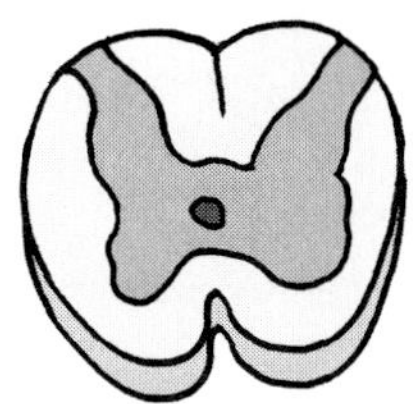
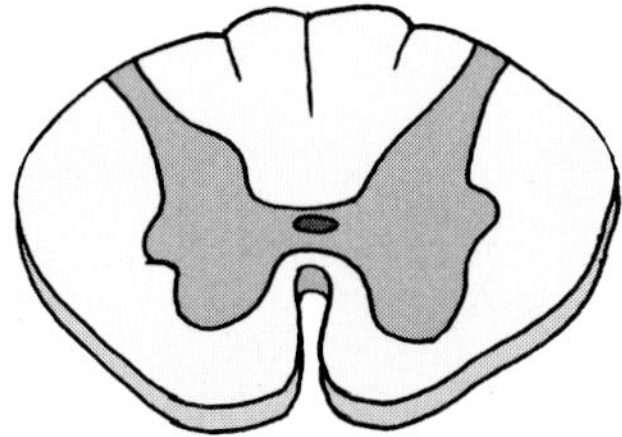

62.11. The lower cervical cord is a flattened oval in transverse section, while sections at still lower levels have a more ____________ shape. The cord segments with the smallest anterior horns are at ____________ levels.

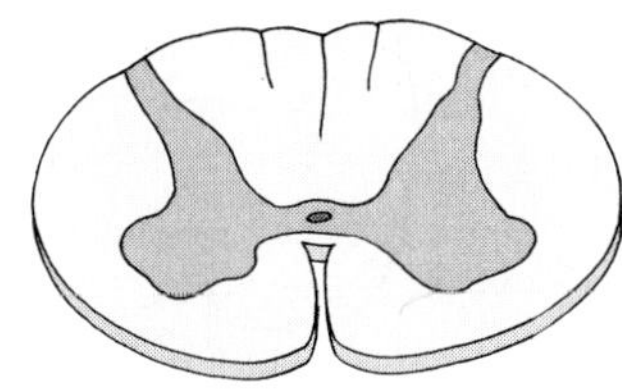
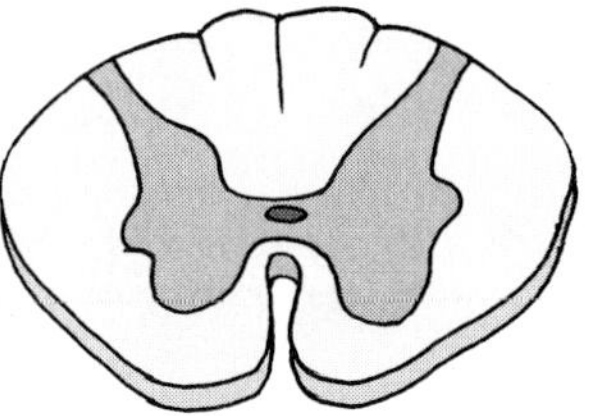
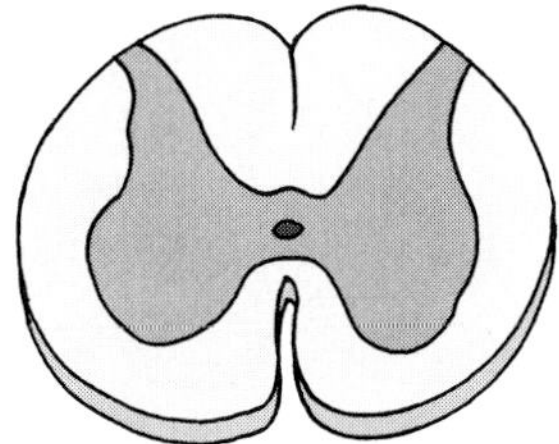
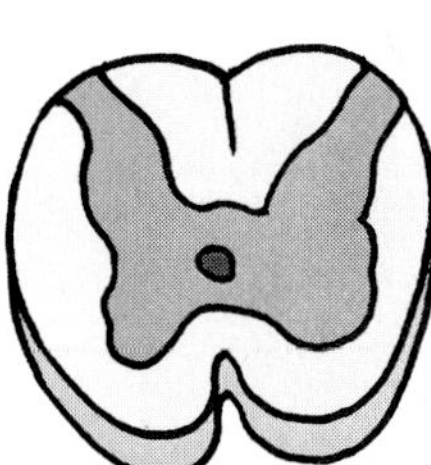

62.12. Label the cervical (C) and thoracic (T) cord sections.

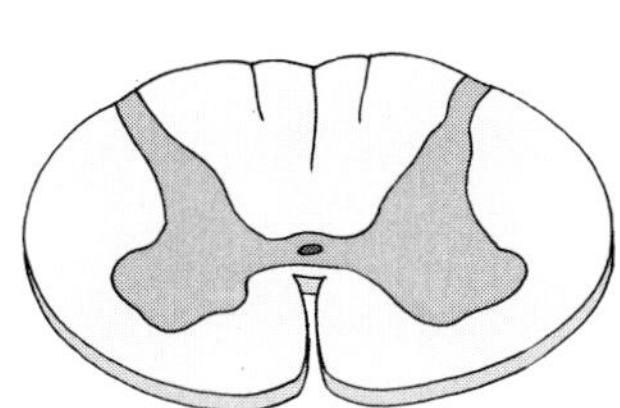
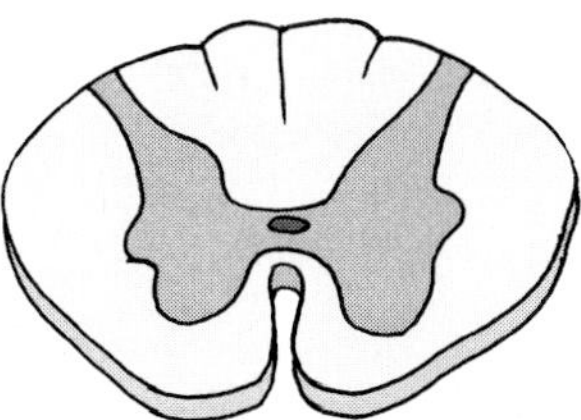
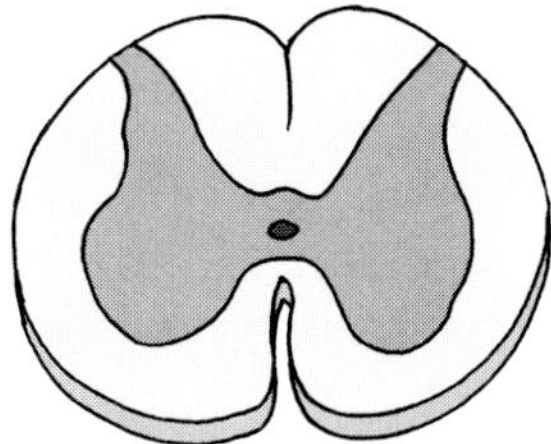
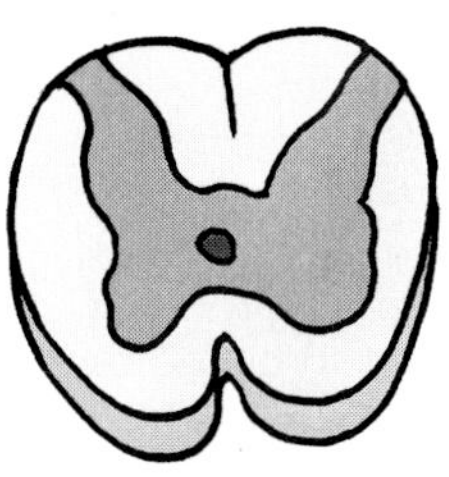

62.9A. lumbosacral

62.10A.

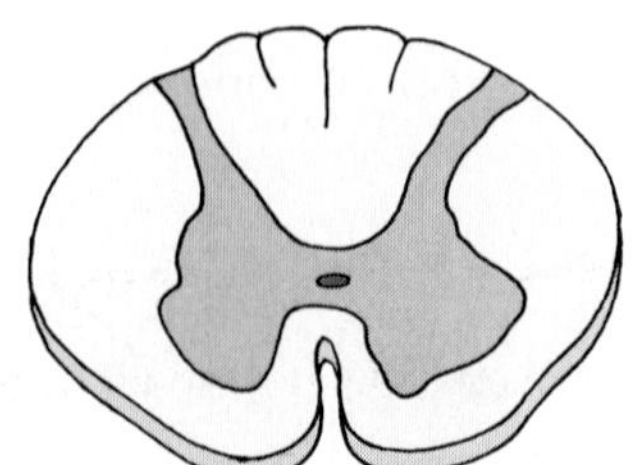

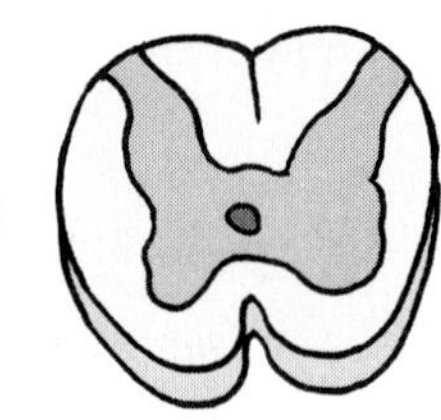

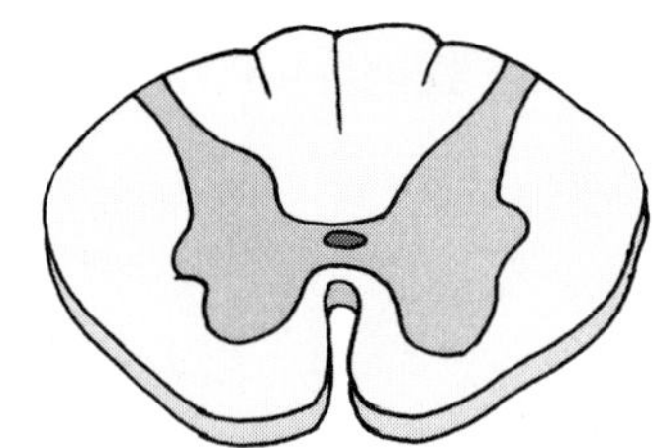

62.11A. circular; thoracic

62.12A.

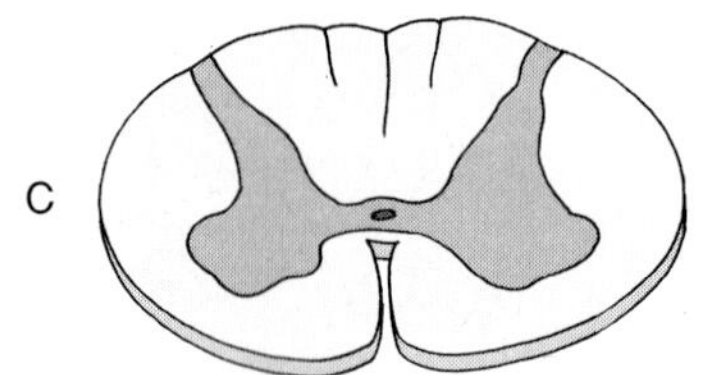

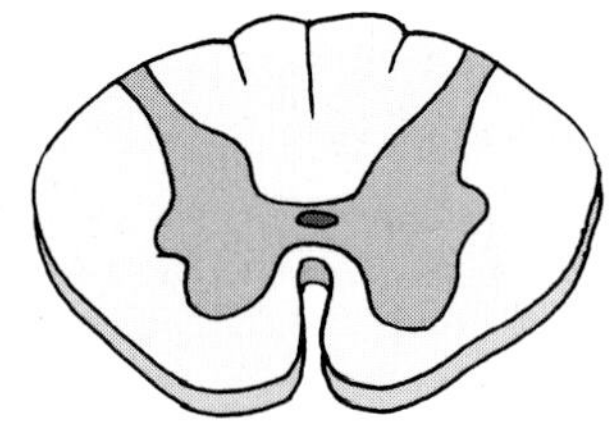

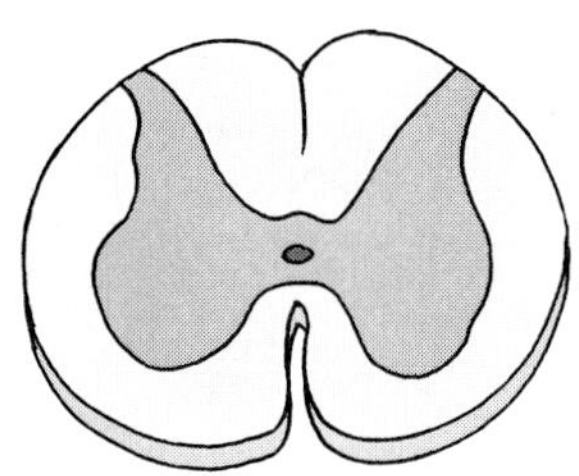

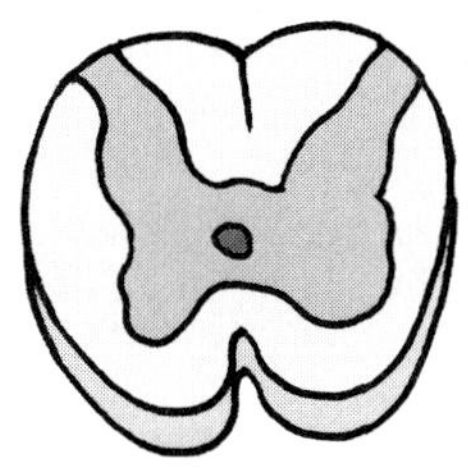

62.13. Comparing cervical and lumbar cord levels, there are fewer corticospinal fibers in the ______ matter at __________ levels; there are fewer kinesthetic, touch, and pressure fibers in the ______ matter of the __________ levels; both levels of the cord have many cells in the ______ matter of the anterior horns; and there is a smaller amount of white matter relative to gray matter at the __________ levels.

Cervical

Lumbar

62.14. Check the features found in the lumbar but not cervical segments:

a. intermediolateral cell column

b. long slender posterior horns

c. small amount of white matter relative to gray matter

d. fasciculus cuneatus

62.15. Label each of the following sections as cervical (C), thoracic (T), lumbar (L), or sacral (S).

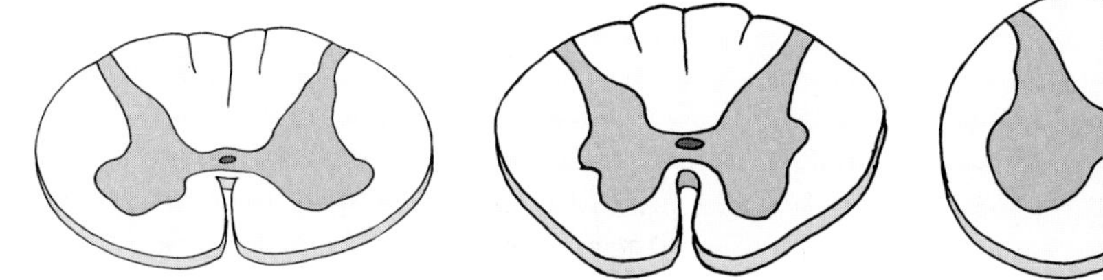

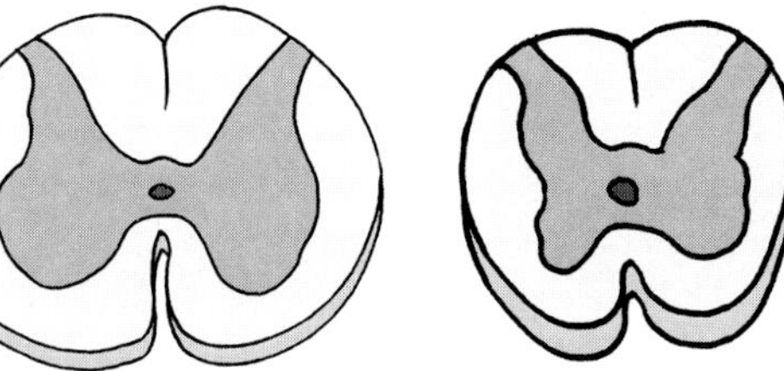

62.16. Name the two cord regions that contain the fewest final common path neurons in the anterior horns: __________ and __________

62.13A. white; lumbar; white; lumbar; gray; lumbar

62.14A.

a. intermediolateral cell column✓

b. long slender posterior horns

c. small amount of white matter relative to gray matter✓

d. fasciculus cuneatus

62.15A.

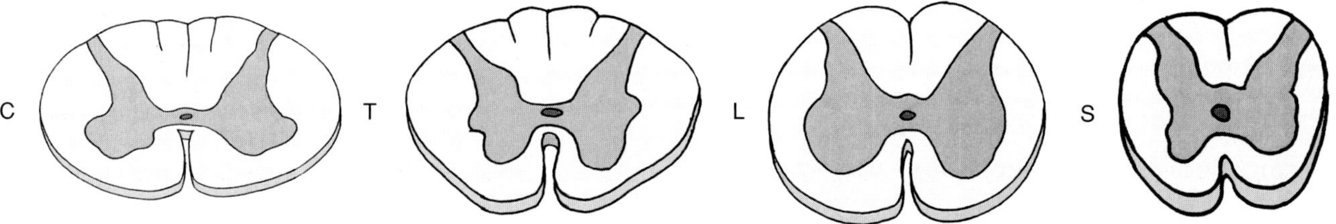

62.16A. thoracic; sacral

62.17. At all cord levels, the white matter immediately adjacent to the gray matter (crosshatched in the image) is called the fasciculus ____________.

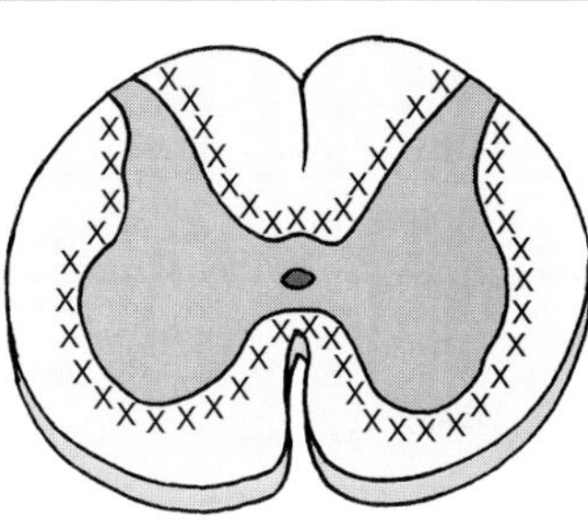

62.18. Proprius means proper to or belonging to. Fibers of the fasciculus proprius arise and terminate within the cord. Proprius fibers are found completely ____________ the spinal cord.

62.19. Short ascending and short descending tracts are found at all levels of the cord, immediately surrounding the gray matter, in the ____________________ ____________. These myelinated axons conducting impulses between nearby cord segments belong not to primary motor or sensory neurons but to ______nuncial neurons.

62.20. The encircled motor tracts are the ____________ ____________________ and the ____________ ____________________ tracts. The size of the encircled tracts ______creases as we pass down the cord. The tract not represented at the lower thoracic and lumbar levels is the ____________ corticospinal tract.

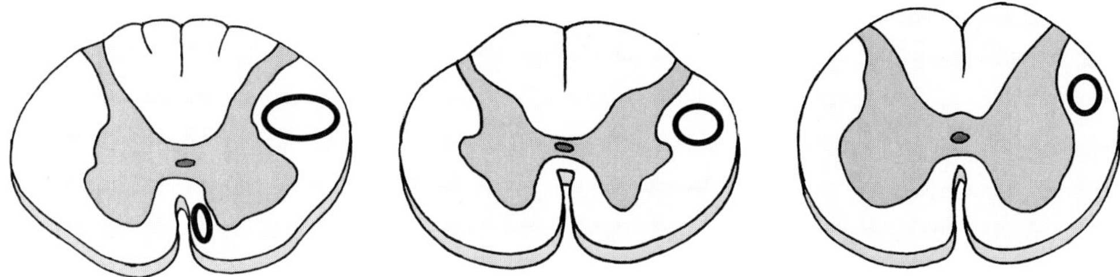

62.21. The anterior corticospinal tract usually ends in the upper thoracic cord. Encircle the lateral and anterior corticospinal tracts, where appropriate, on the right side of the diagram at each cord level.

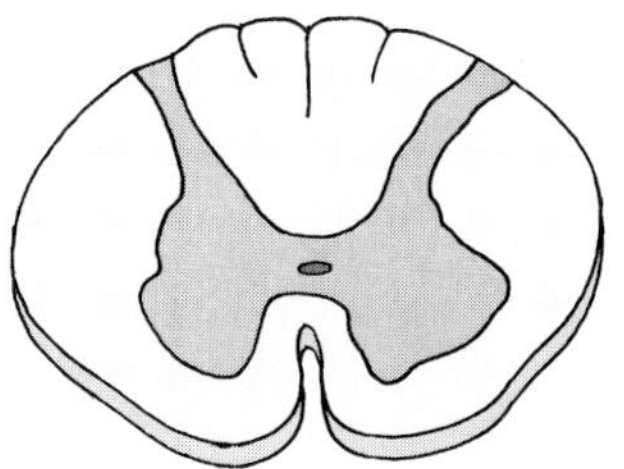
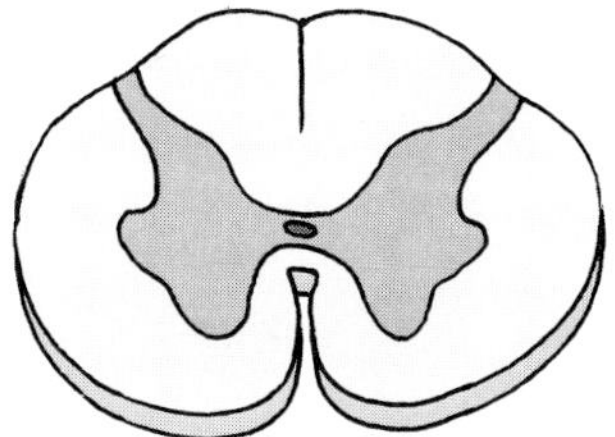
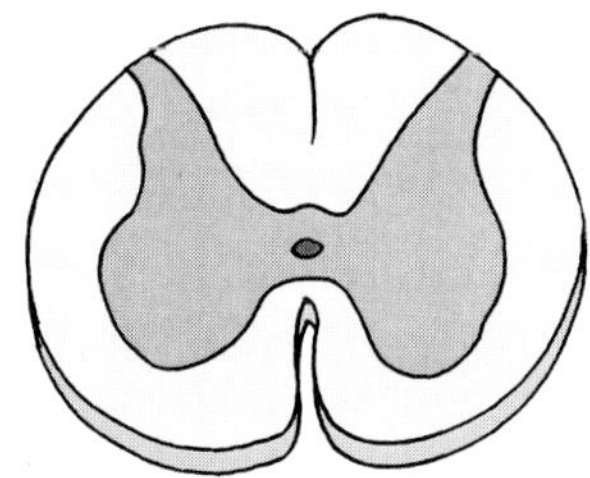

62.17A. proprius

62.18A. within

62.19A. fasciculus proprius; internuncial

62.20A. lateral corticospinal; anterior corticospinal; decreases; anterior

62.21A.

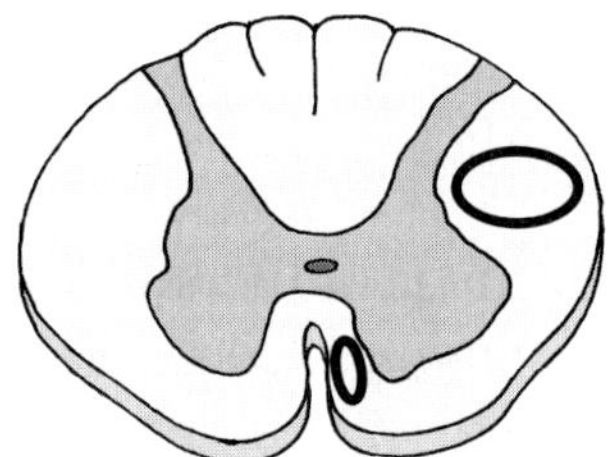
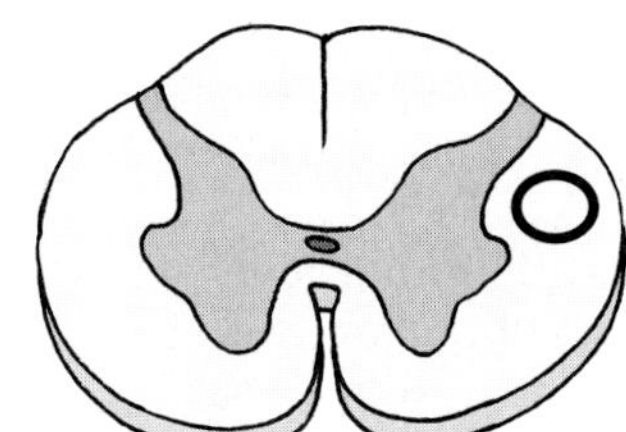
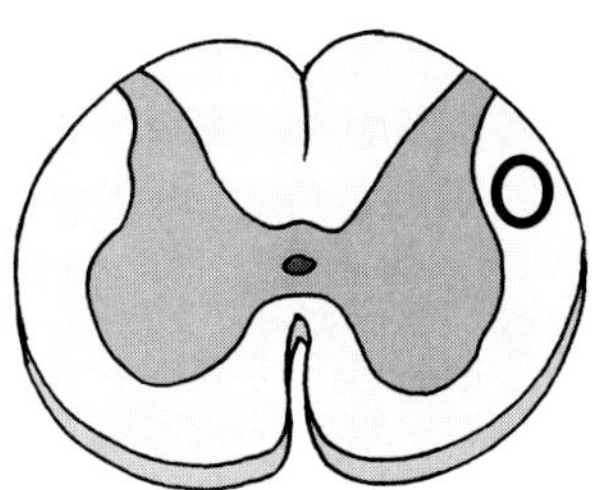

62.22. The white matter that separates the lateral corticospinal tract from the spinal gray matter is the f____________ ____________. The fasciculus gracilis and fasciculus cuneatus occupy the ____________ columns of white matter. The more medial at all levels of the cord is the fasciculus ____________. The fasciculus ____________ is nonexistent at the lower level cord.

62.23. The encircled tract is the fasciculus ____________. Within the encircled tract in the section at C4, write the part of the body represented.

62.24. The encircled tract is the fasciculus ____________. Of the three cord levels illustrated, this tract is not represented at the ____________ level. At progressively higher levels, this tract becomes progressively _______er. The right hand picture illustrates a section at a high level of the ____________ spinal cord. The encircled tract is separated from the posterior horn by a narrow zone of ______ matter, the ________________ ____________.

62.25. Circle and label the following on the right side of the appropriate sections: fasciculus gracilis, fasciculus cuneatus, anterior corticospinal tract, lateral corticospinal tract, and central canal.

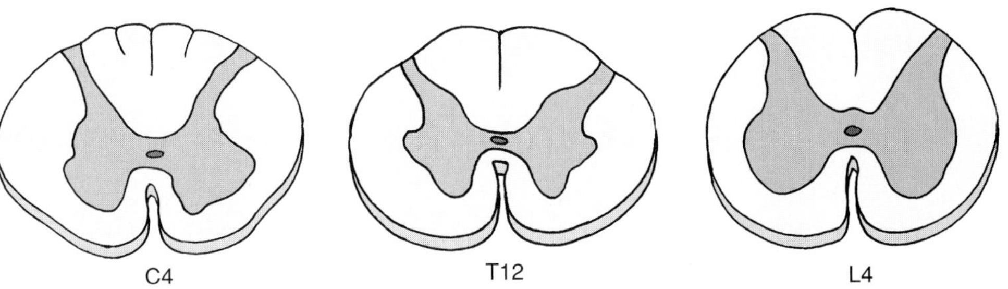

62.22A. fasciculus proprius; posterior (or dorsal); gracilis; cuneatus

62.23A. gracilis

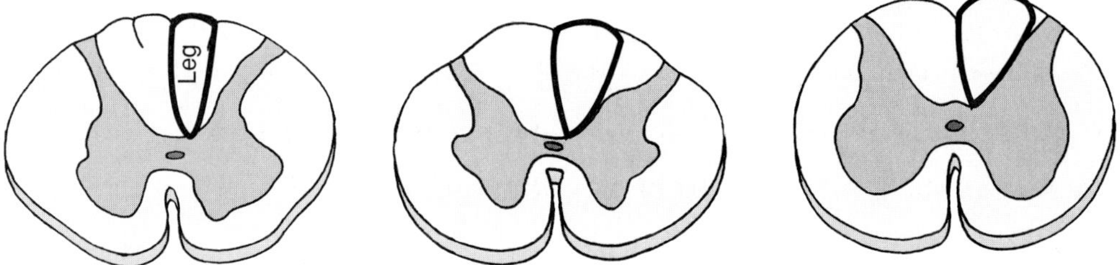

62.24A. cuneatus; lumbar; larger; cervical; white; fasciculus proprius

62.25A.

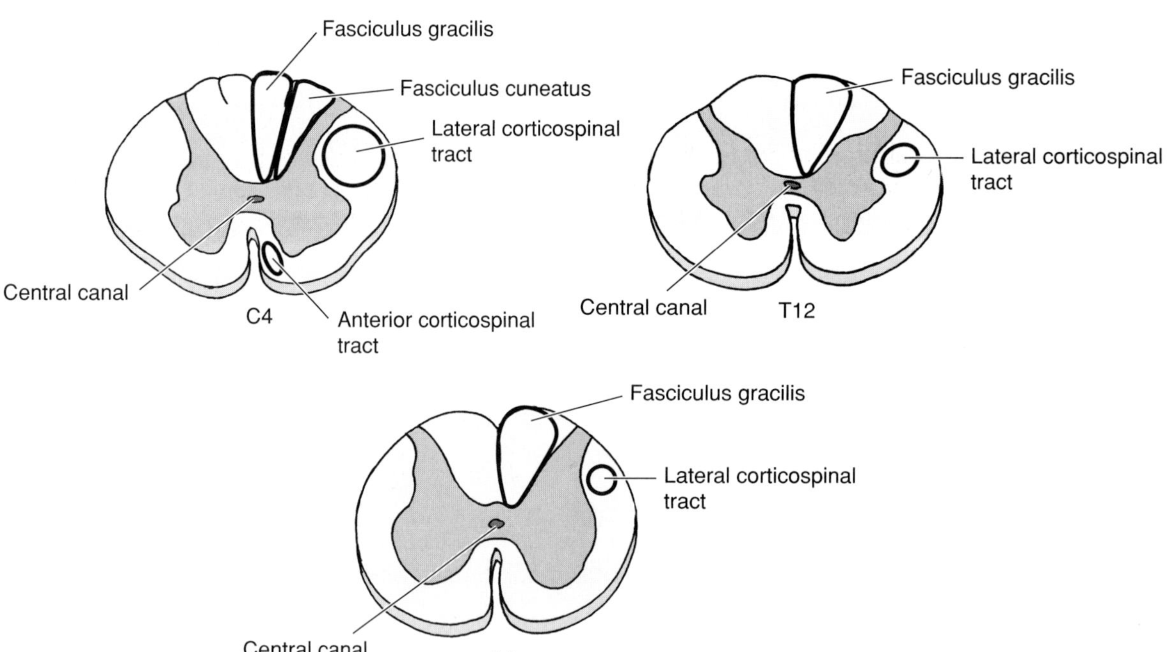

63 White and Gray Matter of the Spinal Cord and Location of Corticospinal Tracts

63.1. The outer substance of the spinal cord consists predominantly of myelinated nerve fibers. The "H"-shaped central area on the image is the ______ matter of the cord.

63.2. The outermost part of the cerebral cortex is ______ matter; the outer part of the spinal cord is ______ matter. In the center of the gray matter of the spinal cord is a tiny ____________ ______.

Central canal

63.3. The gray matter on each side of the spinal cord is roughly divisible into an anterior gray column, an intermediolateral ______ ____________, and an elongated ____________ ______ column. Label the three gray columns on the image.

63.4. White matter is divisible into three zones called funiculi. On the right side of the picture, label the posterior, lateral, and anterior funiculi of white matter as "P", "L," and "A," respectively.

63.5. Motor neurons form a massive column running the length of the spinal cord on each side. A cross section of this column is referred to as the ______ior ______.

63.6. The anterior gray column is more commonly called the anterior horn, and the posterior gray column is called the ____________ h______. Place an "A" on each of the two anterior horns on the diagram.

63.7. The fibers of the pyramidal tract pass from the medulla directly into the ____________ level of the spinal cord.

63.1A. gray

63.2A. gray; white; central canal

63.3A. gray column; posterior gray

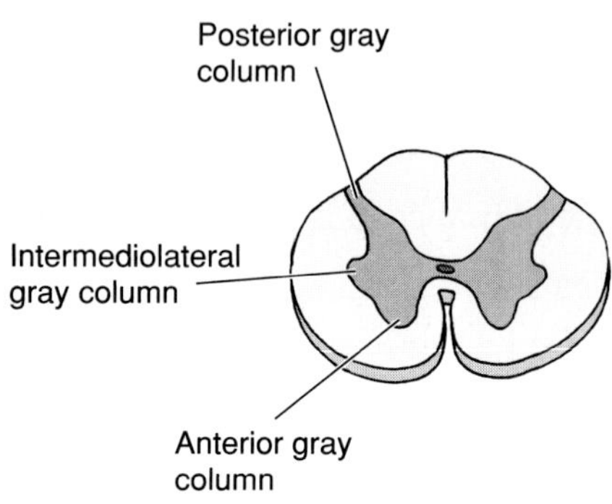

63.4A.

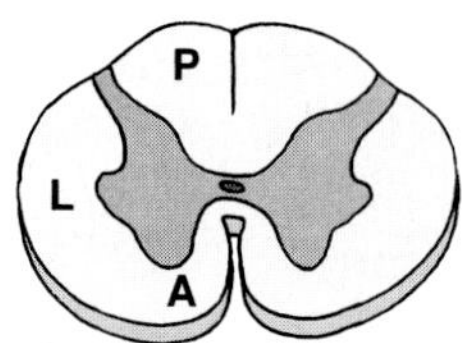

63.5A. anterior; horn

63.6A. posterior horn

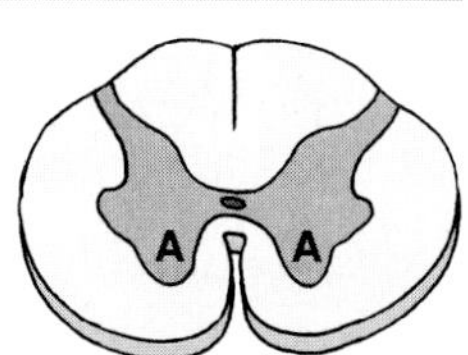

63.7A. cervical

63.8. As the decussating fibers of the pyramidal tract pass from the medulla to the cervical spinal cord, they change from an ____________ position to a posterior and ____________ position on the ________________ side. In the cord, the fibers that have not decussated maintain their ______ior position.

63.9. The lateral corticospinal tract occupies a position in the ______ matter lateral and ____________ to the anterior horn. The anterior corticospinal tract lies medial to the ____________ horn.

63.10. Label the two circled tracts. Place an "X" inside the one whose cell bodies of origin lie on the same side.

63.11. Draw circles on the section to represent the lateral and anterior corticospinal tracts whose fibers originate in the right cerebral hemisphere.

R L

63.12. Most fibers of the anterior corticospinal tract do cross the midline before terminating. They obey the rule that the motor centers of one cerebral hemisphere influence movement of limbs on the ________________ side of the body.

63.13. Bundles of fibers crossing the midline are called commissures. Fibers of the anterior corticospinal tract are thought to cross the midline in the anterior ________________ of the spinal cord and synapse in the ____________ horn on the ________________ side.

63.14. One of the most reliable rules in clinical neurology is that lesions of the corticospinal system above the level of the ________________ of the pyramids affect limbs on the ________________ side.

63.15. Many cell bodies of axons in the right lateral corticospinal tract are in the ________________ gyrus of the ________________ side.

63.8A. anterior; lateral; contralateral; anterior

63.9A. white; posterior; anterior

63.10A.

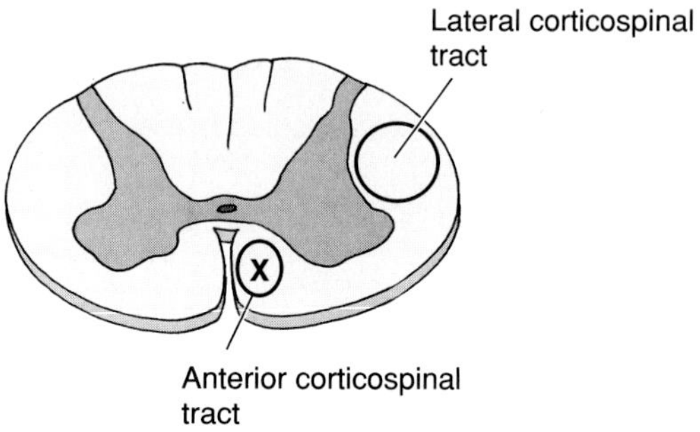

63.11A.

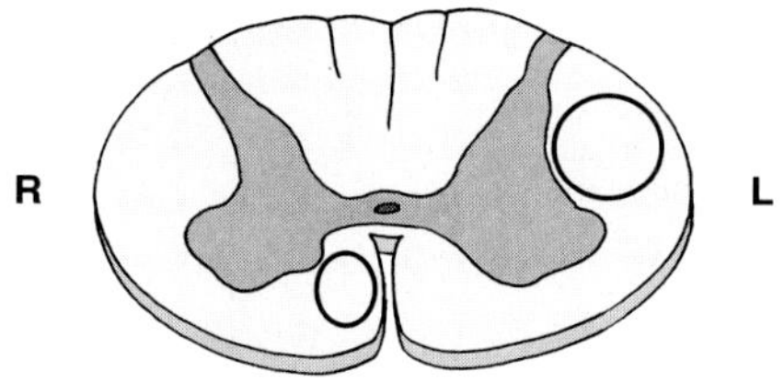

63.12A. contralateral

63.13A. commissure; anterior; contralateral

63.14A. decussation; contralateral

63.15A. precentral; contralateral

63.16. "X" is in the ___________ corticospinal tract; "Y" is in the ___________ corticospinal tract. Fibers at "X" come from the pyramid on the ___________ side. A lesion at "X" has the same effect on voluntary movement of the limbs as a lesion of the basis pedunculi on the ___________ side. A lesion at "X" influences voluntary movement of the ___________ side of the body.

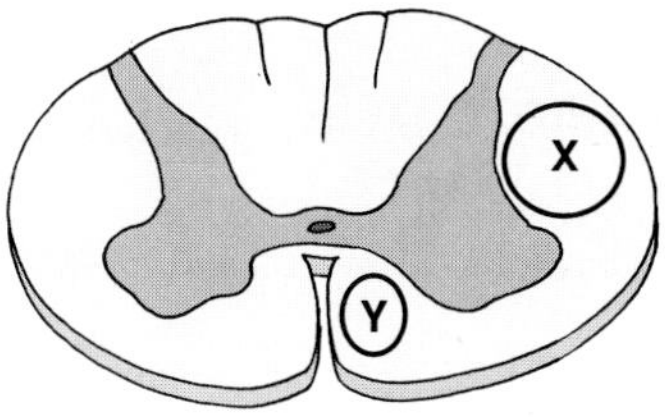

X

Y

63.17. As the diagram indicates, large anterior horn cells send their axons outward in the ___________ root. Encircle the anterior horn cells in the diagram and label the anterior root.

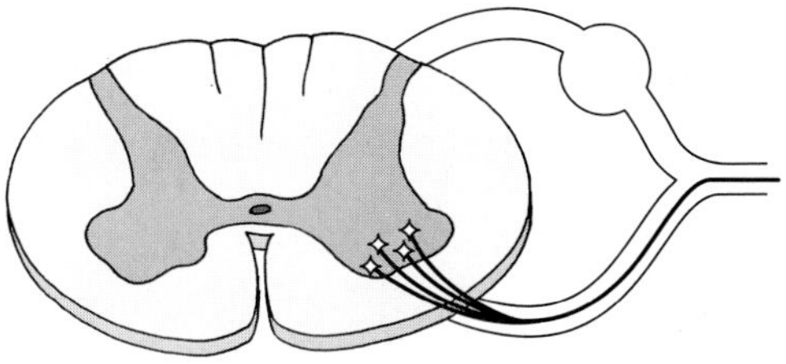

63.18. To effect voluntary movement of an arm, impulses must eventually reach a lower motoneuron. On the left side of the picture, draw a small circle to indicate one such cell body in its proper location. Place an "X" on the lateral corticospinal tract on the side that influences that cell body and a "Y" on the anterior corticospinal tract that influences that cell body.

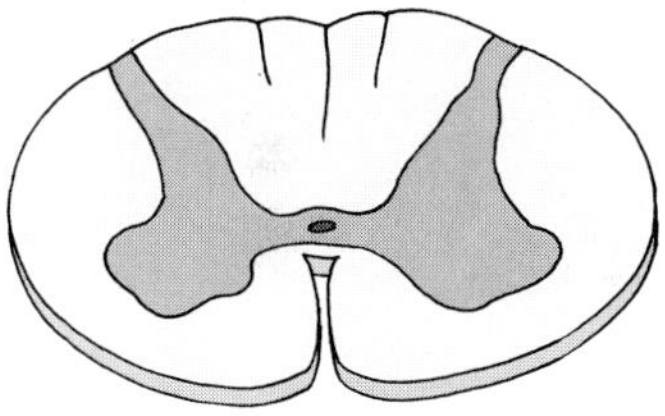

63.19. The arrows indicate the direction of impulse conduction. Place "X"s along the lower motoneuron's course that leads out to the muscles.

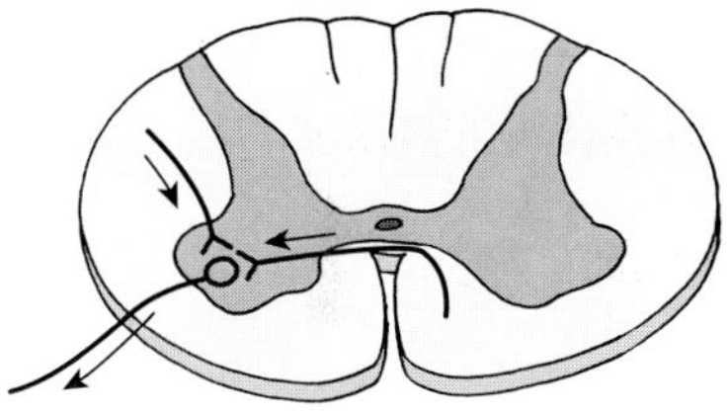

63.20. As the lateral corticospinal tract passes down the spinal cord, fibers leave it and enter the ______ matter. During its passage down the cord, the tract ___________ in size.

63.21. The lateral corticospinal tract is largest in the ___________ segments of the spinal cord. Use the size of the lateral corticospinal tract as a criterion and label the sections as cervical (C) or lumbar (L).

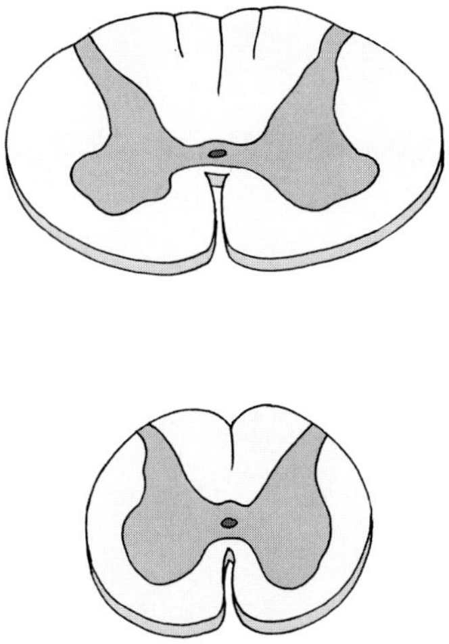

63.16A. lateral; anterior; contralateral; contralateral; ipsilateral

63.17A. anterior

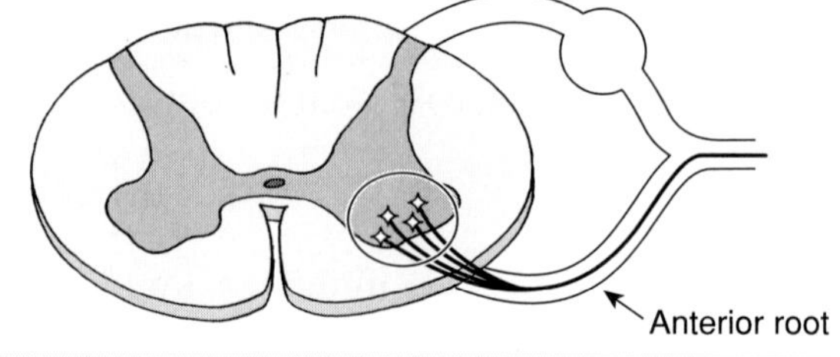

63.18A.

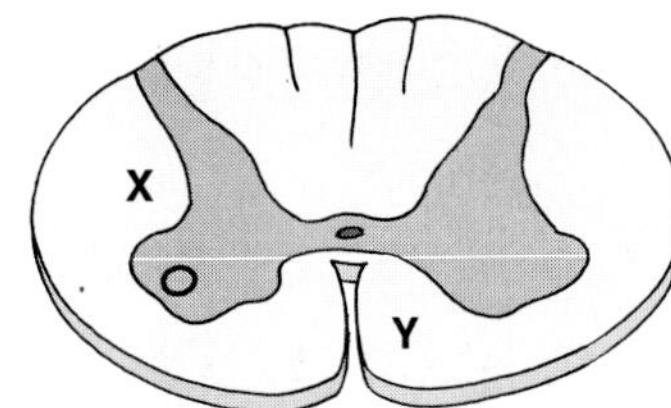

63.19A.

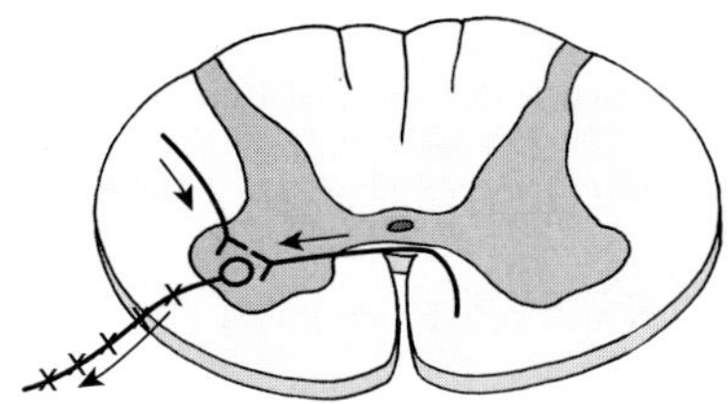

63.20A. gray; decreases

63.21A. cervical

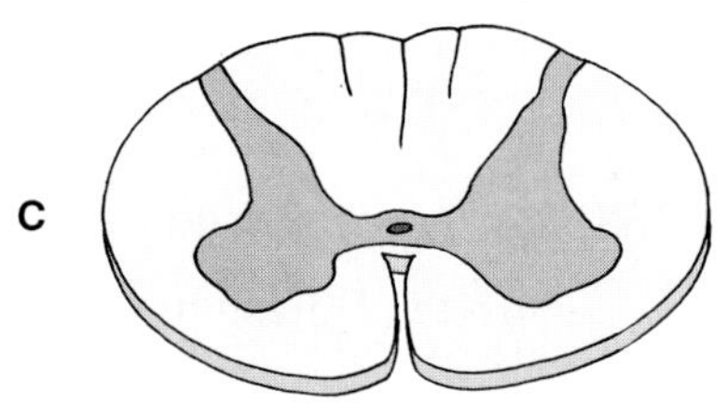

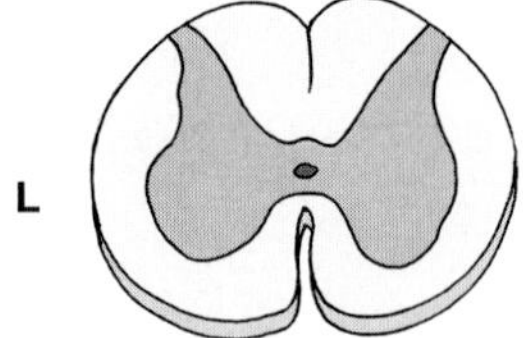

63.22. Muscles of the extremities are innervated mainly by neurons in the __________ and __________ segments of the cord.

63.23. The more muscles supplied, the __________ in size is the anterior horn. Label the thoracic cord segment.

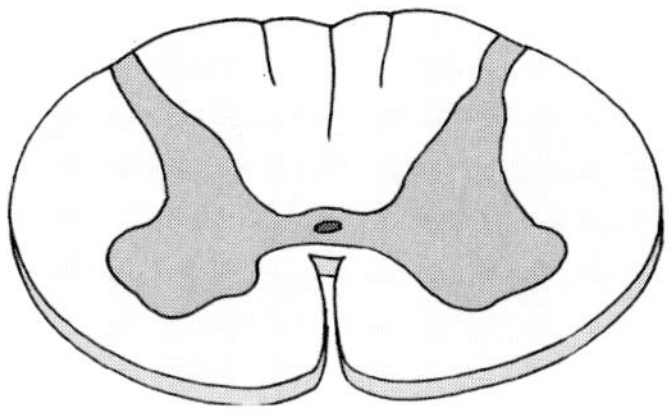

63.24. This section is recognizable as lumbar and not thoracic because the anterior horn has a __________ size.

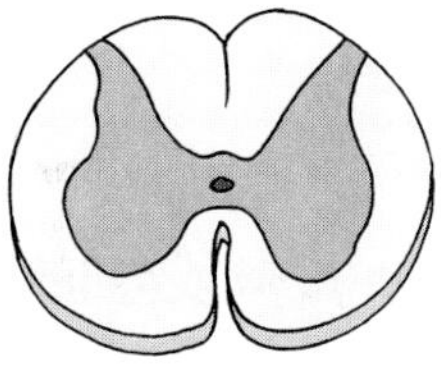

63.25. At the level of this section, the anterior column of cell bodies is __________ in size.

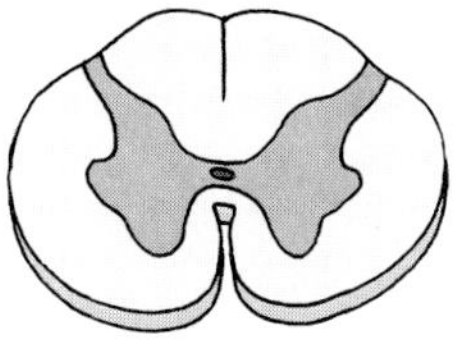

63.26. Label each section as "T" for thoracic or "L" for lumbar.

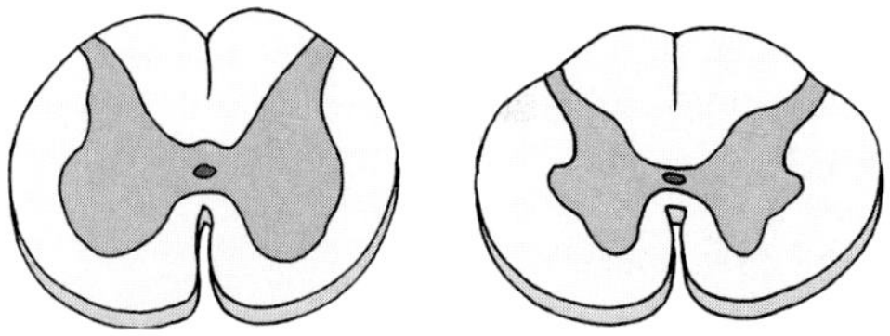

63.27. Number these transverse sections as 1, 2, and 3, with 1 closest to the medulla and 3 closest to the cauda equina.

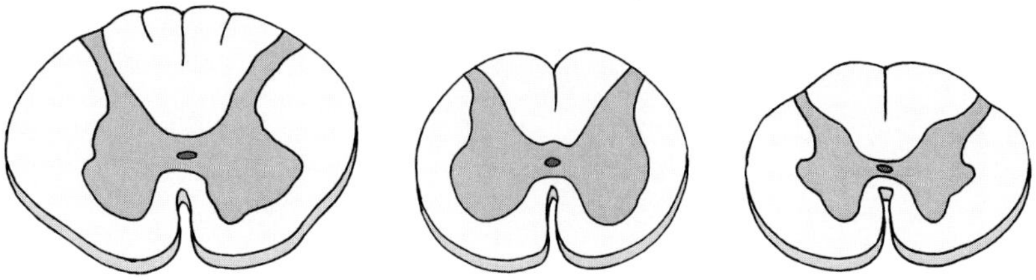

63.22A. cervical; lumbar

63.23A. larger

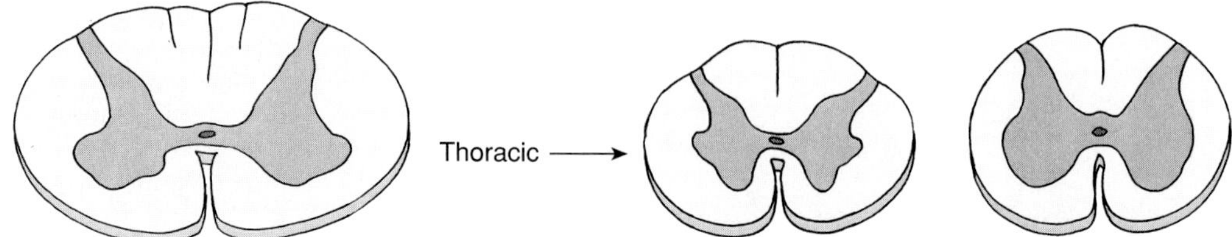

63.24A. larger

63.25A. smaller

63.26A.

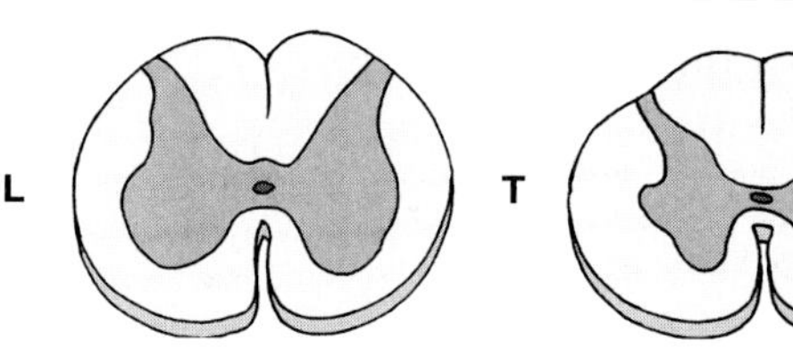

63.27A.

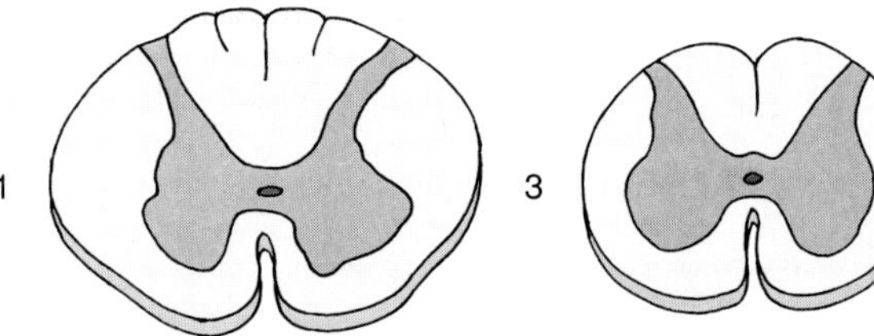

63.28. Within the anterior horn, peripheral muscle territories are represented somatotopically. The most distal parts of the body are represented most ____________ly in position.

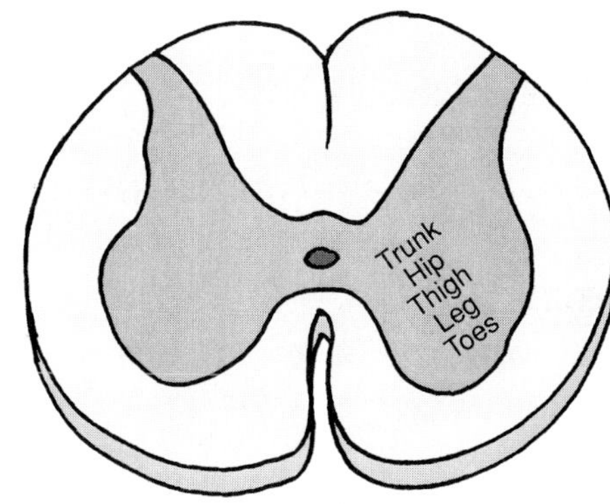

63.29. On the anterior horn, label the neurons that innervate the thigh with a 1, those that innervate the toes with a 2, and those that innervate the trunk with a 3.

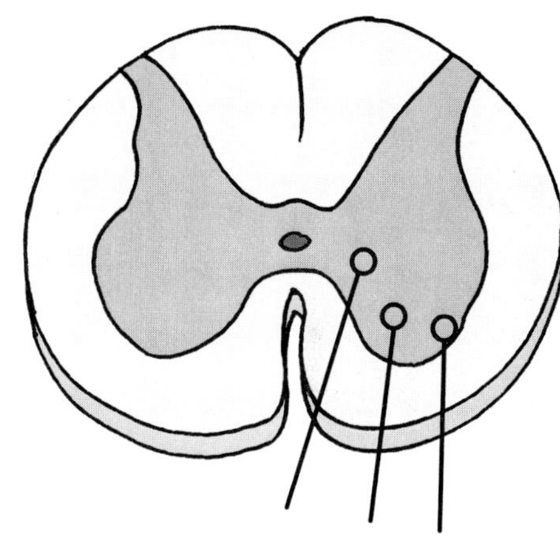

63.30. Neurons innervating flexor muscles lie ______ to neurons innervating ____________ muscles.

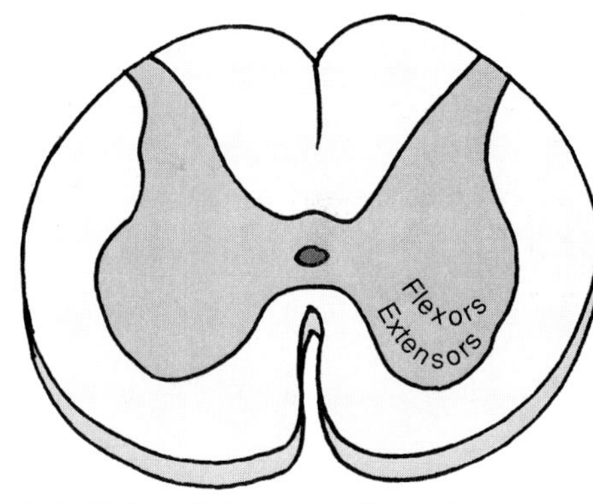

63.31. The adjective polio refers to gray matter. Myelin means spinal cord. The ending –itis means "inflammation of." Anterior poliomyelitis is a disease featuring ________________ of the ______ matter of the ____________ ______.

63.32. The upper limb is innervated by neurons in the ____________ segments of the cord. On the diagram, mark with "X"s a few affected cell bodies of motor neurons in a patient with anterior poliomyelitis and paralysis of the finger muscles.

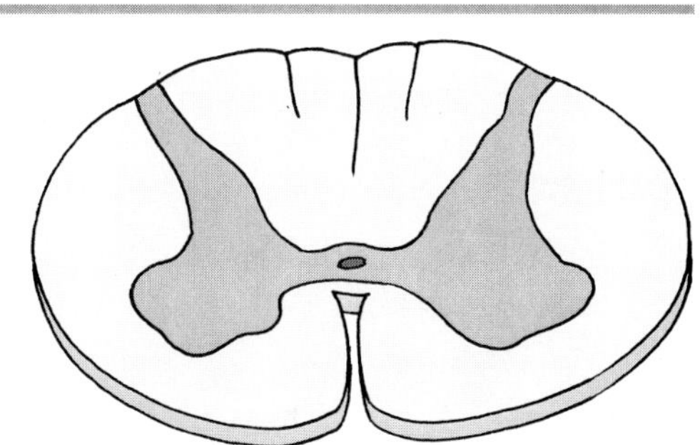

63.28A. laterally

63.29A.

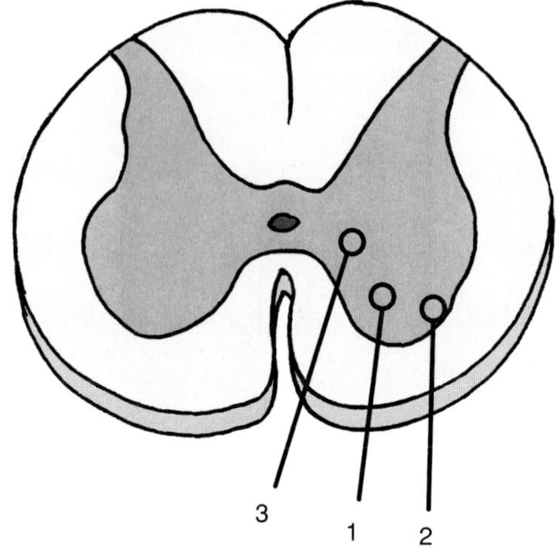

63.30A. deep; extensor

63.31A. inflammation; gray; spinal cord

63.32A. cervical

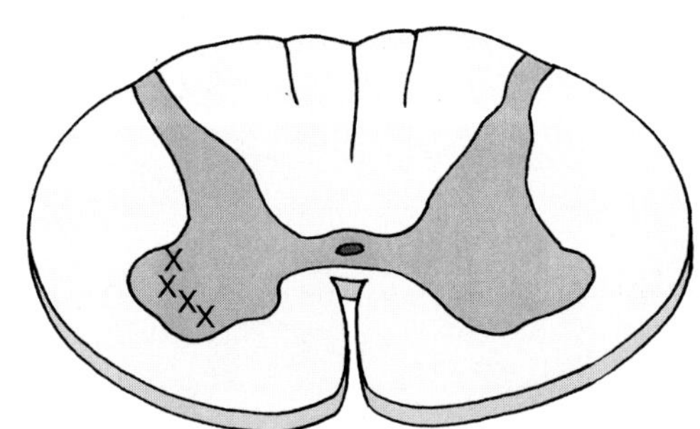

64 The Types of Somesthetic Sensation: Relations Between Peripheral Sensory Pathways and Spinal Cord

64.1. The general senses of the body (soma) are classified as the ______esthetic senses. These senses include touch, pressure, position (joint) sense, temperature senses (hot and ______), and ______.

64.2. The categories of special sensation are: tasting, smelling, hearing, and __________. The categories of general body sensation (the ______________ senses) are: ______, __________, position (joint) sense, temperature senses (______ and ______), and pain.

64.3. If an arm is lightly stroked with a wisp of cotton, the subject reports sensations that we classify as ______. If the flat surface of a ruler is applied gently but firmly to the skin, the subject reports a sense of ______. Recognition of position or movement of a body part involves participation of receptors located in the j______s.

64.4. Three terms meaning the same thing are position sense, kinesthetic sense, and j______ sense. We sense movement of the forearm relative to the upper arm when receptors in the ______ joint are stimulated. "Kinesthetic sense" means "sense of movement." It may seem paradoxical that position sense and ______esthetic sense should be synonymous. Actually, recognition of movement is recognition of a temporal sequence of changing __________s.

64.5. Information about the somesthetic senses arises mainly in encapsulated nerve endings of the skin and __________.

64.6. Touch, pressure, and kinesthetic senses are classified together as one somesthetic group because impulses for these senses are transmitted along similar pathways. The other somesthetic senses—the two ______________ senses and ______—are classed as a different group because a __________ pathway is used for them.

64.7. Another group of impulses, transmitted along a third pathway, arises in sensory receptors of skeletal muscles and tendons. These impulses contribute to the regulation of __________ tone.

64.1A. somesthetic; cold; pain

64.2A. seeing; somesthetic; touch; pressure; hot; cold

64.3A. touch; pressure; joints

64.4A. joint; elbow; kinesthetic; positions

64.5A. joints

64.6A. temperature; pain; different (or second, separate, etc.)

64.7A. muscle

64.8. Proprioception encompasses information coming from skeletal muscle, tendons, and joints. The last of these differs from the others in reaching consciousness. Joint sense is best considered to be one of the five ____________ic senses.

64.9. Pain and temperature senses are considered separately from touch, ____________, and joint sense because information about the two groups of senses travels along ____________ anatomical pathways.

64.10. Three groups of afferent pathways are to be considered. In the following list, circle the items closely allied anatomically and functionally to touch; cross out the item that does not ordinarily enter consciousness.

Touch	Pain
Muscle and tendon, afferents	Pressure
Kinesthetic sense	Temperature senses

64.11. The cell bodies of almost all primary sensory (afferent) neurons lie in the spinal ____________, ______side the CNS.

64.12. The cell bodies of ____________ ____________ ____________, which lie in the spinal ganglia, receive their blood primarily from radicular arteries.

64.13. Label the arteries indicated.

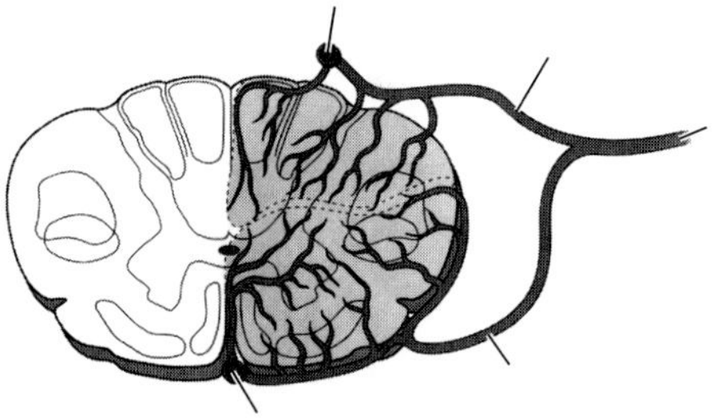

64.14. The primary sensory (afferent) neuron sends a process along the ____________ root. Shortly after entering the spinal cord, the process bifurcates into two branches, one ______scending and one ______scending, via the dorsolateral fasciculus.

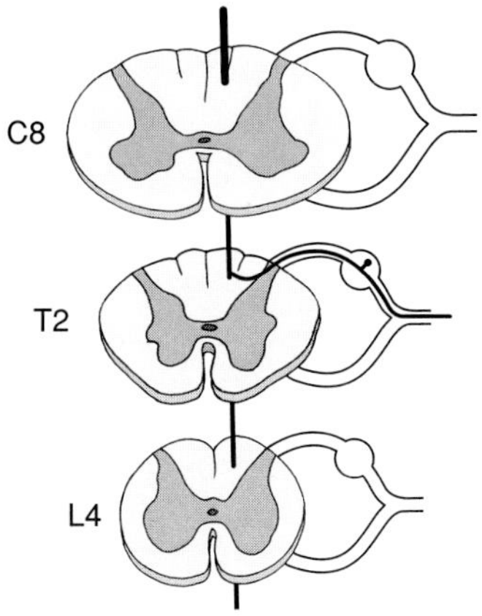

C8

T2

L4

64.8A. somesthetic

64.9A. pressure; separate

64.10A.

Touch
Muscle and tendon afferents
Kinesthetic sense
Pain
Pressure
Temperature senses

64.11A. ganglion; outside

64.12A. primary sensory neurons

64.13A.

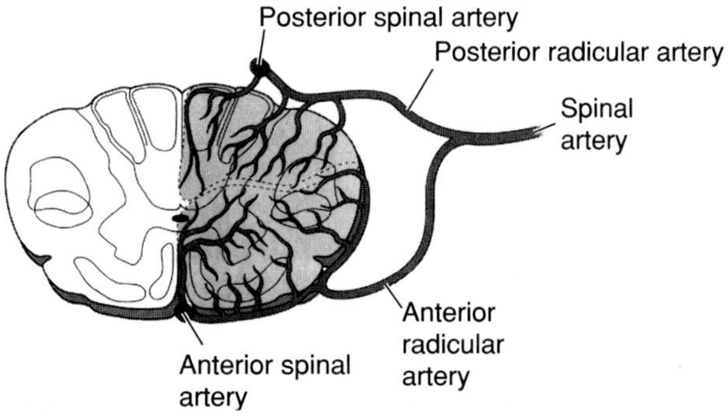

Posterior spinal artery
Posterior radicular artery
Spinal artery
Anterior radicular artery
Anterior spinal artery

64.14A. dorsal; ascending; descending

64.15. The processes of the primary sensory (afferent) neuron may first pass a few spinal cord levels up or down, or they may make synaptic contact with other neurons soon after entering the spinal cord. The sensory (afferent) neuron in the diagram has made synaptic contact with the cell body of a ______ neuron in the gray matter of the ____________ ______ of the spinal cord.

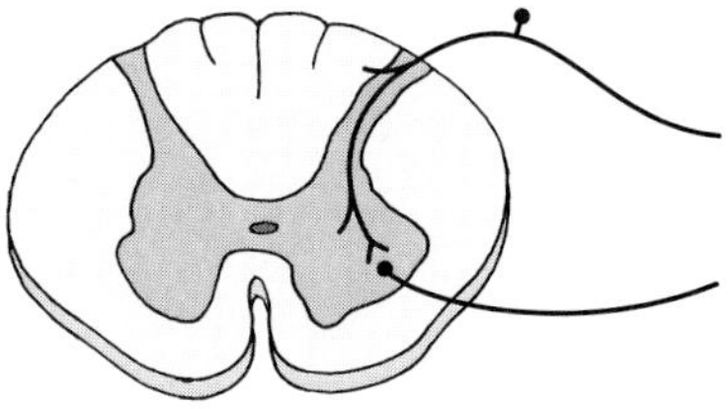

64.16. Within the spinal cord, branches of one primary sensory (afferent) neuron may ascend and/or descend via the ____________________ ____________________ and make synaptic contacts at several levels.

64.17. The sensory (afferent) neuron and neuron "A" form the simplest reflex arc, consisting of only ______ neurons. The reflex arc in the cervical section consists of ______ neurons.

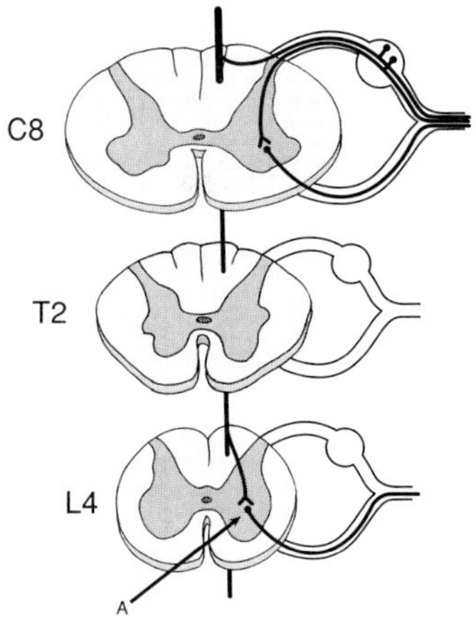

C8

T2

L4

A

64.18. For sensory (afferent) pathways arising in receptors below the neck, the primary sensory cell body lies in a spinal ____________ and transmits impulses from a sense organ into the ____________ nervous system. The ____________ sensory (afferent) neuron participates in local reflex circuits and also may be the first in a chain of ascending neurons. The cell body of the second neuron in the afferent chain lies in the ______ matter of spinal cord or brainstem. The secondary neuron may transmit impulses all the way to the thalamus. A tertiary neuron then transmits from the site of the cell body in the ____________ to the ____________ ____________.

64.19. Somesthetic sensory systems have cell bodies of their primary neurons in ____________ and cell bodies of their tertiary neurons in the ____________. In somesthetic pathways, the minimum number of neurons that can bring information from peripheral sense organs to the cerebral cortex is ______.

64.20. A basic principal is that neurons transmit across synapses in only ______ direction.

64.15A. motor; anterior horn

64.16A. dorsolateral fasciculus

64.17A. 2; 2

64.18A. ganglion; central; primary; gray; thalamus; cerebral cortex (or cerebral hemisphere, postcentral gyrus, parietal lobe, primary sensory cortex)

64.19A. ganglia; thalamus; 3

64.20A. one

64.21. Unlike the diagrams you have been viewing, a given primary neuron in an afferent pathway may make contact with hundreds of ____________ neurons. To further complicate the network, any given secondary neuron may make synaptic contact with many ____________ neurons and also (directly or indirectly) with ______ferent neurons. The response of any given neuron at any given moment results from the net effect of many ex______atory and ____________ory influences.

64.22. Mixed peripheral nerves contain efferent and afferent nerve fibers. When a circumscribed region of the body shows loss of motor function *and* impairment of sensory modalities, the lesion is likely to be in the ____________________ nervous system.

64.23. In the peripheral nervous system, the same fibers carrying information about different sensory modalities lie ____________ to each other. In the central nervous system, as diagrammed, the same fibers may be ____________ from each other.

T2

L4

64.24. The peripheral nerve illustrated contains many fibers that innervate the left foot. A patient was unable to move his left foot or to recognize position or movement, touch, pain, or other sensations in the foot. Movement and sensation in other parts of the body were normal. The site of his disease was probably ______side the CNS.

C8

T2

L4

64.25. All fibers in a given mixed peripheral nerve come from one region of the body. The nerve usually contains many afferent fibers responsive to different types of physical change in the environment. Therefore, a lesion of a peripheral nerve is likely to affect ____________ modalities of sensation, but all from the ______ region of the body.

64.26. Primary sensory neurons send fibers into the ____________ nervous system. The central pathways differ for different modalities. The sensation of pain, for example, might be affected and kinesthetic sense spared in a lesion of the ____________ nervous system; more than one modality is likely to be affected in a lesion of the ____________________ nervous system.

64.21A. secondary; tertiary; efferent; excitatory; inhibitory

64.22A. peripheral

64.23A. adjacent; separate

64.24A. outside

64.25A. several; same

64.26A. central; central; peripheral

65 Location of Sensory Pathways in the White Matter of the Spinal Cord

65.1. Myelinated axons of secondary neurons in sensory systems occupy somewhat different (though often overlapping) territories as they ascend in the _____ matter of the spinal cord.

65.2. Sensory fibers systems are actually less discrete than typical diagrams indicate. The sensory pathways in the white matter are diagrammed on both sides of the picture but are more realistically positioned on the _____ hand side.

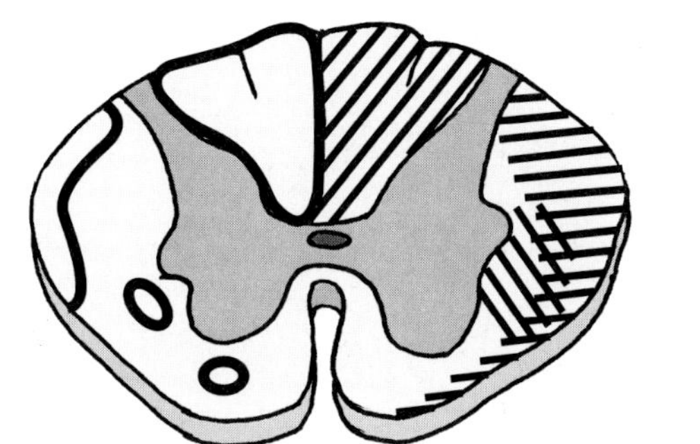

65.3. The central canal occupies a central position in the spinal cord. Structures labeled "anterior" are therefore __________ to the central canal; those labeled "lateral" are __________ to it; etc.

65.4. Among the encircled spinal cord tracts are the right anterior and lateral corticospinal tracts. Indicate them with arrows labeled "A" for anterior and "L" for lateral.

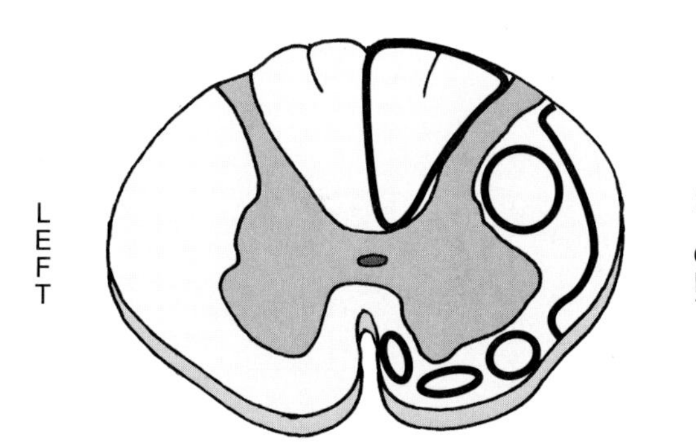

65.5. Label the anterior and lateral spinothalamic tracts on the right side of the picture.

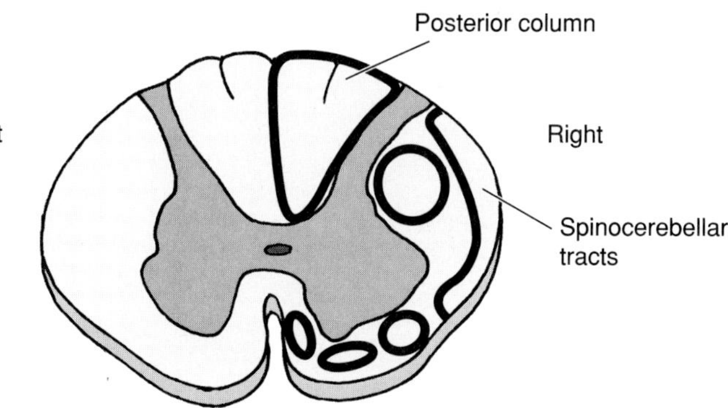

65.1A. white

65.2A. right

65.3A. anterior; lateral

65.4A.

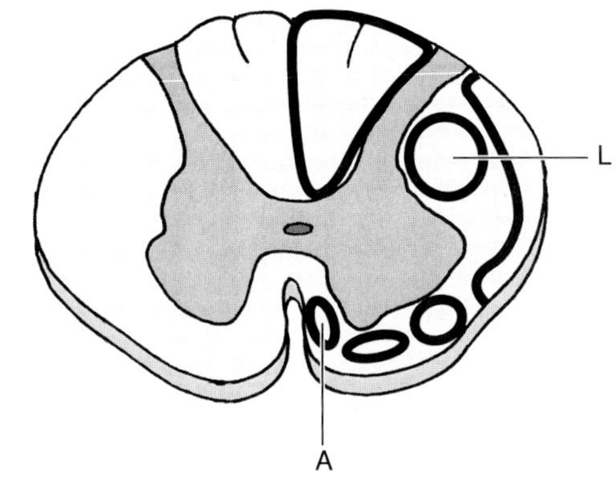

65.5A.

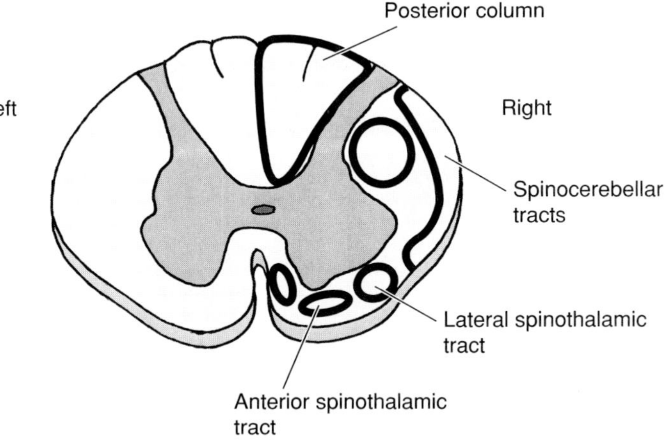

65.6. The lateral and anterior corticospinal tracts are ______fferent with respect to the brain and are named for their origin in the ____________ and their terminus in the ____________ ______. The lateral and anterior spinothalamic tracts are afferent with respect to the brain and take their names from their origin in the ____________ ______ and their terminus in the ____________.

65.7. The white matter on each side of the cord is divisible into posterior, lateral, and anterior funiculi. The anterior funiculus contains the anterior ____________________ and anterior ____________________ tracts; the lateral funiculus contains the lateral corticospinal and lateral spinothalamic tracts as well as the ____________________ tracts; the posterior funiculus contains the ____________ ____________ of white matter.

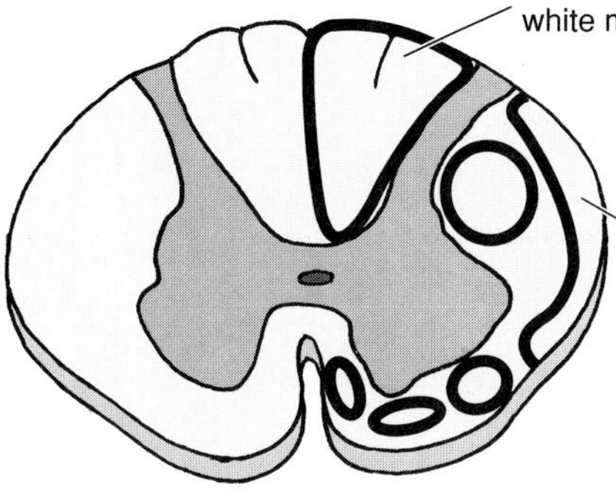

65.8. Blood supply to the posterior funiculi is from branches of the ____________ spinal artery, while blood supply to the lateral and anterior funiculi is from branches of the ____________ spinal artery.

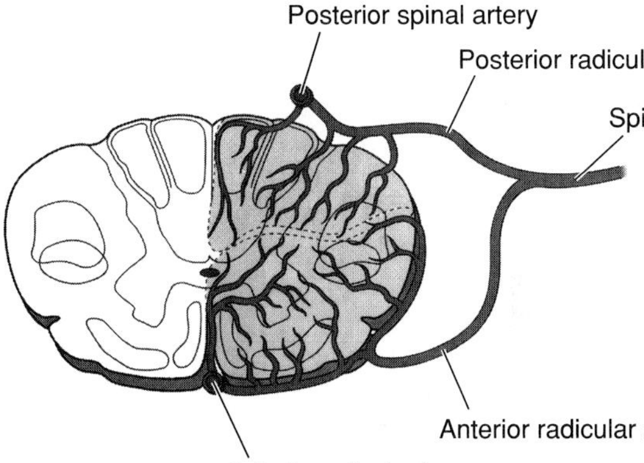

65.9. Blockage of the posterior spinal artery would have the greatest affect on the ____________ ____________.

65.10. Shade the area that receives blood from the anterior spinal artery on the cross section.

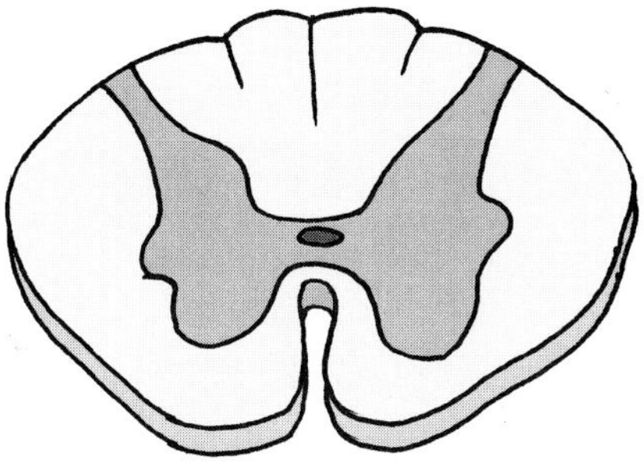

65.6A. efferent; cortex; spinal cord; spinal cord; cortex

65.7A. corticospinal; spinothalamic; spinocerebellar; posterior columns

65.8A. posterior; anterior

65.9A. posterior columns

65.10A.

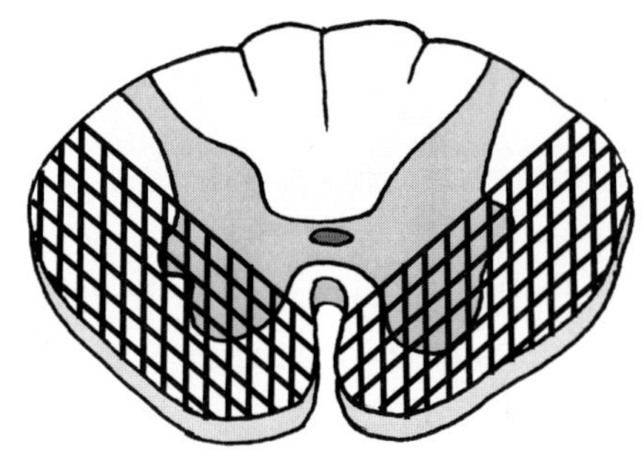

65.11. Circle the name of the tract(s) that would be least affected by blockage of the anterior spinal artery.

Anterior spinothalamic tract

Anterior corticospinal tract

Lateral corticospinal tract

Lateral spinothalamic tract

Posterior column

Spinocerebellar tract

65.12. A lack of pain and temperature information ascending up the spinal cord would most likely result from blockage of the ____________ spinal artery.

65.13. Originating in the spinal cord and terminating in the cerebellum are the ____________ tracts.

65.14. Connect the labels with the appropriate encircled areas.

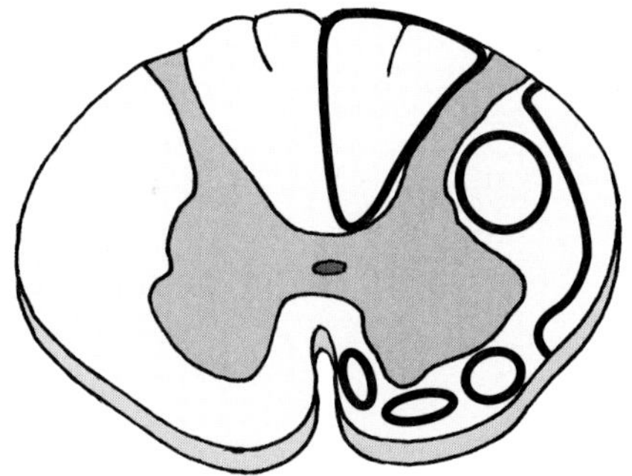

Posterior white column

Lateral corticospinal tract

Spinocerebellar tracts

Lateral spinothalamic tract

Anterior spinothalamic tract

Anterior corticospinal tract

65.15. Four of the areas encircled on the right side consist mainly of sensory fibers. Encircle and label these four areas on the *left* side.

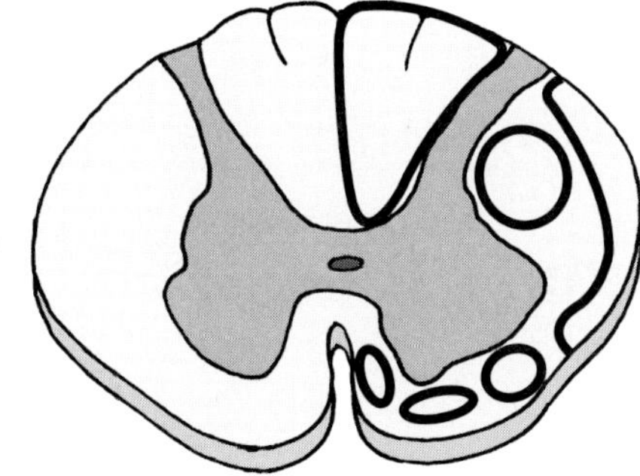

65.11A.

Anterior spinothalamic tract

Anterior corticospinal tract

Lateral corticospinal tract

Lateral spinothalamic tract

Posterior column

Spinocerebellar tract

65.12A. anterior

65.13A. spinocerebellar

65.14A.

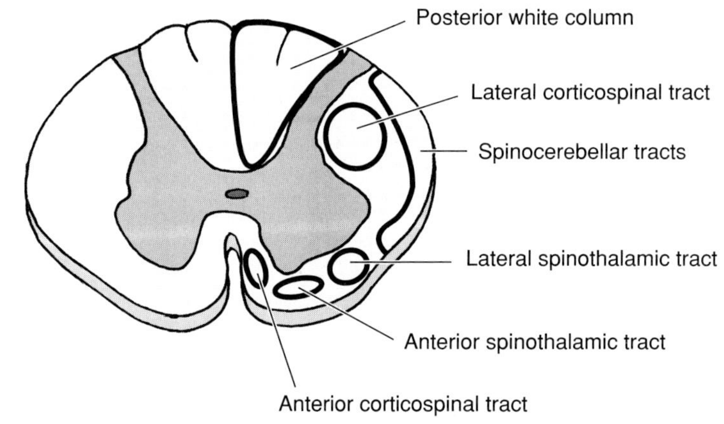

65.15A.

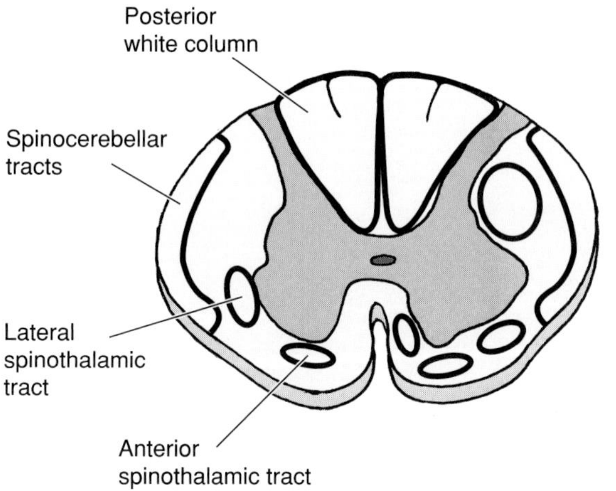

65.16. The posterior column on each side of the cord is divided into two bundles of fibers, or fascicles. The more slender or *gracile* fascicle lies in the more ____________ position.

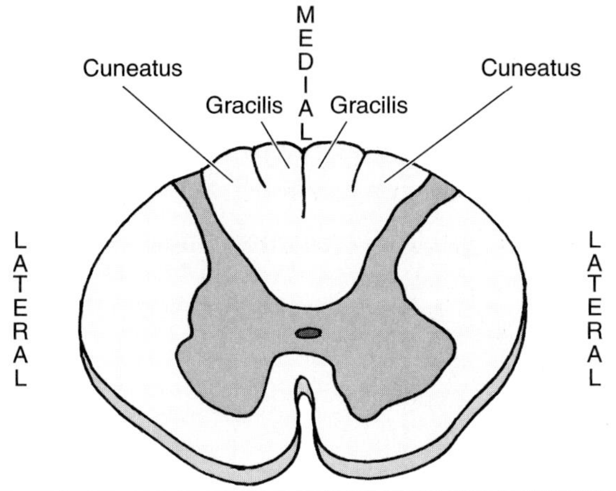

MEDIAL
Cuneatus
Gracilis
Gracilis
Cuneatus
LATERAL
LATERAL

65.17. The slender or *gracile* fascicle receives the formal name, *fasciculus* ____________is. Indicate it on the figure with arrows on *both* sides. The more lateral bundle of fibers in the posterior white column has a "cuneate" or wedge shape and is formally called the ____________________ ____________.

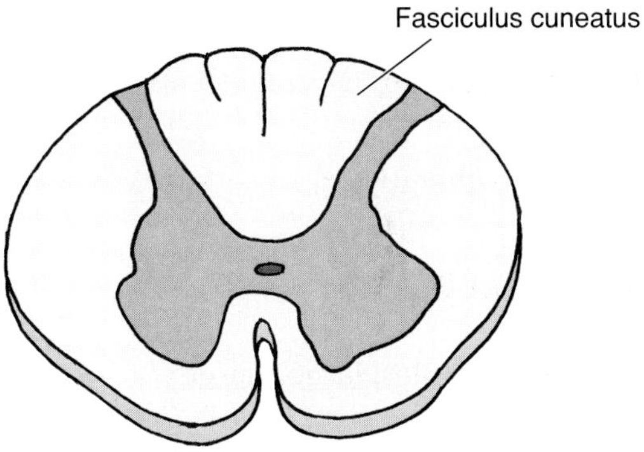

Fasciculus cuneatus

65.18. The fasciculus ____________ is shaded on the diagram.

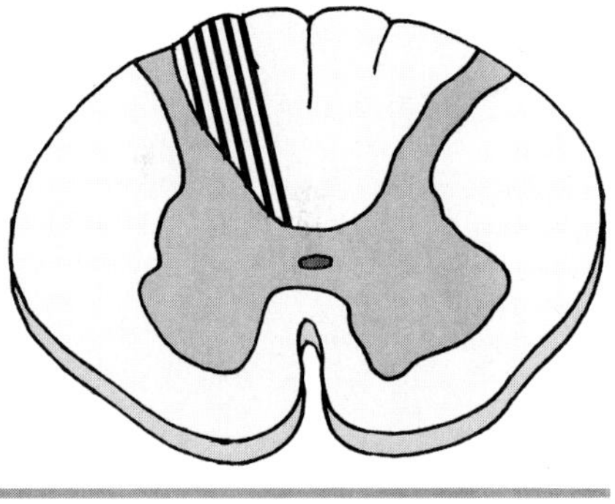

65.19. As the motor tracts descend, their fibers leave the cord, and the tracts become ______er in size. As the sensory tracts ascend within the cord, more fibers join them, and the tracts become ______er in size. The posterior columns of white matter in the cervical cord are ______er in size than the posterior columns in the lumbar cord.

65.16A. medial

65.17A. gracilis; fasciculus cuneatus

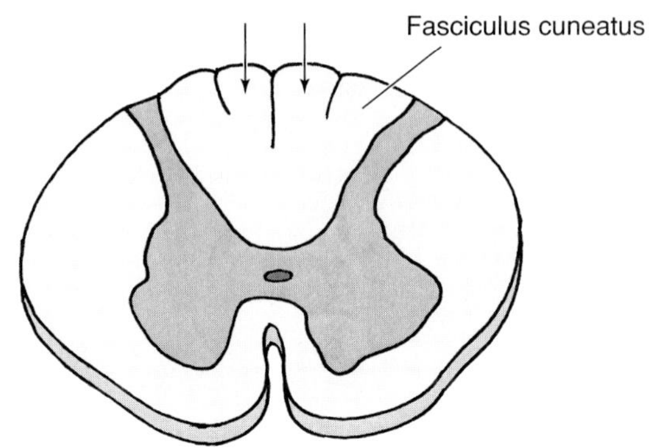

65.18A. cuneatus

65.19A. smaller; larger; larger

65.20. The posterior column is indicated on the right side in two of the pictures. Circle it on *both* sides of all three pictures. Label each picture with the initial letter of the cord region in which it lies—"L," "T," or "C."

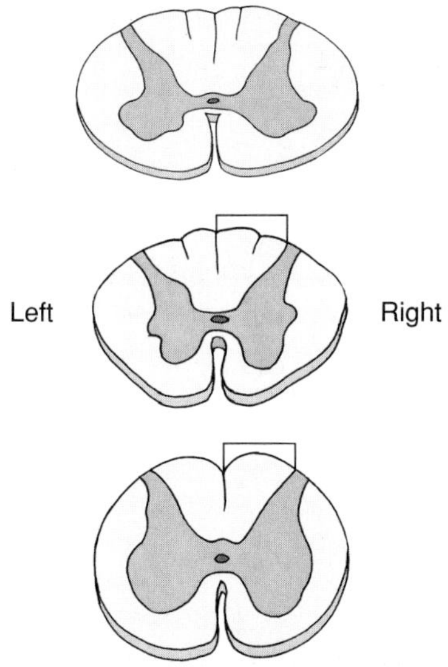

Left

Right

65.21. The diagrams show that, within the posterior columns, fibers from the skin and joints of the legs lie ____________ to fibers from the trunk. Fibers from the upper parts of the body lie most ____________.

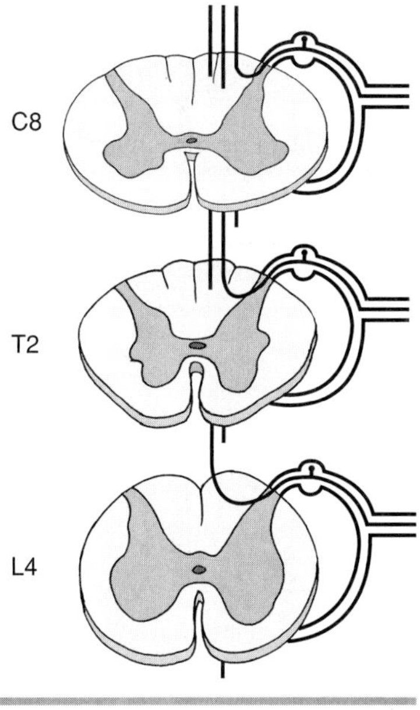

C8

T2

L4

65.22. As one examines sections at progressively higher cord levels, the posterior white columns become progressively ______er. Indicate the approximate position of "arm," "trunk," and "leg" fibers in the posterior column at C8.

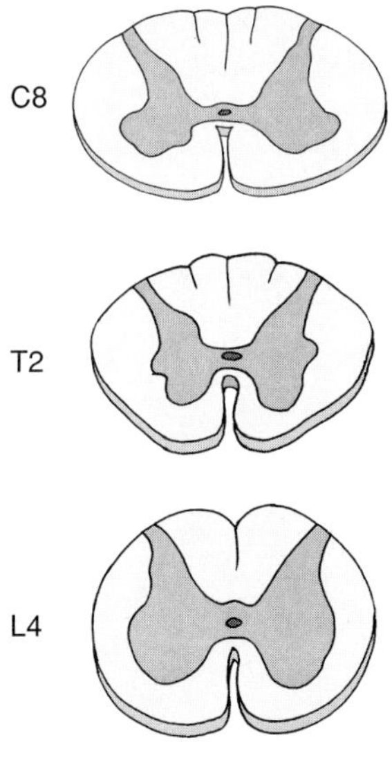

C8

T2

L4

65.20A.

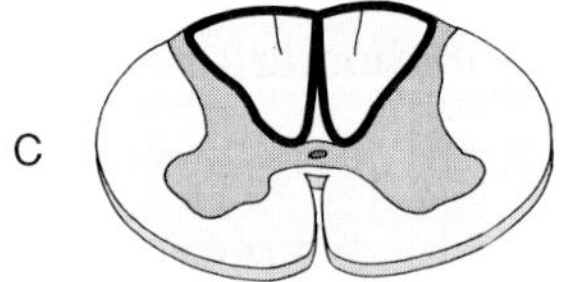

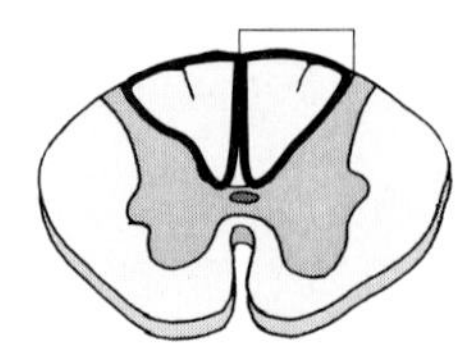

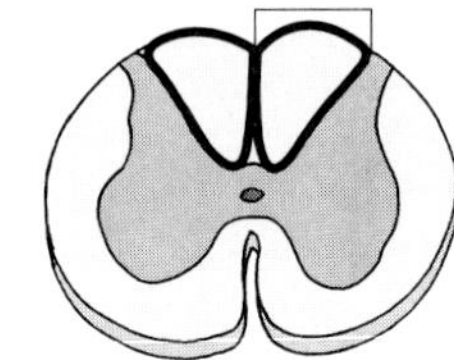

65.21A. medial; lateral

65.22A. larger

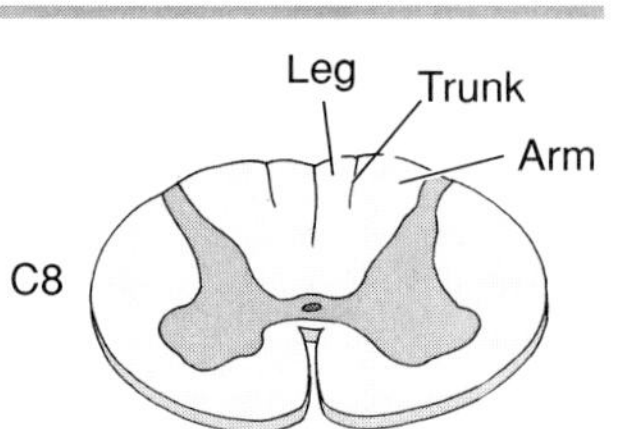

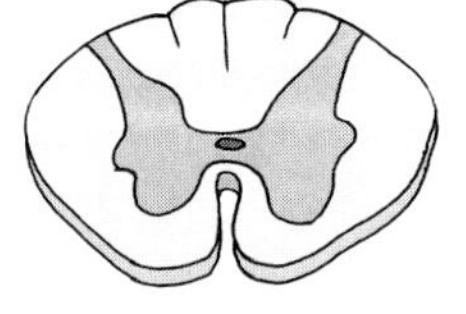

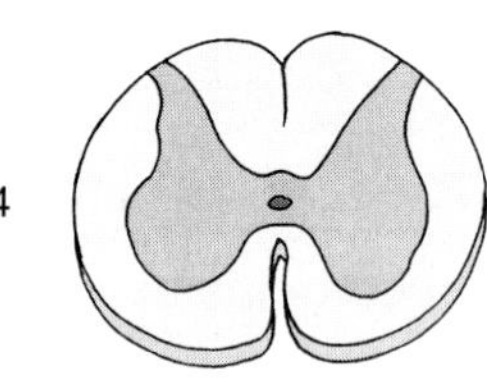

65.23. The posterior white column on each side at the lumbar level contains only fasciculus ________.

65.24. The secondary neurons for pain and temperature convey impulses up a *lateral* column of white matter and eventually reach the tertiary neuron cell body in the *thalamus*. On the *right* side of the picture, encircle and label this tract.

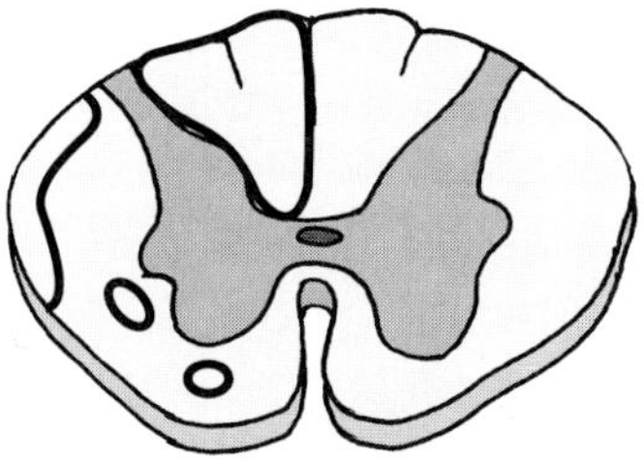

65.25. Information about pain and temperature is carried up the spinal cord in the ________ ____________ tract.

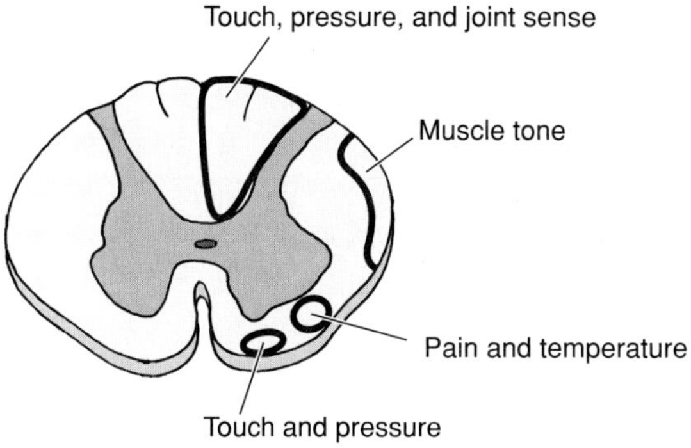

65.26. The secondary sensory axons in the anterior spinothalamic tract convey information about _____ and ________. Encircle the tract carrying these axons on the left side of the picture.

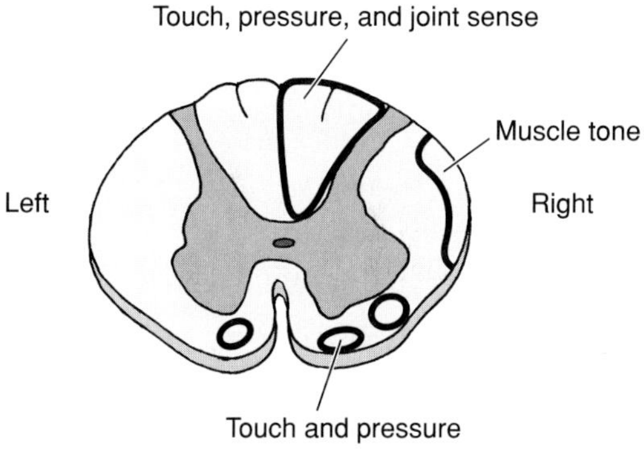

65.27. Information about the somesthetic senses other than pain and temperature is carried in widely separated white matter paths: the ________ white columns on the _____ side and both ________ ____________ tracts. A spinal cord lesion that would abolish all aspects of touch sensation would have to be a very _____ lesion.

65.23A. gracilis

65.24A.

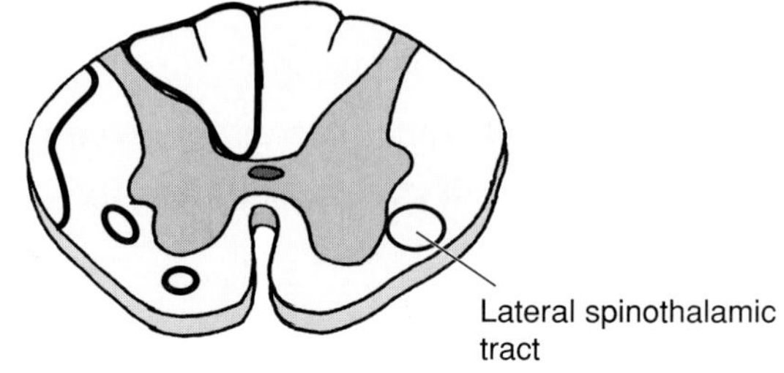

65.25A. lateral spinothalamic

65.26A. touch; pressure

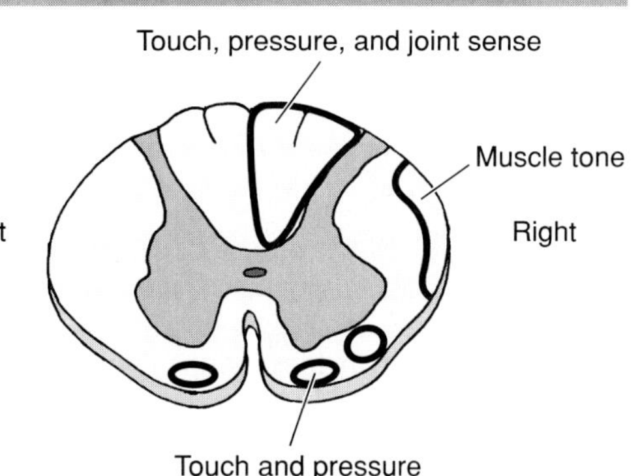

65.27A. posterior; same; anterior spinothalamic; large

65.28. The recognition of position and movement of a body part is called position sense (or ______ sense or ________________ sense). Clinical evidence indicates that this sense is particularly impaired in diseases affecting the ___________ white ___________ of the spinal cord.

65.29. A common clinical test for the integrity of the posterior white columns of the spinal cord is to press the handle of a vibrating tuning fork against the skin overlying a bony prominence such as at the ankle, shin, or hip. This complex stimulus generates impulses for all of the previously described modalities carried in the posterior white columns: touch, ___________, and ___________ sense.

65.30. Whether the impulses arise in touch or pressure receptors of the skin or in receptors of the joints, they travel together along the ___________ ______ ___________ of the spinal cord. Impulses from the lower limbs are transmitted in the fasciculus ___________, which lies ___________ to the fasciculus ___________.

65.31. Even in the presence of completely destructive lesions in the posterior white columns, the senses of touch and pressure are fairly well preserved because of impulses transmitted in the ___________ white columns, particularly in the left and right ___________ ________________ tracts.

65.32. An ischemic event (lack of blood supply) or lesion affecting only the *lateral* white columns of the cord would interfere with sensations of ______ and ________________. Conscious recognition of position and movement in the upper limbs is impaired by a lesion at a high cervical level in the fasciculus ___________.

65.33. Give the sensory modalities conveyed in each of the circled tracts on the diagram.

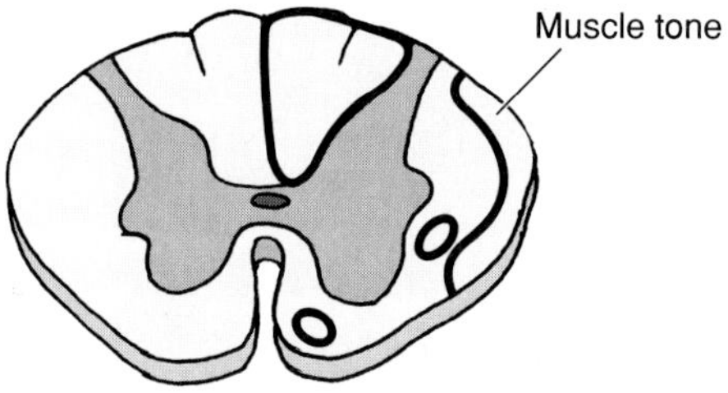

Muscle tone

65.28A. joint; kinesthetic; posterior; columns

65.29A. pressure; position

65.30A. posterior white columns; gracilis; medial; cuneatus

65.31A. anterior; anterior spinothalamic

65.32A. pain; temperature; cuneatus

65.33A.

Touch, pressure, and joint sense
Muscle tone
Pain and temperature
Touch and pressure

65.34. On the figure, label the blood supply to each of the indicated tracts.

__________ spinal artery

__________ spinal artery

__________ spinal artery

__________ spinal artery

65.35. Axons of secondary neurons in the afferent pathway from muscle and tendon receptors run from the *spinal* cord to the *cerebellum*. The tracts carrying these axons are the sp______c__________ar tracts.

65.36. The spinocerebellar tracts are often classified as the anterior and posterior spinocerebellar tracts, with somewhat different origins and routes from the spinal cord to the ______________. For practical purposes, however, they may be lumped together as one pathway, mediating information that contributes to the regulation of muscle ______.

65.37. Draw lines between the two columns to pair appropriate items.

Lateral spinothalamic tract	Touch, pressure, and kinesthetic sense
Spinocerebellar tracts	Pain and temperature
Anterior spinothalamic tract	Touch and pressure
Posterior white column	Muscle tone

65.38. Touch is almost always preserved in focal lesions of the spinal cord because the pathways are multiple and widely separated. The major routes up the cord for touch impulses are the ______________ tracts and the __________ ______ __________ .

65.39. A lesion destroying the anterior half of the cord would severely impair ______ and ______________ senses. The lesion would have a __________ effect on touch because information for this sense would still be conveyed in the intact __________ ______ __________.

65.34A.

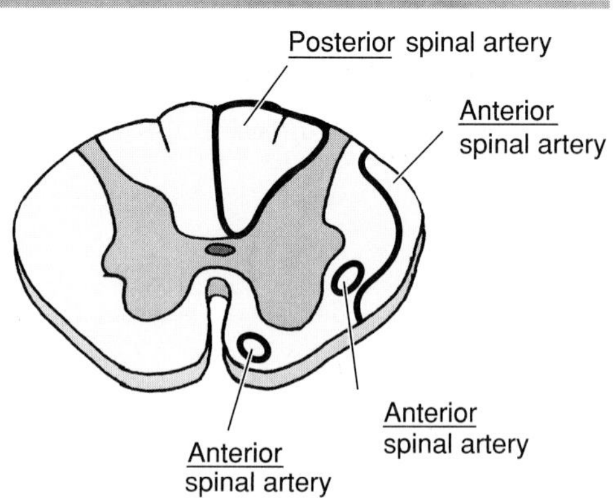

65.35A. spinocerebellar

65.36A. cerebellum; tone

65.37A.

Lateral spinothalamic tract	Touch, pressure, and kinesthetic sense
Spinocerebellar tracts	Pain and temperature
Anterior spinothalamic tract	Touch and pressure
Posterior white column	Muscle tone

65.38A. spinothalamic; posterior white columns

65.39A. pain; temperature; lesser; posterior white columns

65.40. Name the encircled tracts and write in parentheses the types of information conveyed in each.

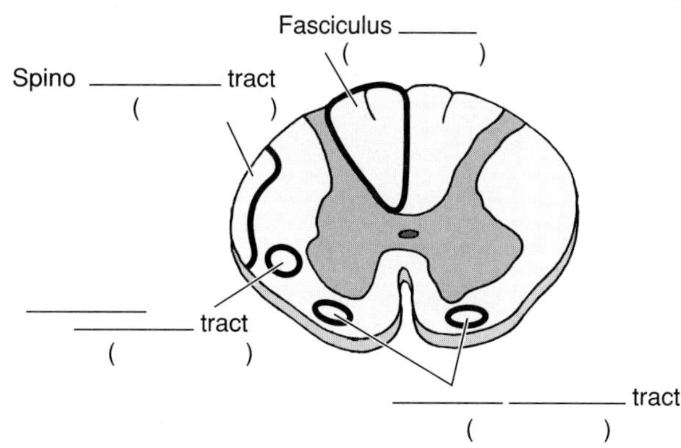

65.40A.

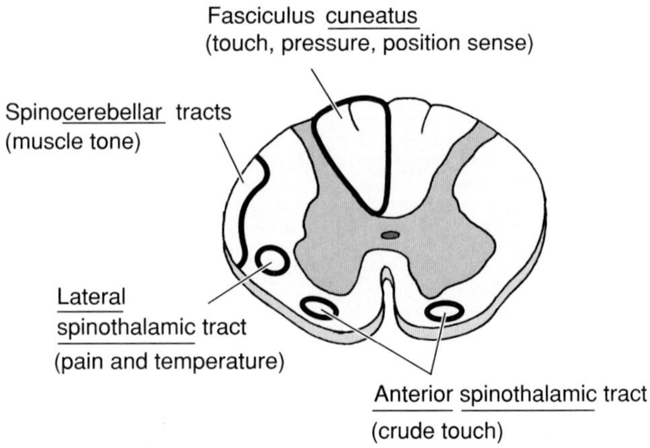

Fasciculus cuneatus
(touch, pressure, position sense)
Spinocerebellar tracts
(muscle tone)
Lateral
spinothalamic tract
(pain and temperature)
Anterior spinothalamic tract
(crude touch)

66 Synapses in Sensory Pathways: Lateral and Anterior Spinothalamic Tracts

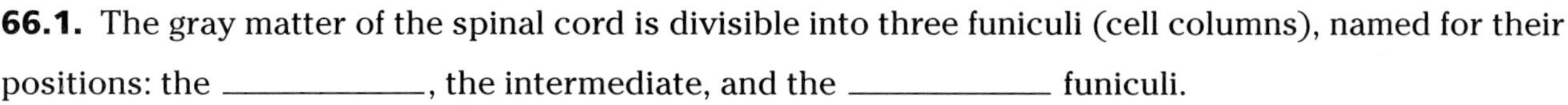

66.1. The gray matter of the spinal cord is divisible into three funiculi (cell columns), named for their positions: the ____________, the intermediate, and the ____________ funiculi.

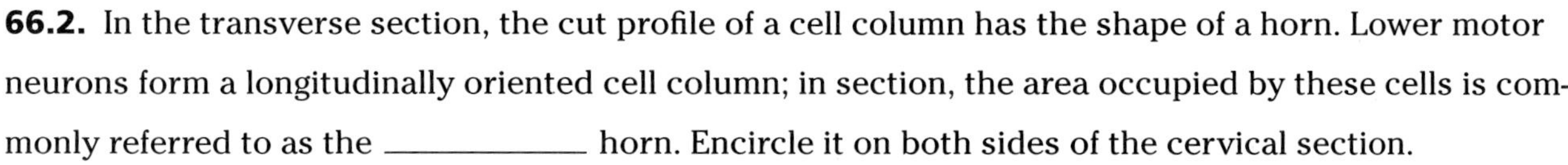

66.2. In the transverse section, the cut profile of a cell column has the shape of a horn. Lower motor neurons form a longitudinally oriented cell column; in section, the area occupied by these cells is commonly referred to as the ____________ horn. Encircle it on both sides of the cervical section.

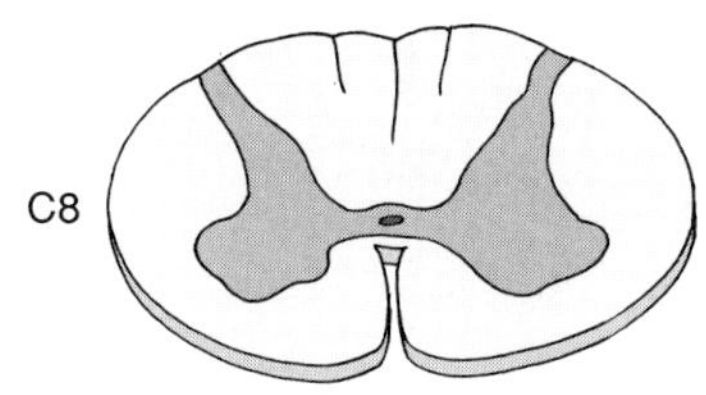

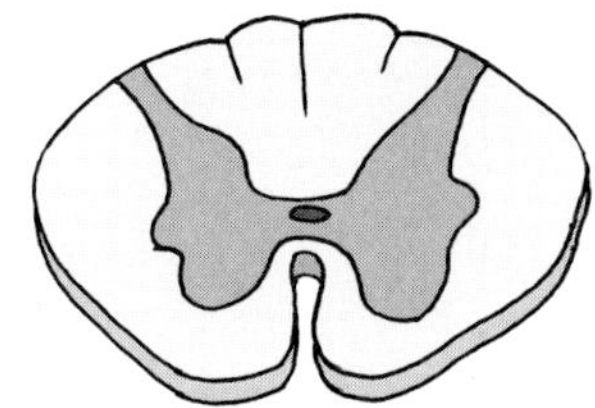

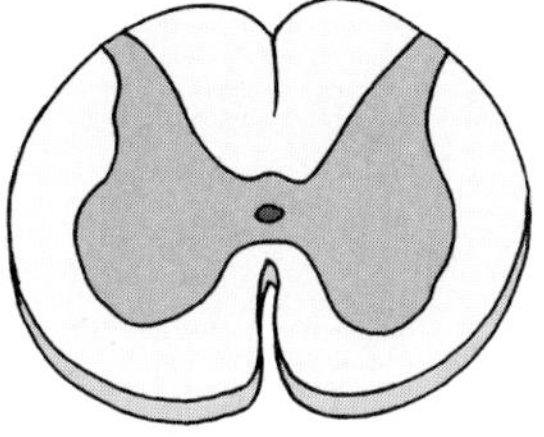

66.3. On the left side of the picture, label the three horns of the gray matter. On the right side, label the three funiculi of white matter with their general names and draw boundary lines between the columns.

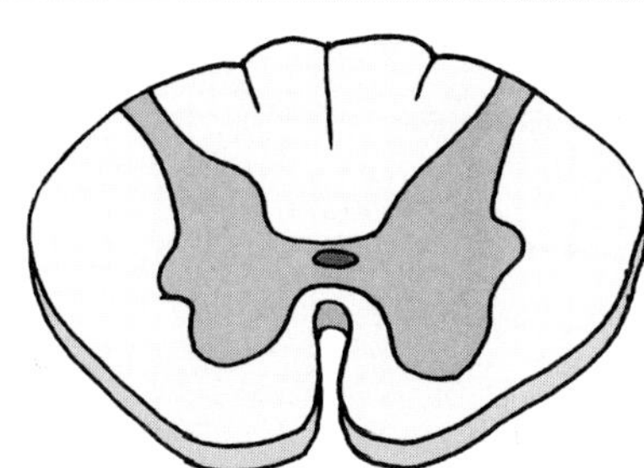

66.4. The anterior horns contain cell bodies of ______fferent neurons; the posterior horns contain cell bodies of ______fferent neurons. Synapses occur almost exclusively in the ______ matter.

66.1A. anterior; posterior

66.2A. anterior

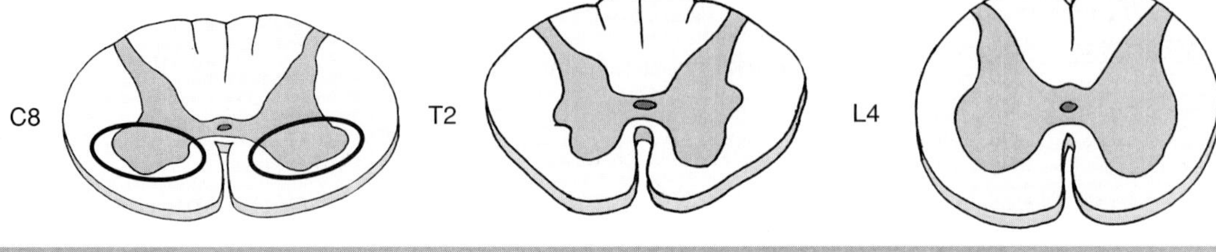

66.3A.

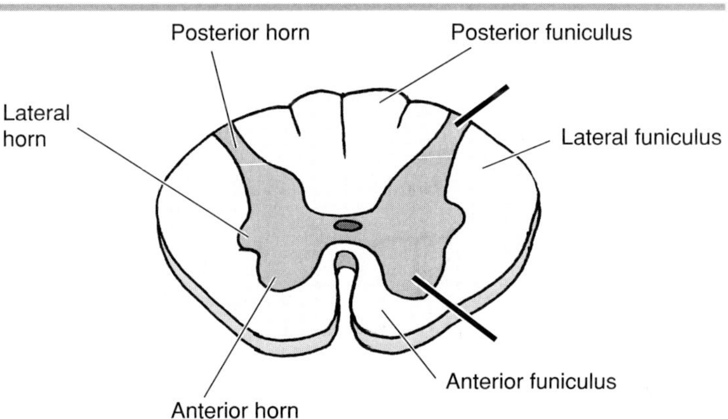

66.4A. efferent; afferent; gray

66.5. The peripheral receptors in the pain pathway are free, naked nerve endings. In the pain pathway, the cell body of the primary neuron lies ______side the spinal cord in a spinal __________. The cell body of the secondary neuron lies in the __________horn. Are the cell bodies of primary and secondary neurons on the same side of the cord? ______ The axon of the __________ary neuron in the pain pathway crosses the midline and ascends the spinal cord in the contralateral __________ __________________ tract.

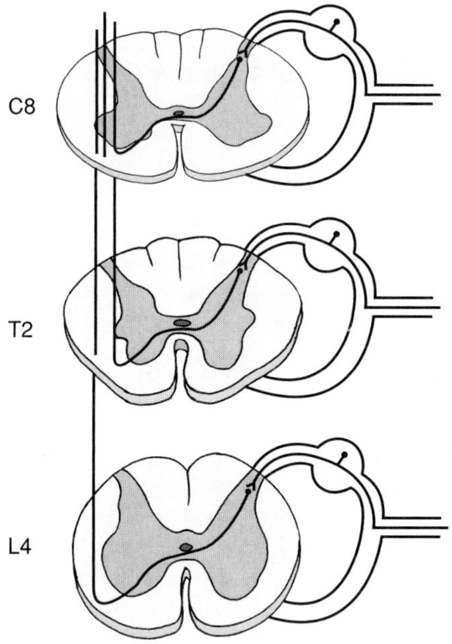

C8

T2

L4

66.6. Any sensory pathway can be analyzed anatomically in terms of (1) the location of synapses and (2) the course of its fibers. Thus, the first synapse in the pain pathway is found in the ______ matter of the cord on the ______ side as the stimulus. The axon of the secondary neuron carries impulses to the contralateral __________ funiculus of the spinal cord.

66.7. Connect the fiber of the illustrated *primary* neuron to its cell body. Draw the *cell body* of the secondary neuron with which the primary neuron synapses.

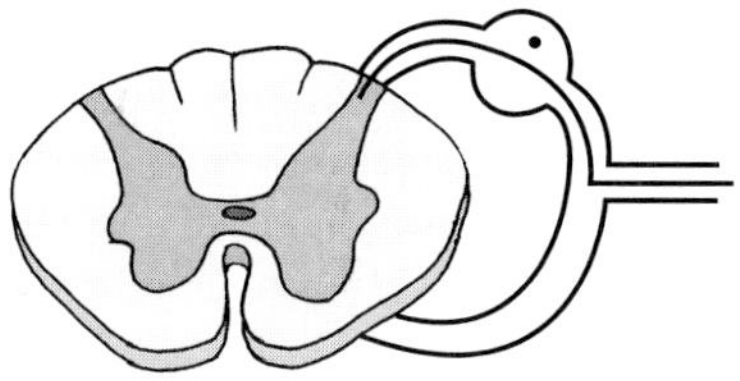

66.8. In the pain pathway—as in *all* sensory pathways—the cell bodies of the primary and secondary neurons lie on the ______ side.

66.9. Axons of almost all primary sensory neurons branch after entering the spinal cord. One branch of the "pain fiber" in the diagram passes directly into the anterior horn and makes synaptic contact with an internuncial neuron, which in turn contacts a ______ neuron; the other branch contacts a __________ary sensory neuron whose axon crosses the midline. Like axons of the anterior corticospinal tract, axons of secondary neurons in the pain and temperature pathways cross the midline in the __________ com__________ just __________ to the central canal.

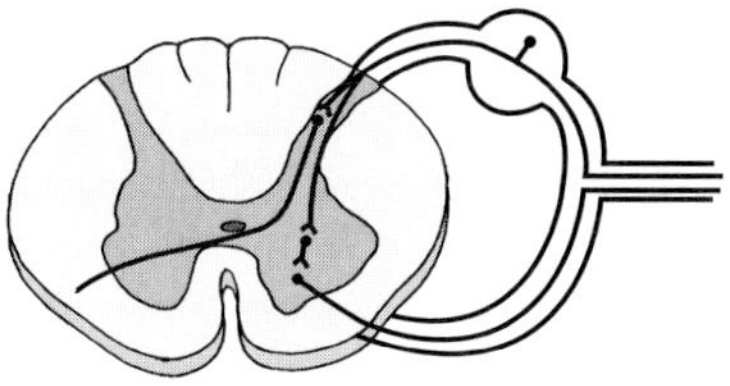

66.5A. outside; ganglion; posterior; Yes; secondary; lateral spinothalamic

66.6A. gray; same; lateral

66.7A.

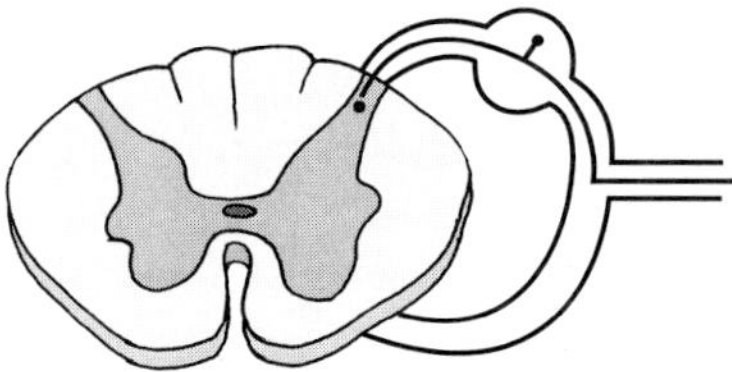

66.8A. same

66.9A. motor; secondary; anterior commissure; anterior

66.10. Draw an arrow to indicate the anterior commissure.

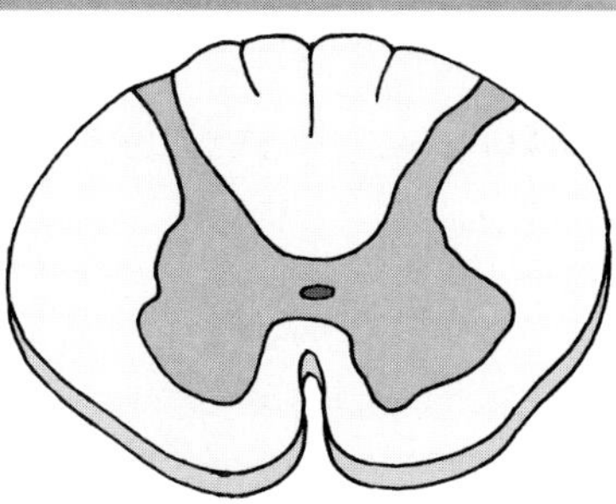

66.11. Like most sensory neurons, the cell bodies of the primary neurons in the pain and temperature pathway are outside the CNS, in the ____________ ____________. The cell bodies of the primary and secondary neurons are on the ______ side of the cord, and the ______ of the secondary pain and temperature neuron crosses the midline. The left lateral spinothalamic tract is occupied by axons of ____________ary sensory neurons whose cell bodies are in the posterior horn on the ______ side.

66.12. Segments of an axon in the pain pathway are drawn on the picture. Draw the cell body in its proper location and add the part of the axon between the cell body and the arrow. This axon terminates in synaptic contact with a tertiary neuron in the ____________.

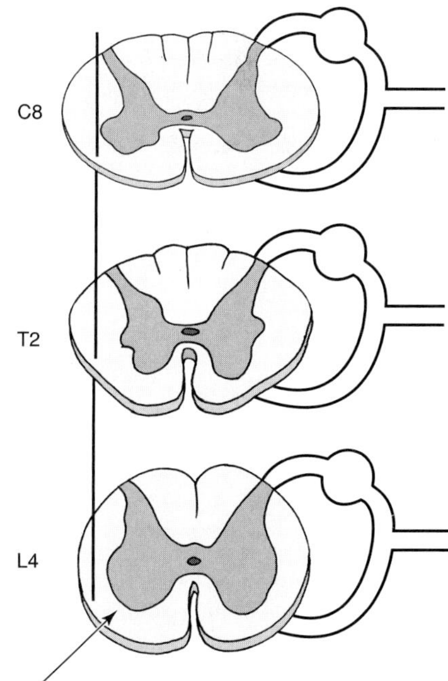

66.13. Draw a secondary *pain* nerve cell body on the left side of the lumbar cord and another on the right side of the thoracic cord. Draw the axons of each to reach the cervical cord and indicate the direction of impulse conduction with arrows on each axon.

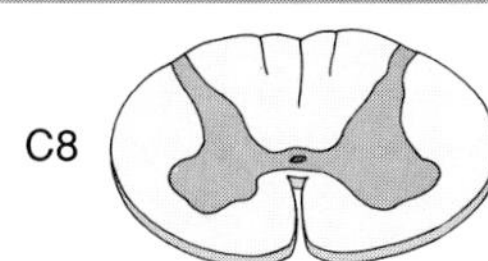

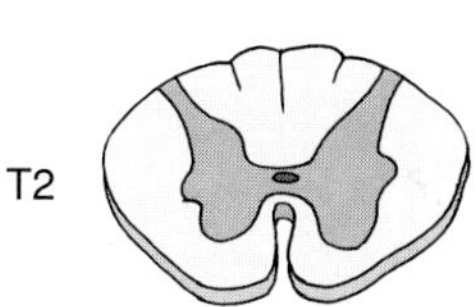

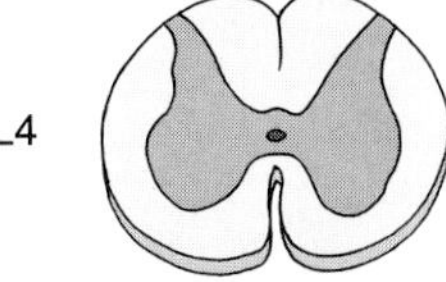

66.10A.

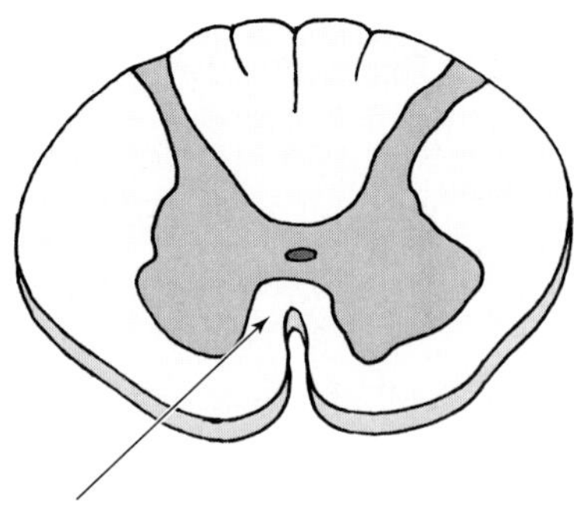

66.11A. spinal ganglion; same; axon; secondary; right

66.12A. thalamus

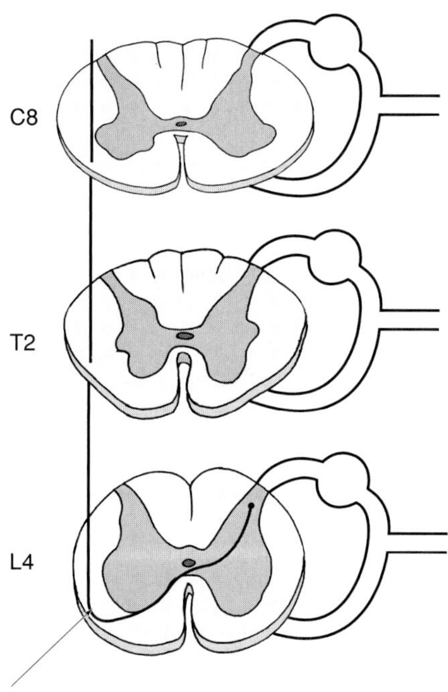

66.13A.

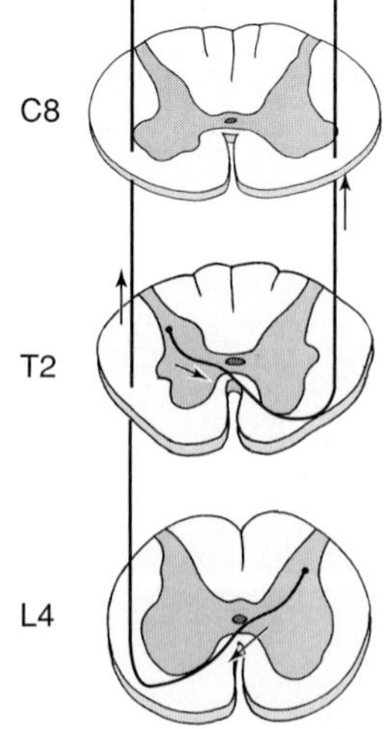

66.14. Axons of primary neurons conveying information about pain and temperature enter the cord and branch. The branches synapse with secondary sensory neurons in the gray matter of the ____________ horn. Some branches serve in local reflex circuits by making synaptic contacts with the inter______ial neurons, which in turn directly or indirectly contact ______ neurons.

66.15. Axons actually ascend one to two cord segments as they cross. The axons cross just ______erior to the central canal and collect on the opposite side as the ____________ ____________________ ______ .

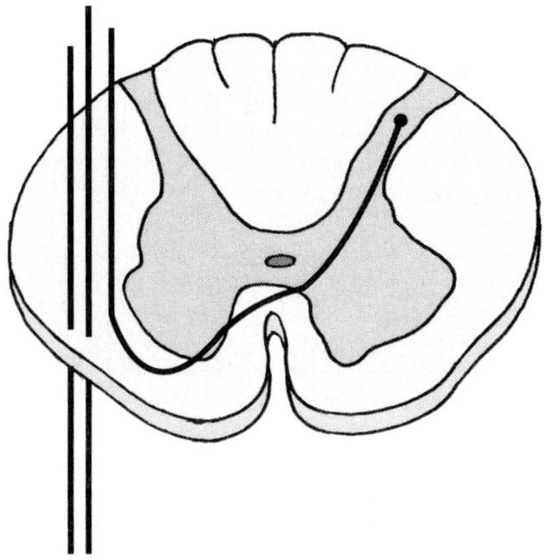

66.16. For convenience, we have been representing the branches of the *primary* sensory fibers as synapsing in the same plane of section as their cell body. Actually, the branches may ascend and/or descend *one* or *two* segments before synapsing with ____________ sensory neurons.

66.17. The nerve impulses generated by a pinprick in the *left* great toe enter the cord via a ____________ root on the ______ side. A synapse is made with a secondary neuron whose axon ascends in the ____________ funiculus on the ______ side.

66.18. The axons of the ____________ary neurons cross in the ____________ ____________________ and travel in the contralateral ____________ ____________________ tract all the way to the ____________.

66.14A. posterior; internuncial; motor

66.15A. anterior; lateral spinothalamic tract

66.16A. secondary

66.17A. posterior; left; lateral; right

66.18A. secondary; anterior commissure; lateral spinothalamic; thalamus

66.19. Impulses mediating the sensation of pain travel along fibers intermingled with those for hot and cold. Encircle the area containing the cell bodies of *secondary* neurons in the pathway transmitting information about heat applied to the *left leg*. The axons of these neurons ______scend one to two segments as they cross the midline. On the other cord section, place an "X" on the tract that contains the axons of the encircled "heat" neurons.

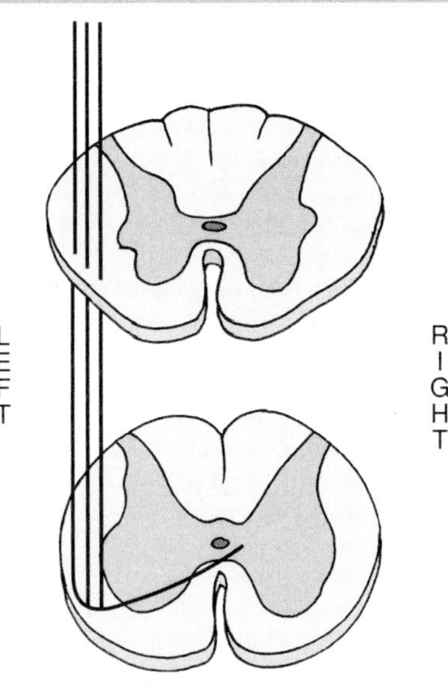

66.20. A given sensory pathway typically crosses the midline only once. The cell bodies of origin are in the ______ matter at a ______er level of the cord on the ________________ side.

66.21. Reports in the touch, pressure, or kinesthetic categories are obtained on stimulation of the __________ gyrus.

66.22. The conventional categories of somesthetic senses are: hot, ______, ______, ______, __________, and __________ sense.

66.23. This diagram shows cells and processes that transmit sensory information of ______ and __________.

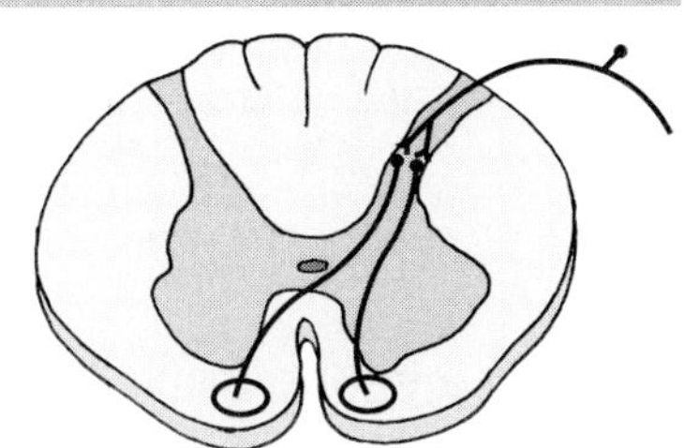

66.24. Primary touch fibers synapse both with secondary neurons whose axons cross the midline to the __________ spinothalamic tract on the contralateral side of the cord and with secondary neurons whose axons ascend on the ________________ side of the cord.

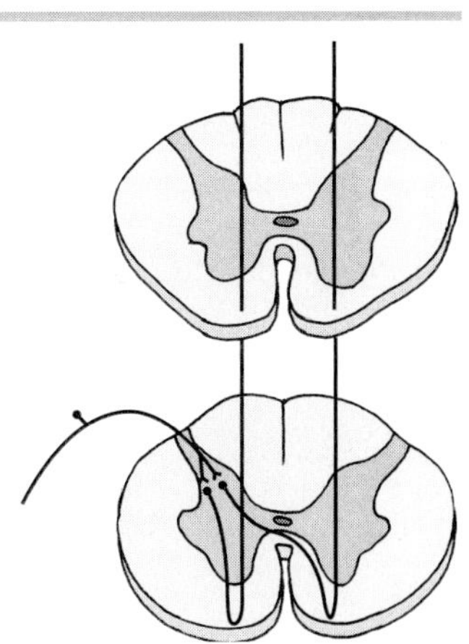

66.19A. ascend

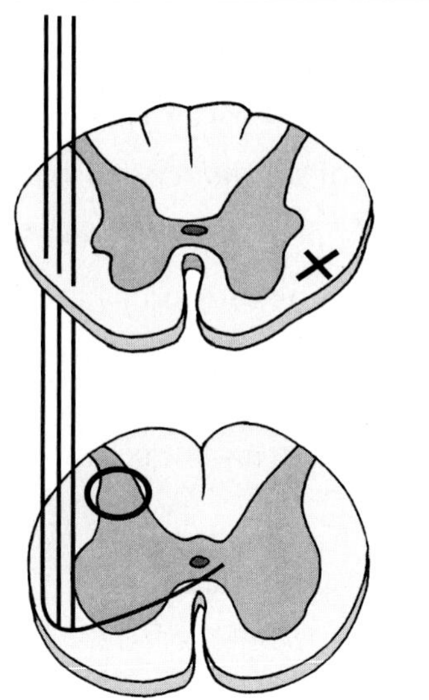

66.20A. gray; lower; contralateral

66.21A. postcentral

66.22A. cold; pain; touch; pressure; position (or joint or kinesthetic)

66.23A. touch; pressure

66.24A. anterior; ipsilateral

66.25. By strict definition, a bundle of axons crossing the midline and connecting two equivalent, symmetrically placed structures is called a *commissure*. A different term is used for a bundle of axons crossing the midline between different structures; for example, fibers passing between the left pyramidal tract in the ____________ and the right ____________ corticospinal tract constitute the pyramidal ____________________.

66.26. In common practice, *any* bundle of axons that crosses the midline may be called a com____________. All secondary pain and temperature axons and many of the secondary pressure and ______ axons cross the midline in the ____________ ____________________ of the cord. Other secondary touch and pressure axons ascend in the ____________ ____________________ tract on the ____________________ side.

66.27. On the diagram, draw the two missing secondary sensory cell bodies in the touch pathways.

66.28. On the diagram, draw the missing secondary sensory fiber in the touch and pressure pathway. The missing fiber crosses the cord in the ____________ ____________________.

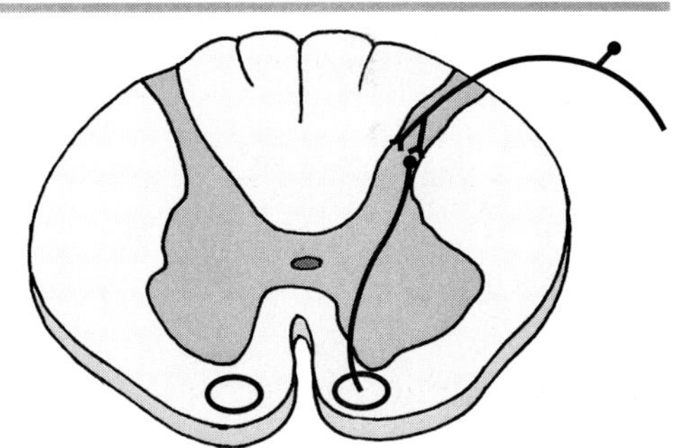

66.29. On the schematic diagram, draw the missing secondary sensory axon. "A" is the cell body of a ________ary sensory neuron.

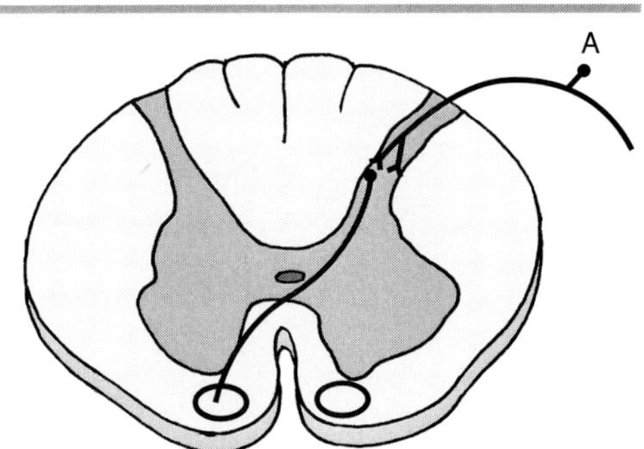

66.25A. medulla; lateral; decussation

66.26A. commissure; touch; anterior commissure; anterior spinothalamic; ipsilateral

66.27A.

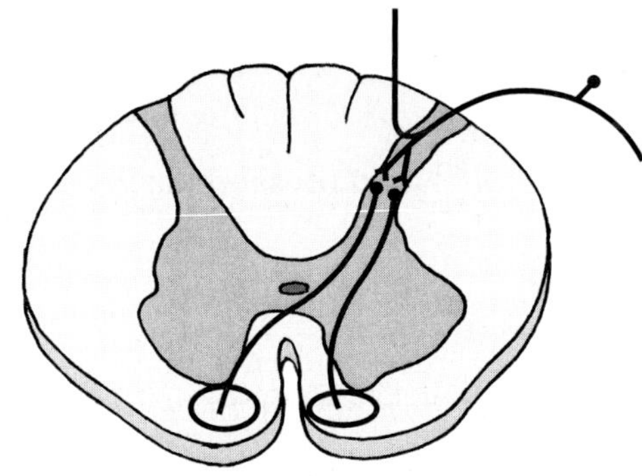

66.28A. anterior commissure

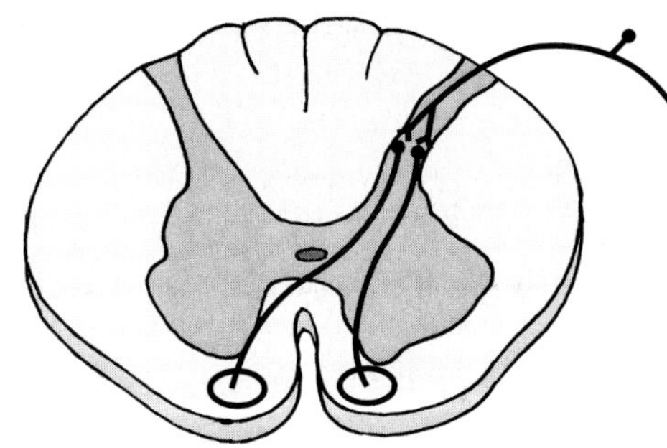

66.29A. primary

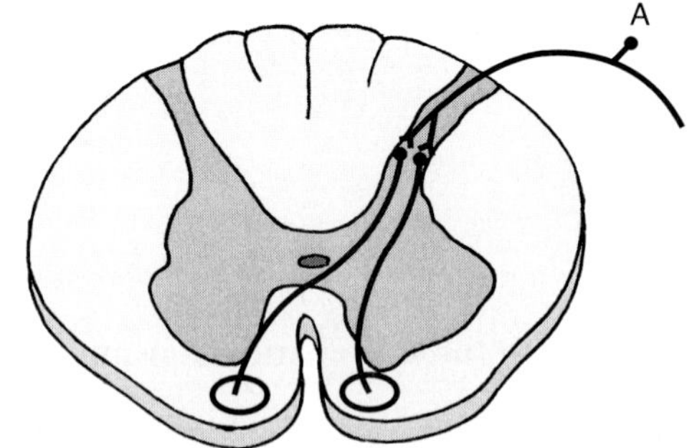

66.30. On the right side of the diagram, draw a *primary* cell body and axon in the touch pathway. Circle both anterior spinothalamic tracts. Draw the missing secondary cell bodies and axons in the touch pathway. These pathways would also serve to represent the sensation of ___________.

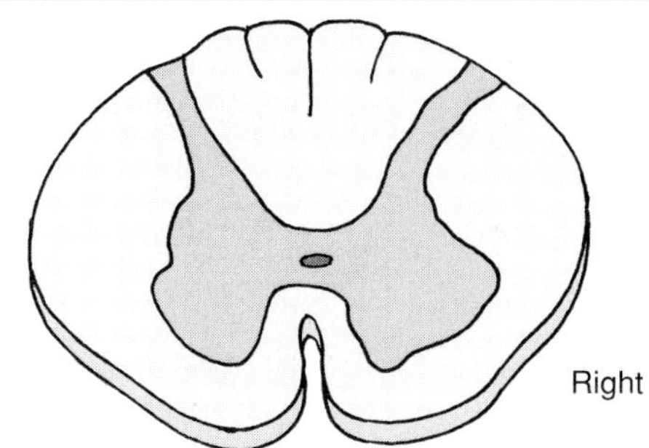

66.31. Fibers from *one* posterior horn pass into *both* anterior spinothalamic tracts. Fibers in one anterior spinothalamic tract are derived from ______ posterior horns. The anterior spinothalamic tracts receive blood primarily from the ___________ spinal artery.

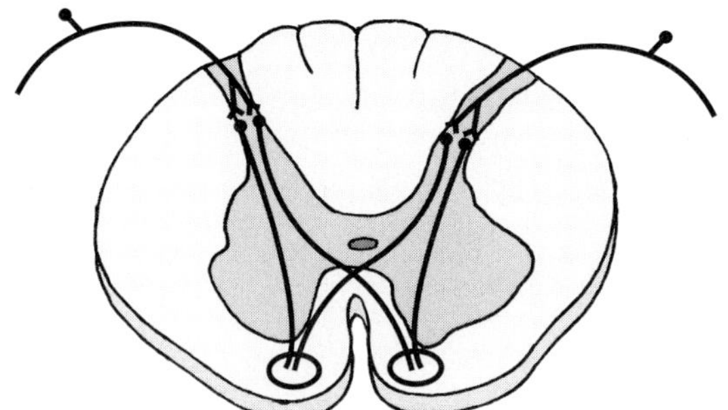

66.32. Circle the *right* anterior spinothalamic tract on the diagram. On *each* side of the cord, draw in a cell body of an axon entering the *encircled* tract. Label the encircled tract with the modalities of sensation that it mediates.

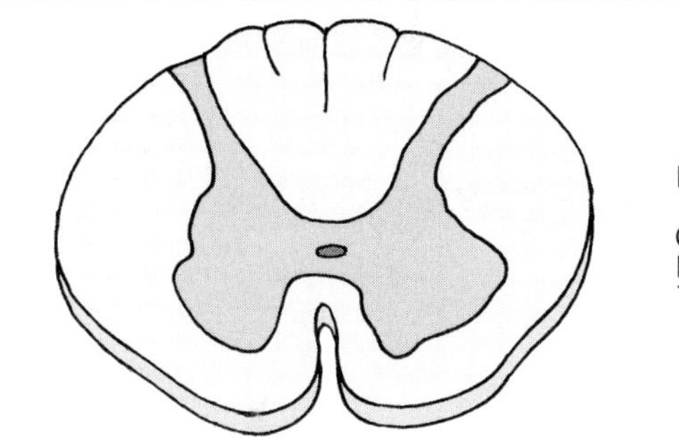

66.30A. pressure

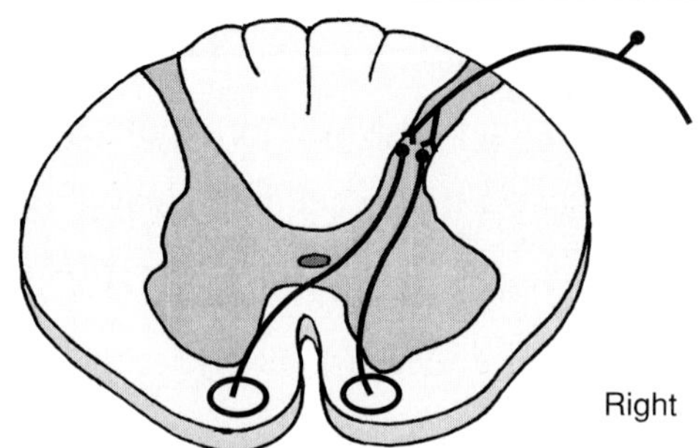

66.31A. both; anterior

66.32A.

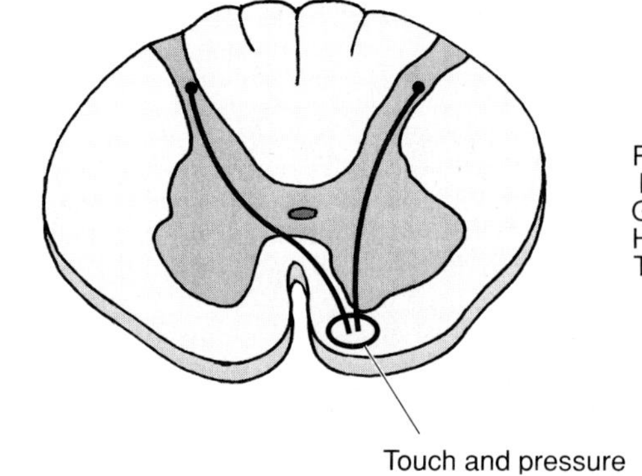

67 Synapses in Sensory Pathways: Posterior Columns and Spinocerebellar Tracts

67.1. Touch pathways are widely distributed in the spinal cord. Impulses from a given area of skin travel in the anterior spinothalamic tracts of both sides, along axons of ___________ary sensory neurons. Other touch impulses from the same area of skin ascend in the posterior columns of the same side. These impulses have not yet reached a synapse; they are traveling in the ___________ white ___________ along axons of the ______ary sensory neurons.

67.2. Which one of the numbered fibers does *not* convey information about the sense of touch? Fiber ______. Information about joint sense might be carried along fiber ______.

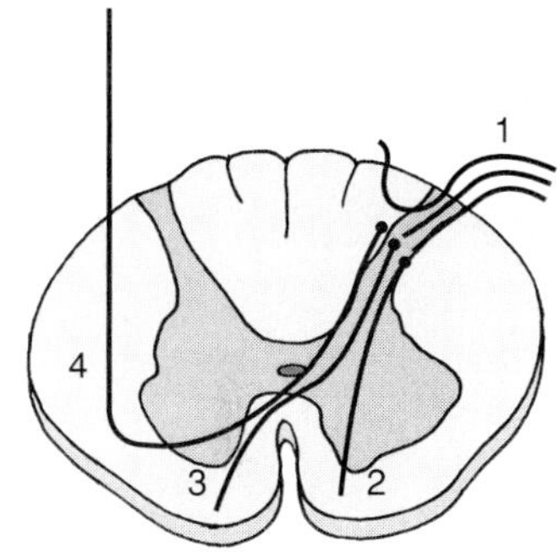

67.3. *Medial* and *lateral* are relative terms. The medial part of the posterior root is at the ______al margin of the posterior white column. Fibers for kinesthetic (joint) sense enter the cord from the *medial* part of the posterior root. On the diagram, indicate such a fiber with an arrow.

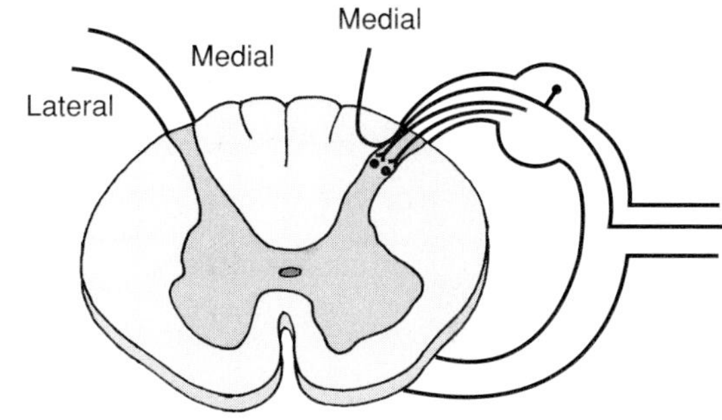

67.4. The medial part of the posterior root contains fibers about to enter the ___________ ______ column. The lateral part of the root contains fibers that are about to enter the ________________ ________________ and then make ___________ic contact with internuncial neurons and secondary neurons in the ______ matter.

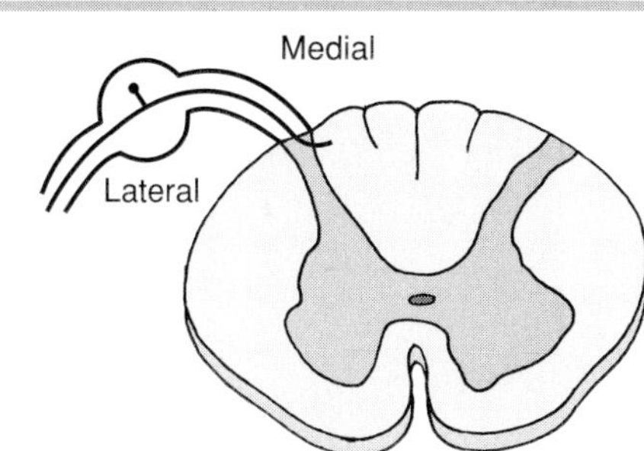

67.5. Primary neuron cell bodies for kinesthetic sense are in the ___________ ___________. Draw one such cell body on the diagram. As its axon passes centrally toward the cord, it lies in the medial part of the ___________ root. Draw such an axon traversing the root.

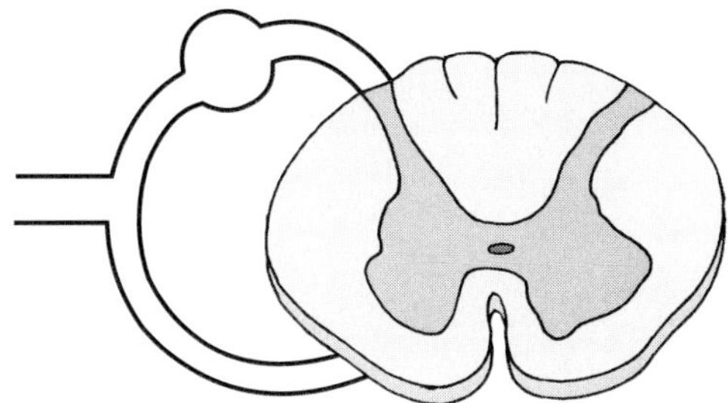

67.1A. secondary; posterior; columns; primary

67.2A. 4; 1

67.3A. lateral

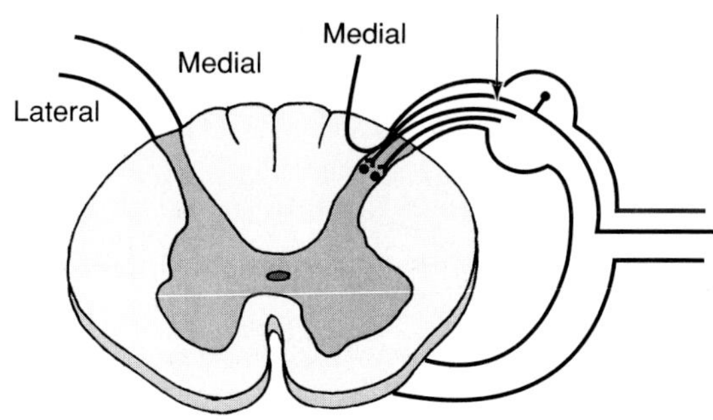

67.4A. posterior white; dorsolateral fasciculus; synaptic; gray

67.5A. spinal ganglion; posterior

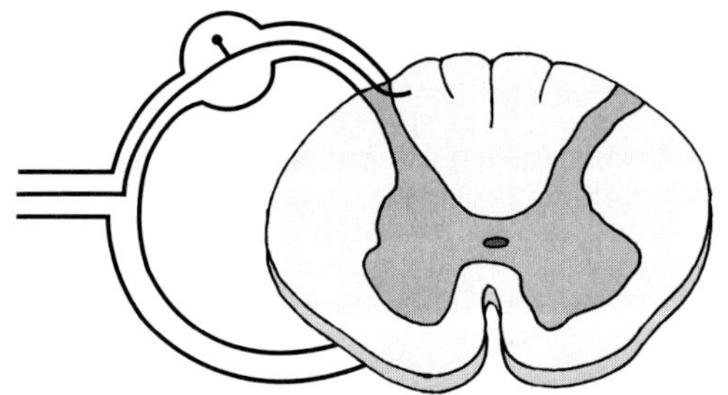

67.6. On the diagram, encircle the synapses of pain and touch neurons. The posterior columns, unlike tracts in the lateral and anterior funiculi, contain mainly axons of ______ary afferent neurons.

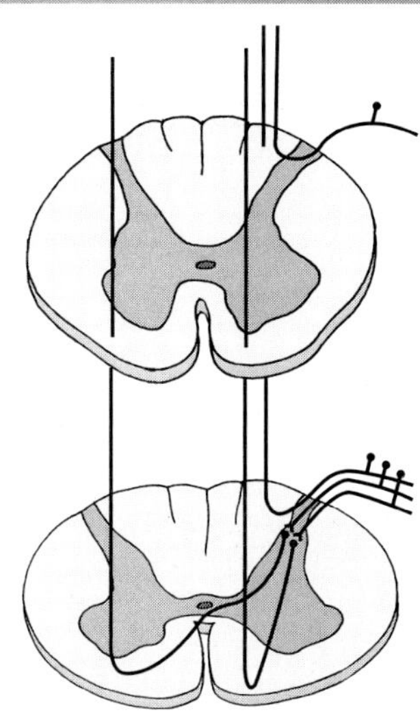

67.7. Axons of some primary afferent neurons ascend all the way to the medulla in the __________ funiculi before making synaptic contact (in the nuclei gracilis and cuneatus) with __________ary afferent neurons. The first two afferent cell bodies always are on the ______________ side.

67.8. Peripheral nerve lesions may abolish the sense of touch in a given region. Spinal cord lesions are less likely to do so because impulses conveying tactile information for a given region are transmitted in widely separated paths: the __________ __________ of the same side and both __________ ______________ tracts.

67.9. Each kinesthetic fiber enters the __________ __________ and splits into two or more branches. The ascending branch reaches the medulla before making a __________. The __________ing branch makes spinal reflex connections with __________ial neurons at lower cord levels.

67.10. *All* secondary sensory fibers in the __________ ______________ tract have crossed the cord. About *half* of the secondary sensory fibers in the __________ ______________ tract have crossed the cord. *None* of the primary sensory fibers in the __________ funiculus have crossed the cord.

67.11. *All* secondary sensory fibers concerned with _____ and ______________ cross the cord. Some of the secondary fibers concerned with the modalities of _____ and __________ cross the cord. *No* synapses with secondary sensory fibers are made in the cord by primary sensory fibers concerned with __________ sense.

67.6A. primary

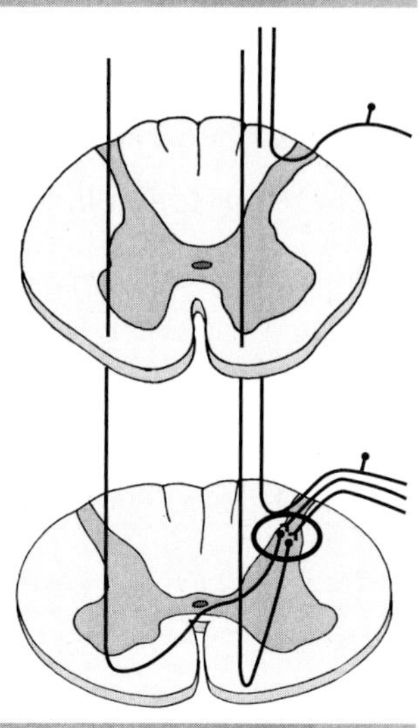

67.7A. posterior; secondary; ipsilateral

67.8A. posterior columns; anterior spinothalamic

67.9A. posterior funiculus; synapse; descending; internuncial

67.10A. lateral spinothalamic; anterior spinothalamic; posterior

67.11A. pain; temperature; touch; pressure; position

67.12. On the diagram, the fasciculus __________ is encircled. The central ends of the encircled axons are in the medulla. The cell *bodies* are in __________ __________, and the peripheral ends are in skin or ______s of the ______er limb on the ______________ side.

LEFT RIGHT

67.13. Pain and temperature impulses from all regions of the body below the neck enter the spinal cord and cross the midline in the __________ ______________; kinesthetic impulses and those touch impulses traveling with them cross the midline above the spinal cord in the __________.

67.14. In the chain of afferent nerves mediating position sense and some degree of pressure and touch from the left thumb, the secondary neuron cell bodies lie in the ______ side of the __________ and, as in the pain and temperature afferent chain, send their axons up the ______________ side of the brainstem to the __________.

67.15. Axons in the posterior columns convey impulses that eventually reach the postcentral gyrus of the parietal lobe. In all, the impulses travel over a chain containing a minimum of ______ neurons.

67.16. Almost all primary sensory neurons have their cell bodies in __________ __________. The gray matter of the posterior *horn* contains the cell bodies of secondary sensory neurons concerned with the modalities of ______, ______________, __________, and ______ but not __________ sense.

67.12A. gracilis; spinal ganglia; joints; lower; ipsilateral

67.13A. anterior commissure; medulla

67.14A. left; medulla; contralateral; thalamus

67.15A. 3

67.16A. spinal ganglia; pain; temperature; pressure; touch; position

67.17. Beside each tract, place the numbers of the appropriate items below: lateral spinothalamic tract ________________; anterior spinothalamic tract ________________; posterior white columns ________________; lateral corticospinal tract ________________; anterior corticospinal tract ________________.

1. Cells of origin and fibers of tract on same side as each other
2. Cells of origin and fibers of tract on opposite sides from each other
3. Primary axons in the dorsolateral fasciculus
4. Primary axons in ascending spinal cord tract
5. Secondary cell bodies in posterior horn of spinal cord
6. Secondary cell bodies in the medulla
7. Secondary axons in ascending spinal cord tract
8. Crosses over in the anterior commissure
9. Crosses over in the pyramidal decussation
10. Crosses over in the medulla or contacts a secondary neuron with axons that cross in the medulla

67.18. Neurons of the lateral and anterior cortico*spinal* tracts synapse in the spinal cord. Neurons of the lateral and anterior spino*thalamic* tracts synapse in the ____________. Neurons of the posterior columns synapse in the ____________. Neurons of the spinocerebellar tracts synapse in the ________________.

67.19. Many impulses influencing muscle tone are relayed through the cerebellum via the ________________ tracts. Impulses mediating position sense, by contrast, reach all the way to the __________ __________.

67.20. Impulses from sense organs need not "reach consciousness"; such impulses are not literally "sensory," but they are ______ferent components of reflex circuits. Spinocerebellar impulses, from receptors in skeletal __________ and tendons, give unconscious information about muscle ______.

67.21. *Proprioception* is divided into two components, complete the table.

		Impulses Rise in	Information
Proprioception	__________sense	__________	reaches consciousness
	__________tone	__________ and __________	remains __________

67.17A.

lateral spinothalamic tract 2, 3, 5, 7, 8

anterior spinothalamic tract 1, 2, 3, 5, 7, 8

posterior (white) columns 1, 3, 4, 6, 10

lateral corticospinal tract 2, 9, 10

anterior corticospinal tract 1, 8

67.18A. thalamus; medulla; cerebellum

67.19A. spinocerebellar; cerebral cortex

67.20A. afferent; muscles; tone

67.21A.

Proprioception	position sense	Impulses Rise in joints	Information reaches consciousness
	muscle tone	muscles and tendons	remains unconscious

67.22. Like neurons that influence joint sense, primary neurons influencing muscle tone send axons into the CNS via the ______al part of the posterior root.

67.23. The only afferent system in which virtually all of the cell bodies and fibers influencing a given body part remain on the same side is the system conveying information about ____________ ______. The *secondary* afferent fibers in this system originate in the ____________ horn of the spinal cord and terminate by making synaptic contacts in the ________________.

67.24. On the diagram, add an arrowhead to each of the four arrows to indicate the direction of impulse conduction. Label the encircled nucleus.

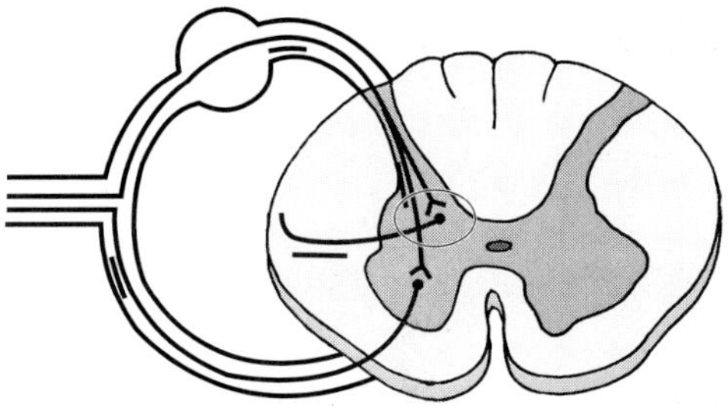

67.25. The same primary sensory neuron may send one branch to synapse in the dorsal horn (which transmits impulses to the ________________) and another branch to synapse *directly* with a *motor* neuron in the ____________ horn. The latter reflex pathway may involve only ______ neurons.

67.26. The two-neuron spinal reflex arc is called the *stretch* reflex. The afferent neuron is stimulated when the skeletal muscle ____________es. The efferent neuron runs from the cord back out to the ____________.

67.27. In the pathway contributing to the control of muscle tone, the axons of neurons with cell bodies in the right ____________ horn of the spinal cord gray matter travel up the cord in the ________________ tract of the ________________ side.

67.28. Complete the entries in the table.

Tract	Mediate Impulses Concerned With:	Axons Arise from Cell Bodies on Which Side: Left, Right, or Both?	Cell Bodies Located in:
Right lateral spinothalamic	______ and ________________	______	____________ horn
Right anterior spinothalamic	______ and ____________	______	____________ horn
Right posterior white columns	____________	______	____________ ____________
Left spinocerebellar	____________ ______	______	n. ____________

67.22A. medial

67.23A. muscle tone; posterior; cerebellum

67.24A.

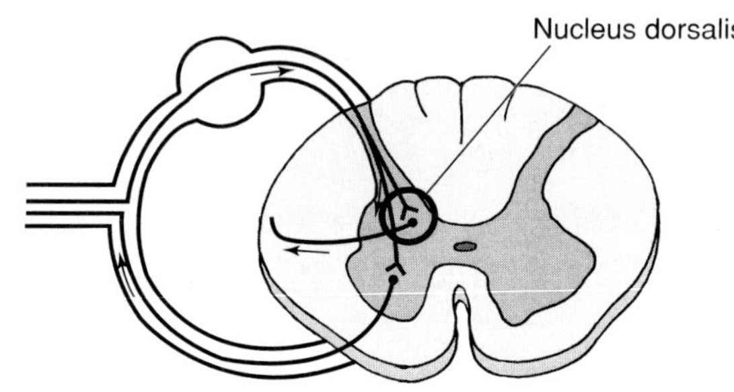

67.25A. cerebellum; anterior; two

67.26A. stretches; muscle

67.27A. posterior; spinocerebellar; ipsilateral

67.28A.

Tract	Mediate Impulses Concerned with:	Axons Arise from Cell Bodies on Which Side: Left, Right, or Both?	Cell Bodies Located in:
Right lateral spinothalamic	pain and temperature	left	posterior horn
Right anterior spinothalamic	touch and pressure	both	posterior horn
Right posterior white columns	position	right	spinal ganglia
Left spinocerebellar	muscle tone	left	n. dorsalis

67.29. The *lateral* funiculus contains one large *eff*erent tract, the ___________ ________________ tract, which receives blood from the ___________ ________________ artery. It also contains two main groups of afferent tracts, the spinocerebellar tracts and the ___________ ________________ tract. All of which receive blood from the ___________ ___________ artery.

67.30. A lesion interrupting all fibers in both *anterior* (white) funiculi of the spinal cord at C4 would not destroy touch sensation because ascending fibers are still intact in the ___________ columns. Are the lateral corticospinal tracts still intact? _____ Would involuntary control of limb movements be retained? _____

67.31. The ___________ corticospinal tract crosses the midline in the decussation of the pyramids. The structure in which the anterior corticospinal tract crosses the midline is the ___________ ________________ of the cord. The axons of the left lateral corticospinal tract arise mainly in neurons on the _____ side of the ___________ *lobe* of the cerebral cortex. Axons of the left *anterior* corticospinal tract arise in cell bodies on the _____ side of the brain.

67.32. Label the structures indicated.

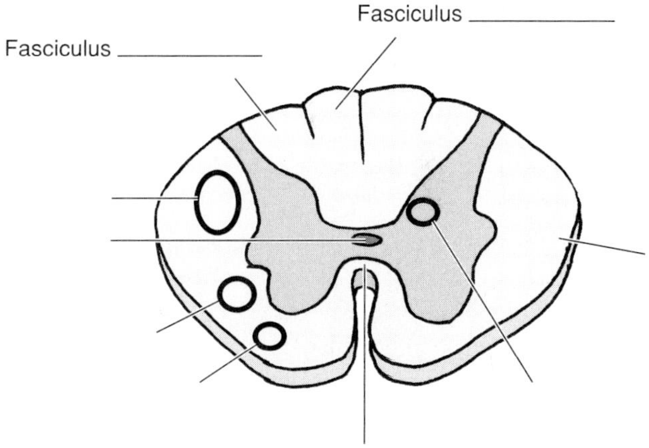

Fasciculus ___________

Fasciculus ___________

67.33. Complete the table.

	Tissues in Which Impulses Arise	First Synapse in	Impulses Ascend Spinal Cord
_____sense	___________	nuclei gracilis and cuneatus of medulla	___________ ___________ ___________ ___________ of ___________ columns
___________ tone	___________ and ___________	___________ ___________	___________ tracts

67.29A. lateral corticospinal; anterior spinal; lateral spinothalamic; anterior spinal

67.30A. posterior; Yes; Yes

67.31A. lateral; anterior commissure; right; frontal; left

67.32A.

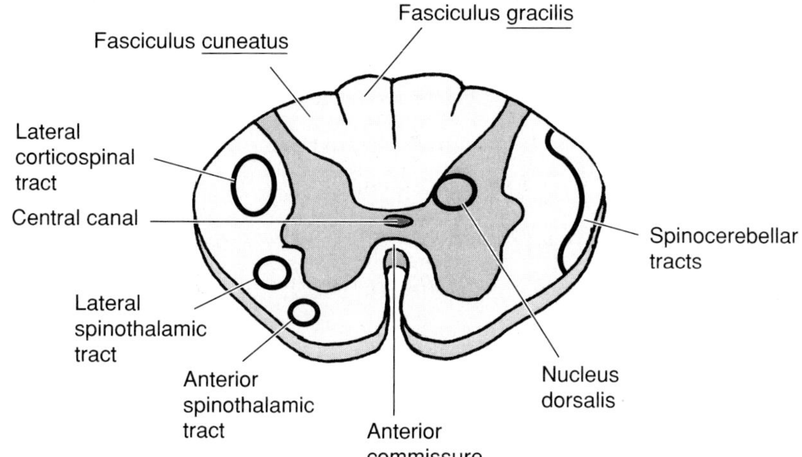

67.33A.

	Tissues in Which Impulses Arise	**First Synapse in**	**Impulses Ascend Spinal Cord**
joint sense	joints	nuclei gracilis and cuneatus of medulla	fasciculus gracilis and fasciculus cuneatus of posterior columns
muscle tone	muscles and tendons	nucleus dorsalis	spinocerebellar tracts

68 Reflexes as Indications of Motor Disease

68.1. Sensory nerve fibers in muscle are activated when a specific type of muscle fiber is stretched. The sensory receptor is called a ______tch receptor.

68.2. Stretch receptors generate impulses when they are mechanically deformed. One of the simplest relations between sensory and motor systems is demonstrated by the knee jerk reflex. The number of neurons involved is ______; one neuron is afferent and the other ____________.

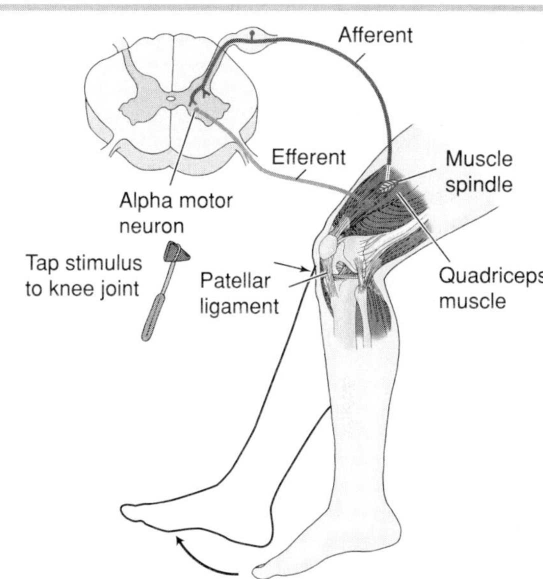

68.3. When the patellar tendon at the knee is struck, the leg jerks forward (extends at the knee); this reflex is called the knee ______. Similarly, when the Achilles tendon behind the ankle is struck, the foot extends (plantarflexes); this reflex is commonly called the ______ jerk.

68.4. Stretch receptors are ordinarily fired when muscle is made to contract by efferent nerve stimulation, not when a reflex hammer is used to tap on a ____________.

68.5. The nucleus pulposis of the intervertebral disk may rupture out and press against nerve roots—a ruptured disc. When nerve roots are damaged in this way, stretch reflexes may be diminished. A ruptured disc at the level indicated would cause pain radiating down the back of one lower limb (sciatica) and loss of the ______ jerk.

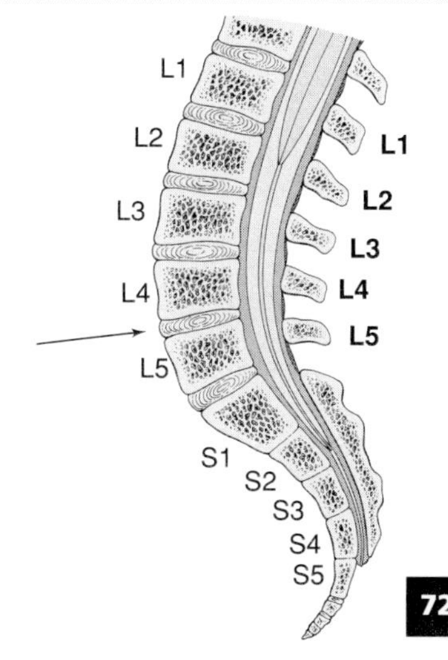

68.1A. stretch

68.2A. 2; efferent

68.3A. jerk; ankle

68.4A. tendon

68.5A. ankle

68.6. A certain amount of activity or tension normally persists in muscle at all times. The amount of tension reflects the net balance of firing in muscle afferents and efferents. In other words, muscle tone (tension) is determined largely by net activity in str______ reflex circuits.

68.7. The persistent state of tension in muscle, determined largely by fiber systems that influence the activity of __________ reflexes, is designated as muscle t______.

68.8. Corticospinal impulses normally inhibit muscle tone. Increased muscle tone is accompanied by increased activity of stretch reflexes. A patient with a stroke usually shows impaired voluntary movement, plus ______creased muscle tone and ______creased stretch reflexes. If the lesion is on one side of the brain above the decussation of the pyramids, the abnormalities are found in the limbs on the ________________ side.

68.9. Increased tone in muscles of the leg is accompanied by increased tendon reflexes. Both phenomena are consequences of lesions in the ________________ tract.

68.10. Abnormally increased resistance to passive movement of a limb reflects increased muscle ______. Tendon reflexes in the same limb would be ______er than normal.

68.11. A state of decreased reflex activity is referred to as a hyporeflexia. A state of increased reflexes is referred to as ______reflexia. Corticospinal tract lesions result in __________ muscle tone and __________flexia.

68.12. The alternate and repeated contraction of antagonist muscles is called clonus. An example of cl______ is a result of alternate contractions of __________ and flexor muscles around the knee joint. The presence of clonus indicates a change in the normal regulation of stretch reflex activity in the direction of hyp______activity.

68.13. The clinical term spasticity describes the combination of increased muscle tone and ______reflexia. Spasticity may also be expressed by the phenomenon called __________.

68.6A. stretch

68.7A. stretch; tone

68.8A. increased; increased; contralateral

68.9A. corticospinal

68.10A. tone; greater

68.11A. hyperreflexia; increased; hyperreflexia

68.12A. clonus; extensor; hyperactivity

68.13A. hyperreflexia; clonus

68.14. Three signs of corticospinal tract damage are ______creased muscle tone, ______reflexia, and cl______. These are summed up in the term __________ity.

68.15. Flaccidity is the opposite of ______________. A flaccid limb shows __________ muscle tone and ______reflexia. Absence of activity in stretch reflexes is detectable as __________ity.

68.16. Draw lines between the two columns to pair the appropriate items:

flaccidity	internal capsule lesion
spasticity	anterior root lesion

68.17. The cell body of the upper motor neuron is in the brain, somewhere above the foramen __________. The cell body of the lower motor neuron is likely to be in the __________ horn of the __________ ______. Spasticity is a clinical sign of damage to the axon of the ______er motor neuron. Does the damage produce loss of reflex movements? ______

68.18. A patient with a severe lesion of the left pyramidal tract in the medulla cannot voluntarily move his ______ arm and leg. However, even reflex movements are lost after lesions of cell bodies or axons of ______ motor neurons.

68.19. After each item, place a "W" for white matter or a "G" for gray matter:

Anterior horn: ______	Anterior corticospinal tract: ______
Posterior horn: ______	Intermediolateral cell column: ______
Lateral corticospinal tract: ______	Internal capsule: ______

68.20. Spasticity in the left leg, with normal stretch reflex activity in the arms, strongly suggests the presence of a lesion in the ______ matter at the __________ level of the spinal cord on the ________________ side.

68.21. The most important and useful reflex sign of corticospinal damage is called, in honor of the Polish neurologist who described it, the ______ski sign.

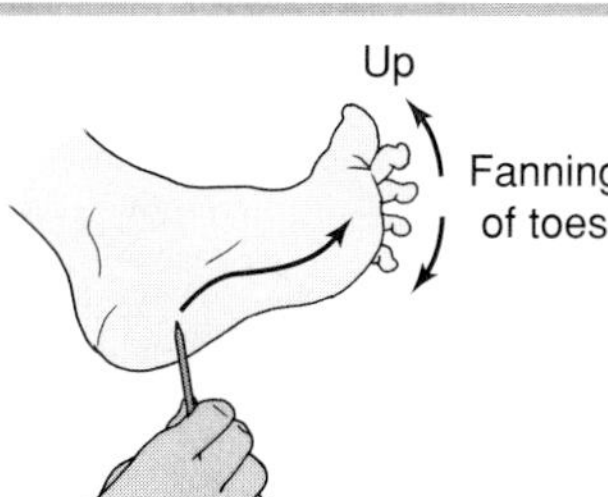

68.14A. increased; hyperreflexia; clonus; spasticity

68.15A. spasticity; decreased; hyporeflexia; flaccidity

68.16A.

flaccidity — anterior root lesion
spasticity — internal capsule lesion

68.17A. magnum; anterior; spinal cord; upper; No

68.18A. right; lower

68.19A. G; G; W; W; G; W

68.20A. white; thoracic; ipsilateral

68.21A. Babinski

68.22. The normal adult response when the outer border of the foot is stroked with a blunt instrument, is downward (plantar) flexion of all the toes. In the B__________ sign, the four outer toes spread apart, and the big toe moves ______ward.

68.23. A positive Babinski sign involves dorsiflexion of the big toe. Dorsiflexion describes ______ward movement of the big toe.

68.24. The normal infant in the first few months after birth shows a positive Babinski sign. But after the ________________ tract matures and establishes its normal functional contacts, stroking of the outer border of the foot leads to ______ward flexion of the toes, toward the plantar surface of the foot. The normal adult response is p__________ flexion.

68.25. After a lesion of the lateral corticospinal tract at T6 on the right side of the cord, dorsiflexion of the big toe is found on stroking the outer border of the ______ foot. Tendon reflexes are __________ in the right arm, __________ in the left leg, and __________ in the right leg.

68.26. You have traced the corticospinal system from the cortex to muscle, starting with the giant ______ cells in the precentral gyrus and ending with a nerve–muscle combination called a ______ ______. The initial neuron of the chain always terminates in the ________________ side of the spinal cord. After passing through the three brainstem levels—consecutively, the __________, ______, and __________—70–90% of the corticospinal fibers cross in the __________ ________________ and travel down the cord in the __________ corticospinal tract. The other 10–30% travel down in the __________ corticospinal tract and cross over in the __________ ________________ of the spinal cord.

68.27. The number of corticospinal fibers within the cord is greatest in the segments of the __________ level and least in the __________ segments. Most corticospinal fibers synapse in the __________ horn of the cord. Sensory fibers enter the cord via the __________ root. Sympathetic nerve cell bodies lie between the anterior and posterior horns, in the ________________ cell column, at the __________ and __________ cord levels; their axons leave the cord via the __________ nerve roots.

68.22A. Babinski; upward

68.23A. upward

68.24A. corticospinal; downward; plantar

68.25A. right; normal; normal; increased

68.26A. Betz; motor unit; contralateral; midbrain; pons; medulla; pyramidal decussation; lateral; anterior; anterior commissure

68.27A. cervical; sacral; anterior; posterior; intermediolateral; thoracic; lumbar; anterior

69 The Sympathetic Nervous System in the Spinal Cord

69.1. Presynaptic sympathetic cell bodies occupy the ________________ cell column in the lumbar and ___________ segments of the spinal cord.

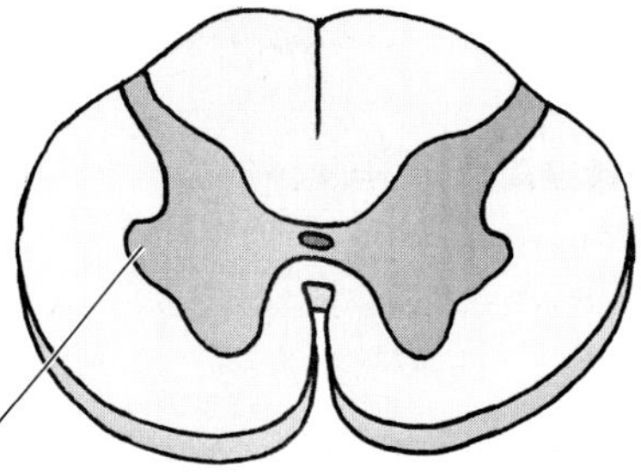

Intermediolateral cell column

69.2. On the diagram, label the intermediolateral cell column, which lies intermediate between the anterior and posterior columns of gray matter. The sympathetic division of the nervous system is sometimes called the _____aco_____ar system due to its location in the thoracic and lumbar regions of the cord.

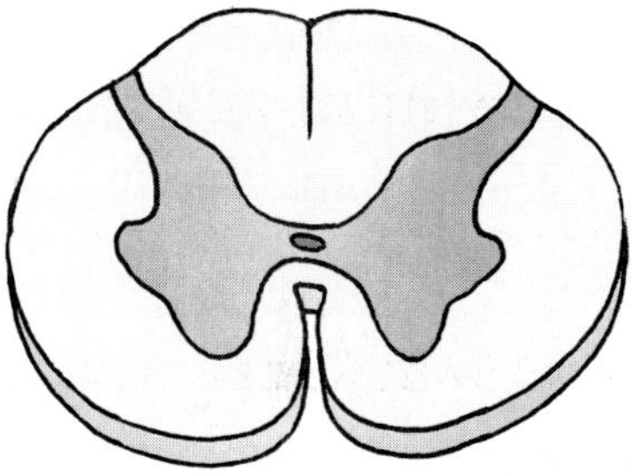

69.3. The intermediolateral cell column is found only in the _____ matter of the ___________ and ___________ segments of the cord. It is a column of cells belonging to the ________________ system.

69.4. Sympathetic neurons, like the anterior horn cells, conduct _____fferent impulses.

69.5. The final common path for all efferent neurons of the cord is the ___________ root. On the left side of the cord, draw one anterior horn cell body supplying hip muscle, one sympathetic nerve cell body, and the axons of both cells in the appropriate root.

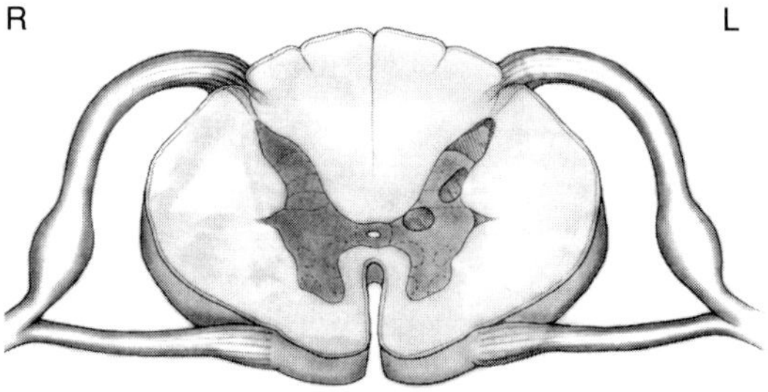

R L

69.1A. intermediolateral; thoracic

69.2A. thoracolumbar

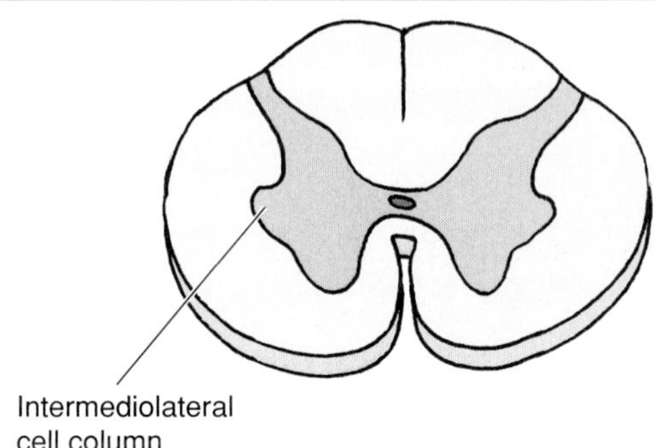

69.3A. gray; thoracic; lumbar; sympathetic

69.4A. efferent

69.5A. anterior

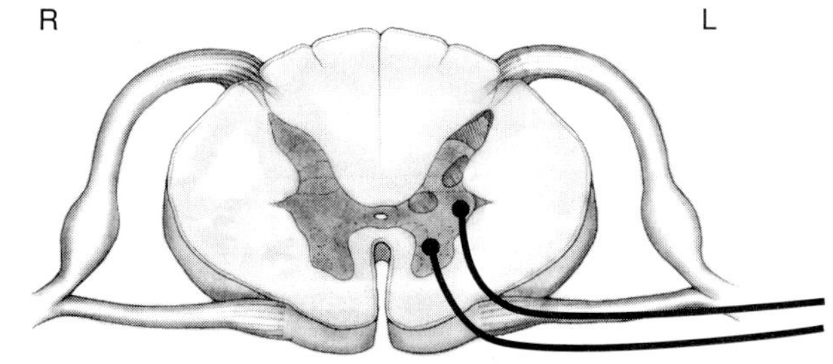

69.6. As the picture shows, the axon of the presynaptic sympathetic neuron makes synaptic contact with postsynaptic sympathetic neurons in the ________________ ____________. In the efferent chain of sympathetic neurons, the one that precedes the ganglion is called the ______synaptic neuron, and the one with an axon leaving the ganglion is the ________________ neuron.

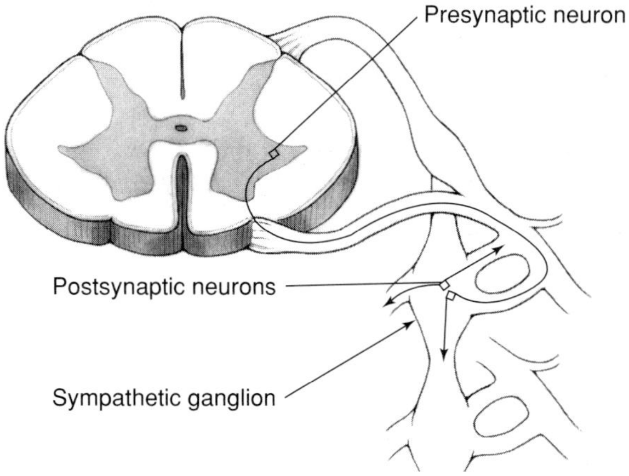

Presynaptic neuron

Postsynaptic neurons

Sympathetic ganglion

69.7. In the sympathetic system, the ______synaptic neuron cell body is in the ________________ cell column of the __________ and __________ segments of the spinal cord.

69.8. Label the cord levels. Place an "F" on cell bodies that directly innervate muscles of the fingers, and place an "S" on the sympathetic nerve cell bodies.

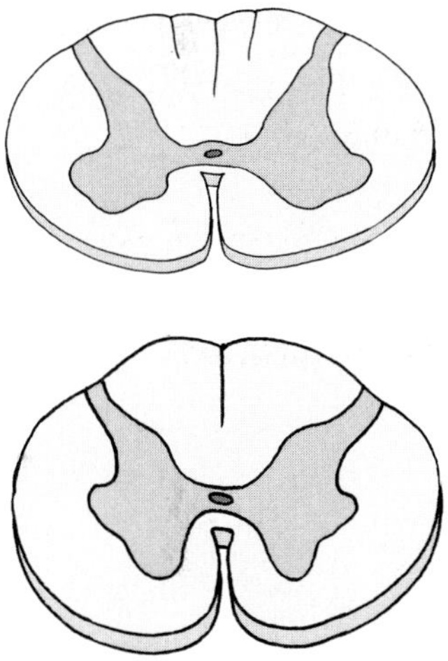

69.9. Several efferent tracts have cell bodies in the brainstem and run from the brainstem to the spinal cord. The encircled tracts arise in vestibular neurons of the medulla and are called the left and right ______ibulo__________ tracts.

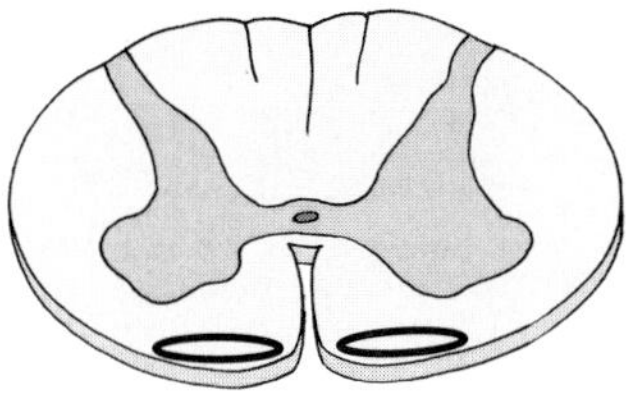

69.6A. sympathetic ganglion; presynaptic; postsynaptic

69.7A. presynaptic; intermediolateral; thoracic; lumbar

69.8A.

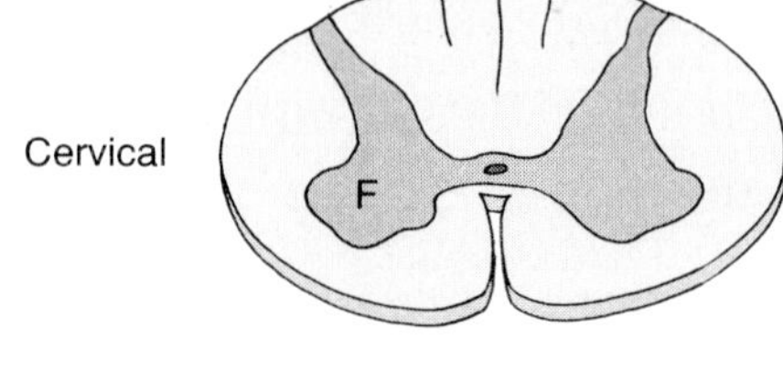

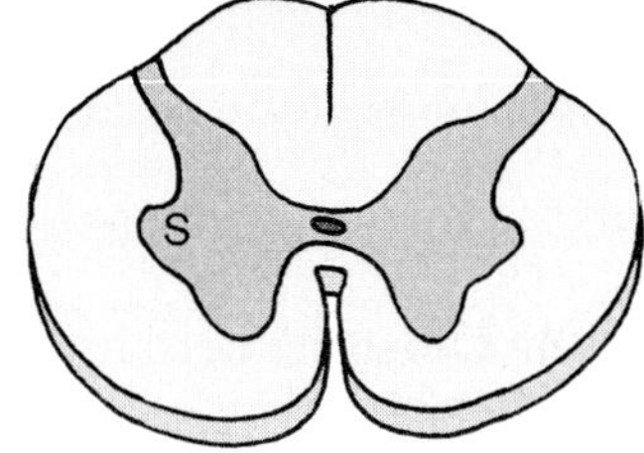

69.9A. vestibulospinal

69.10. Motor control is effected mainly via the cortico__________ system. Most fibers in this system cross the midline in the ______________ of the pyramids.

69.11. Complete the labels on the diagram.

69.12. On the sections, encircle and label, where appropriate, the right lateral corticospinal tract, left anterior corticospinal tract, and left intermediolateral cell column.

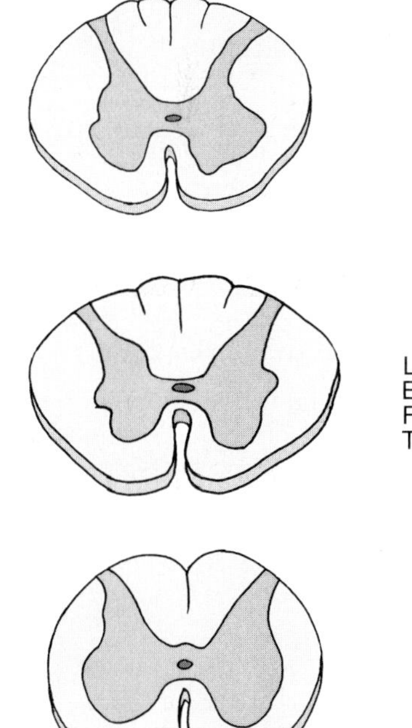

69.10A. corticospinal; decussation

69.11A.

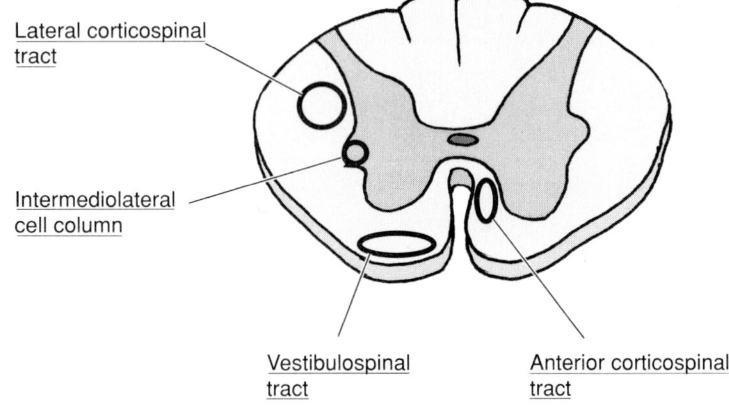

69.12A.

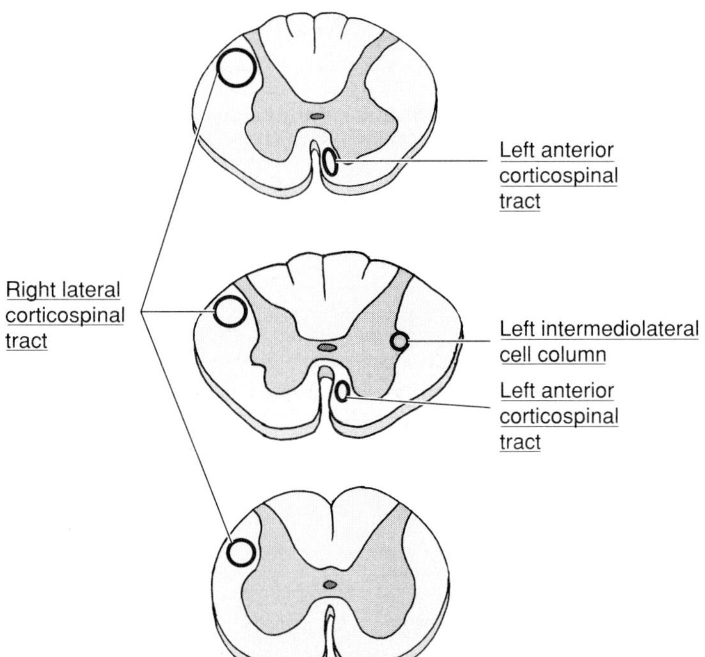

70 Review of Spinal Pathways: Clinical Examples

70.1. The axon is a specialized cytoplasmic process of the nerve cell. Survival of the axon depends on the continuous reception of materials from the trophic center of the cell—the cell body. If the cell body is destroyed, the axon will ______. The part of the axon most distant from the cell body shown in the picture is marked with the letter ______. If the axon is damaged at point "B," the segment of axon between "A" and "B" may survive, but the portion distal to "B" (between "B" and "C") is isolated from vital nutrients. Will the segment between "B" and "C" survive? ______

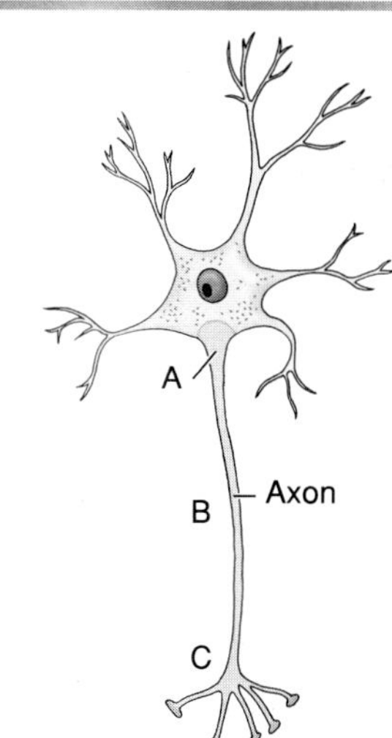

70.2. The myelin sheath is composed of sheets of Schwann cell (in peripheral nerve) or oligodendroglia (in CNS) surface membrane wrapped concentrically around the ______.

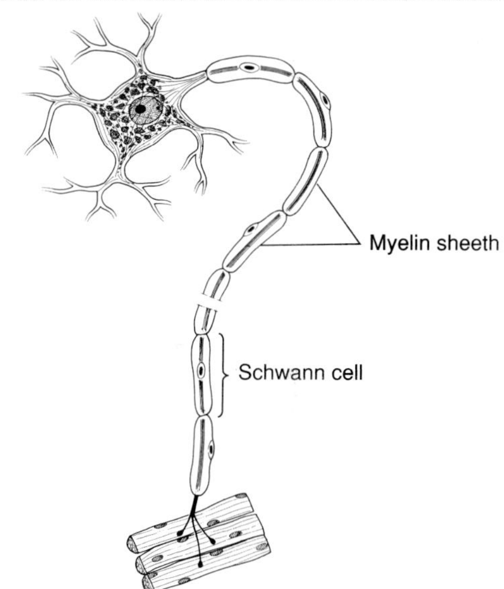

70.3. Even though myelin is part of the ____________ cell (in the peripheral nervous system) or the ______dendroglia (in the CNS) and is not directly part of the neuron, myelin is not maintained when the axon enclosed within it degenerates. Place a series of "X"s on the parts of this branched myelinated axon that degenerates following an injury at the arrow.

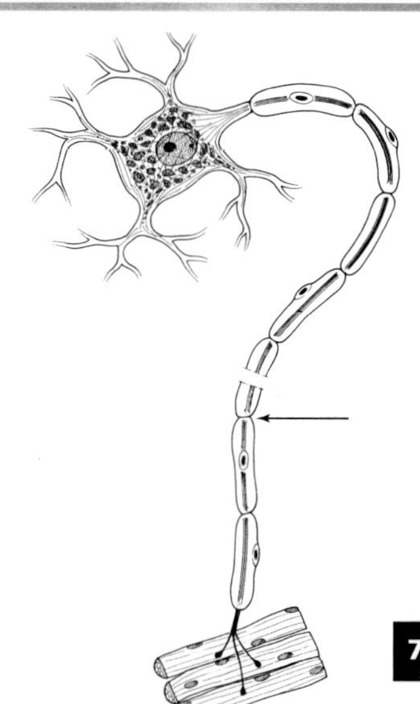

70.1A. die; C; No

70.2A. axon

70.3A. Schwann; oligodendroglia

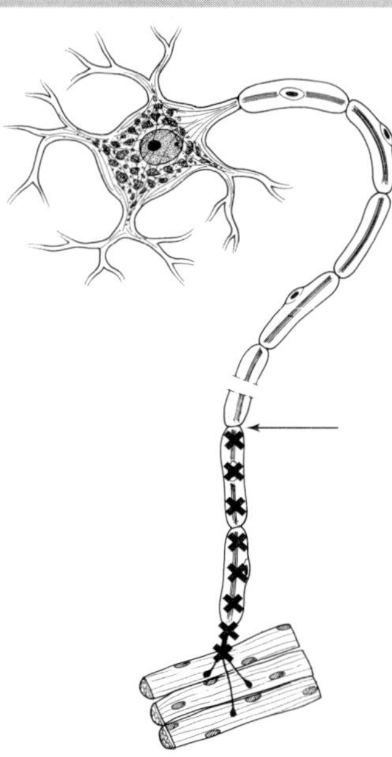

70.4. In order to cut off part of a myelinated axon from its trophic center, the damage must be between the site showing loss of myelin and the cell ______.

70.5. Nerve fibers are not continuous across a synapse. Look at "X," "A," and "B" on the diagram. A lesion at "X" will produce nerve (Wallerian) degeneration at ______.

Neuron 1
X
B
Synapse
Neuron 2
A

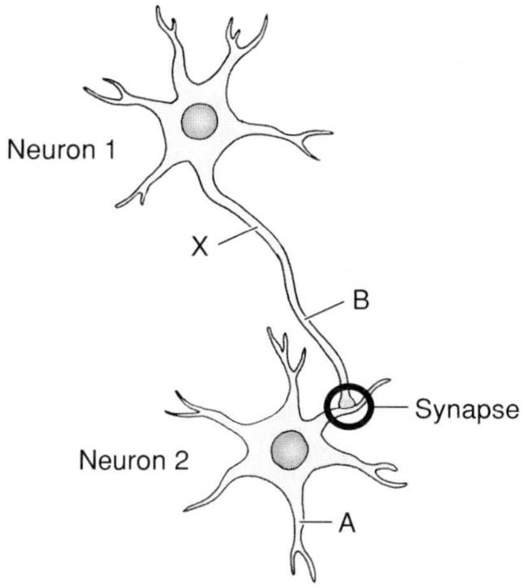

70.6. Many secondary afferent axons pass all the way from the spinal cord to the thalamus without synapsing. If such axons are damaged, they show __________ degeneration from the site of injury up to the __________. Wallerian degeneration is a well-described sequelae of events and characteristics in nerve degeneration.

70.7. Hemisection means transection of the left or right half of the spinal cord. After hemisection of the cord, Wallerian degeneration is located in motor tracts ______ the lesion and in sensory tracts ______ the lesion.

70.8. Sensory fibers innervating the leg enter the spinal cord at lumbar levels. The lumbar segments lie just below the __________ segments and just above the __________ segments. A soldier's spinal cord was completely transected at T10 by a shell fragment. He died 4 months later. Sections of his spinal cord showed Wallerian degeneration at L4 in all __________ tracts and at C4 in all __________ tracts.

70.9. In humans, motor control is effected mainly via the cortico__________ system. Most fibers in this system cross the midline in the ________________ of the pyramids.

70.10. A large lesion in the left parietal lobe, left side of the thalamus, or left side at almost any brain-stem level impairs sensation in the limbs and trunk on the ______ side.

70.4A. body

70.5A. B

70.6A. Wallerian; synapse

70.7A. below; above

70.8A. thoracic; sacral; efferent; afferent

70.9A. corticospinal; decussation

70.10A. right

70.11. Following a complete cord transection at T10, the patient was anesthetic (loss of all sensation) in dermatomes supplied by cord segments beginning at or slightly below the injury. Draw crosshatch lines across the anesthetic skin on the diagram.

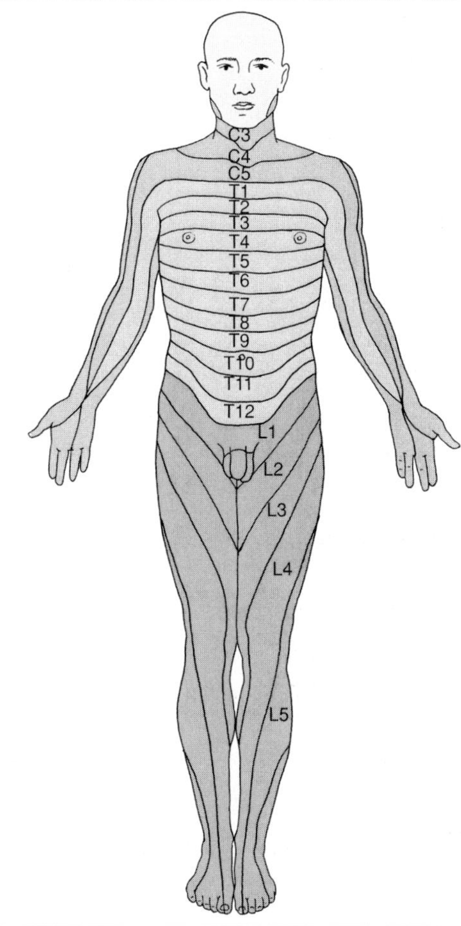

70.12. In terms of clinical testing, it is customary to speak of "pain and temperature" sense. Generally, a spinal cord lesion affecting the sense of pain will also affect ______ and ______ sensations. In one sentence or phrase explain why this is so.

____

70.13. The secondary neurons in the pain and temperature pathway have cell bodies in the ____________ horn on the ______ side as the primary neuron. The axons of the secondary neurons ascend a segment or two while they are crossing in the ____________ ________________ of the cord, and then these axons enter the ____________ ________________ tract. Thus, transection of this tract on the left side of the cord at T6 abolishes pain and temperature sensibility in skin innervated from about T7/T8 and below, on the ______ side.

70.14. The lesion crosshatched on the diagram would abolish pain and temperature sense beginning one or two segments below the lesion on the ________________ side of the body.

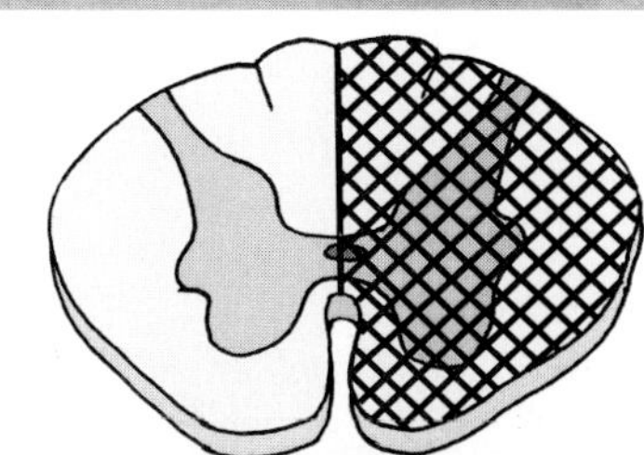

70.11A.

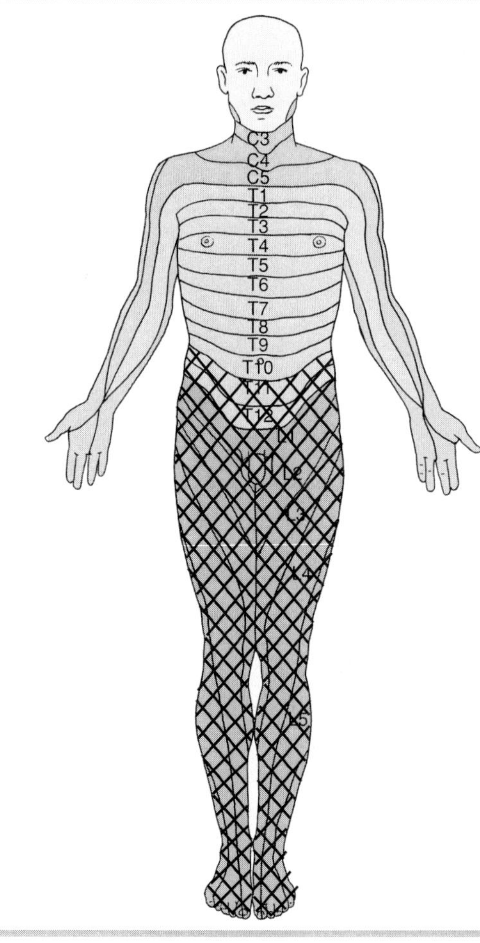

70.12A. hot; cold; They ascend the cord in the same tract—the lateral spinothalamic tract.

70.13A. posterior; same; anterior commissure; lateral spinothalamic; right

70.14A. contralateral

70.15. A patient was found to have lost sensitivity to pain, heat, and cold in his entire left leg, as indicated by the crosshatching on the diagram. His lesion was probably located about one spinal cord segment higher at L_____, on the _____ side of the cord.

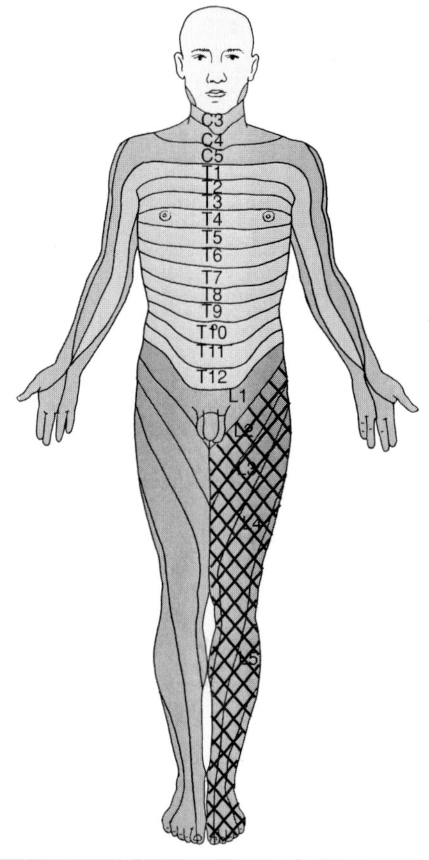

70.16. Analgesia means loss of pain sensation. Anesthesia means loss of all sensation. A patient with complete cord transection at T4 has lost _____ sensation below the level of the nipples. The patient is __________ic below the transection. A patient with hemisection of the cord at T10 on the left side is an______ic and has loss of temperature sense below the __________ (name the body part) on the _____ side.

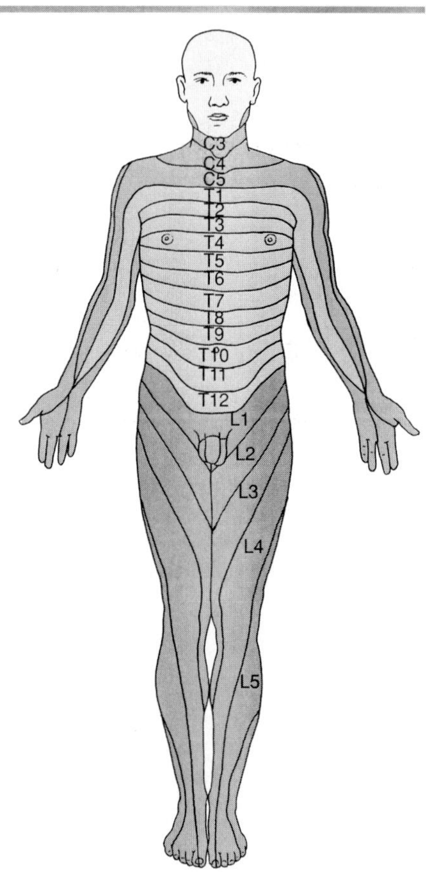

70.15A. L1; right

70.16A. all; anesthetic; analgesic; umbilicus; right

70.17. The prefix hypo means diminished, reduced, or under. The "o" may be omitted. For example, diminished pain sensibility is called ______algesia.

70.18. Hypalgesia means diminished sensibility to ______. Analgesia means absent sensibility to ______. Hypesthesia means ____________ sensibility to all somesthetic modalities. Anesthesia means ________ sensibility to all ________ modalities.

70.19. Anesthesia is produced by complete transection of the cord or, in the peripheral nervous system, by complete transection of a nerve. In the former case, anesthesia is found in all parts of the body ______ the level of the transection. Anesthesia in a restricted part of the body would more likely reflect severe disease localized to a ______.

70.20. Sensibility to touch in a given part of the body is influenced by impulses in widely separated parts of the cord—the left and right ________ ____________ tracts and the ipsilateral (same side as receptor) ________ column. Therefore, a spinal lesion causing complete loss of touch would have to be very ______ in size and would have to involve ______ sides of the cord.

70.21. According to the diagram, a lesion in the posterior columns of white matter in the cord impairs ________ ______ but does not affect the sense of ______.

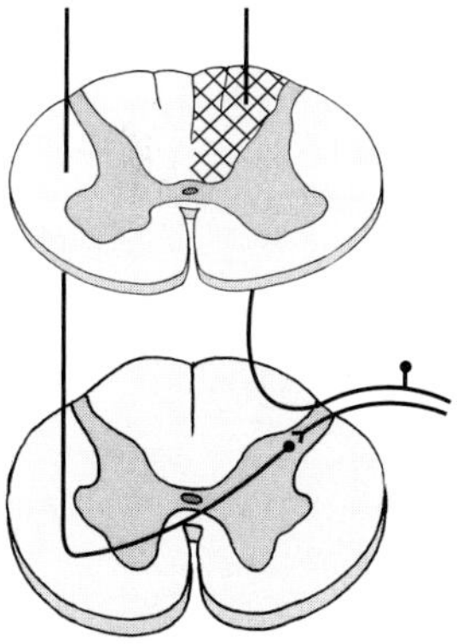

70.22. A lesion in the posterior columns of the spinal cord on the right side impairs ________ sense on the ______ side but spares the other modality whose pathway is diagrammed, ______ sense. A lesion at "X" would impair ______ modalities in the ______ leg.

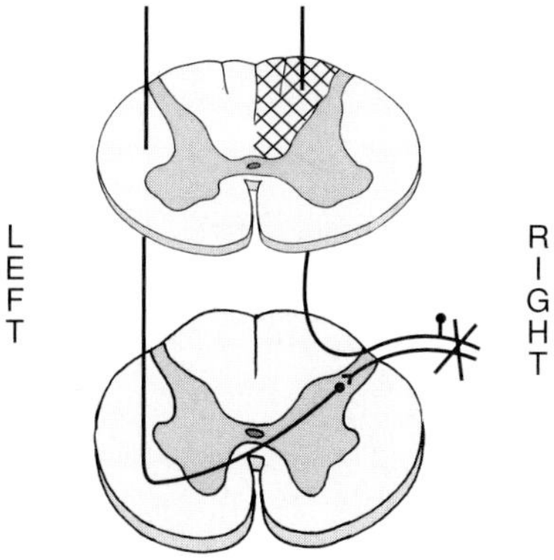

LEFT

RIGHT

70.17A. hypalgesia

70.18A. pain; pain; diminished; absent; sensory

70.19A. below; nerve

70.20A. anterior spinothalamic; posterior; large; both

70.21A. position sense; pain

70.22A. position; right; pain (or temperature); both; right

70.23. Impulses mediating kinesthetic sense in the whole left lower limb are cut off by a lesion in the fasciculus ___________ on the _____ side. This impairment would result from such a lesion at any level of the spinal cord above the ___________ segments.

70.24. Wallerian degeneration is confined to the myelinated part of the injured neuron beyond the site of the injury; it does not extend across synapses. If afferent fibers are interrupted as they ascend the cord, Wallerian degeneration will occur at all levels _____ the point of interruption, until a ___________ is reached. Following section of a posterior root (between ganglion cell bodies and spinal cord), Wallerian degeneration is seen in the posterior columns on the _____ side but not in the spino___________ and _____cerebellar tracts because these tracts contain axons of ___________ary neurons, whereas the lesion affected _____ary neurons.

70.25. If the left fasciculus gracilis fails to stain in myelin preparation at C8 but stains normally at T12, the disorder must lie in the ___________ segments of the cord on the _____ side.

70.26. Draw an axon of the thoracic spinal ganglion cell from point "A," through the posterior columns (fasciculus ___________), upward to point "B." Suppose that a disease causes inflammation and destructive damage at point "A." Place a series of "X"s on the part of the diagrammed neuron that shows Wallerian degeneration.

B

A

70.27. Wallerian degeneration at a given spinal cord level in a descending (efferent) tract indicates disease at a _____er level of the cord or brain. Wallerian degeneration in an ascending (afferent) tract indicates disease at a _____er level of the cord.

70.28. The large amount of _____ matter relative to _____ matter shows that this section is at a high ___________ level. The posterior roots in this patient are affected at the lumbar level bilaterally and at no other level. Encircle and crosshatch the fiber bundles that ought to show Wallerian degeneration.

70.23A. gracilis; left; lumbar

70.24A. above; synapse; same; spinothalamic; spinocerebellar; secondary; primary

70.25A. thoracic; left

70.26A. gracilis

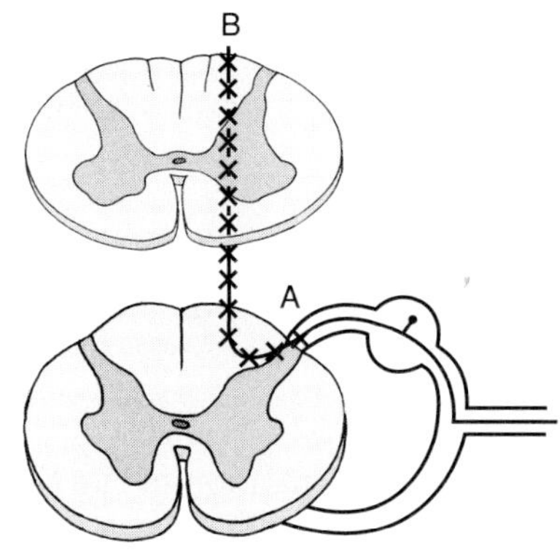

70.27A. higher; lower

70.28A. white; gray; cervical

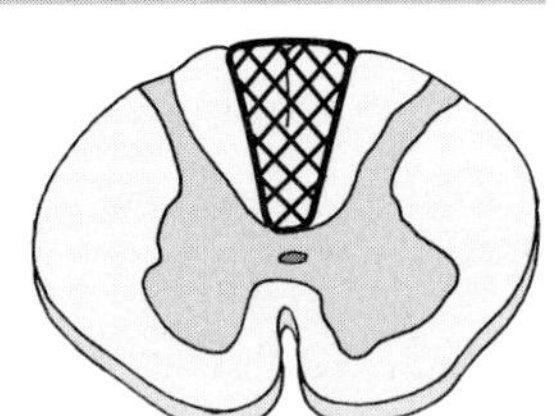

71 Review of Spinal Pathways: Further Clinical Examples

71.1. The somesthetic senses have been classified into five modalities: ______, ________________, ______, ____________, and ____________ sense.

71.2. Draw lines from items in the center column to appropriate items in the other columns. (An item may be used once, more than once, or not at all).

	Touch	
Posterior white columns	Pressure	Anterior spinothalamic tract
	Joint sense	
Spinocerebellar tracts	Pain	Lateral spinothalamic tract
	Temperature	

71.3. Label the tracts indicated on the diagram.

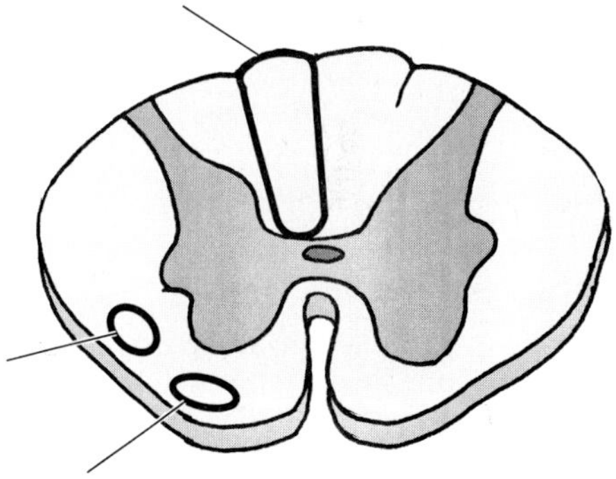

71.4. Information about touch and pressure is said to be conveyed bilaterally in the ____________ ____________________ tracts and ipsilaterally (on the ______ side as the stimulus) in the ____________ ____________. A single cord lesion smaller than a hemisection is unlikely to cause complete loss of touch sensation below the level of the lesion because information about touch is conveyed along (complete the sentence in a few words)____.

71.5. Lesions of the posterior (dorsal) columns do not abolish the sense of touch but do impair some of its qualities. Patients with such lesions have difficulty recognizing exactly where they are being touched or with what. Similarly altered is the sense of ____________, whereas ____________ sense may be severely diminished or absent.

71.6. Recognition of the location of touch or pressure stimulus, the size of the skin area stimulated, the stimulating material, etc., is summarized in the terms discriminative or fine touch. Information about these qualities is conveyed in the ____________ ____________.

71.1A. pain; temperature; touch; pressure; position

71.2A.

Posterior white columns — Touch, Pressure, Joint sense

Anterior spinothalamic tract — Touch, Pressure

Spinocerebellar tracts

Lateral spinothalamic tract — Pain, Temperature

71.3A.

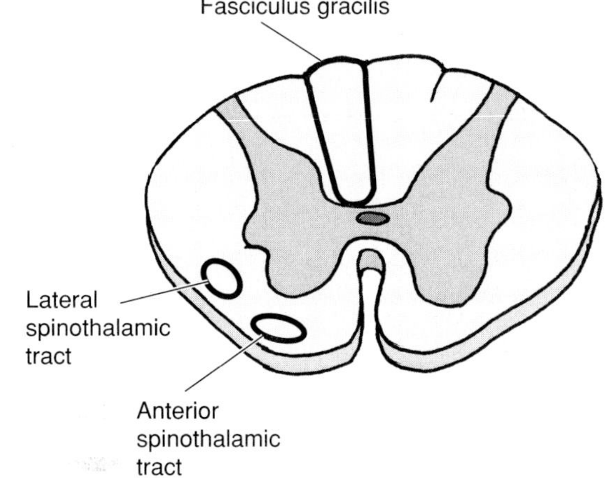

71.4A. anterior spinothalamic; same; posterior (or dorsal) columns; widely separated pathways

71.5A. pressure; position

71.6A. posterior (or dorsal) columns

71.7. A patient with tabes dorsalis (a form of syphilis of the nervous system) recognized neither the vibrations of a tuning fork placed on his legs or feet nor the positions of his toes when the examiner moved them. He had good motor power in his legs and feet. Pain, temperature, and some touch sensation were present. Where in the spinal cord white matter would one expect to find degenerated fibers? ________ ________

71.8. A patient with pernicious anemia (vitamin B_{12} deficiency) was found to have: 1) impaired position (conscious proprioceptive) and vibratory sense, and 2) mild spasticity of the limbs and a positive Babinski sign. This central nervous system disease affects: 1) a sensory system in the ________ ________, and 2) a ______ system in the nearby lateral columns—the ________ ________ tract.

71.9. Patients with tabes dorsalis or with vitamin B_{12} deficiency may have similar sensory deficits, the former because of disease ______side the CNS, in the posterior ______, and the latter because of disease ______side the CNS, in the ________ ______ ________ of the spinal cord.

71.10. A lower motor neuron has its cell body in the ________ horn of the cord. The motor tracts descending through the cord contain axons of the ______er motor neurons.

71.11. Lateral corticospinal fibers are axons of upper motor neurons. When they are damaged, the patient has spastic weakness of the limbs below the level of the injury. Deep tendon reflexes (stretch reflexes) in the affected limbs are ______creased. Upper motor neuron lesions produce weakness (or paralysis) and ________ of the limbs. Lower motor neuron lesions produce muscle atrophy, flaccidity, and ________.

71.12. Damage involving the right lateral corticospinal tract causes increased reflexes and spastic weakness in the ________ lower limb. The same disorder in the same leg would be caused by damage to the pyramidal tract on the ________ side of the rostral medulla.

71.13. In addition to its effect on long tracts in the white matter, a hemisection is likely to destroy some lower motor neurons located at the site of the lesion. The signs would be flaccid tone, ________, and ________ of some muscles.

71.7A. Posterior (or dorsal) columns

71.8A. posterior (or dorsal) columns; motor; lateral corticospinal

71.9A. outside; roots; inside; posterior white columns

71.10A. anterior; upper

71.11A. increased; spasticity; weakness

71.12A. ipsilateral; contralateral

71.13A. weakness; atrophy

71.14. The patient with a left hemisection at T10 shows spasticity, or ______creased deep tendon (stretch) reflexes, in the left leg. When the lateral edge of the sole of the left foot is stroked, the great toe dorsiflexes, and the other toes fan out, demonstrating a positive ____________ sign.

71.15. The anterior corticospinal tract has no influence on motor function detectable by ordinary clinical methods. A patient with a left hemisection at C8 has spastic paralysis of the ______ leg. Motor function in the right leg is ____________.

71.16. The indicated lesion, drawn with crossed lines, involves the area of the central canal. The lesion transects the ____________ ____________________ of the cord and interrupts all fibers carrying information about ______ and ____________________ senses.

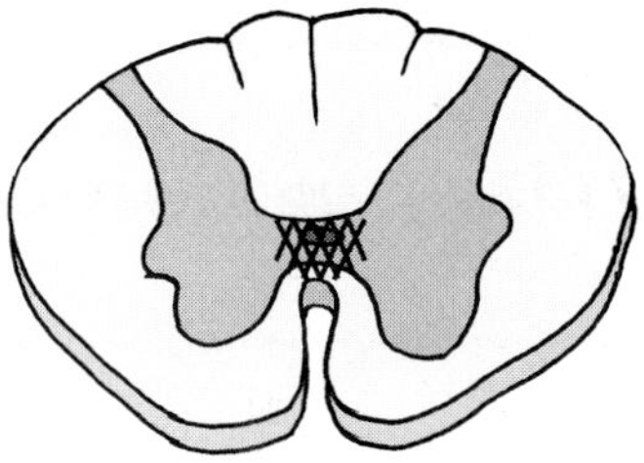

71.17. The lesion drawn affects pain and temperature but only over one or a few dermatomes in the ______er limbs. Information about these sensations from lower bodily levels continues to be transmitted normally in the intact ____________ ____________________ tracts.

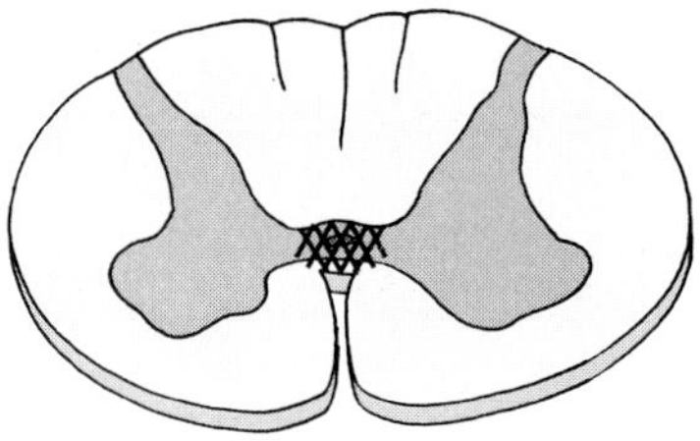

71.18. A man repeatedly burned his fingers on both hands while cooking because he seemed not to recognize when the pots were too hot to handle. His fingers were not painful even though they were injured enough to be badly scarred. He had no other symptoms. Place an "X" at the one possible site for his lesion on the diagram.

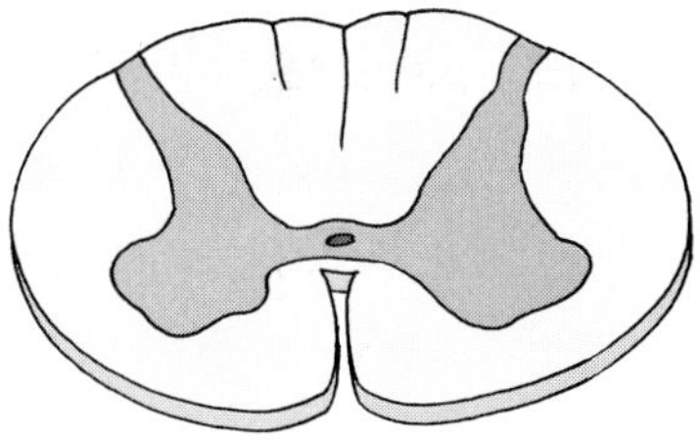

71.19. The man's disease is called syringomyelia; it begins with destruction of spinal cord tissue around the central ______ and spreads irregularly outward. Pain and temperature senses were unaffected below the arms because the ____________ ____________________ tract, transmitting impulses from lower levels, was intact bilaterally. Circle the approximate position of this tract bilaterally.

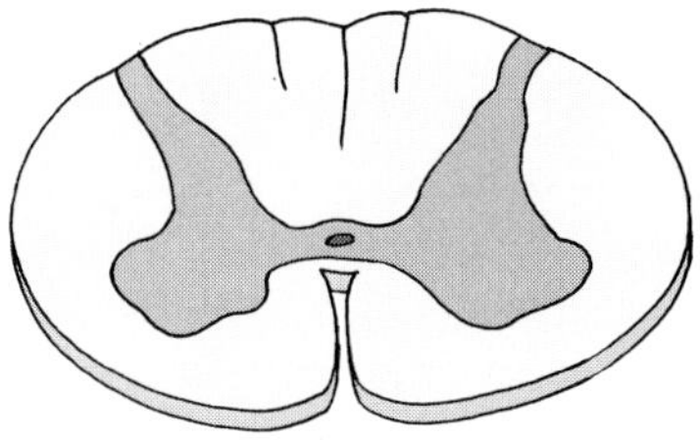

71.14A. increased; Babinski

71.15A. left; normal

71.16A. anterior commissure; pain; temperature

71.17A. upper; lateral spinothalamic

71.18A.

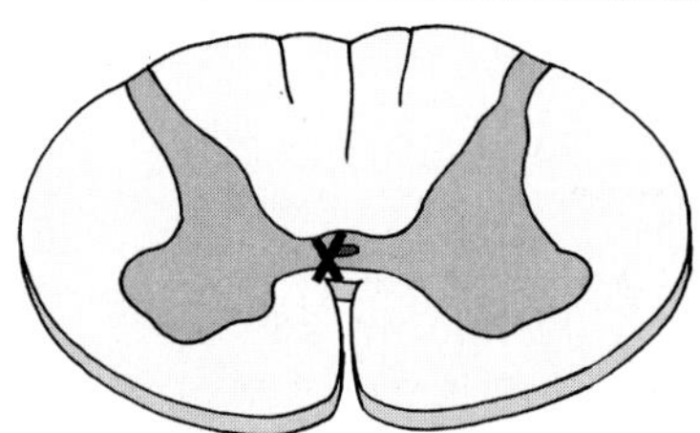

71.19A. canal; lateral spinothalamic

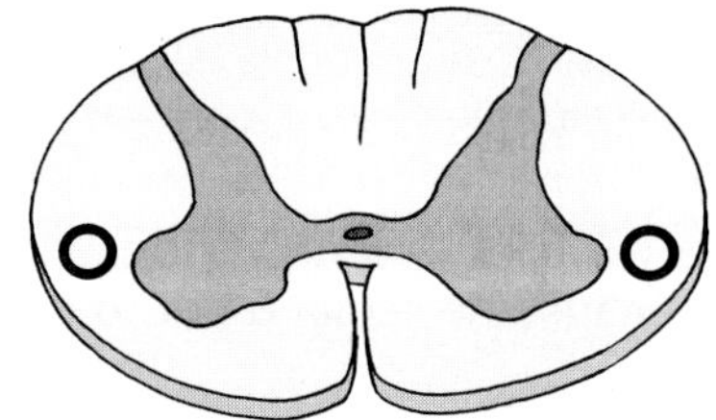

71.20. A single small lesion causing loss of pain and temperature sense bilaterally in the territory of one or a few segments probably involves fibers located in the __________ ________________ of the cord, near the central canal.

71.21. When all tissue elements are destroyed in a region of the central nervous system, a cavity (syrinx) may be left. Myelon means marrow. The spinal cord is the marrow of the vertebral column. Syrinx formation in the myelon is indicated by the term __________myelia.

71.22. A patient with this lesion would light a match and sometimes allow it to burn down until his fingers were singed. He had normal pain and temperature sensation in his legs because the lesion did not affect the lumbar region or the __________ ________________ tracts. His disease is called ________________.

71.23. On the right side of the picture, indicate the boundaries between the posterior, lateral, and anterior funiculi. Label the indicated tracts.

LEFT

RIGHT

71.24. Touch is usually not lost in syringomyelia because the ascending touch pathways are diffusely distributed in the cord. Touch impulses from the left hand travel up the cervical cord in the left and right __________ ________________ tracts and in the fasciculus __________ on the ______ side.

71.25. Place a check by the correct findings in the list in a patient with a left-sided hemisection at C8.

a. Increased deep tendon reflexes in the left leg

b. Anesthesia in the right thigh

c. Analgesia in the left leg

d. Inability to recognize direction of movement in left great toe when eyes are closed

71.20A. anterior commissure

71.21A. syringomyelia

71.22A. lateral spinothalamic; syringomyelia

71.23A.

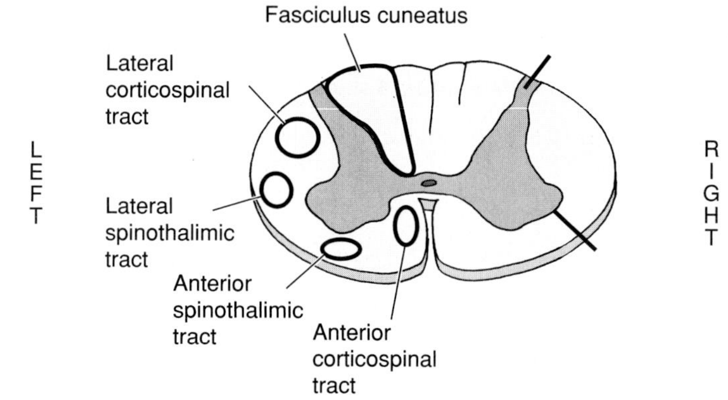

Fasciculus cuneatus

Lateral corticospinal tract

Lateral spinothalimic tract

Anterior spinothalimic tract

Anterior corticospinal tract

LEFT

RIGHT

71.24A. anterior spinothalamic; cuneatus; same (or left)

71.25A.

a. Increased deep tendon reflexes in the left leg ✓

b. Anesthesia in the right thigh

c. Analgesia in the left leg

d. Inability to recognize direction of movement in left great toe when eyes are closed ✓

71.26. A lesion destroying the right half of the cord would not abolish touch from the right foot because some of the secondary axons ______ the midline and ascend in the left __________ __________________ tract.

71.27. A hemisection of the cord abolishes the sensation of pain below the level of the lesion on the __________________ side of the body. The hemisection does not abolish touch sensation at any body site because the axons of secondary neurons in this pathway ascend ______ sides of the cord.

71.28. Place a check by the correct findings in the list in a patient with a left-sided hemisection at C8.

a. Babinski reflex (dorsiflexion of great toe) on the right side

b. Atrophy and flaccid paralysis of ulnar muscles in left hand (innervated by anterior horn cells at C8)

c. Spasticity and voluntary paralysis of the left lower limb

d. Absent touch sensation in right side of chest

e. Analgesia in right leg and right side of abdomen and chest

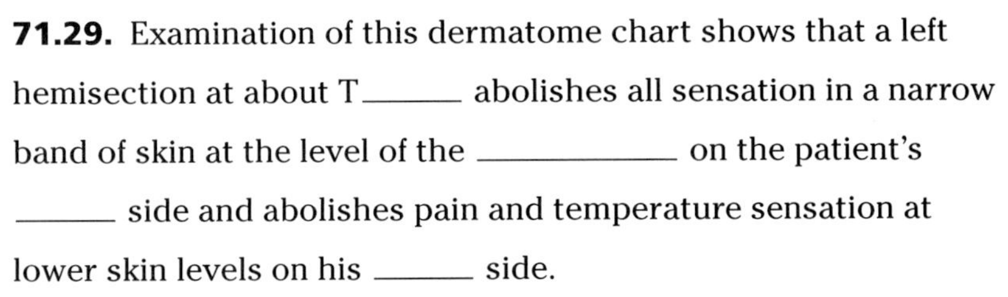

71.29. Examination of this dermatome chart shows that a left hemisection at about T______ abolishes all sensation in a narrow band of skin at the level of the __________ on the patient's ______ side and abolishes pain and temperature sensation at lower skin levels on his ______ side.

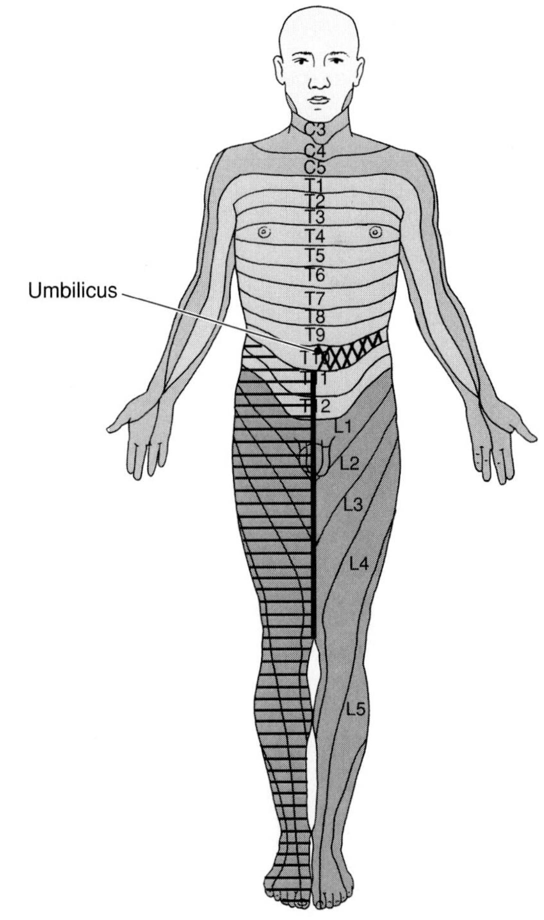

71.26A. cross; anterior spinothalamic

71.27A. contralateral; both

71.28A.

a. Babinski reflex (dorsiflexion of great toe) on the right side

b. Atrophy and flaccid paralysis of ulnar muscles in left hand (innervated by anterior horn cells at C8) ✓

c. Spasticity and voluntary paralysis of the left lower limb ✓

d. Absent touch sensation in right side of chest

e. Analgesia in right leg and right side of abdomen and chest ✓

71.29A. T10; umbilicus; left; right

71.30. The sensory findings in a patient are charted in the diagram. He has a ______section of the cord at about the ______ segment on his ______ side. The vertical lines represent loss of afferent information carried along fibers of the ____________ columns.

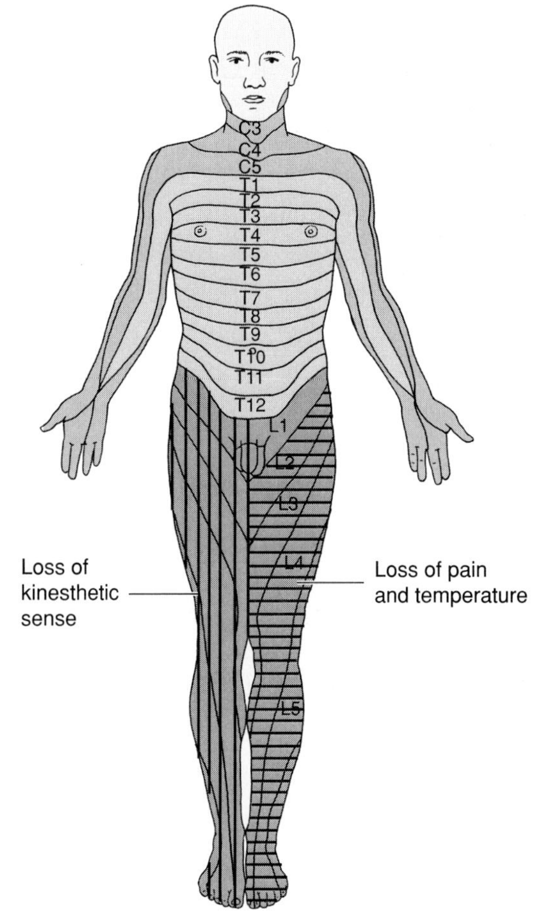

71.31. Encircle the left posterior white columns and the left spinocerebellar tracts. Does the information carried on these tracts originate mainly on the same side of the body as the tracts? ______ Is this true of any other afferent spinal tracts? ______

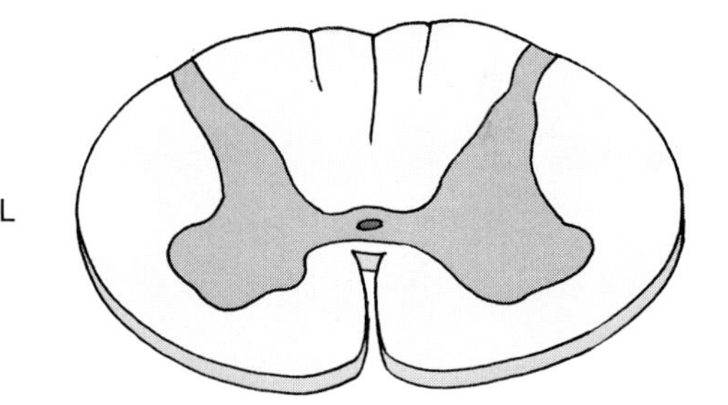

71.32. A patient had a right-sided hemisection at T4. The lesion interrupted fibers transmitting information that originated in the right foot—posterior column fibers and spino________________ fibers. In the left foot, he failed to perceive sensations of ______ and ________________.

71.30A. hemisection; T12 (or L1); right; posterior (or dorsal)

71.31A. Yes; No

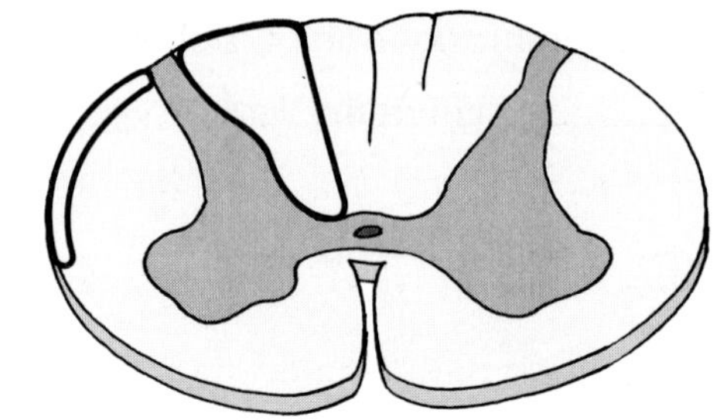

71.32A. spinocerebellar; pain; temperature

71.33. In the following list, place an "X" beside those tracts in which the axons are on the opposite side from their cell bodies, a check mark beside those in which the axons come from cell bodies of both sides, and a zero beside those in which axons and their cell bodies are on the same side.

Lateral spinothalamic tract

Fasciculus cuneatus

Spinocerebellar tracts

Lateral corticospinal tract

Anterior spinothalamic tract

Fasciculus gracilis

71.34. A patient was found to have hyperactive reflexes, a Babinski sign, and voluntary paralysis of the left leg. With her eyes closed, she could not recognize whether the examiner was moving her great toe up or down in the left foot, and she could not distinguish a pencil point from the flat side of a ruler pressed against her left leg. Her right leg was analgesic. Her lesion was probably a ____________________ of the ______ side of the cord.

71.33A.

Lateral spinothalamic tract	✗	Lateral corticospinal tract	✗
Fasciculus cuneatus	0	Anterior spinothalamic tract	✓
Spinocerebellar tracts	0	Fasciculus gracilis	0

71.34A. hemisection; left

72 Lesions of the Spinal Cord

72.1. Spinal cord lesions result from a variety of pathologies, such as vascular insufficiencies, degenerative disorders, or space-occupying lesions including tumors, just to name a few. With spinal cord lesions, both ______ and ______ matter may be affected, including funiculi and their ascending and descending ___________. Well-defined functional deficits occur depending on the location of the lesion.

72.2. For illustrative purposes, we will consider the effects of lesions that affect the ___________ing and ___________ing white matter tracts. Lesions affecting the gray matter typically manifest themselves as altered reflexes and decreased muscle tone, which, due to considerable functional and structural overlap in these systems, are less easily discernible.

72.3. There are two major descending white matter tracts that originate in the primary motor cortex—the lateral corticospinal tract, which is found in the ___________ funiculus and the ___________ corticospinal tract, which is found in the anterior funiculus.

72.4. Circle and identify the anterior and lateral corticospinal tracts on the diagram.

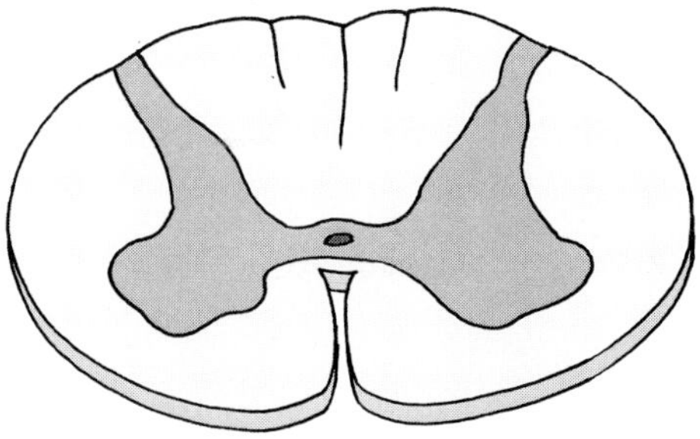

72.5. The fibers forming the ___________ corticospinal tract cross in the caudal ___________ in the pyramidal decussation. The fibers maintain a somatotopic organization, with fibers leading to motor neurons of the anterior horn, controlling the upper limb, most medially located, trunk in the middle and fibers controlling the lower extremities, most lateral.

72.6. Space-occupying lesions that press on the lateral aspects of the spinal cord, which affect the structures in the lateral funiculus, may impinge upon the fibers of the lateral corticospinal tract. Functional loss will *first* appear as ______lateral motor problems in the ______ extremities.

72.1A. gray; white; tracts

72.2A. ascending; descending

72.3A. lateral; anterior

72.4A.

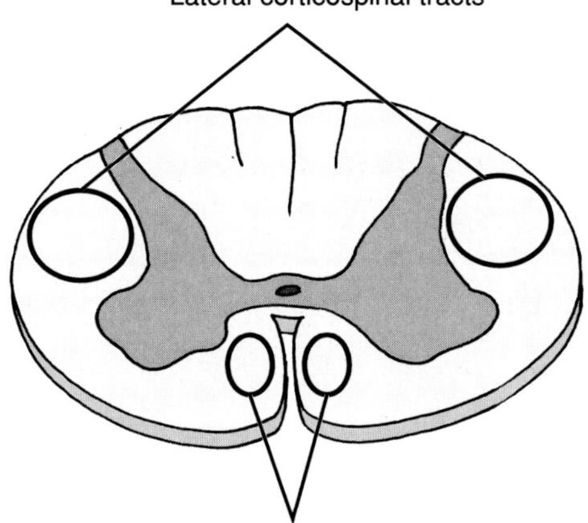

72.5A. lateral; medulla

72.6A. ipsilateral; lower

72.7. In addition to the many descending spinal cord tracts, one of which—the lateral corticospinal—was discussed earlier, there are a multitude of ascending, or ______ory, tracts that can be affected in cases of spinal cord damage.

72.8. On the following spinal cord cross section, identify the tracts indicated.

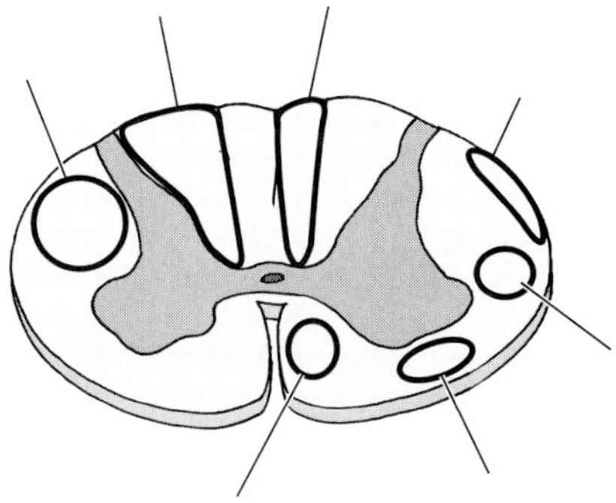

72.9. The lateral spinothalamic tract carries ______ and ____________ information from the ____________lateral body to the thalamus.

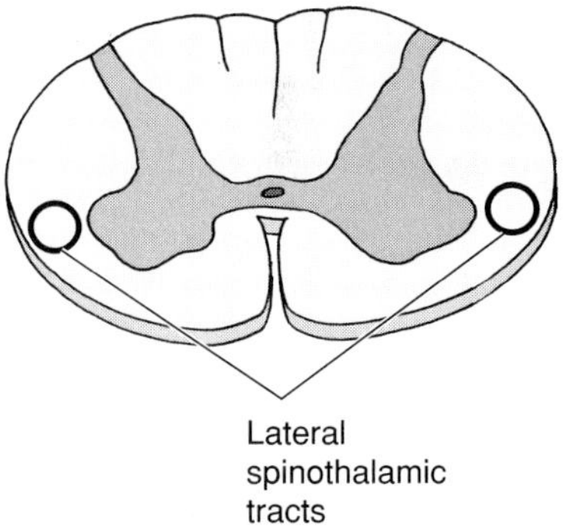

Lateral spinothalamic tracts

72.10. The lateral spinothalamic tract exhibits a ____________topic organization, with fibers conveying pain and temperature information from the lower extremities being most lateral, the trunk being in the middle, and pain and temperature fibers from the ______ extremities being most medial.

72.11. Pressure on the ____________ aspect of the cord, from a tumor or bone spur, will first affect pain and temperature from the lower extremities contralateral to the lesion.

72.12. The anterior spinothalamic tracts are found in the ____________ funiculus and carry crude or general touch information from the ____________lateral side of the body. Lesion of this tract is difficult to appreciate if the ______ touch system located in the posterior (dorsal) columns is still intact.

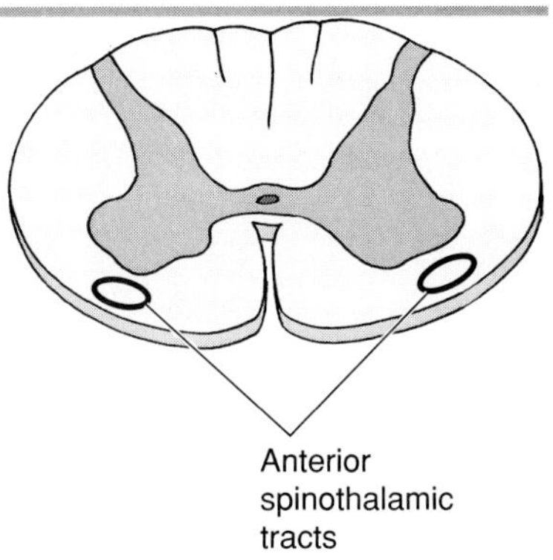

Anterior spinothalamic tracts

72.7A. sensory

72.8A.

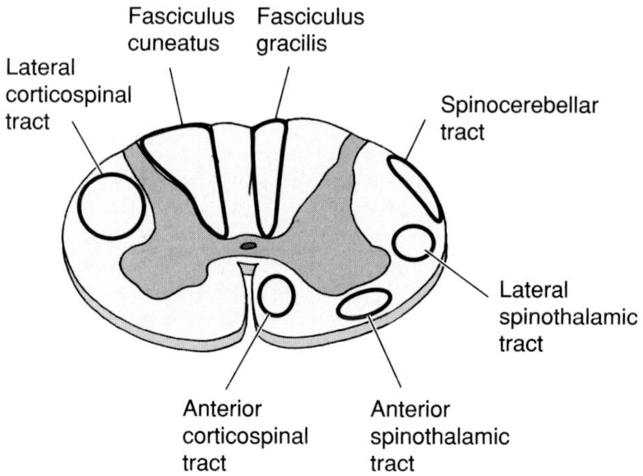

Fasciculus cuneatus
Fasciculus gracilis
Lateral corticospinal tract
Spinocerebellar tract
Lateral spinothalamic tract
Anterior corticospinal tract
Anterior spinothalamic tract

72.9A. pain; temperature; contralateral

72.10A. somatotopic; upper

72.11A. lateral

72.12A. anterior; contralateral; fine (or discriminatory)

72.13. The posterior (dorsal) white columns carry information on ______ touch, position sense, and ____________ ory sense. The fibers are uncrossed in the spinal cord.

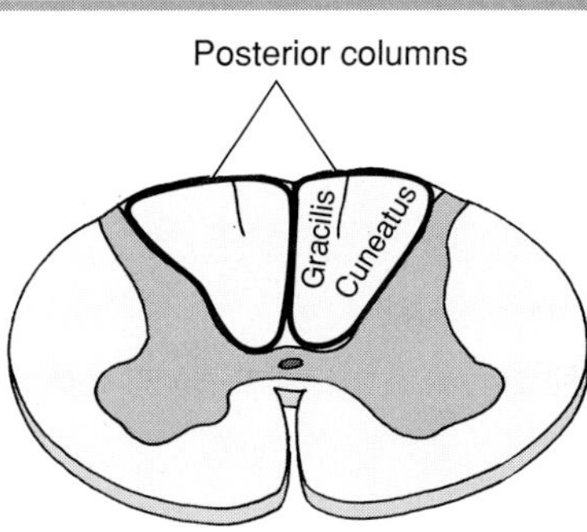

72.14. The posterior (dorsal) columns also exhibit a ____________topic organization, with fibers from lower levels being located most ____________, unlike the lateral corticospinal and lateral spinothalamic tracts. Therefore, compression of the cord affecting this tract will first manifest itself as a lack of sensation ipsilateral to the lesion affecting the upper extremities first, assuming that the lesion is at a high enough cord level that the fasciculus ____________ is present.

72.15. Unconscious or reflex proprioception is carried in ______cerebellar tracts; damage to these tracts leads to problems determining the position of the limbs in space (____________ spinocerebellars) or difficulty with the ability to maintain coordinated posture with the axial musculature (____________ spinocerebellars).

72.16. The area affected in the lesion will result in which of the following being affected? Place a check next to all that will be affected.

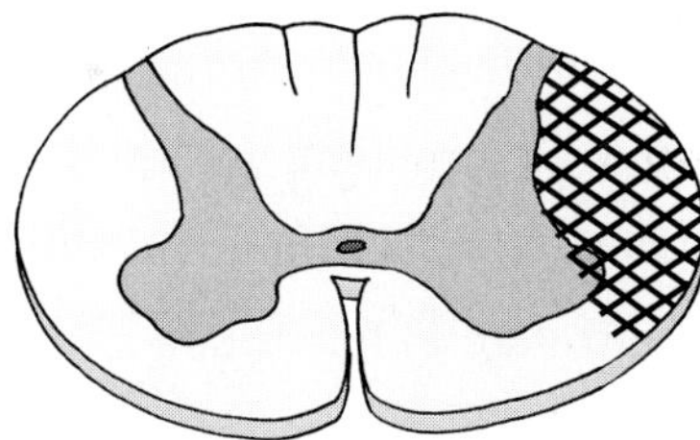

Ipsilateral pain and temperature
Contralateral pain and temperature
Ipsilateral fine touch and vibratory sense
Contralateral fine touch and vibratory sense
Ipsilateral motor control of muscles
Contralateral motor control of muscles
Ipsilateral crude touch
Contralateral crude touch

72.17. The area affected in the lesion will result in which of the following being affected? Place a check next to all that will be affected.

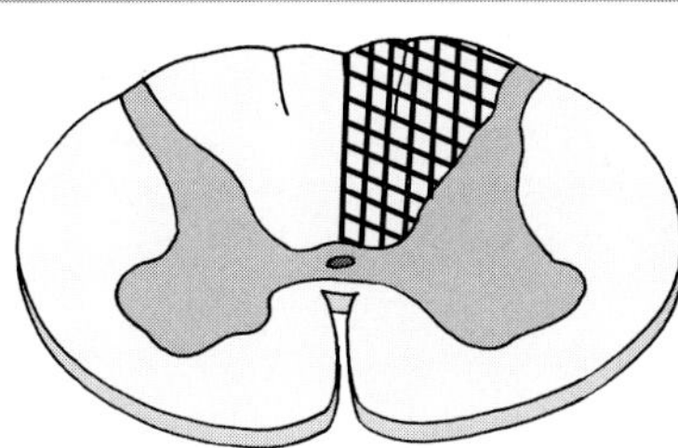

Ipsilateral pain and temperature
Contralateral pain and temperature
Ipsilateral fine touch and vibratory sense
Contralateral fine touch and vibratory sense
Ipsilateral motor control of muscles
Contralateral motor control of muscles
Ipsilateral crude touch
Contralateral crude touch

72.13A. fine (or discriminatory); vibratory

72.14A. somatotopic; medial; cuneatus

72.15A. spinocerebellar; posterior; anterior

72.16A.

Ipsilateral pain and temperature
Contralateral pain and temperature ✓
Ipsilateral fine touch and vibratory sense
Contralateral fine touch and vibratory sense

Ipsilateral motor control of muscles ✓
Contralateral motor control of muscles
Ipsilateral crude touch
Contralateral crude touch

72.17A.

Ipsilateral pain and temperature
Contralateral pain and temperature
Ipsilateral fine touch and vibratory sense ✓
Contralateral fine touch and vibratory sense

Ipsilateral motor control of muscles
Contralateral motor control of muscles
Ipsilateral crude touch
Contralateral crude touch

73 Membranes of the Spinal Cord

73.1. Like the brain, the spinal cord is covered by a pia-arachnoid membrane. This membrane is formed by two layers, the ______ mater and the ____________ mater.

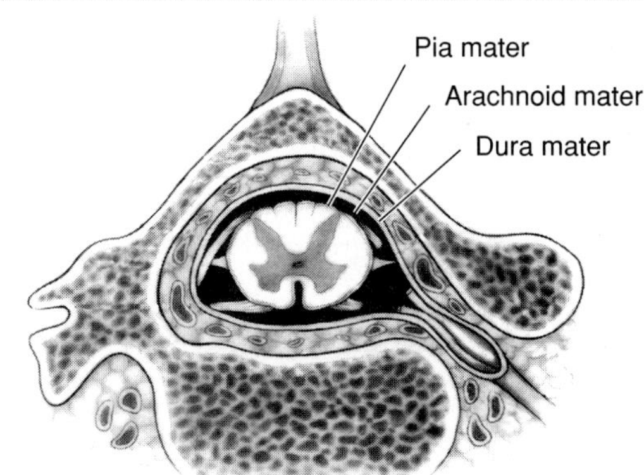

73.2. Superficial to the pia mater is a fluid-filled space. This fluid separates the pia from the ____________. The ______ contains blood vessels and is closely applied to the surface of the spinal cord.

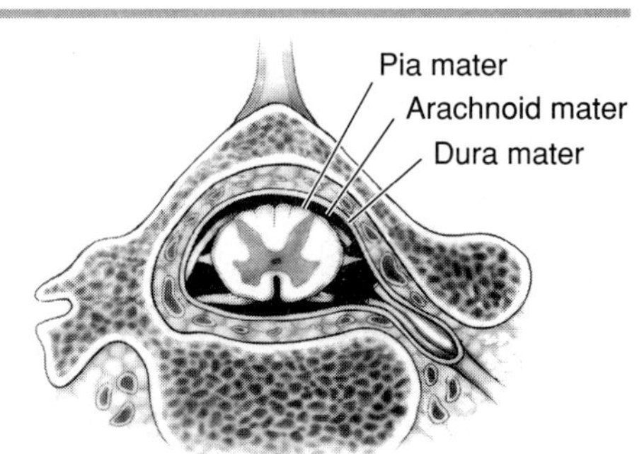

73.3. Because of its position deep to the arachnoid membrane, this space is called the sub____________ sp______.

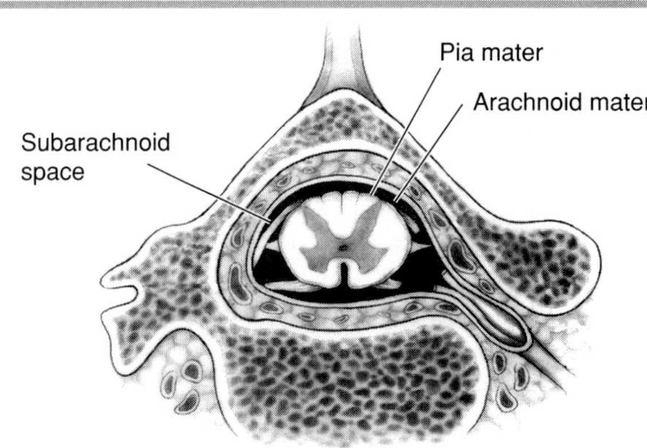

73.4. The clear, watery fluid in the subarachnoid space is called *c*erebro*s*pinal *f*luid, commonly abbreviated as C______F. As the name suggests, cerebrospinal fluid is continuous from the ____________ hemispheres to the ____________ ______.

73.1A. pia; arachnoid

73.2A. arachnoid; pia

73.3A. subarachnoid; space

73.4A. S; cerebral; spinal cord

73.5. Draw a hypodermic needle passing between L3 and L4 vertebrae. Your needle punctures the arachnoid membrane and taps the ______ in the ______arachnoid space.

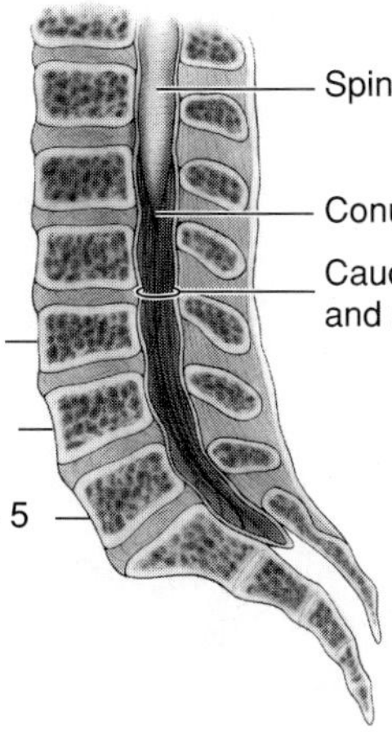

Spinal cord
Conus medullaris
Cauda equina (roots of lumbar and sacral nerves)
LV - 3
LV - 4
LV - 5

73.6. A needle passing between T8 and T9 vertebrae to penetrate the subarachnoid space would likely pierce the ____________ ______. A needle could not be passed between two sacral vertebrae because sacral vertebrae are ______ed.

73.7. In order to tap cerebrospinal fluid without injuring the spinal cord, the needle enters between two of the lower ____________ vertebrae and punctures the arachnoid. The procedure is commonly called an LP, or a l______ p____________.

73.8. The nerve roots of the c______ e______ are enclosed within the ____________ space. The roots are immersed directly in ______.

73.9. A thicker, tougher connective tissue membrane called the dura mater lies superficial to the arachnoid. The space between the arachnoid and pia is the ____________________ space. The space between the dura and arachnoid is the ______dural space.

73.10. The dural and arachnoid membranes are virtually fused. The potential space between them is called the sub______al space.

73.5A. CSF; subarachnoid

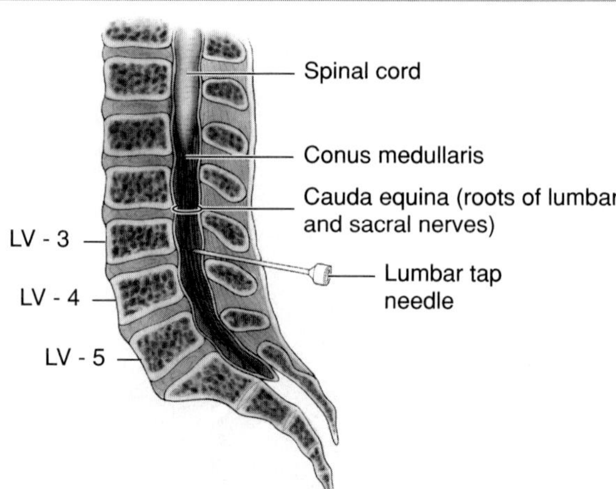

73.6A. spinal cord; fused

73.7A. lumbar; lumbar puncture

73.8A. cauda equina; subarachnoid; CSF

73.9A. subarachnoid; subdural

73.10A. subdural

73.11. In this posterior view of the spinal cord, the vertebrae have been removed. Over spinal cord segments T4 to T7, the thick ______ mater has been incised and pulled to either side, exposing the membrane deep to it. Over spinal cord segments T6–T7, this more filmy ____________ membrane has been completely removed to expose the ______ membrane with its blood vessels visible. Label the three membranes (dura mater, arachnoid mater, and pia mater).

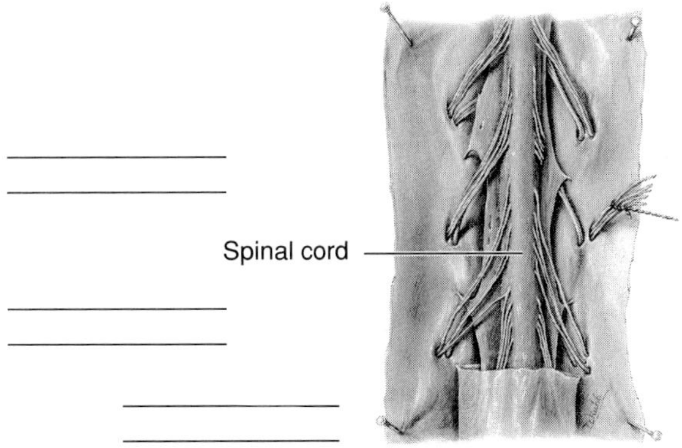

Spinal cord

73.12. The subarachnoid space is ______ternal to the potential subdural space. Label the two spaces indicated. A third space, between the dura and vertebrae (see diagram), is the ____________ space.

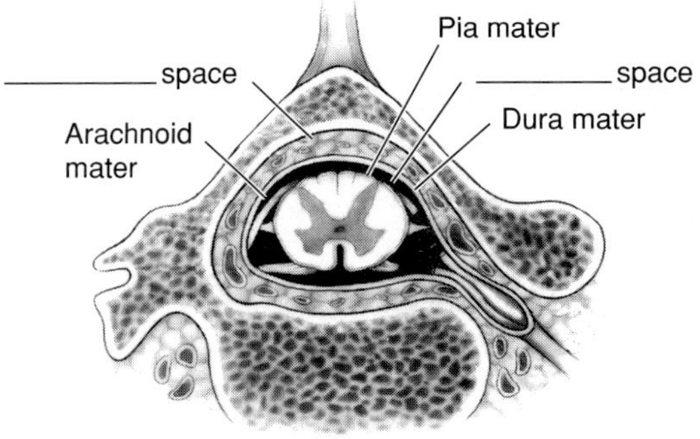

Pia mater
__________ space
__________ space
Arachnoid mater
Dura mater

73.13. Deep to the dura is a potential space called the ____________ space, and outside the dura is the ____________ space.

73.14. Adipose tissue partially fills the ____________ space and probably helps to cushion the spinal cord from the ____________ that enclose it.

73.15. Each posterior root breaks up into a series of rootlets as its reaches the spinal cord. The rootlets are directly covered by the ____________ membrane. The rootlets are bathed in ______.

73.16. At one point bilaterally in each segment of cervical and thoracic spinal cord, the pia, ____________, and dura are fused, and the spinal cord is thus anchored to the dura. These points of attachment, illustrated in the figure, are called the ____________________ ligaments.

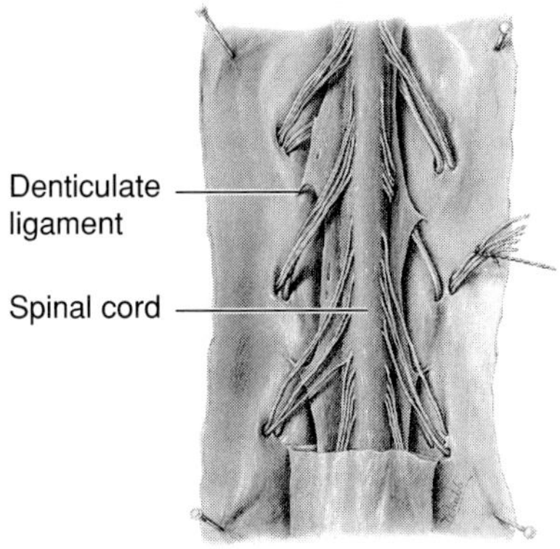

Denticulate ligament
Spinal cord

Posterior View

73.11A. <u>dura</u>; <u>arachnoid</u>; <u>pia</u>

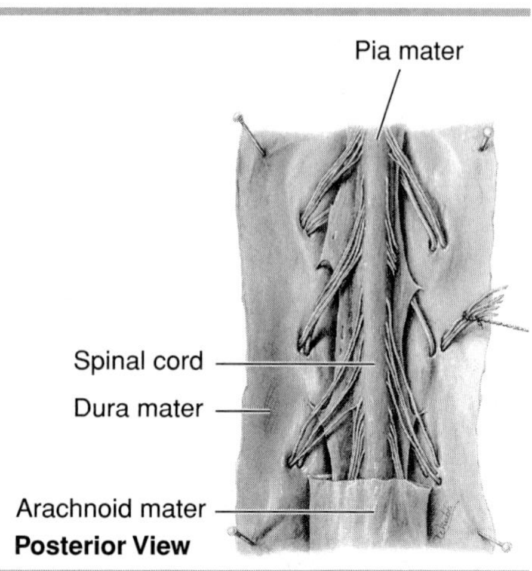

73.12A. <u>in</u>ternal; <u>epidural</u>

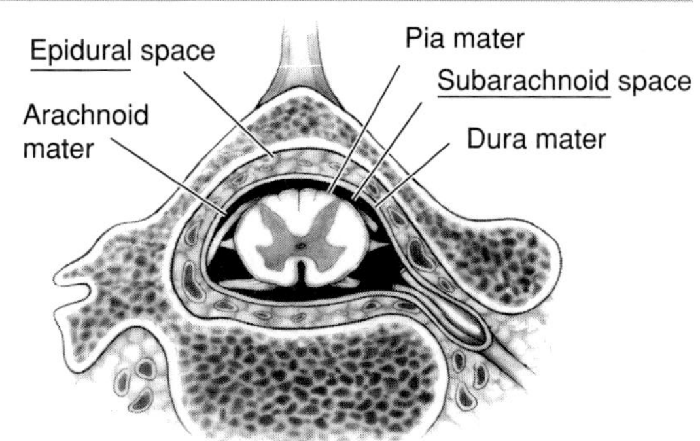

73.13A. <u>subdural</u>; <u>epidural</u>

73.14A. <u>epidural</u>; <u>vertebrae</u>

73.15A. <u>arachnoid</u>; <u>CSF</u>

73.16A. <u>arachnoid</u>; <u>denticulate</u>

Animations

1. **Pain and Temperature** (Chapters 64, 65, 66)
2. **Crude Touch** (Chapters 64, 65, 66)
3. **Fine Touch** (Chapters 64, 65, 67)
4. **Reflex Proprioception** (Chapters 64, 65)
5. **Reflex Withdrawal** (Chapters 64 and 65)
24. **Sympathetic** (Chapter 69)
31. **Spinocerebellum** (Chapter 67)

VII SPECIAL SENSES

74 Visual System

74.1. The special sense of sight or vision begins in the retina. Special photoreceptor cells—rods and cones—transduce light energy into a signal that stimulates the cells that form the ______ nerve (CN II).

74.2. The optic nerve is composed of the axons of the ganglion cells of the retina. As may be expected given their name, the ganglion cells form the ______lion cell layer of the retina. The optic nerve is a central nervous system tract, not an actual nerve, and as such is surrounded by the same three ____________ as the rest of the central nervous system.

74.3. The fibers forming the ______ nerve pass posteriorly out of the eye to the lateral geniculate body of the ____________. However, as they pass posteriorly, a clever crossing of fibers occurs in the optic chiasm, such that visual information from the left visual field of both eyes ends up in the same lateral geniculate body; the same is true for visual information from the right visual fields of both eyes.

74.4. In the optic ____________, the fibers from the temporal side of each retina do not cross, whereas fibers from the nasal side of the retina do ______, thereby matching the information from the same visual field of each eye.

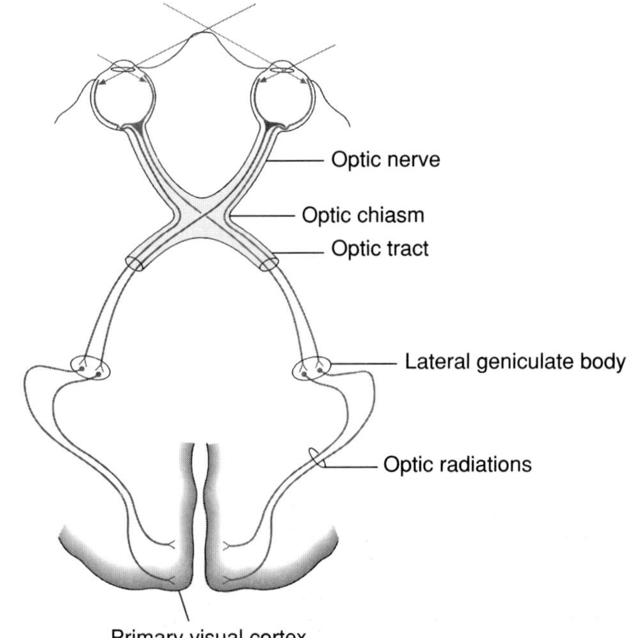

74.1A. optic

74.2A. ganglion; meninges

74.3A. optic; thalamus

74.4A. chiasm; cross (or decussate)

74.5. In the following schematic, trace the fibers conveying information from the right visual field of both eyes (indicated with an "X") to their emergence from the optic chiasm.

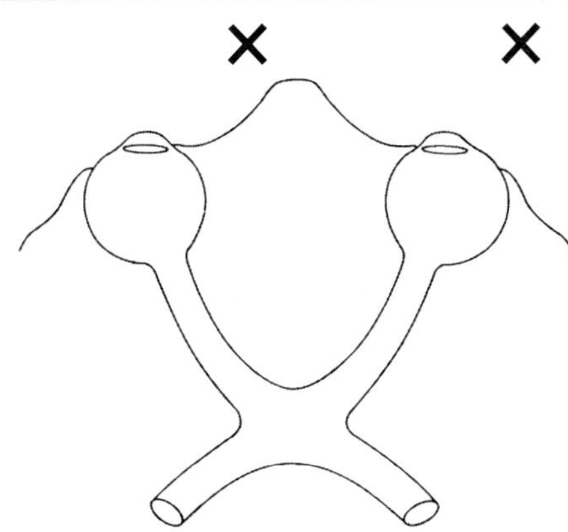

74.6. Fibers leaving the optic __________ form the optic tract. Each optic tract projects to the ______lateral lateral __________________ body of the thalamus and to the superior colliculus of the ______brain. The superior colliculus mediates audiovisual reflexes in conjunction with the inferior colliculus.

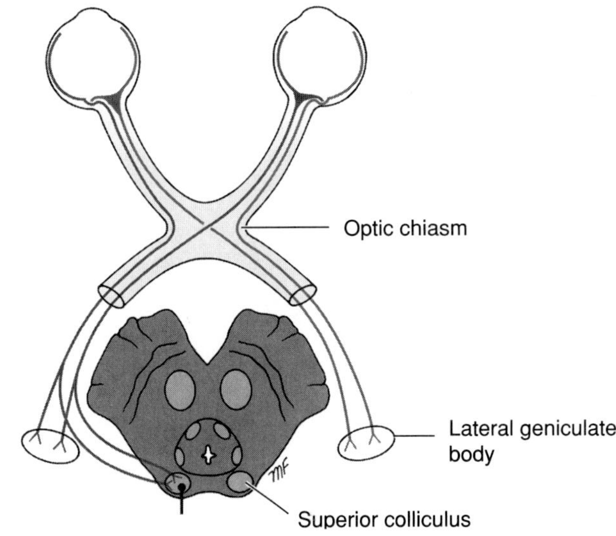

74.7. The lateral geniculate body is a __________ relay nucleus, like most thalamic nuclei. It gives rise to the optic radiations or geniculocalcarine tract. Calcarine is in reference to the primary visual cortex, which lies on the banks of the calcarine sulcus of the occipital lobe.

74.8. The ______ radiations may be divided into an upper and lower division, with the upper division conveying information from the inferior visual field (upper retina) of both eyes to the cuneate gyrus of the occipital lobe (on the superior side of the calcarine sulcus), and the lower division carrying information from the __________ visual field (______ retina) of both eyes to the lingual gyrus of the occipital lobe (on the __________ side of the __________ sulcus).

74.5A.

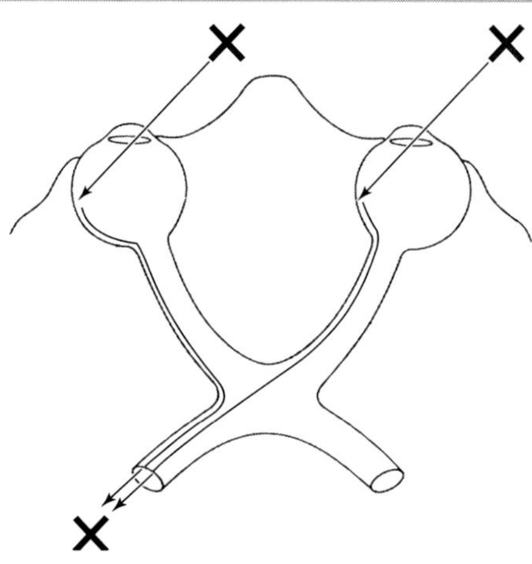

74.6A. chiasm; ipsilateral; geniculate; midbrain

74.7A. sensory

74.8A. optic; superior; lower; inferior; calcarine

74.9. The optic radiations maintain a specific retinotopic organization as they pass posteriorly. The inferior-most fibers of the lower division loop far into the temporal lobe, forming Meyer's loop. Damage to ____________ loop results in a visual field loss ____________lateral to the lesion in both eyes affecting the ______ior visual fields.

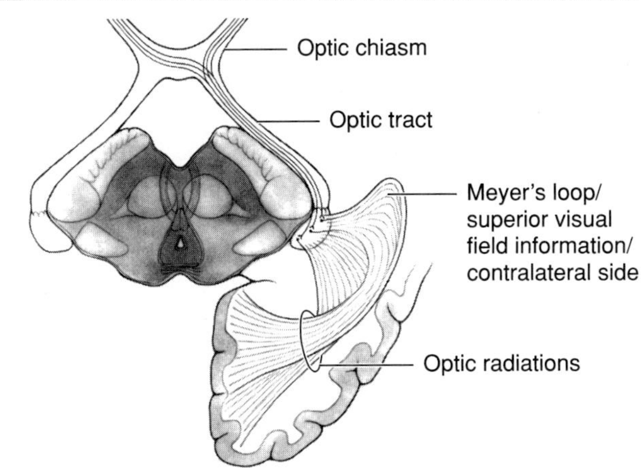

74.10. The primary visual cortex (striate cortex, which is named for its striated appearance), Brodmann's area 17, is found along the superior and inferior banks of the calcarine sulcus. On the following diagram, label the calcarine sulcus, cuneate gyrus, and lingual gyrus.

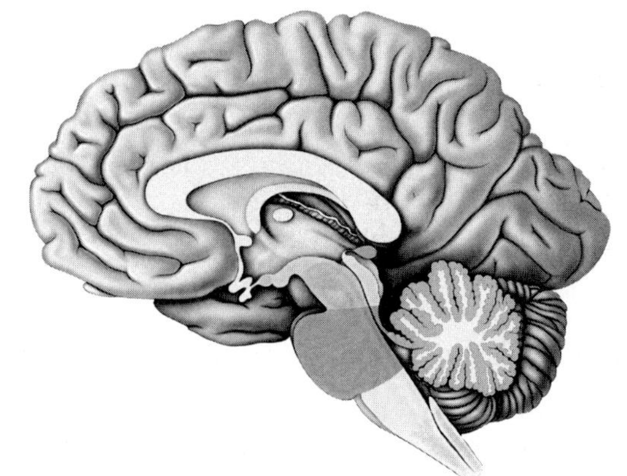

74.11. The most posterior aspect of the ____________ visual cortex is concerned with visual information from the most central aspects of the retina. As one moves anteriorly along the visual cortex, information is concerned with progressively more peripheral aspects of the retina.

74.12. Place an "X" on the part of the primary visual cortex that receives information from the central and superior aspect of the *retina*. Place an "O" on the area of the primary visual cortex that deals with the superior and peripheral *visual field*.

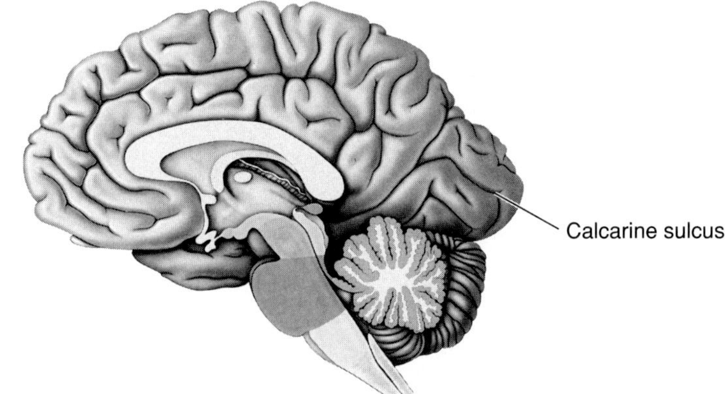

74.9A. Meyer's; contralateral; superior

74.10A.

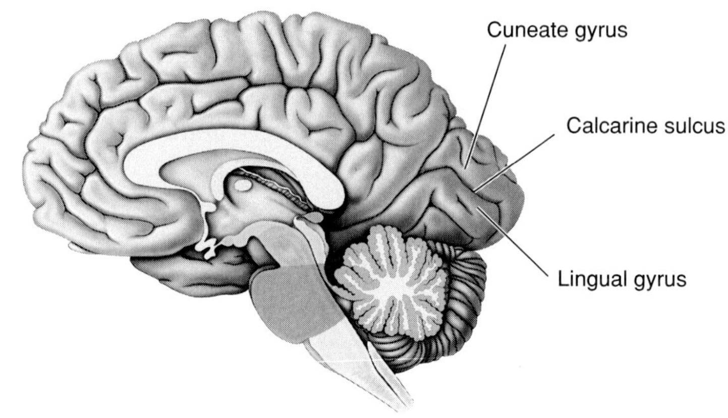

74.11A. primary

74.12A.

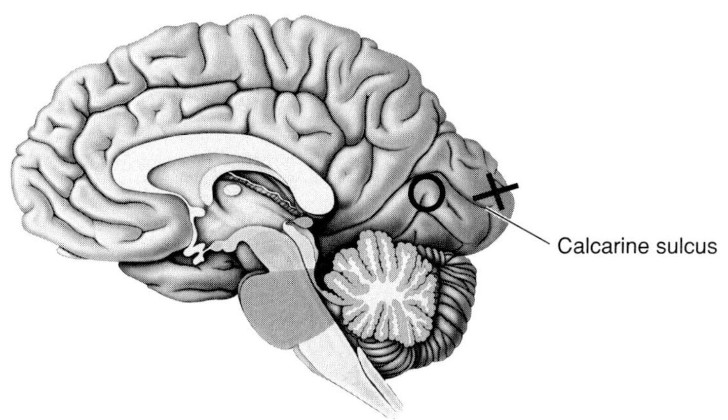

74.13. Consider the lesion indicated in the following diagram. Cross out the incorrect information to accurately complete the statements.

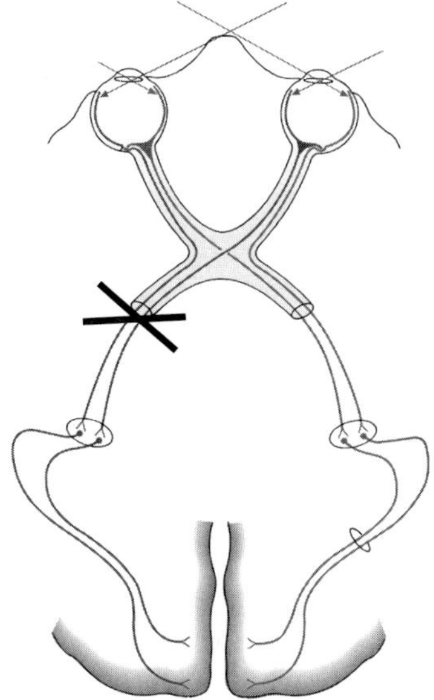

The lesion would cause loss of visual information in both/one eye(s).

The visual loss would be in the visual field contralateral/ipsilateral to the lesion.

74.13A.

The lesion would cause loss of visual information in both eyes.

The visual loss would be in the visual field contralateral to the lesion.

75 Chemical Senses

75.1. Both the sense of smell (olfactory sense) and taste (gustatory sense) involve the interpretation of chemicals and their concentrations dissolved in fluid (i.e., saliva or nasal mucous) to stimulate the systems. The central nervous system interprets the chemicals as specific smells or tastes. Because both taste and smell involve chemical receptors, they are often referred to as the __________ senses.

75.2. The olfactory receptor cells lie in the nasal mucosa along the superior aspect of the nasal cavity. Their central processes extend superiorly through the cribriform plate of the ethmoid bone and constitute the __________ nerve (CN I).

75.3. Axons of the __________ receptor cells synapse in the olfactory bulb on __________-order sensory neurons called mitral cells.

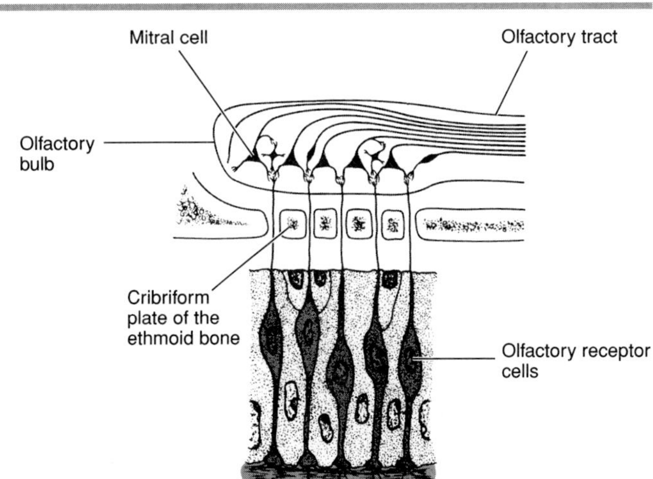

75.4. Label the olfactory receptor cells, mitral cells, and the olfactory bulb on the following diagram. Write a "1" beside the primary afferent cell and a "2" beside the secondary afferent cell.

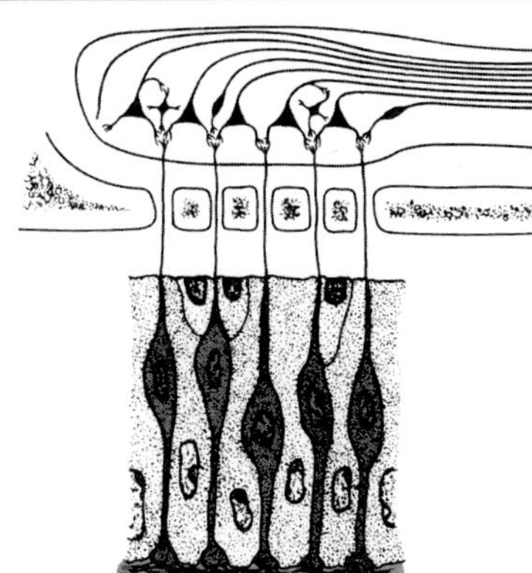

75.1A. chemical

75.2A. olfactory

75.3A. olfactory; second-order

75.4A.

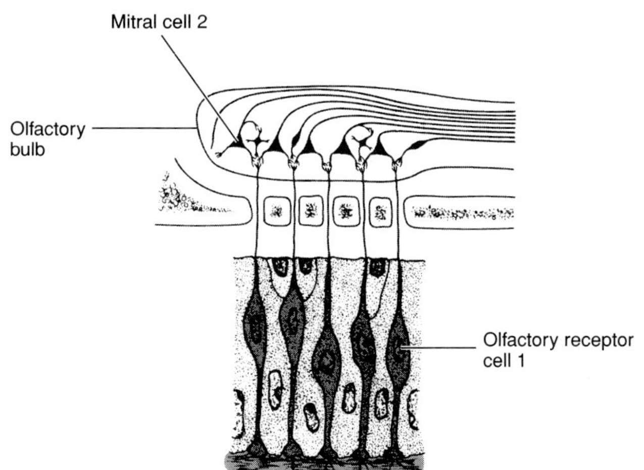

75.5. Axons of the ____________ cells form the olfactory tract. In an obvious exception to all other ______ory systems of the body, the olfactory system does not relay in the thalamus; instead, the mitral cells project directly to the primary olfactory cortex.

75.6. Primary ____________ cortex is found along the parahippocampal gyrus. It projects to structures of the diencephalon—the thalamus (which in turn projects to the frontal cortex for interpretation of smells) and hypothalamus—and to parts of the limbic system for memory formation and emotional and visceral responses to smells.

75.7. The receptor cells associated with taste are located in the ______ buds of the tongue. Due to the fact that the tongue is derived from several pharyngeal arches, each with a different innervation, taste sensation is carried on several different cranial nerves.

75.8. Taste from the anterior two-thirds of the tongue is associated with CN VII, the ____________ nerve, the cell bodies of which are found in the geniculate ganglion. CN IX, the ____________________ nerve, carries taste from the posterior one-third of the tongue, the cell bodies of which are located in the petrosal ganglion. The most posterior aspects of the oral cavity, including the epiglottis, possess taste buds associated with CN X, the ______ nerve, the cell bodies of which are located in the nodose ganglion.

75.9. All three nerves carrying taste project via the solitary tract to the ____________ nucleus. In this way, all taste is brought together in one place centrally.

75.10. The solitary nucleus conveys taste information to the ventral posterior medial nucleus of the ____________, which projects to primary gustatory cortex (Brodmann's area 43). Here, taste is interpreted and sent to the limbic system for memory formation and emotional response.

75.11. What makes the olfactory sense different from taste (and all sensory systems) centrally?

75.5A. mitral; sensory

75.6A. olfactory

75.7A. taste

75.8A. facial; glossopharyngeal; vagus

75.9A. solitary

75.10A. thalamus

75.11A. It does not send fibers to the thalamus.

76 Auditory and Vestibular Systems

76.1. Although the auditory and vestibular systems mediate very different senses, their receptor organs are remarkably similar. Both systems involve specialized ciliated cells called hair cells, which, when stimulated through bending of the "hairs," depolarize the primary __________ nerve endings of CN VIII, the ________________ nerve, which are in contact with the base of the receptors cells.

76.2. The __________ division of the vestibulocochlear nerve conducts information regarding hearing into the pons, where it synapses on the cochlear nuclei. The cochlear nuclei project bilaterally via the lateral lemniscus to the superior olivary nucleus and the inferior colliculus on each side.

76.3. The _____lateral projections to the superior olivary nuclei have a function in sound localization and sound dampening. Projections from the superior olivary nuclei to the facial motor nucleus and the trigeminal motor nucleus cause contraction of the stapedius and tensor tympani, respectively. Both muscles connect to ossicles of the middle ear cavity; their contraction inhibits the vibration of the ossicles to protect the hearing apparatus of the inner ear—the organ of Corti.

76.4. Rostral projections from the inferior colliculus connect it to the superior colliculus, which is associated with the __________ system, to mediate audiovisual reflexes, and to the medial geniculate body of the __________.

76.5. The __________ serves as a sensory relay for auditory information, forwarding the information to the primary auditory cortex—Brodmann's areas 41 and 42—along the superior temporal gyrus (the transverse gyri of Heschl).

76.6. The primary auditory cortex maintains an organization based on sound frequency identical to that of the auditory receptor system of the _____ ear. This tonotopic arrangement is thus maintained throughout the auditory pathway.

76.1A. afferent; vestibulocochlear

76.2A. cochlear

76.3A. bilateral

76.4A. visual; thalamus

76.5A. thalamus

76.6A. inner

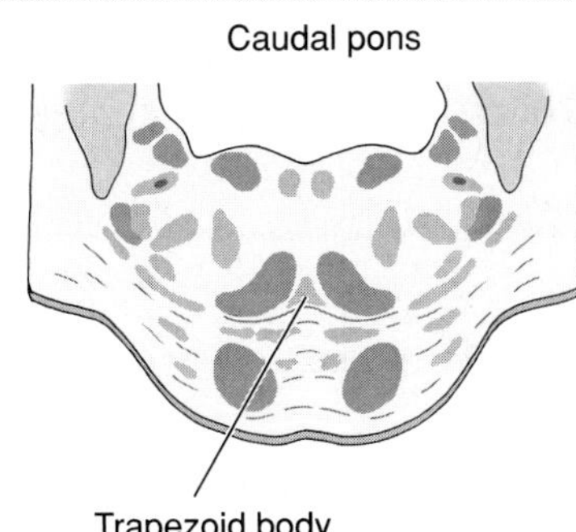

76.7. Due to the ______lateral nature of the auditory pathway for all connections "upstream" of the cochlear nuclei, damage to the pathway above the cochlear nuclei does not result in deafness. To cause deafness in an ear, damage must occur in the cochlear nuclei before they project across the midline (crossing fibers form the trapezoid body), the ________________ nerve, or the inner, middle, or external ear.

76.8. Stimulation of the hair cells associated with balance and equilibrium works in much the same way as stimulation of the hair cells associated with hearing, resulting in stimulation of the primary ______fferents of the vestibular division of the ________________ nerve (CN VIII).

76.9. The cell bodies of the primary afferents conducting ____________ and ________________ information are located in the vestibular or Scarpa's ganglion.

76.10. CN VIII ______fferents project to the vestibular nuclei of the brainstem. The vestibular nuclei have large and diverse connections within the brainstem.

76.11. The vestibular nuclei project to the: 1) cerebellum via the inferior cerebellar peduncle; 2) spinal cord as medial (bilateral to cervical cord levels) and lateral (ipsilateral to all cord levels) vestibulo____________ tracts; 3) motor nuclei of CN III (________________ nucleus), CN IV (____________ nucleus), and CN VI (____________ nucleus); 4) thalamus; 5) contralateral vestibular nuclei; 6) reticular formation; and 7) labyrinth.

76.12. Label the targets indicated on the following diagram.

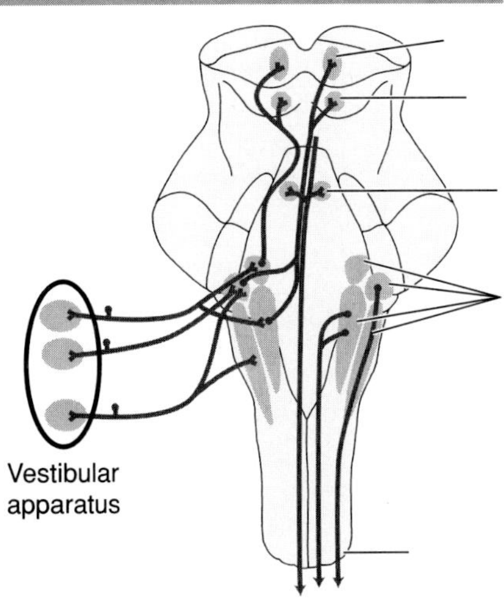

76.7A. <u>bi</u>lateral; <u>vestibulocochlear</u>

76.8A. <u>a</u>fferents; <u>vestibulocochlear</u>

76.9A. <u>balance</u>; <u>equilibrium</u>

76.10A. <u>e</u>fferents

76.11A. vestibulo<u>spinal</u>; <u>oculomotor</u>; <u>trochlear</u>; <u>abducens</u>

76.12A.

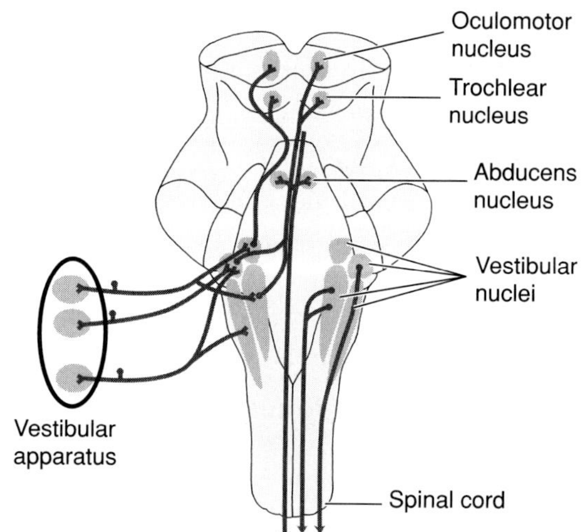

76.13. On the diagram, draw arrows indicating the pathways out of the vestibular nuclei to the targets indicated, and label the medial (bilateral) and lateral (ipsilateral) vestibulospinal tracts.

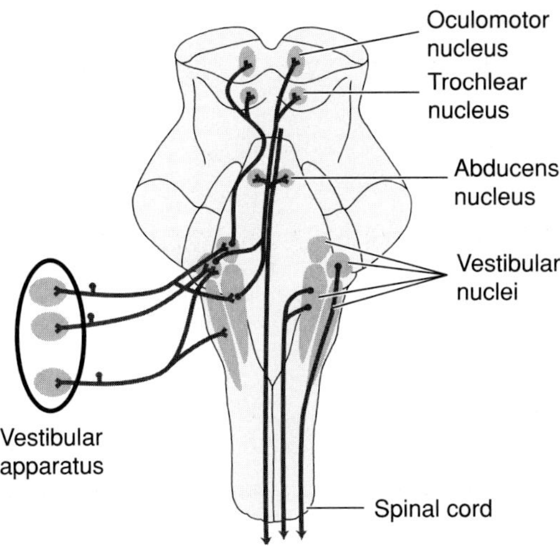

76.14. Next to each of the seven targets listed below, write a brief explanation of the purpose of each connection.

1. Cerebellum–
2. Spinal cord–
3. Motor nuclei of CN III, IV, and VI–
4. Thalamus–
5. Contralateral vestibular nuclei–
6. Reticular formation–
7. Labyrinth–

76.13A.

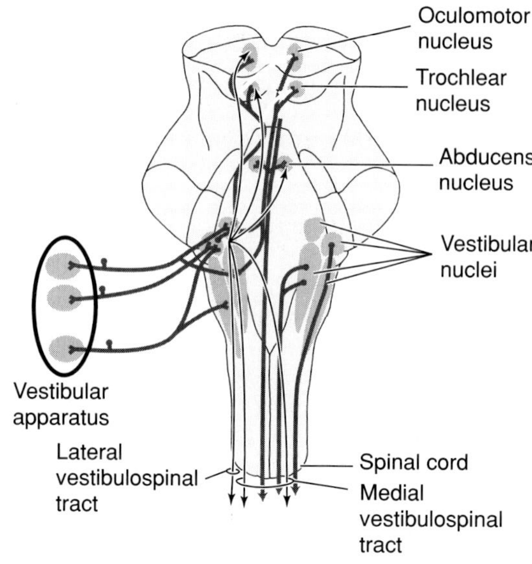

76.14A.

1. Cerebellum–to coordinate head movement with the rest of the motor system
2. Spinal cord–to help maintain balance and stability during head movement
3. Motor nuclei of CN III, IV, and VI–to coordinate eye and head movement
4. Thalamus–to cerebral cortex for conscious appreciation of head movement
5. Contralateral vestibular nuclei–to coordinate with the opposite decrease or increase in activity from the contralateral receptor organs
6. Reticular formation–to visceral centers, as evidenced by sea sickness
7. Labyrinth–to fine tune the receptor system

Animations

26. Auditory (Chapter 76)
27. Vestibular (Chapter 76)
28. Olfactory (Chapter 75)
29. Taste (Chapter 75)
33. Higher Association Visual (Chapter 74)
34. Higher Association Language (Chapter 76)
35. Higher Association Frontal Lobes (Chapter 75)
37. Visual (Chapter 74)

Credits

Figure Acknowledgments

Specific acknowledgment is made for permission to use the following material in either original or modified reproductions.

Agur AMR, Dalley AF: Grant's Atlas of Anatomy, 11th ed. Baltimore: Lippincott Williams & Wilkins, 2005. For **Figures 17.1, 17.5, 17.6, 17.7, 17.7A, 17.12, 17.12A, 17.13, 17.14, 17.14A, 17.16, 17.22, 17.22A, 17.24, 17.24A, 18.4, 18.14, 22.12, 60.3, 60.3A, 60.12, 60.12A, 60.13, 60.13A, 73.11, 73.11A,** and **73.16.**

Baily P: Intracranial Tumors, 2nd ed. Springfield, IL: Charles C. Thomas, 1948. For **Figures 6.2** and **6.6.**

Barr ML, Kiernan JA: The Human Nervous System, 6th ed. Philadelphia: Lippincott Williams & Wilkins, 1993. For **Figures 39.4, 39.4A, 39.5, 39.9, 39.10, 39.12, 39.12A, 39.14, 39.15, 39.16, 39.16A, 39.17,** and **39.19.**

Bear MF, Connors BW, Paradiso MA: Neuroscience: Exploring the Brain, 3rd ed. Baltimore: Lippincott Williams & Wilkins, 2007. For **Figures 1.1, 1.2, 1.3, 1.3A, 1.4, 1.4A, 1.8, 1.10, 1.15, 1.15A, 1.16, 1.16A, 1.18, 1.19, 1.19A, 1.21, 1.27, 1.28, 1.28A, 1.30, 1.30A, 1.32, 1.32A, 1.33, 1.33A, 1.34, 1.34A, 1.35, 1.35A, 2.1, 2.1A, 2.3, 2.4, 2.4A, 2.5, 2.6, 2.7, 2.9, 2.10, 2.11, 2.12, 2.13, 2.14, 2.15, 2.15A, 2.16, 2.16A, 2.17, 2.17A, 2.18, 2.18A, 2.20, 2.20A, 2.21, 2.23, 2.23A, 2.25, 2.26, 2.26A, 2.27, 2.28, 2.30, 2.30A, 2.32, 2.32A, 2.34, 2.35, 2.35A, 2.40, 2.40A, 2.41, 2.41A, 5.1, 5.1A, 5.3, 5.4, 5.5, 5.6, 5.7, 5.8, 5.9, 5.10, 5.10A, 6.7, 6.8, 6.8A, 14.32, 15.8, 15.8A, 15.11, 15.11A, 16.21, 16.21A, 16.22, 16.22A, 22.6, 22.6A, 27.1, 27.1A, 27.2, 27.2A, 27.3, 27.3A, 40.1, 40.1A, 43.3A, 43.12, 43.12A, 43.13, 43.13A, 46.19, 46.20, 46.21, 46.21A, 46.22, 47.11, 47.11A, 48.20, 48.20A, 74.10, 74.10A, 74.12,** and **74.12A.**

Bear MF, et al.: Neuroscience: Exploring the Brain, 2nd ed. Baltimore: Lippincott Williams & Wilkins, 2001. For **Figures 3.3, 3.4, 3.5, 70.11, 70.15, 71.29,** and **71.30.**

Kingsley RE: Concise Text of Neuroscience, 2nd ed. Baltimore: Lippincott Williams & Wilkins, 2000. For **Figures 3.1, 5.11, 5.11A, 5.13, 5.13A, 5.14, 5.22, 5.22A, 27.9, 27.9A, 27.10, 27.10A, 33.1, 33.2, 33.3, 33.4, 33.6, 33.6A, 33.7, 33.7A, 38.3, 38.4A, 38.8, 38.19, 38.25, 40.2, 40.2A, 40.3, 45.2, 45.2A, 45.12, 45.12A, 46.14, 46.14A, 46.22A, 46.24, 46.24A, 64.13, 64.13A, 64.14, 64.15, 64.17, 64.23, 64.24,** and **65.8.**

Siegel A, Sapru HN: Essential Neuroscience. Baltimore: Lippincott Williams & Wilkins, 2006. For **Figures 2.37, 2.38, 2.38A, 2.39, 2.41, 2.41A, 3.3, 3.4, 3.5, 3.6, 3.20, 3.21, 5.15, 5.15A, 5.20, 5.20A, 5.23, 5.24, 5.25, 5.25A, 5.26, 5.27, 5.27A, 7.20, 7.20A, 7.21, 7.21A, 7.22, 7.22A, 7.23, 7.23A, 7.24, 7.24A, 7.25, 7.25A, 7.26, 7.26A, 7.27, 7.28, 7.28A, 7.55, 7.55A, 11.11, 11.20, 11.26, 11.27, 12.17, 14.23, 14.23A, 19.12, 19.12A, 20.11, 20.12, 21.1, 21.1A, 21.2, 21.3, 21.5, 21.6, 21.7, 21.7A, 21.12, 21.15, 22.4, 22.10, 22.14, 22.21, 22.22, 23.2, 23.2A, 23.3, 23.3A, 24.1, 25.1, 25.8, 26.3, 26.4, 26.5, 26.6, 26.7, 26.7A, 26.8, 26.11, 27.4, 27.4A, 27.5, 27.6, 27.6A, 27.7, 27.7A, 27.8, 28.1, 28.2, 28.4, 31.2, 31.2A, 31.8, 31.8A, 31.9, 31.9A, 32.7, 32.7A, 36.4, 36.11, 36.17, 36.20, 36.20A, 36.21, 36.21A, 36.22, 36.23, 37.1, 37.1A, 37.2, 37.3, 37.5, 37.6, 37.8, 37.10, 37.12, 37.16, 37.17, 37.17A, 39.19, 37.20, 37.21, 37.21A, 37.22, 38.2, 38.2A, 38.14, 38.18, 38.20, 38.20A, 38.22, 39.18, 40.4, 40.5, 40.5A, 43.14, 43.16, 43.16A, 43.20, 43.20A, 43.21, 43.21A, 43.22, 43.23, 43.24, 43.24A, 43.29, 43.29A, 44.1, 44.1A, 44.2, 44.2A, 44.3, 44.3A, 44.4, 44.4A, 44.5, 44.5A, 44.6, 44.6A, 44.7, 44.7A, 44.11, 44.11A, 44.12, 44.12A, 44.15, 44.15A, 44.19, 44.19A, 45.4, 45.4A, 45.5, 45.5A,**

45.6, 45.6A, 45.9, 45.9A, 45.10, 45.10A, 46.5, 46.5A, 46.9, 46.9A, 46.12, 46.12A, 46.13, 46.13A, 46.15, 46.17, 46.27, 46.28, 46.28A, 46.29, 46.29A, 46.30, 46.30A, 47.4, 47.4A, 47.6, 47.6A, 47.10, 47.10A, 47.14, 47.14A, 47.15, 47.15A, 47.21, 47.21A, 47.22, 47.22A, 47.23, 47.24, 47.24A, 47.25, 47.28, 47.33, 47.33A, 47.34, 47.38, 47.38A, 47.39, 47.39A, 48.1, 48.1A, 48.2, 48.3, 48.3A, 48.4, 48.5, 48.5A, 48.9, 48.12, 48.14, 48.14A, 48.15, 48.15A, 48.17, 48.17A, 48.18, 48.18A, 48.20, 48.20A, 48.22, 48.23, 48.23A, 48.24, 48.26, 49.1, 49.3, 52.1, 52.2, 52.3, 52.3A, 52.4, 52.4A, 53.1, 53.1A, 53.3, 53.5, 53.5A, 53.6, 53.6A, 53.7, 53.7A, 53.9, 53.9A, 53.10, 53.10A, 53.11, 53.11A, 53.12A, 54.1, 54.1A, 54.2, 54.2A, 54.4, 54.4A, 54.6, 54.6A, 54.8, 54.8A, 54.9, 54.9A, 54.10, 54.10A, 54.11, 54.11A, 54.12, 54.12A, 54.13, 54.17, 54.17A, 54.19, 54.19A, 54.20, 54.20A, 54.21, 54.21A, 54.22, 54.22A, 54.23, 54.25, 54.25A, 54.26, 54.26A, 54.27, 54.27A, 54.28, 54.28A, 54.29, 54.29A, 54.31, 54.31A, 54.32, 54.33, 54.33A, 54.34, 54.34A, 54.35, 54.36, 54.36A, 54.37, 54.37A, 54.38, 54.39, 54.40, 54.40A, 55.9, 55.12, 55.13, 55.13A, 55.14, 55.14A, 55.16, 55.16A, 55.17, 55.17A, 55.21, 55.22, 55.22A, 55.31, 55.31A, 55.32, 55.35, 55.36, 55.36A, 56.3, 56.4, 56.4A, 56.7, 56.7A, 56.8, 56.11, 56.11A, 56.14, 56.14A, 56.16, 56.17, 56.21, 56.31, 56.32, 57.9, 57.9A, 57.11, 57.11A, 57.13, 57.13A, 58.3, 58.4, 58.4A, 58.5, 58.5A, 58.6, 58.6A, 58.8, 58.8A, 58.9, 58.9A, 58.10, 58.11, 58.11A, 58.14, 58.15, 58.15A, 58.16, 58.16A, 58.20, 58.20A, 58.22, 58.23, 58.23A, 60.1, 60.2, 60.6, 60.8, 60.10, 60.10A, 60.11, 60.14, 60.14A, 60.16, 60.17, 60.18, 60.19, 60.20, 60.20A, 61.3, 61.3A, 61.4, 61.4A, 62.1, 62.1A, 62.3, 62.3A, 62.4, 62.4A, 62.7, 62.10, 62.10A, 62.11, 62.12, 62.12A, 62.13, 62.15, 62.17, 62.20, 62.21, 62.21A, 62.22, 62.23, 62.23A, 62.24, 62.25, 62.25A, 63.1, 63.2, 63.3, 63.3A, 63.4, 63.4A, 63.6, 63.6A, 63.9, 63.10, 63.10A, 63.11, 63.11A, 63.16, 63.17, 63.17A, 63.18, 63.18A, 63.19, 63.19A, 63.21, 63.21A, 63.23, 63.23A, 63.24, 63.25, 63.26, 63.26A, 63.27, 63.27A, 63.28, 63.29, 63.29A, 63.30, 63.32, 63.32A, 65.2, 65.4, 65.4A, 65.5, 65.5A, 65.7, 65.10, 65.10A, 65.14, 65.14A, 65.15, 65.15A, 65.16, 65.17, 65.17A, 65.18, 65.20, 65.20A, 65.21, 65.22, 65.22A, 65.24, 65.24A, 65.25, 65.26, 65.26A, 65.33, 65.33A, 65.34, 65.34A, 65.37, 65.37A, 65.40, 65.40A, 66.2, 66.2A, 66.3, 66.5, 66.7, 66.7A, 66.9, 66.10, 66.10A, 66.12, 66.12A, 66.13, 66.13A, 66.15, 66.19, 66.19A, 66.23, 66.24, 66.27, 66.27A, 66.28, 66.28A, 66.29, 66.29A, 66.30, 66.30A, 66.31, 66.32, 66.32A, 67.2, 67.3, 67.3A, 67.4, 67.5, 67.5A, 67.6, 67.6A, 67.12, 67.24, 67.24A, 67.32, 67.32A, 68.2, 68.5, 68.21, 68.22, 69.1, 69.2, 69.2A, 69.8, 69.8A, 69.9, 69.11, 69.11A, 69.12, 69.12A, 70.1, 70.5, 70.14, 70.16, 70.21, 70.22, 70.26, 70.26A, 70.28, 70.28A, 71.3, 71.3A, 71.16, 71.17, 71.18, 71.18A, 71.19, 71.19A, 71.22, 71.23, 71.23A, 71.31, 71.31A, 72.4, 72.4A, 72.8, 72.8A, 72.9, 72.12, 72.13, 72.16, 72.17, 76.7, 76.12, 76.12A, 76.13, and **76.13A.**

Smith CG: Serial Dissections of the Human Brain. Baltimore: Urban & Schwarzenberg, Inc., and Toronto: Gage Publishing Ltd., 1981. For **Figures 9.14, 9.14A, 9.15, 9.16, 9.16A, 9.17, 9.17A, 9.18, 9.18A, 9.19, 9.19A, 9.20, 9.20A, 10.6, 10.6A, 10.7, 10.7A, 10.21, 10.21A, 10.22, 10.22A, 12.5, 12.8, 12.12, 12.12A, 12.14, 12.14A, 12.19, 12.19A, 13.6, 13.7, 13.7A, 13.8, 13.16, 14.20, 14.20A, 15.2, 23.6, 23.6A, 23.9, 23.10, 43-11, 43-11A, 46.22, 46.22A, 46.23, 46.23A, 46.25, 46.25A, 46.26, 46.26A, 47.11,** and **47.11A.**

Snell RS: Clinical Neuroanatomy, 6th ed. Baltimore: Lippincott Williams & Wilkins, 2006. For **Figures 4.1, 5.17, 5.17A, 5.19, 5.19A, 5.21, 5.21A, 8.1, 9.21, 9.21A, 9.22, 9.22A, 9.23, 9.23A, 9.24, 9.24A, 10.5, 10.5A, 10.11A, 30.1, 30.4, 30.5, 30.5A, 30.6, 30.6A, 30.13, 30.13A, 30.14, 30.21, 30.23, 30.23A, 30.24, 30.24A, 30.25, 30.25A, 34.2, 35.2, 35.4, 35.4A, 35.6, 35.6A, 35.8, 35.8A, 36.6, 36.6A, 36.7, 36.7A, 36.8, 36.12, 36.12A, 36.16, 36.16A, 36.19, 37.14, 37.14A, 39.1, 57.4, 74.4, 74.5, 74.5A, 74.6, 75.3, 75.4,** and **75.4A.**

Young PA, Young PH: Basic Clinical Neuroanatomy. Baltimore: Lippincott Williams & Wilkins, 1997. For **Figures 3.2, 3.2A, 3.7, 3.8, 3.8A, 3.9, 3.11, 3.11A, 3.14, 3.14A, 3.15, 3.15A, 3.17, 3.18, 3.19, 3.22, 3.23, 3.23A, 3.25, 3.25A, 3.26, 3.26A, 3.27, 3.27A, 3.28, 3.28A, 3.29, 3.29A, 3.30, 3.32, 3.33, 4.1A, 4.2, 4.3, 4.4, 4.4A, 4.5, 4.5A, 4.6, 4.6A, 4.7, 4.7A, 4.8, 4.8A, 4.9, 4.11, 4.12, 4.13, 4.13A, 6.3, 6.4, 6.7, 6.9, 6.9A, 6.10, 6.11, 6.12, 6.13, 6.14, 7.22, 7.22A, 7.24, 7.24A, 7.25, 7.25A, 7.26, 7.26A, 7.27, 7.28, 7.28A, 7.29, 7.30, 7.30A, 7.31, 7.33, 7.36, 7.36A, 7.56, 11.2, 11.22, 15.1, 19.1, 19.2A, 19.3, 19.4, 19.5, 19.5A, 19.6, 19.6A, 19.7, 19.7A, 19.8, 19.8A, 19.9, 19.9A, 19.10, 19.10A, 19.11, 19.11A, 23.7, 24.2, 24.5, 24.6, 24.7, 24.7A, 24.8, 24.11, 24.11A, 8.8, 8.9, 30.17, 30.17A, 35.3, 35.5, 35.11, 36.1, 36.1A, 36.2, 36.3, 36.5, 36.10, 36.14, 36.15, 36.15A, 36.18, 36.18A, 36.24, 36.25, 36.25A, 38.6, 38.20A, 38.24, 40.6, 40.6A, 57.7, 57.7A, 60.5, 60.5A, 69.5, 69.5A, 69.6, 70.2, 70.3, 70.3A, 73.1, 73.2, 73.3, 73.5, 73.5A, 73.12, 73.12A, 74.9,** and **74.13.**